T0135278

Difficult Decisions in Surgery: An Evidence-Based Approach

Series Editor
Mark K. Ferguson, Department of Surgery
University of Chicago
Chicago, IL, USA

The complexity of decision making in any kind of surgery is growing exponentially. As new technology is introduced, physicians from nonsurgical specialties offer alternative and competing therapies for what was once the exclusive province of the surgeon. In addition, there is increasing knowledge regarding the efficacy of traditional surgical therapies. How to select among these varied and complex approaches is becoming increasingly difficult. These multi-authored books will contain brief chapters, each of which will be devoted to one or two specific questions or decisions that are difficult or controversial. They are intended as current and timely reference sources for practicing surgeons, surgeons in training, and educators that describe the recommended ideal approach, rather than customary care, in selected clinical situations.

More information about this series at http://www.springer.com/series/13361

Vassyl A. Lonchyna • Peggy Kelley
Peter Angelos

Editors

Difficult Decisions in Surgical Ethics

An Evidence-Based Approach

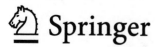 Springer

Editors
Vassyl A. Lonchyna
The University of Chicago Medicine
University of Chicago
Chicago, IL, USA

Peggy Kelley
Providence Children's Surgical Services
St. Vincent Hospital
Portland, OR, USA

Peter Angelos
Department of Surgery
MacLean Center for Clinical Medical Ethics
The University of Chicago
Chicago, IL, USA

ISSN 2198-7750   ISSN 2198-7769   (electronic)
Difficult Decisions in Surgery: An Evidence-Based Approach
ISBN 978-3-030-84627-5   ISBN 978-3-030-84625-1   (eBook)
https://doi.org/10.1007/978-3-030-84625-1

© The Editor(s) (if applicable) and The Author(s), under exclusive license to Springer Nature Switzerland AG 2022
This work is subject to copyright. All rights are solely and exclusively licensed by the Publisher, whether the whole or part of the material is concerned, specifically the rights of translation, reprinting, reuse of illustrations, recitation, broadcasting, reproduction on microfilms or in any other physical way, and transmission or information storage and retrieval, electronic adaptation, computer software, or by similar or dissimilar methodology now known or hereafter developed.
The use of general descriptive names, registered names, trademarks, service marks, etc. in this publication does not imply, even in the absence of a specific statement, that such names are exempt from the relevant protective laws and regulations and therefore free for general use.
The publisher, the authors and the editors are safe to assume that the advice and information in this book are believed to be true and accurate at the date of publication. Neither the publisher nor the authors or the editors give a warranty, expressed or implied, with respect to the material contained herein or for any errors or omissions that may have been made. The publisher remains neutral with regard to jurisdictional claims in published maps and institutional affiliations.

This Springer imprint is published by the registered company Springer Nature Switzerland AG
The registered company address is: Gewerbestrasse 11, 6330 Cham, Switzerland

We dedicate this book to

Mark and Anna Siegler
Your guidance of hundreds of Clinical
Ethics Fellows
through their time at the MacLean Center for
Clinical Medical Ethics,
and your collective enthusiasm, warmth, and
dedication
to the study of clinical medical ethics
have inspired this book.

Foreword

The complexity of decision making in medicine, and in surgery in particular, is growing exponentially. As new technology is introduced, physicians from nonsurgical specialties offer alternative, competing, and sometimes superior therapies for what was once the exclusive province of the surgeon. The increasingly frequent use of institutional databases and national databases has provided information regarding the efficacy of standard surgical therapies. Similar levels of scrutiny regarding nonsurgical therapies have not been achieved in many instances, making comparisons among different approaches to conditions challenging. The lack of relevant outcomes data for a variety of procedural approaches for a specific condition makes discussing interventions with patients and their families challenging.

Concepts such as shared decision making are growing in stature, offering patients and their families more input and autonomy in the acceptance of surgery as a remedy. Surgeons are learning to become less dogmatic and paternalistic. Instead, they are providing information to patients and their families and offering tools such as decision aids to help patients express their wishes. These recent changes in the clinical landscape offer seemingly endless possibilities for treatment decisions based on risks, complications, prognosis, and quality of life. How to navigate among these varied and complex approaches is becoming increasingly challenging.

In response to these needs, a series of books was launched in 2007 titled "Difficult Decisions in Surgery: An Evidence-Based Approach," designed to assist surgeons and other medical professionals in decision making. The first two volumes were focused on thoracic surgery. The success of these volumes prompted development of a broader overview of challenging surgical situations, and now includes a number of surgery-related specialty and subspecialty areas.

The editors for each volume are selected from individuals who have a current or prior important relationship to The University of Chicago, particularly the Department of Surgery. This institution is regularly named among the top 10 universities world-wide and is associated with perhaps the largest number of Nobel laureates of any in the world. This history, and the thoughtful process of faculty recruitment, imbue the medical school faculty with a considered approach to clinical science. This approach is particularly true of the editors of this volume, who are highly skilled clinical surgeons. In addition, they are well-trained and experienced in clinical medical ethics, and thus are able to approach the field of clinical ethical decision making with an informed rigor.

This volume was conceived of and developed in a unique setting. The University of Chicago is noted for transforming the work of theoretical bioethicists in the 1970s to bring focus to applications of ethics in clinical practice. Led by Dr. Mark Siegler, these efforts were formalized with the founding of the MacLean Center for Clinical Medical Ethics in 1984. This Center has helped develop guidelines in clinical medical ethics, pioneered the inpatient Ethics Consultation service, and has long been associated with the field of Surgical Ethics. The MacLean Center developed a Clinical Medical Ethics Fellowship program, which has graduated nearly 500 fellows. This includes the lead editor for this volume, Dr. Vassyl Lonchyna, one of over 80 surgeon graduates, who, as a Fulbright Scholar, developed an ethics curriculum in Ukraine. The Center currently has a number of American College of Surgeons grantees who are pursuing a one-year program in surgical ethics and Dr. Peggy Kelley, a pediatric ENT specialist, was one of the first of these ACS selectees. Dr. Peter Angelos, one of the first surgeons to complete the Fellowship, is a prolific author in surgical ethics and the current Associate Director of the MacLean Center.

To date, previous Difficult Decisions publications include the following subspecialty volumes: bariatric, cardiothoracic critical care, colorectal, endocrine, head and neck oncology, hepatobiliary/pancreatic, thoracic, trauma, and vascular. The current volume on Surgical Ethics is unique to the series. Rather than being developed based on PICO formatted statements, the chapters focus on the four pillars of ethics: beneficence, non-maleficence, autonomy, and justice. The editors of this volume have compiled a dizzying array of clinical situations and populated the author list with internationally recognized experts. Together, they sort through the challenges these scenarios offer and provide wise counsel that every reader can benefit from. This volume is unique in the Difficult Decisions series and is unique in the history of biomedical publication.

Department of Surgery   Mark K. Ferguson 🆔
The University of Chicago,   mfergus@bsd.uchicago.ed
Chicago, IL, USA

Contents

Part IX   Do Not Resuscitate/Palliative Care/End of Life

Part X   Global Surgery

Part XI   Covid-19 Pandemic of 2020

Part XII   Surgical Innovation/Research

Contributors

Ciro Andolfi Section of Urology, Department of Surgery, The University of Chicago Medical Center, Chicago, IL, USA

Peter Angelos Department of Surgery and MacLean Center for Clinical Medical Ethics, The University of Chicago, Chicago, IL, USA

Megan K. Applewhite Department of Surgery, Alden March Bioethics Institute, Albany Medical College, Albany, NY, USA

Maya A. Babu Cleveland Clinic Martin Health, Port Saint Lucie, FL, USA

Erica C. Bennett Department of Surgery, Division of Otolaryngology – Head and Neck Surgery, University of New Mexico, Albuquerque, NM, USA

Todd D. Beyer Department of Surgery, Albany Medical College, Albany, NY, USA

Margret Bock Congenital Anomalies of the Kidney and Urinary Tract Program, Fetal Genitourinary Anomalies Working Group, Children's Hospital Colorado, Aurora, CO, USA

Pediatric Nephrology, University of Colorado School of Medicine, Aurora, CO, USA

Douglas Brown Department of Surgery, Center for Humanism and Ethics in Surgical Specialties, Washington University in St. Louis School of Medicine, St. Louis, MO, USA

Darren S. Bryan Department of Surgery, Brigham and Women's Hospital, Boston, MA, USA

Paul Burcher Wellspan, York Hospital, York, PA, USA

Pennsylvania State University College of Medicine, Drexel University College of Medicine, York, PA, USA

T. Johelen Carleton Hospice & Palliative Medicine, Phoenix, AZ, USA

Erica M. Carlisle Division of Pediatric Surgery, Department of Surgery, University of Iowa Carver College of Medicine, University of Iowa Hospitals and Clinics, Iowa City, IA, USA

Leah Conant Washington University in Saint Louis School of Medicine, Saint Louis, MO, USA

Eric M. Curto University of North Dakota School of Medicine and Health Sciences, Grand Forks, ND, USA

Karen Devon, MDCM Women's College Hospital, University Health Network, Toronto, ON, Canada

Department of Surgery, University of Toronto, Toronto, ON, Canada

Brian C. Drolet Department of Plastic Surgery, Department of Biomedical Informatics and Center for Biomedical Ethics and Society, Vanderbilt University Medical Center, Nashville, TN, USA

Assunta Fabozzo Department of Cardio-Thoracic and Vascular Sciences and Public Health, Hospital-University of Padova, Padova, Italy

Erin Fennern Department of Surgery, The Mount Sinai Hospital, New York, NY, USA

Alberto R. Ferreres Department of Surgery, University of Buenos Aires, Buenos Aires, Argentina

Department of Surgery, University of Washington, Seattle, WA, USA

R. Matthew Galocy Section of Urology, Department of Surgery, The University of Chicago Medical Center, Chicago, IL, USA

Sabha Ganai, MD, PhD University of North Dakota School of Medicine and Health Sciences, Grand Forks, ND, USA

Sanford Clinic, Fargo, ND, USA

Gino Gerosa Department of Cardio-Thoracic and Vascular Sciences and Public Health, Hospital-University of Padova, Padova, Italy

Eric Grossman Cottage Hospital, Santa Barbara, CA, USA

Kristina Guyton Department of Surgery, University of Iowa, Iowa City, IA, USA

Jason J. Han Division of Cardiothoracic Surgery, Department of Surgery, Hospital of the University of Pennsylvania, Philadelphia, PA, USA

Tracilyn Hall Dan L Duncan Comprehensive Cancer Center, Baylor College of Medicine, Houston, TX, USA

Annie Hess Washington University School of Medicine, St. Louis, MO, USA

Norman D. Hogikyan Department of Otolaryngology-Head and Neck Surgery, Center for Bioethics and Social Sciences in Medicine, Michigan Medicine, Ann Arbor, MI, USA

Claire Hoppenot Dan L Duncan Comprehensive Cancer Center, Baylor College of Medicine, Houston, TX, USA

Catherine Hunter Division of Pediatric Surgery, Department of Surgery, University of Oklahoma, Norman, OK, USA

Scott J. Hunter Section of Neuropsychology, Department of Psychiatry and Behavioral Neuroscience, Institutional Review Board, Biological Sciences Division, The University of Chicago Medical Center, Chicago, IL, USA

Lulia A. Kana University of Michigan Medical School, Ann Arbor, MI, USA

Peggy Kelley Providence Children's Surgical Services, St. Vincent Hospital, Portland, OR, USA

Piroska Kopar Department of Surgery, Center for Humanism and Ethics in Surgical Specialties, Washington University in St. Louis School of Medicine, St. Louis, MO, USA

Hannah Kornfeld Cottage Hospital, Santa Barbara, CA, USA

Kelly C. Landeen Department of Otolaryngology – Head and Neck Surgery, Vanderbilt University Medical Center, Nashville, TN, USA

Alexander Langerman Department of Otolaryngology—Head and Neck Surgery, Department of Radiology and Radiological Sciences, Center for Biomedical Ethics and Society, Vanderbilt University Medical Center, Nashville, TN, USA

Amy G. Lehman The Lake Tanganyika Floating Health Clinic, Chicago, IL, USA
Iroko Health, Kalemie, Democratic Republic of the Congo

Barron H. Lerner Department of Medicine, NYU Langone Health, New York, NY, USA
Department of Cardiothoracic Surgery, NYU Langone Health, New York, NY, USA

Samara Lewis Division of Pediatric Surgery, Department of Surgery, University of Oklahoma, Norman, OK, USA

Bernard Lo School of Medicine, University of California San Francisco, San Francisco, CA, USA

Chen Lin Department of General Surgery, Chinese Academy of Medical Sciences, Peking Union Medical College Hospital, Beijing, China

Vassyl A. Lonchyna MacLean Center for Clinical Medical Ethics, University of Chicago, Chicago, IL, USA
Institute for Bioethics, Ukrainian Catholic University, Lviv, Ukraine

Jessica G. Y. Luc Division of Cardiovascular Surgery, Department of Surgery, University of British Columbia, Vancouver, BC, Canada

Boris D. Lushniak University of Maryland School of Public Health, College Park, MD, USA

Robert M. MacGregor Department of Surgery, Washington University School of Medicine, Barnes Jewish Hospital, St. Louis, MO, USA

Alan T. Makhoul Vanderbilt University School of Medicine, Nashville, TN, USA

Fabien Maldonado Departments of Thoracic Surgery, Department of Pulmonology, Center for Biomedical Ethics and Society, Vanderbilt University Medical Center, Nashville, TN, USA

Emily Marchiano Department of Otolaryngology-Head and Neck Surgery, Michigan Medicine, Ann Arbor, MI, USA

Pringl Miller Department of Medical Education, Physician Just Equity, San Francisco, CA, USA

Michael Millis Department of Surgery, University of Chicago Medicine, Chicago, IL, USA

Ross Milner Division of Vascular Surgery, Department of Surgery, The University of Chicago Medicine & Biological Sciences, Chicago, IL, USA

Karishma B. Mistry Sanford Clinic, Fargo, ND, USA

Brian Mitzman Division of Cardiothoracic Surgery, University of Utah, Salt Lake City, UT, USA

Department of Cardiothoracic Surgery, NYU Langone Health, New York, NY, USA

Elisheva T. A. Nemetz Faculty of Medicine, University of Toronto, Toronto, ON, Canada

Christian Fernandez Olortegui Department of Radiation Oncology, Thomas Jefferson University Hospital, Philadelphia, PA, USA

Ethan Paddock Department of Surgery, Division of Otolaryngology – Head and Neck Surgery, University of New Mexico, Albuquerque, NM, USA

Xavier Pereira Department of Surgery, Montefiore Medical Center, New York City, NY, USA

Maria Urdaneta Perez Division of Pediatric Surgery, Department of Surgery, University of Oklahoma, Norman, OK, USA

Lauren McLendon Postlewait Division of Surgical Oncology, Department of Surgery, Emory University School of Medicine, Atlanta, GA, USA

Nicola Pradegan Department of Cardio-Thoracic and Vascular Sciences and Public Health, Hospital-University of Padova, Padova, Italy

Jaishankar Raman University of Melbourne, Fitzroy North, VIC, Australia

Deakin University, Melbourne & Geelong, VIC, Australia

University of Illinois at Urbana-Champaign, Champaign, IL, USA

Oregon Health & Science University, Portland, OR, USA

James Cook University, Townsville, Queensland, Australia

St Vincent's Hospital, Melbourne, VIC, Australia

Shuddhadeb Ray Department of Surgery, Washington University School of Medicine, St. Louis, MO, USA

Samantha Ratner University of Michigan, Ann Arbor, MI, USA

Samuel Reis-Dennis Alden March Bioethics Institute, Albany Medical College, Albany, NY, USA

Robert M. Sade Division of Cardiothoracic Surgery, Department of Surgery, Institute of Human Values in Health Care, Medical University of South Carolina, Charleston, SC, USA

Baddr A. Shakhsheer Division of Pediatric Surgery, Department of Surgery, Washington University School of Medicine, St. Louis, MO, USA

Arieh L. Shalhav Section of Urology, Department of Surgery, The University of Chicago Medical Center, Chicago, IL, USA

Michael Shapiro Department of Surgery, Rutgers New Jersey Medical School, University Hospital, Newark, NJ, USA

Andrew G. Shuman Department of Otolaryngology-Head and Neck Surgery, Center for Bioethics and Social Sciences in Medicine, Michigan Medicine, Ann Arbor, MI, USA

Mark Siegler The MacLean Center for Clinical Medical Ethics, Chicago, IL, USA

The Bucksbaum Institute for Clinical Excellence, The University of Chicago, Chicago, IL, USA

Eric A. Singer Section of Urologic Oncology, Rutgers Cancer Institute of New Jersey and Rutgers Robert Wood Johnson Medical School, New Brunswick, NJ, USA

Puneet Singh Department of Breast Surgical Oncology, Division of Surgery, University of Texas MD Anderson Cancer Center, Houston, TX, USA

Kinga B. Skowron Olortegui Section of Colon & Rectal Surgery, Department of Surgery, MacLean Center for Clinical Medical Ethics, University of Chicago Medicine, Chicago, IL, USA

Mindy B. Statter Department of Surgery, Montefiore Medical Center, New York City, NY, USA

Robert P. Sticca University of North Dakota School of Medicine and Health Sciences, Grand Forks, ND, USA

Malini D. Sur Northside Hospital Cancer Institute, Atlanta, GA, USA

Ashley Suah Department of Surgery, University of Chicago Medicine, Chicago, IL, USA

Giuliano Testa, MD, MBA, FACS Annette C. and Harold C. Simmons Transplant Institute, Baylor University Medical Center, Dallas, TX, USA

Chad M. Teven, MD Division of Plastic and Reconstructive Surgery, Department of Surgery, Mayo Clinic, Phoenix, AZ, USA

Vijaya Vemulakonda Pediatric Urology, University of Colorado School of Medicine, Aurora, CO, USA

Congenital Anomalies of the Kidney and Urinary Tract Program, Fetal Genitourinary Anomalies Working Group, Children's Hospital Colorado, Aurora, CO, USA

Anji Wall, MD, PhD, FACS Annette C. and Harold C. Simmons Transplant Institute, Baylor University Medical Center, Dallas, TX, USA

Peipei Wang Peking Union Medical College Hospital, Beijing, China

Sean C. Wightman Division of Thoracic Surgery, Keck School of Medicine, University of Southern California, Los Angeles, CA, USA

M. Jeanne Wirpsa Northwestern Memorial Hospital, Chicago, IL, USA

MacLean Center for Clinical Ethics, University of Chicago, Chicago, IL, USA

Bin Wu Peking Union Medical College Hospital, Beijing, China

Rolla Zarifa Division of Vascular Surgery, Department of Surgery, The University of Chicago Medicine & Biological Sciences, Chicago, IL, USA

Part I
In the Beginning

Chapter 1
Introduction

Bernard Lo

Abstract "A surgeon is a physician and more." This declaration by one of my surgery professors could serve as a motif for this book on surgical ethics. In several ways, surgical ethics is more than clinical ethics in other specialties. This introduction places the chapters of this comprehensive multi-authored book into a broader perspective by discussing several themes that cut across the chapters.

Keywords Patient trust · Adverse events · Surgical innovation
Surgical learning · Disclosure · Artificial intelligence

"A surgeon is a physician and more."

1.1 Special Features of Surgical Ethics

Like all physicians, surgeons follow the ethical principles of respect for patients and their autonomy, acting in the patient's best interests, optimizing the balance between benefits and harms of interventions, and distributing resources and benefits justly. In addition, all physicians, including surgeons, should act with compassion, trustworthiness, integrity, and self-reflection. However, surgery differs from other specialties in important clinical ways, which lead to differences in the weight and interpretation of ethical guidelines, as well how surgeons respond to specific clinical situations and dilemmas [1].

Surgery has several distinctive clinical features. First, surgeons intentionally cause short-term injury to patients in order to achieve long-term therapeutic goals. Although all medical interventions involve risk, many surgical adverse effects are certain and occur before any benefit can be realized. All surgical patients undergo

B. Lo (✉)
School of Medicine, University of California San Francisco, San Francisco, CA, USA
e-mail: Bernard.Lo@ucsf.edu

© The Author(s), under exclusive license to Springer Nature
Switzerland AG 2022
V. A. Lonchyna et al. (eds.), *Difficult Decisions in Surgical Ethics*, Difficult
Decisions in Surgery: An Evidence-Based Approach,
https://doi.org/10.1007/978-3-030-84625-1_1

operative risks, experience post-operative pain, and emerge with scars. Second, patients give the surgical team control of their bodies in the operating room [2]. Neither patients, their families, nor their primary care or referring physicians know what happens in the operating room. Third, operations are not standardized like standard dosages and regimens for pharmaceuticals. The surgeon's technical skill, judgment, experience, and confidence influence patient outcomes. It is challenging for non-surgeons to assess the quality of surgical care. Surgeon-specific outcomes, or even hospital-specific outcomes, for a procedure are generally not available; even when they are, it is challenging to account for case mix and severity of illness.

These distinctive clinical characteristics of surgery have important ethical implications [1], as subsequent chapters in the book discuss in detail. Acting in *the patient's best interests* takes on heightened importance in surgery because patients are completely dependent on the surgical team during operations. In other specialties, a patient who is strongly dissatisfied with a physician's care and outcomes can switch to another doctor who can alter the plan of care if necessary. But once an operation commences, a patient remains in the surgeon's hands until the procedure is completed. Because patients are so dependent during the operation, it is important that they feel able to trust their surgeon, as we discuss at the end of the introduction.

The *informed consent procedure and shared decision-making* are especially important because surgery is a major bodily invasion. Some operations, such as mastectomy, colostomy, or amputation, dramatically alter the patient's body image, sense of self, or daily functioning. Patients differ in what surgical risks they are willing to accept in return for what prospect of benefit. For example, patients might place different weight on the trajectory of returning to full activities or on the size of the post-operative scar.

Surgical innovation, research, and lifelong learning is important but challenging.

During the careers of current surgeons, major innovations have been introduced into surgery, including laparoscopic and robotic surgery. Rigorous assessment of surgical interventions has grown. Randomized controlled trials (RCTs) in surgery are important because they control for baseline differences between patients in the intervention and control arms. However, RCTs are difficult to carry out because the surgeons' techniques, judgment, skills, and experience with the procedure need to be similar in the intervention and control arms. Moreover, it may be misleading to carry out a trial too soon after an operation or approach is introduced, because over time operations evolve and outcomes improve. Despite such challenges, during the past decade well-designed RCTs have clarified the safety and effectiveness of surgery for common operations such as bariatric surgery for diabetes, percutaneous valve replacement, discectomy for persistent sciatica, and fundoplication for refractory heartburn.

Learning in surgery is a lifelong process. Five chapters discuss surgical training during residency. Learning procedural skills can be more challenging than learning cognitive skills. More experienced physicians can supervise medical decision making by trainees in ways that reduce the risks and consequences of mistakes. A trainee can propose a plan for care on rounds, and the resident or attending physician can provide feedback, suggestions, and modifications before the plan is implemented. During an operation, however, the trainee has manual control of the procedure, and there is the possibility of a significant mistake before the supervising surgeon can intervene.

After their residency and fellowship, surgeons must continue to learn new technologies and new procedures after they are in practice. Surgical procedures have a learning curve [3], and high-volume hospitals and high-volume surgeons are associated with better outcomes [4]. For laparoscopic procedures, initially complication rates are higher than with open techniques and operating times are longer. As surgeons get more experience, complication rates become comparable to those of open procedures. Thus, when practicing surgeons learn new procedures, their early patients are at risk for adverse outcomes. However, practicing surgeons have few extended opportunities for learning new procedures under supervision and mentoring. When surgeons are learning a new procedure, ethical dilemmas arise regarding disclosure to patients.

Many patients consider it important to know a surgeon's experience with a new technique [5]. However, such information is generally not readily available. Moreover, surgeons might be reluctant to discuss their personal experience because of concerns that patients who learn that they are inexperienced with a procedure will not trust them to do the operation, making it more difficult for them to master new skills.

Responsibility of Individual Surgeons Surgeons feel deep personal responsibility for the outcomes of surgery because of their "hands-on" involvement in care [2], as the chapters on surgical errors discuss. When perioperative complications and deaths occur, surgeons must discuss in morbidity and mortality conferences why they operated and how the case was managed [6]. Colleagues scrutinize whether the surgeon erred in judgment or technique. Such personal responsibility is ethically praiseworthy.

As later chapters carefully describe, during the COVID-19 pandemic, surgeons and other front-line health care workers extended their responsibilities to very long hours and new or heightened clinical responsibilities, despite serious personal risks. These risks included COVID-19 infection and death and serious mental health problems. An overlooked but important ethical issue is how an individual surgeon can act ethically when policies and resources fall short. It seems unfair to expect front-line health care workers to be heroes, to do whatever it takes to care for a surge of patients when hospitals, public health agencies, and government officials have not developed fair, evidence-based policies to meet a public health crisis, provided adequate personal protective equipment, and addressed workers' emotional and mental health needs.

1.2 Ethical Issues on the Horizon

1.2.1 Artificial Intelligence in Surgery

Artificial intelligence (AI) pervades everyday life. AI runs Internet search engines, opens cell phones using facial recognition, recommends movies to watch and merchandise to purchase, and corrects spelling errors. AI algorithms also recommend which loan applicants to approve, which job applicants to interview and hire, and which detainees receive bail or probation.

In medicine, AI algorithms have been developed to make diagnoses from radiology images, retinal scans, or skin photographs and identify patients at increased risk for critical care or hospital readmission. In surgery, AI can make intraoperative histopathological diagnoses in near real time, allowing neurosurgeons to optimally reduce cancer burden while preserving neurological functions [7]. Future uses for AI in surgery may include autonomous robotic surgery and assessment of surgical risk.

AI algorithms may be biased. Bias can occur if the algorithm was derived or validated on datasets that are not representative of the populations where it will be applied. For instance, facial recognition is less accurate with persons of color because they were underrepresented in training datasets. Bias in machine learning algorithms can also occur if the training dataset contained biased decisions. Historically Black loan and job applicants were less successful even when they are equally qualified. Such discrimination can be perpetrated in algorithms. In health care, the Institute of Medicine found that bias, stereotyping, and prejudice may contribute to racial and ethnic disparities in health care [8]. Disparities continue to occur in surgery. Blacks and Hispanics have lower rates of total hip replacement than non-Hispanic Whites, higher surgical complication rates, and longer lengths of stay, even after preoperative and perioperative factors were controlled [9]. Finally, bias may occur if AI algorithms are not assessed in terms of clinically significant outcomes [10].

Physicians can play important roles to make AI equitable and clinically meaningful. First, surgeons can identify meaningful opportunities where AI might improve surgical care. Second, physicians can train and validate clinical AI algorithms on data sets that represent the full range of patients for whom the algorithm will be used. Third, physicians can evaluate AI algorithms in terms of clinically meaningful outcomes and impact on workflow before they are introduced into practice. Fourth, surgeons can plan how to explain the use of AI to patients and address their concerns. Finally, since machine learning algorithms are designed to change over time, physicians can make sure that their outcomes—both beneficial and harmful—are continually assessed in the context of the institution and patient population.

1.2.2 The Surgeon and Ethical Issues in Society

Surgeons live and work within societal and institutional contexts. Although the focus of this book is primarily on the individual clinical decisions surgeons make with individual patients, several chapters show how surgeons' options are shaped by and constrained by societal policies, for example laws and regulations regarding brain death, surrogate decision-making, medical malpractice, and crisis standards of care during a pandemic. The five chapters on the COVID-19 pandemic illustrate how ethical decisions for individual patients depend on public health and institutional policies and resources.

Physicians can address ethical issues in society by helping to shape health care policies in institutions and society, particularly when their expertise, experience, and perspective is lacking in discussions. In particular, physicians can call attention to gaps and inconsistencies in policies, failure to take into account the best available evidence, disparities between formal policies and on-the-ground implementation, and unintended adverse outcomes of policies.

1.2.3 The Importance of Trust

Earlier we noted that surgical patients, who are completely dependent on the surgeon in the operating room, need to trust their surgeon and the surgical team. Several personal anecdotes underscore the difficulty of obtaining information about surgeons and the importance of trust. As a general internist, I often am asked to recommend a surgeon for a particular procedure. Usually, I ask a faculty surgeon whom they would recommend and why. Rather than immediately suggesting names, some thoughtful colleagues first ask a senior resident who has been in the operating room with attending surgeons recently and managed their patients post-operatively. Even eminent surgeons are not familiar with how their colleagues operate on, interact with, and manage their patients, except if they cross-cover a patient or hear a discussion at a morbidity and mortality conference. Only the team that works with the attending surgeon on a daily basis—the fellows, residents, and nurses—know this crucial information.

As a family member, I have seen how decisions about choosing a surgeon are highly individualized. My mother had a breast biopsy by a surgeon renowned for her expertise in breast cancer, patient advocacy, and interactions with patients. At each step of the biopsy the surgeon explained what she was going to do and provided reassurance. Afterwards, my mother announced that she wanted another surgeon: "She talks too much. She should concentrate more on what she is doing." For mastectomy, my mom chose a surgeon who was much more directive and told her what he was going to do, with little consideration of her preferences.

Several chapters address the importance of communication in building trust. Shared decision-making is preferred by most patients today. However, some patients prefer other decision-making styles [11]. For her operation, my mother preferred a paternalistic approach and biomedical communication style, in which the surgeon demonstrated medical authority and decisiveness, presented information clearly, and made decisions with little patient input. At the other end of the spectrum, in a "consumerist" approach, the patient makes decisions and the physician's role is to provide medical information. A patient's preferred decision-making and communication styles might vary depending on the clinical situation, the nature of the surgery, and the stage of illness.

Although physicians should generally employ shared decision-making, they can also individualize their approach to the patient. Early in a patient visit, the physician might ask about the patient's preferred role in decision-making and style of communication. Whatever the patient's preferred style, it can be helpful for the physicians to first listen to the patient's concerns and values before giving recommendations that take those into account.

In summary, this book showcases the growing scholarship by surgeons on ethical issues in surgery. The chapters address scenarios that all physicians will recognize and provide thoughtful approaches to important ethical issues.

References

1. Lo B. Ethical issues in surgery. In: Resolving ethical dilemmas: a guide for clinicians. 6th ed. Wolters Kluwer; 2020. p. 276–83.
2. Angelos P. Surgical ethics and the future of surgical practice. Surgery. 2018;163(1):1–5. https://doi.org/10.1016/j.surg.2017.09.018.
3. Hopper AN, Jamison MH, Lewis WG. Learning curves in surgical practice. Postgrad Med J. 2007;83(986):777–9. https://doi.org/10.1136/pgmj.2007.057190.
4. Morche J, Mathes T, Pieper D. Relationship between surgeon volume and outcomes: a systematic review of systematic reviews. Syst Rev. 2016;5(1):204. https://doi.org/10.1186/s13643-016-0376-4.
5. Lee Char SJ, Hills NK, Lo B, Kirkwood KS. Informed consent for innovative surgery: a survey of patients and surgeons. Surgery. 2013;153(4):473–80. https://doi.org/10.1016/j.surg.2012.08.068.
6. Bosk CL. Forgive and remember: managing medical failure. University of Chicago Press; 1979.
7. Hollon TC, Pandian B, Adapa AR, et al. Near real-time intraoperative brain tumor diagnosis using stimulated Raman histology and deep neural networks. Nat Med. 2020;26(1):52–8. https://doi.org/10.1038/s41591-019-0715-9.
8. Institute of Medicine. Unequal treatment: confronting racial and ethnic disparities in health care. National Academy Press; 2003. https://doi.org/10.17226/10260.
9. Ezomo OT, Sun D, Gronbeck C, Harrington MA, Halawi MJ. Where do we stand today on racial and ethnic health disparities? An analysis of primary total hip arthroplasty from a 2011–2017 national database. Arthroplast Today. 2020;6(4):872–6. https://doi.org/10.1016/j.artd.2020.10.002.
10. Obermeyer Z, Powers B, Vogeli C, Mullainathan S. Dissecting racial bias in an algorithm used to manage the health of populations. Science. 2019;366(6464):447–53. https://doi.org/10.1126/science.aax2342.
11. Swenson SL, Zettler P, Lo B. 'She gave it her best shot right away': patient experiences of biomedical and patient-centered communication. Patient Educ Couns. 2006;61(2):200–11. https://doi.org/10.1016/j.pec.2005.02.019.

Chapter 2
The Importance of Formal Education and Training in Clinical Medical Ethics for the 21st Century

Mark Siegler

Abstract In 1972, soon after I started the first medical intensive care unit (MICU) at the University of Chicago, a unit whose patients raised multiple, serious ethical issues, I created the new field of Clinical Medical Ethics (CME) in the Department of Medicine at the university. In my view, both in 1972 and today, CME is an intrinsic part of medicine, surgery and all medical disciplines, and is not a branch of bioethics or philosophical ethics or legal ethics or theoretical ethics. Rather, it is a central component of clinical care that must be practiced and applied by licensed clinicians in their routine, daily encounters with patients. Although bioethicists may provide theoretical insights to clinicians, bioethicists cannot practice medicine or examine patients or provide care to patients. During the past 49 years, CME has become a transformative field in medicine and surgery that aims to improve both the clinical and ethical quality of care and outcomes that clinicians provide their patients (Singer et al., BMC Med Ethics 2:1, 2001). In ordinary clinical practice, CME addresses many clinical ethical issues, including truth-telling, informed consent, confidentiality, surrogate decision-making, the risks, benefits and alternatives to surgical or medical procedures, end-of-life care, and also encourages personal, humane, compassionate, and fair interactions between doctor and patient.

The goals of CME are to improve patient care and outcomes by helping physicians, surgeons and other health professionals identify and respond to clinical-ethical challenges that arise in the ordinary care of patients. As Edmund Pellegrino, Peter A. Singer and I wrote 30 years ago: "The central goal of CME is to improve the quality of patient care by identifying, analyzing and contributing to the resolution of ethical problems that arise in the routine practice of clinical medicine" (Siegler et al., J Clin Ethics 1:5–9, 1990). Similar to cardiology and oncology con-

M. Siegler (✉)
The MacLean Center for Clinical Medical Ethics, Chicago, IL, USA

The Bucksbaum Institute for Clinical Excellence, The University of Chicago, Chicago, IL, USA
e-mail: msiegler@medicine.bsd.uchicago.edu

© The Author(s), under exclusive license to Springer Nature Switzerland AG 2022
V. A. Lonchyna et al. (eds.), *Difficult Decisions in Surgical Ethics*, Difficult Decisions in Surgery: An Evidence-Based Approach,
https://doi.org/10.1007/978-3-030-84625-1_2

sultations, ethics consultations are a small component of a much larger field, just as the consultations in cardiology and oncology or CME are certainly not at the core of cardiology, oncology or Clinical Medical Ethic.

This article will discuss the following five topics: the origins of the field of CME; the goals and methods of CME; the relationship between the larger field of CME and the narrower practice of ethics consultations; the contributions of the MacLean Center at the University of Chicago in developing the fields of Clinical Medical Ethics; and how CME has improved the practice of medicine and surgery (Siegler, J Clin Ethics 30:17–26, 2019).

Keywords Clinical Medical Ethics · MacLean Center for Clinical Medical Ethics Doctor-patient accommodation · Shared decision-making · Truth-telling · Informed consent · Confidentiality · Surrogate decision-making

2.1   Introduction

I launched the field of Clinical Medicine Ethics in 1972 in the Department of Medicine at the University of Chicago [1]. Clinical Medicine Ethics is an intrinsic part of daily medical and surgical practice. CME is not a branch of bioethics or philosophical ethics or legal ethics or theoretical ethics. Rather, it is a central component of clinical care that must be practiced and applied by licensed medical and surgical clinicians in their ordinary encounters with patients. During the past 49 years, CME has become integrated into medical education and medical practice. CME has become a transformative field in medicine and surgery that aims to improve the clinical and ethical quality of routine care and outcomes that clinicians provide to their patients. Although bioethicists may offer theoretical insights to clinicians, bioethicists are not licensed or trained to practice medicine or examine patients or provide care to patients. In daily practice, CME addresses clinical ethical issues such as truth-telling, informed consent, confidentiality, surrogate decision-making, the risks and benefits and alternatives of surgical and medical practice, end-of-life care, while also encouraging personal, humane, compassionate and socially fair interactions between doctor and patient.

In this chapter, I will discuss the following issues relating to Clinical Medical Ethics (CME):

  I. What were the origins of the field of Clinical Medical Ethics? When was the field named CME? And when did the term "CME" first appear in the medical literature?
 II. What are the goals and methods of CME?
III. What is the relationship between the larger field of Clinical Medical Ethics and the far more limited practice of doing clinical medical ethics consultations?
IV. How has the MacLean Center at The University of Chicago contributed to developing the fields of clinical medical ethics and surgical ethics?
 V. How has CME improved the practice of medicine?

2.2 Discussion

- **SECTION I. What were the origins of the field of Clinical Medical Ethics? When was the field named CME? And when did the term "Clinical Medical Ethics" first appear in the medical literature?**

In 1972, when I joined the University of Chicago faculty, the Chair of Medicine, Dr. Alvin Tarlov, asked me to establish and direct our hospital's first Medical Intensive Care Unit (MICU). I did this within our recently established academic section of General Internal Medicine. In those days, there were very few MICUs, in part because there were very few effective ventilators, and the specialty of critical care medicine did not yet exist. In fact, the first American Board of Internal Medicine certification exam in Critical Care Medicine was not held until 1987, 15 years after we had opened our MICU. In time, MICUs would become one of the great medical and technological advances that saved many lives, prolonged many lives, and in the process raised new ethical questions that clinicians had never before faced.

Directing the MICU from 1972 to 1977 changed my career and encouraged me to establish the field of Clinical Medical Ethics. Our seven-bed MICU received the sickest adult patients in the hospital. Our mortality rate was over 60% [2]. Each day, my team and I confronted ethical issues such as rationing beds, negotiating informed consent, deciding when we needed surrogate consent, deciding whether it was ethically acceptable to stop a treatment once we had started it, and communicating a truthful prognosis to the patient or the family. My previous training in medicine had not prepared me for this set of problems, problems that arose every day in the MICU.

Faced with these recurring issues, I soon discovered that there was no place to send my housestaff and students to find answers. The medical literature and textbooks did not discuss these matters. Although there was a new, emerging literature in biomedical ethics, written largely by non-clinicians—that is, by philosophers, theologians, legal scholars and social scientists—this literature rarely addressed the practical concerns faced in the MICU by medical students, residents, nurses and physicians. The language of biomedical theory was different from the language of clinicians, and bioethical theory was often not helpful in resolving the practical dilemmas clinicians faced while caring for sick and dying patients. One repeated clinical ethical challenge in our 7-bed Intensive Care Unit involved when, if ever, was it clinically and ethically appropriate to remove a patient already in the MICU because a new patient had a better chance of benefiting and surviving in the unit. Because MICUs were so new at that time, there was little advanced clinical guidance for such daily clinical ethical challenges. Furthermore, in the early 1970s, very few clinicians were even aware of the bioethics movement, and those who were often reacted negatively and sometimes with hostility to bioethics and to non-physician bioethicists.

At that time in 1972, I first realized that if we were to improve the care of patients in the MICU and throughout the hospital, it was essential that doctors, nurses, other health professionals, patients and families become more closely involved in discussions about these new and difficult clinical and ethical questions. Physicians and patients needed help to better understand the ethical issues in daily clinical practice so that they could incorporate ethical analysis into their clinical decisions. It was these insights that led me to change my career goals. In addition to caring for patients, which I have now done for 53 years, I would also devote my career to develop and expand the new field of Clinical Medical Ethics. I would do so by involving practicing physicians and surgeons, nurses and patients in the goal of improving medical care and patient outcomes.

I was fortunate that in the mid-1970s, four distinguished pioneering bioethicists were working at the University of Chicago: James Gustafson (Theology), Richard McCormick (Theology), Stephen Toulmin (Philosophy and The Committee on Social Thought), and Leon Kass (The Committee on Social Thought). I found myself frequently seeking guidance about ethical dilemmas from these experts, especially from Jim Gustafson and Stephen Toulmin. In all of these encounters, I was struck by how relevant for medical practice these new bioethical insights were, while at the same time, I was troubled deeply by the general absence of clinicians from these discussions and by the widespread ignorance among clinicians about the fields of bioethics and about the recently established field of Clinical Medical Ethics. I believe the creation of Clinical Medical Ethics in 1972 at last encouraged clinicians to become involved and aware of ethical challenges that arise in routine clinical situations.

I came to realize that Clinical Medical Ethics could not be an elective area of study for physicians and surgeons. Rather, it was an essential field that physicians had to learn in order to practice good medicine. I also soon realized that Clinical Medical Ethics was far more closely aligned to clinical practice than it was to bio-ethical theory.

My central point is that intensive care physicians and, in fact, physicians in general, routinely encounter many clinical-ethical issues and that dealing with these clinical-ethical issues is an intrinsic part of reaching clinical decisions and providing good clinical care to patients. For this reason, it was imperative that we create, develop and expand the new field of Clinical Medical Ethics, a field that prepared and assisted clinicians who were caring for patients and making clinical-ethical decisions each day.

In 1996, the late Daniel Callahan, the co-founder of The Hastings Center, attacked the field of Clinical Medical Ethics in an article published in The Hastings Center Report. The article was entitled "Does Clinical Ethics Distort the Discipline?" Callahan wrote:

> In one of my first articles on bioethics, I wrote that the principal aim of the field should be to help the medical practitioner deal with concrete cases. While I would hardly want to overlook the needs of the practitioner, I now wonder if that is the right place to center our attention…. Does reality lie in the particularity of individual cases where most clinicians think it does—or in a more general, abstract and universal realm no less real but just more hidden [3].

Dan Callahan's views of reality certainly differed in a major way from the goals of Clinical Medical Ethics that I had stated: that is, I encouraged clinicians to improve the routine care and outcomes of individual patients.

In 1997, a year after Callahan's article was published, The Lancet published an editorial that strongly endorsed my 1972 views about CME and directly challenged Callahan's views. The Lancet editorial stated:

> Ethics needs to be rooted in clinical practice and not in armchair moral philosophy. Debate on ethical matters is as much an integral part of everyday doctoring as choosing the best treatment for patients. Departments of ethics that are divorced from the medical profession, wallowing in theory and speculation, are quaintly redundant [4].

I changed my career goals during the 5 years that I directed the MICU and dedicated my career both to developing and to improving the care of patients by training physicians, surgeons and other clinicians to apply the concepts of CME in their daily work and to expand the new field of Clinical Medical Ethics. I would dedicate my career to training physicians and other clinicians to apply the concepts of Clinical Medical Ethics in their routine patient encounters in order to improve our care of patients.

The first paper I wrote related precisely to an important issue in clinical medical ethics, that is, telling the truth to patients and their family members. The paper was entitled, "Pascal's Wager and the Hanging of Crepe," and referred to the fact that my younger associates in the intensive care unit had been telling all patients who had been admitted to the ICU or the patient's family or surrogates that the patient would certainly die during this admission. When I first learned of this situation, I quickly corrected it and then wrote a paper highlighting that the routine deceit of patients and families violated the central rule of CME and was clinically unacceptable [5].

In the spring of 1973, Alvan Feinstein, MD, the late renowned clinician-scholar and Sterling Professor of Medicine at Yale University, reinforced my choice of the term "Clinical Medical Ethics" when he and I met at the annual ASCI/AAP medical meetings in Atlantic City. Dr. Feinstein called his own work "*Clinical* Judgment" and "*Clinical* Epidemiology," because, unlike traditional studies, his clinical and epidemiology studies were based directly on his clinical care of patients. Similarly, Dr. Feinstein regarded the work that I had started at the MICU at the University of Chicago as "*Clinical* Medical Ethics," which he vigorously distinguished from what he called theoretical, ivory-tower, biomedical ethics. Beginning in 1973, Dr. Feinstein considered my program at The University of Chicago to be the birthplace of the new field of Clinical Medical Ethics.

In 1974, James Gustafson, Ann Dudley Goldblatt and I wrote a grant to the Department of Health Education and Welfare (DHEW) entitled "Clinical Ethics and Human Values." As far as I know, this was the first grant application, federal or otherwise, that used the term "clinical ethics." The grant was approved, and we received three years of federal support to develop a multi-disciplinary program in Clinical Medical Ethics at the University of Chicago.

In 1978, I published a paper in *The Journal of the American Medical Association (JAMA)* entitled "A Legacy of Osler: Teaching Clinical Ethics at the Bedside" [6]. This was probably the first use of the term "clinical ethics" in the medical literature. This article noted that the advantages of teaching clinical ethics at the bedside included dealing with actual cases to maximize the physician's personal accountability; reinforcing the relationship between clinical practice and ethical decisions; and helping to decrease the widespread resistance at that time of the medical profession to bioethics. The following year (1979), I started the first section of Clinical Medical Ethics in an American medical journal, the American Medical Association's *Archives of Internal Medicine* [7].

In 1979 and 1981, I proposed a new model for health care in the United States. The model I proposed was called "doctor-patient accommodation," a model that was soon accepted in 1982 by the President's Commission under their term "shared decision-making" [8–10].

In 1983, Hanna H. Gray, President of the University of Chicago, gave her approval to Arthur Rubenstein, MD, the chair of the Department of Medicine, and me to organize a Center for Clinical Medical Ethics at the University, a center that is now beginning its 39th year of operation. In 1984, I published a paper on the evolution of Clinical Ethics [11]. With encouragement from President Gray, Dr. Rubenstein and I developed a clinical, research and financial plan for the new center. We secured initial funding for the Center from several leading foundations, including the Andrew W. Mellon Foundation, the Henry J. Kaiser Family Foundation, and the Pew Family Trust. I am also deeply indebted to the late Dorothy Jean MacLean and to Barry and the late Mary Ann MacLean, and to the MacLean family, for their continuous support of our program and their unwavering commitment since 1984 to the MacLean Center and its goals.

This early support enabled us initially to train fifteen physician-leaders from the US and Canada in the new field of Clinical Medical Ethics and to launch our CME Fellowship Training Program. Twelve of our early leading physician-fellows— Susan Tolle (Oregon), Peter A. Singer (Toronto), Alvin Moss (West Virginia), Jay Jacobson (Utah), Robert Walker (South Florida), the late Douglas Kinsella (Calgary), Joel Howell (Michigan), Eric Kodish (The Cleveland Clinic), Christine McHenry (Cincinnati Children's), Robert Orr (Loma Linda), John LaPuma (University of Califonia), and Laura Roberts (New Mexico)—returned to their home institutions to become the founding directors of other Clinical Medical Ethics programs around the US and Canada.

- **SECTION II. What is Clinical Medical Ethics (CME) and what are its goals and methods?**

As noted in the introduction, Clinical Medical Ethics (CME) is a new *medical and surgical* field, an intrinsic part of clinical care. The goals of CME are to improve patient care and outcomes by helping physicians, surgeons and other health professionals identify and respond to clinical-ethical challenges that arise in the daily care of patients. As Drs. Edmund Pellegrino, Peter A. Singer and I observed 30 years ago:

"The central goal of CME is to improve the quality of patient care by identifying, analyzing and contributing to the resolution of ethical problems that arise in the routine practice of clinical medicine" [12]. The doctor-patient relationship along with the nurse-patient relationship are at the heart of CME. The central focus of CME is individual patient-physician decision-making. CME helps patients, families, physicians, and other health professionals reach good clinical decisions by taking into account:

- the *medical facts* of the situation (including the differential diagnosis, proposed diagnostic and therapeutic interventions, and treatment choices);
- the patient's *personal preferences* and values for diagnostic interventions and therapeutic management;
- *ethical considerations* involving family wishes, financial concerns, and research and teaching activities in academic institutions.

Unlike biomedical ethics, clinical medical ethics is not a theoretical undertaking; rather, it must be practiced and applied every day, by licensed clinicians (rather than by unlicensed bioethicists, humanists or social scientists) in order to provide excellent clinical and ethical care to patients.

In 1982, Albert Jonsen (who died in 2020), William Winslade and I wrote a book entitled *Clinical Ethics: A Practical Approach to Ethical Decisions in Clinical Medicine* [13]. The book, now in its eighth edition, with a ninth edition being prepared for publication in 2021, strongly supported the practical application of CME to patient care and the regular use of clinical medical ethics to help patients and physicians make good decisions relating to the care of the patient. The book stated, "Clinical ethics is inextricably linked to the physician's primary task, deciding on and carrying out the best clinical care for a particular patient in a particular set of circumstances" [13]. As Albert Jonsen wrote in 1988: "[The book] *Clinical Ethics* proposed a method of analysis that was closer to the reasoning of clinicians than to the speculation of philosophers" [14].

The foreword to the first edition of *Clinical Ethics* was written by the late Dr. Robert Petersdorf, one of the most powerful and influential medical leaders of his generation. In the foreword, Dr. Petersdorf wrote: "Despite the increasing importance of ethics in medicine, few clinicians spend the time and effort it takes to read a book on ethics. All too often, these books have been couched in weighty philosophy and abstruse theory. This little book handles ethical problems in medicine quite differently. Jointly authored by an ethicist, a clinician and a lawyer, it attacks ethical problems in real-life terms. …. This is a very useful little book, primarily because it is so helpful to the 'working doctor'" [13].

- **SECTION III. What is the relationship between the larger field of Clinical Medical Ethics and the far more limited practice of doing ethics consultation?**

Beginning in the mid-1970s, The University of Chicago medical faculty pioneered the development of ethics consultations to assist patients, families, physicians, and the health team. MacLean Center faculty and fellows wrote much of the early literature on Clinical Ethics consultations [15], including the first book on the topic of ethics consultations [16]. There are some ethicists, especially non-clinician bioethicists, who claim that the core of Clinical Medical Ethics is performing ethics consultations. It is not. Far fewer than one-half of one percent of the 40 million inpatients per year in the U.S. and almost none of the more than 1 billion outpatient visits per year in the U.S. receive an ethics consultation. In contrast to ethics consultations, Clinical Medical Ethics addresses the needs of all inpatients and outpatients and is a critical part of modern clinical practice. When clinicians such as I started the field of CME in the early 1970s, we viewed it as a new and improved approach to clinical medicine that worked to integrate ethical considerations into the _entire_ range of outpatient and inpatient medical and surgical practice. In 2021, to practice good medicine, physicians must know the central elements of CME and regularly apply these elements in their care of patients. For clinicians today, applying CME standards in patient care is no longer an elective matter. Rather, the central principles of CME have now become the clinical, legal and professional standard of patient care. While very few physicians today are formally trained as clinical medical ethicists, all physicians are expected to routinely apply CME elements such as truth telling, informed consent and confidentiality and, when needed, surrogate decision making and end-of-life care, in their regular, daily work with patients.

CME applies to all clinical decisions and not just to ethical dilemmas or conflicts that may generate requests for ethics consultations. In fact, it is important to note that whereas the field of CME started in the early 1970s, ethics consultation played only a minor role in the field until about 15 years later when John Fletcher and Albert Jonsen convened a meeting in Washington, D.C. to form a society called The Society for Bioethics Consultation. As I recall, there were about 60 participants at the meeting, the majority of whom were PhDs with only eight physicians present. While ethics consultations remain a component of the larger field of Clinical Medical Ethics, they are a relatively small component compared to all the other critically important contributions the field of Clinical Medical Ethics makes on a daily basis as an integral part of patient care. I have often thought that the ultimate goal of clinical ethics consultations should be to teach clinicians enough about ethical standards that in the future they can resolve ethical problems by themselves without calling an ethics consultation. Although ethics consultations may be helpful in dealing with some ethical dilemmas or conflicts that arise in the course of medical practice, Clinical Medical Ethics is a much broader field that has important applications not just in terms of relatively infrequent ethics consultations, but rather throughout the entire spectrum of daily medical practice.

The difference between these views about ethics consultations and the broader field of CME can be compared to cardiology consultations or oncology consultations. The practices of cardiology and oncology are much larger and more complex and far more inclusive than merely performing cardiology or oncology consultations. While consultations certainly have a modest role in the fields of cardiology and oncology, consultations clearly do not constitute the central purpose or body of clinical or research practice in these fields. Similarly, the field of CME is much larger and more encompassing and more fundamentally relevant in medical care than the occasional rare request for an ethics consultation.

- **SECTION IV. How has the MacLean Center at The University of Chicago contributed to developing the fields of clinical medical ethics and surgical ethics?**

Beginning in 1972, my colleagues and I at The University of Chicago created, named, developed and led the new field of Clinical Medical Ethics [1]. During the past 49 years, The MacLean Center for CME has continued to advance the field of CME in many important ways [17]. These advances include:

A. Establishing clinical ethics fellowship training.

The MacLean Center's clinical medical ethics fellowship program is the oldest, largest and the most successful clinical ethics fellowship program in the world [1]. Since beginning the fellowship program in 1981, the Center has trained more than 500 fellows, including more than 400 physicians and surgeons [18, 19].

Graduates of the MacLean Fellowship have served as directors of more than 45 ethics programs in the United States, Canada, South America, Europe, the Middle East, Africa, Australia and China. MacLean Center fellowship graduates have held faculty appointments in more than 70 university programs. More than 25 fellowship graduates have held endowed university professorships. MacLean Center former fellows have written more than 200 books and thousands of peer-reviewed journal publications. Many of the graduates of our ethics fellowship program are leaders, scholars and mentors who advance empirical scholarship in Clinical Medical Ethics and who are dedicated to strengthening the patient-physician relationship and to improving patient care. In 2016, the Johns Hopkins Institute of Bioethics presented an award to the MacLean Center that stated: "The training program established by you... [has] had a greater impact than any other clinical ethics training program in the world" [20].

Central components of the MacLean Clinical Ethics Fellowship have included: (1) An annual MacLean Center Fellows' Conference; (2) a five-week intensive summer program for new fellows that includes 70–80 lectures and seminars; and (3) an annual year-long lecture series on topics related to Clinical Medical Ethics. Let me comment briefly on these three programs.

1. The MacLean Center Conference on Clinical Medical Ethics. For the past 32 years, the MacLean Center has organized a two-day conference in mid-November that is named for Dorothy J. MacLean the original founder and supporter of the MacLean Center. D.J. MacLean believed that education was the best way to improve the world and throughout her long life she supported many leading educational institutions in the U.S., including the MacLean Center. The annual MacLean Conference meets on the Friday and Saturday of the second week in November. Speakers are selected from current MacLean Center Faculty and from former MacLean Center Fellowship graduates. Each year, for the past 32 years, this

conference has been the leading clinical ethics conference in the world. In 2020, eleven of the 35 talks will focus on ethical issues related to COVID-19 pandemic. [Appendix 1]

2. The MacLean Center's Summer Clinical Medical Ethics Intensive Program. For the past 30 years, the MacLean Center has begun each fellowship year with a unique summer intensive program. The program consists of 70–80 lectures and seminars taught by more than 30 of the MacLean Center-University of Chicago faculty. The Summer Intensive Program offers "mini-courses" on topics that include: clinical medical ethics; philosophical ethics; health disparities; law and ethics; ethics consultations; end-of-life care; surgical ethics; pediatric ethics; transplantation ethics; reproductive ethics; psychiatric ethics; genetics ethics. [Appendix 2]

3. The MacLean Center's 39th Annual Lecture Series. In 1981, Mark Siegler and Richard Epstein organized a year-long interdisciplinary lecture series on "Medical Innovation and Bad Outcomes: Legal, Social and Ethical Responses." The success of that initial lecture program and of the book based upon the lectures demonstrated that there was great interest at The University of Chicago in creating a sustainable, interdisciplinary forum to discuss health-related subjects with colleagues from across campus. Each year since 1981, the MacLean Center has organized an annual lecture series to examine the ethical aspects of one major health related issue from a cross-section of academic disciplines. Recent annual lecture series topics have included: Organ Transplantation; Pediatric Ethics; Global Health; Reproductive Ethics; Health Care Disparities; Pharmaceutical Innovation and Regulation; End-of-Life Care; Neuro-Ethics; Trauma, Violence and Trauma Surgery; and Improving Value in the US Healthcare System. In 2019, our lecture series was "The Present and Future of the Doctor-Patient Relationship. In 2020, our lecture topic is: Ethics and the COVID-19 Pandemic: Medical, Social and Political Issues." The COVID-19 pandemic is an unprecedented event in our lifetimes, and the extent to which it has permeated our everyday lives obligates us to examine the ethics of contagion. The pervasive and disruptive nature of the pandemic has forced us to reconsider our social interactions and behavior, the limits of our medical response, and our relationships with each other, our local and global communities, and the environment. [Appendix 3]

B. Developing the new field of surgical ethics.

Working in close association with the American College of Surgeons, the MacLean Center has led a national effort to train surgeons in clinical surgical ethics and to encourage research on topics related to surgical ethics. During the past fourteen years under the guidance of Dr. Peter Angelos, who is widely regarded as the leading surgical ethicist in the U.S., the MacLean Center has trained more than 75 surgeons in the new field of surgical ethics.

Surgical ethics focuses on the ethical issues in the care of patients undergoing surgery [21–23]. Although the ethical issues faced by surgeons and surgical patients are not completely different from the ethical issues elsewhere in medical practice, there are nuances and practicalities of the timing of surgical care that warrant specific attention. Informed consent for surgery is not different from informed consent in other areas of medicine, but the increased vulnerability of patients in the operating room demands a greater degree of trust. Furthermore, when caring for a patient in the operating room, a surgeon may be faced with unexpected problems that raise specific ethical issues. The anatomy of a patient may be such that the planned operation is not possible, and the surgeon must utilize an innovative procedure. Such innovation is not allowable in other areas of medical care where, drugs, for example, cannot be tried on patients without FDA approval outside of a clinical trial. In contrast, a surgeon is fully expected to creatively solve his or her patient's problem even if it means doing a procedure that has not previously been described. Alternatively, the unexpected intraoperative findings may force the surgeon to change the planned operation in the middle of the procedure. Surgeons may be faced with deciding whether to proceed in the best interests of the patient to do the different operation or to abort the surgery and discuss with the patient later, or even to speak with the family during the operation to obtain surrogate consent.

The goal of the surgical ethics program is to prepare surgeons for academic careers that combine clinical surgery with scholarly studies in surgical clinical ethics. Surgical ethics fellows receive training in empirical research, teaching and surgical ethics consultations, which are similar to medical consultations except that they are done in surgical situations. Graduates of the MacLean Center's Surgical Ethics Training Program currently work in more than 40 university surgery departments in the United States. Since 2016, the MacLean Center has sponsored a joint surgical ethics fellowship program with the American College of Surgeons (ACS), a program that has now trained 15 surgeons from institutions including Harvard, The University of Michigan, Stanford, UCLA, Duke, The University of Alabama-Birmingham, The University of Wisconsin, The University of North Carolina, Case Western University and The University of Colorado. Also under the auspices of the ACS, a new textbook on surgical ethics was recently published with Peter Angelos as co-editor, with many MacLean Center faculty and former fellows contributing chapters to the book [24].

C. Strengthening the doctor-patient relationship by introducing the concept of shared decision-making.

Clinical Medical Ethics aims to improve patient outcomes by encouraging shared decision-making between patients and physicians. In a 1979 talk to the New York Academy of Medicine and a subsequent paper based upon that talk, I introduced the concept of the Doctor-Patient Accommodation and indicated that it was a preferred alternative to either the old model of physician paternalism or the then prevailing model of patient autonomy [25]. In the 1982 report by the President's Commission for the Study of Ethical Problems in Medicine and Biomedical and Behavioral Research, the President's Commission repeatedly cited my paper on the Doctor-Patient Accommodation as an important basis for their recommendation of a shared decision-making approach in medicine [10]. The President's Commission regarded the term I used, "the doctor-patient accommodation," as similar to the term they used, "shared decision-making." Both the paternalism and autonomy models imply an adversarial relationship between the patient and physician, although the models disagree on whether the ultimate power and control should rest in the doctor's hands or the patient's hands. By contrast, my model of Doctor-Patient Accommodation and the President's Commission model of "shared decision-making" assume that the physician and patient work together as partners or colleagues to achieve a common goal, which is to address the healthcare needs of the patient who has asked the doctor for help. The President's Commission stated in its report:

> The Commission's view is intended to encompass a multitude of different realities, each one shaped by the particular medical encounter and each one subject to change, as the participants move towards patient-physician accommodation through the process of shared decision-making.
>
> In this report, the President's Commission attempts to shift the terms of discussion towards how to foster a relationship between patients and professionals characterized by mutual participation and respect and by shared decision-making [10].

Shared decision-making has become an essential element of the doctor-patient relationship. It was not always so. Over the past 50 years, there has been a vigorous discussion among doctors, patients, lawyers, philosophers, theologians and social scientists about the best way for doctors and patients to make decisions together. The complexities are inherent in the nature of the doctor-patient relationship. Patients often are sick, scared and vulnerable. Doctors have specialized knowledge, societal privileges, and the control of access to medical resources and care. Doctors are supposed to serve their patients, but patients often do not and cannot know what they want or need except through the assistance and guidance of the doctor. The emergence of the field of Clinical Medical Ethics by our team in the early 1970s is closely tied to the development of shared decision-making in the 1980s. Shared decision-making reflects a particular view of doctors' moral obligations to both respect patient autonomy and also to respect their own fundamental commitment to use their medical knowledge to improve the clinical and ethical outcomes for patients.

D. Contributing to the "empirical turn" in ethics research.

Beginning in the 1980s, the MacLean Center and its founding Research Director, the late Carol Stocking, PhD, a distinguished sociologist, played a key role in advancing the "empirical turn" in clinical ethics scholarship. This "turn" refers to the application of the techniques of clinical epidemiology, health services research, decision sciences, and evidence-based outcomes to the study of ethical matters in clinical practice. Empirical research gathers data with survey methods or clinical studies. Empirical data showing that a particular way of ethical practice is better than an alternative helps develop a professional consensus and encourages changes in practice. Previously, ethics research had relied primarily on non-data-based, analytic scholarship done by philosophers, theologians and legal scholars, and such analytic scholarship had less impact on modifying clinical practice than empirical data-driven clinical studies.

E. Introducing the concept of research ethics consultations.

In a landmark article in 1989 in the *New England Journal of Medicine*, the MacLean Center introduced the concept of "research ethics consultations," an innovative approach to the ethics of clinical and translational research [26]. We described research ethics consultations as "…a process in which the ethical issues raised by an innovative therapy are analyzed before a protocol is submitted to the Institutional Review Board. This process has been an essential part of our living liver donor transplantation program in recent years" [26]. Research ethics consultations have now been widely adopted by many research groups, including Clinical and Translation Science Award programs and also by Marian Danis and colleagues at the National Institutes of Health [27].

- **SECTION V. How has CME changed and improved the practice of medicine in the United States?**

In the 1960s and 1970s, the early development of biomedical ethics in the United States was led mainly by non-physician bioethicists—theologians, philosophers, humanists, legal scholars and social scientists. Physicians and other clinicians had minimal involvement in this development and the impact of biomedical ethics on medical practice and medical education was very limited [17].

Clinical Medicine Ethics, by contrast, has succeeded in changing and improving medicine in critical ways that would otherwise be neglected. In contrast to the 1970s, when physicians expressed widespread resistance to biomedical ethics, Clinical Medical Ethics has become so well integrated into current practice that physicians often don't realize they are actually "practicing" clinical medical ethics, which is the goal of all ethics teaching. Applying clinical ethics precepts without being aware of doing so reminds me of the character Monsieur Jourdain from a play by Moliere who was surprised to learn that he had been speaking prose all his life [28]. Physicians are indeed practicing clinical ethics (and speaking prose) every day when they tell patients the truth, or when they break bad news, or when they negotiate informed consent for a procedure or a medication, or when they make decisions based on shared decision-making, or when they decide that a patient lacks decisional capacity and turn instead to surrogate decision-makers. These and other clinical ethical considerations have become so much a part of routine medical practice that they have become widely accepted as the legal and professional "standard of care." While very few U.S. physicians today are formally trained as clinical ethicists, all physicians regularly apply clinical medical ethics approaches in their ordinary, daily work with patients.

I would go so far as to say that these days clinicians cannot practice good medicine—that is, technically competent and ethically appropriate medicine—without some knowledge of and ability to apply the core principles of Clinical Medical Ethics.

Since 1972, the changes brought by clinical medical ethics to medicine have been profound and have occurred without fanfare or drama. In contrast to the 1970s, today almost every medical organization has a code of ethics and an ethics committee. Similarly, every large hospital is required by the Joint Commission to have a mechanism—usually either a hospital ethics committee or an ethics consultation service—to resolve clinical ethical problems when they occur [29, 30]. Publications on clinical ethics issues appear regularly, both in ethics journals that are infrequently read by clinicians, and in medical journals that are widely read by clinicians.

2.3 Concluding Remarks

In contrast to the 1970s, Clinical Medical Ethics discussions have become a part of everyday clinical discourse and of routine clinical decisions in outpatient and inpatient settings across the country. This transition was critical in American medicine and ethics. The physician, not the bioethicist, has the special knowledge as well as the legal and professional responsibility to assist patients in curing or caring for their illness and to assist patients in dealing with the fear, pain and suffering that often accompany ill health. Physicians and nurses are licensed by the state and are professionally, legally and personally accountable to the patient if they fail to adequately integrate clinical ethics into their care of patients.

The field of Clinical Medical Ethics (CME) is now nearly 50 years old. CME, which involves the close integration of ethical principles with everyday clinical practice and requires the commitment and involvement of clinicians, has helped to improve medicine and medical practice. The field has also greatly improved patient care and patient outcomes. As we look toward the future and recognize emerging challenges to humane, compassionate and personalized medical practice, I am confident that Clinical Medical Ethics will remain a vitally essential program that continues to defend and improve clinical medicine and surgery for the benefit of patients.

2.4 Selected References

- Siegler M, Pellegrino ED, Singer PA. Clinical medical ethics. J Clin Ethics. 1990;1:5–9.

  - This was the introductory article for the first issue of the Journal of Clinical Ethics, a journal in continuous publication since 1990.

- Siegler M. Clinical medical ethics: its history and contributions to American medicine. J Clin Ethics. 2019;30:17–26.

  - This article summarizes my views on the origin, evolution and contributions of the MacLean Center to the field of Clinical Medical Ethics.

- Siegler M. Clinical medical ethics. In: Roberts LW, Siegler M, editors. Clinical medical ethics: landmark works of Mark Siegler, MD. Springer; 2017. p. 10–1.

  - This book compiles 45 of my most significant papers in a single volume. Also of note: Introductory essays by leaders in the field.

- Siegler M. Pascal's wager and the hanging of crepe. N Engl J Med. 1975;293:853–7. https://doi.org/10.1056/nejm197510232931705

  - This was my first published article, and it relates closely to my experiences after establishing one of the first Medical Intensive Units in the City of Chicago.

- Siegler M. A legacy of Osler: teaching clinical ethics at the bedside. JAMA. 1978;239:951–6. https://doi.org/10.1001/jama.1978.03280370047023

  - As far as I know, this JAMA article was the first time the phrase "clinical ethics" appeared in a medical journal.

- Siegler M. The physician-patient accommodation: a central event in clinical medicine. Arch Intern Med. 1982;142:1899–902. https://doi.org/10.1001/archinte.1982.00340230145024

  - This article introduced an alternative model to either the paternalism or autonomy models and encouraged "shared decision-making."

- President's Commission for the Study of Ethical Problems in Medicine and Biomedical and Behavioral Research. Making health care decisions. The ethical and legal implications of informed consent in the patient-practitioner relationship. US Government Printing Office; 1982. p. 34–9.

  - This report cited my reference #26 (below) multiple times and linked my idea of the "physician-patient accommodation' to the President's Commission term of "shared decision-making."

- Jonsen AR, Winslade WJ, Siegler M. Clinical ethics: a practical approach to ethical decisions in clinical medicine. McGraw-Hill; 1982.

  - The ninth edition to this book is due to be published in 2021.

- Ferreres AR, Angelos P, Singer EA, editors. Ethical issues in surgical care. American College of Surgeons; 2017.

  - Two of the editors, Angelos and Ferreres, are former MacLean Fellows, as are many of the authors contributing to this book.

- Siegler M. Searching for moral certainty in medicine: a proposal for a new model of the doctor-patient encounter. Bull N Y Acad Med. 1981;57:56–69. PMID: 6937229.

  - The new model of the Doctor-Patient Encounter—an alternative model to either the paternalism or autonomy models—which encouraged "shared decision-making," was discussed at this address. It was subsequently cited by the President's Commission (reference #13) multiple times and linked my idea of the "physician-patient accommodation' to their term of "shared decision-making."

Appendix 1: The 33rd Annual MacLean Fellows Conference on Clinical Medical Ethics. November 12–13, 2021

Each year for the past 33 years, the MacLean Center has hosted a conference at which former MacLean Fellows and current faculty discuss major issues in Clinical Medical Ethics. The MacLean Center for Clinical Medical Ethics at the University of Chicago is the oldest, largest, and most distinguished clinical ethics program in the world. Since the MacLean Center was founded in 1984, the Center has trained more than 625 Clinical Ethics Fellows, and they include more than 500 physicians. In 2016, Dr. Mark Siegler and the MacLean Center received the prestigious Meyerhoff Award from the Johns Hopkins Berman Institute of Bioethics. The award stated, "The training program established by the MacLean Center has had a greater impact than any other Clinical Medical Ethics training program in the world."

This year's MacLean Conference, on November 12–13, will include more than 40 exceptional lectures on the following topics: Clinical Ethics Decision-Making, Covid-19 Clinical Ethics, Health Policy and Health Disparities, Surgical Ethics, Pediatrics and Family Ethics, and End-of-Life Care.

Please refer to this year's brochure and schedule: https://drive.google.com/file/d/1QDVQMYEXu7_rc5pK_rZ_7pwttKrjPXDy/view?usp=sharing

Appendix 2: The 2021–2022 MacLean Center Summer Intensive Program for the Fellowship in Clinical Medical Ethics. July 6–30, 2021

The MacLean Summer Intensive Program is unique and remarkable. This year, it offered fellows a four-week intensive experience that included more than 80 lectures and seminars presented by more than 37 MacLean Center Faculty. This year's summer program offered courses on topics that included: Clinical Medical Ethics, Philosophical Ethics, Ethics Consultation, End-of-Life Care, Health Policy and Health Disparities, Law and Ethics, Surgical Ethics, Pediatrics and Family Ethics, Transplantation Ethics, Reproductive Ethics, Genetic Ethics, and Psychiatric Ethics.

Please refer to this year's brochure and schedule: https://drive.google.com/file/d/1XU_nGvQTn1ZUR469XwoIAq6-hSrVcs9L/view?usp=sharing

Appendix 3: The MacLean Center's 40th Annual Lecture Series. The History of Medicine and Ethics. Wednesdays 12:00–1:30 PM CT

In 1981, Mark Siegler and Richard Epstein organized a year-long, University-wide interdisciplinary lecture series on "Medical Innovation and Bad Outcomes: Legal, Social and Ethical Responses." The success of that initial lecture program and of the book published based upon those lectures, demonstrated that there was great interest at the University of Chicago in creating a sustainable interdisciplinary forum to discuss health-related subjects with colleagues from the entire University campus. Each year since 1981, the MacLean Center for Clinical Medical Ethics has organized an annual lecture series of 20 or more lectures to examine the ethical aspects of one key health-related issue. Recent annual lecture series topics have included: Reproductive Ethics; Organ Transplantation; Pediatric Ethics; Global Health; Health Care Disparities; Pharmaceutical Innovation and Regulation; End-of-Life Care; Neuroethics; Trauma, Violence and Trauma Surgery, and Improving Value in the US Healthcare System. In the past two years, our lecture series topics were "The Present and Future of the Doctor-Patient Relationship" (2019–2020) and "Ethics and the Covid-19 Pandemic: Medical, Social and Political Issues" (2020–2021).

Please refer to this year's brochure and schedule: https://drive.google.com/file/d/11oE4ynx1yclNv2r_3EMx7RJo__mMb891/view?usp=sharing

References

1. Siegler M. Clinical medical ethics. In: Roberts LW, Siegler M, editors. Clinical medical ethics: landmark works of Mark Siegler, MD. Springer; 2017. p. 10–1.
2. Siegler M. Critical illness: the limits of autonomy. Hast Cent Rep. 1977;7:12–5.
3. Callahan D. Does clinical ethics distort the discipline? Hast Cent Rep. 1996;26(6):28–9. PMID: 8970795.
4. Editorial. The ethics industry. Lancet. 1997;350(9082):897. https://doi.org/10.1016/s0140-6736(97)21039-1.
5. Siegler M. Pascal's wager and the hanging of crepe. N Engl J Med. 1975;293:853–7. https://doi.org/10.1056/nejm197510232931705.
6. Siegler M. A legacy of Osler: teaching clinical ethics at the bedside. JAMA. 1978;239:951–6. https://doi.org/10.1001/jama.1978.03280370047023.
7. Siegler M. Clinical ethics and clinical medicine. Arch Intern Med. 1979;139:914–5. https://doi.org/10.1001/archinte.1979.036330450056016.
8. Siegler M. The physician-patient accommodation: a central event in clinical medicine. Arch Intern Med. 1982;142:1899–902. https://doi.org/10.1001/archinte.1982.00340230145024.
9. Siegler M. Decision-making strategy for clinical ethical problems in medicine. Arch Intern Med. 1982;142:2178–9. https://doi.org/10.1001/archinte.1982.00340250144021.
10. President's Commission for the Study of Ethical Problems in Medicine and Biomedical and Behavioral Research. Making health care decisions. The ethical and legal implications of informed consent in the patient-practitioner relationship. US Government Printing Office; 1982. p. 34–9.
11. Siegler M. Annotated bibliography of clinical ethics. Ann Intern Med. 1984;101:268–74. https://doi.org/10.7326/0003-4819-101-2-263.
12. Siegler M, Pellegrino ED, Singer PA. Clinical medical ethics. J Clin Ethics. 1990;1:5–9. PMID: 2131058.
13. Jonsen AR, Winslade WJ, Siegler M. Clinical ethics: a practical approach to ethical decisions in clinical medicine. McGraw-Hill; 1982.
14. Jonsen AR. The birth of bioethics. Oxford University Press; 1998. p. 366.
15. Siegler M, Singer PA. Clinical ethics consultation: godsend or "God Squad?". Am J Med. 1988;85:759–60. https://doi.org/10.1016/s0002-9343(88)80016-0.
16. La Puma J, Schiedermayer D. Ethics consultation: a practical guide. Jones & Bartlett; 1994.

17. Siegler M. Clinical medical ethics: its history and contributions to American medicine. J Clin Ethics. 2019;30:17–26.
18. Pellegrino ED, Siegler M, Singer PA. Teaching clinical ethics. J Clin Ethics. 1990;1:175–80.
19. Siegler M. Training doctors for professionalism: some lessons from teaching clinical medical ethics. Mt Sinai J Med. 2002;69:404–9. PMID: 12429959.
20. Kahn J. Meyerhoff leadership in bioethics award letter. Johns Hopkins Berman Institute of Bioethics; 2016.
21. Angelos P. Surgical ethics and the future of surgical practice. Surgery. 2018;163:1–5. https://doi.org/10.1016/j.surg.2017.09.018.
22. Angelos P. "Clinical" surgical ethics. J Clin Ethics. 2019;30:49–55.
23. Siegler M, Rogers S, editors. Violence trauma and trauma surgery: ethical issues, interventions, and innovations. Springer; 2019.
24. Ferreres AR, Angelos P. In: Singer EA, editor. Ethical issues in surgical care. American College of Surgeons; 2017.
25. Siegler M. Searching for moral certainty in medicine: a proposal for a new model of the doctor-patient encounter. Bull N Y Acad Med. 1981;57:56–69. PMID: 6937229.
26. Singer PA, Siegler M, Whitington PF, et al. Ethics of liver transplantation with living donors. N Engl J Med. 1989;321:620–2. https://doi.org/10.1056/nejm198908313210919.
27. Danis M, Largent E, Grady C, et al. Research ethics consultations: a casebook. Oxford University Press; 2012.
28. Moliere. The Bourgeois Gentleman; 1670.
29. The Joint Commission. 2012 comprehensive accreditation manual for hospitals: the official handbook. Joint Commission Resources; 2011.
30. Singer PA, Pellegrino ED, Siegler M. Clinical ethics revisited. BMC Med Ethics. 2001;2:1. https://doi.org/10.1186/1472-6939-2-1.

Chapter 3
What Makes Surgical Ethics Unique?

Jessica G. Y. Luc ⓘ, **Jason J. Han** ⓘ, **and Robert M. Sade** ⓘ

Abstract In this chapter, we provide an overview of ethical principles as they apply to health care, with a focus on surgical ethics. We discuss why surgical ethics matter and what makes surgical ethics unique, spanning aspects of patient care, professional integrity, research, administration, education, and surgical training and education. We present observations on how surgical ethics can be taught, and, finally, we speculate on the future of ethics in surgery.

Keywords Surgical ethics · Health care ethics · Health care · Education · Surgical education · Surgeon-patient relationship

3.1 Introduction

The word *ethics* is derived from the Greek word *ethos*, which means "character." Ethics is the branch of philosophy that explores the notion of proper conduct, in that it strives to determine right versus wrong and to balance what is good for the individual versus for society. It investigates the nature of obligations or duties that people owe themselves and one another based on a thoughtful understanding of moral

J. G. Y. Luc
Division of Cardiovascular Surgery, Department of Surgery, University of British Columbia, Vancouver, BC, Canada

J. J. Han
Division of Cardiothoracic Surgery, Department of Surgery, Hospital of the University of Pennsylvania, Philadelphia, PA, USA

R. M. Sade (✉)
Division of Cardiothoracic Surgery, Department of Surgery, Institute of Human Values in Health Care, Medical University of South Carolina, Charleston, SC, USA
e-mail: sader@musc.edu

© The Author(s), under exclusive license to Springer Nature   27
Switzerland AG 2022
V. A. Lonchyna et al. (eds.), *Difficult Decisions in Surgical Ethics*, Difficult
Decisions in Surgery: An Evidence-Based Approach,
https://doi.org/10.1007/978-3-030-84625-1_3

responsibility. The field of ethics has many subdivisions, including bioethics (health care and the biological sciences), clinical ethics (bedside), organization ethics (health care leadership), and medical ethics (physicians) [1]. A subcategory of the last is surgical ethics. What sets surgical ethics apart? How is it different from the more general medical ethics? In this chapter, we explain what makes surgical ethics unique and, going a step further, suggest how it can be taught to surgeons and trainees.

3.2 Discussion

3.2.1 Overview of Ethical Principles and its Application to Health Care

In the practice of medicine and surgery, patient care is dictated by technical capabilities and knowledge as well as the exercise of clinical and moral judgment. When decisions must be made in the context of competing choices, no single answer may be apparent. Ethical principles can help in selecting or justifying the most favorable course of action.

Ethical analysis in medicine can take many forms and are generally classified into three frameworks: consequentialism, deontology, and virtue ethics [2]. In general, consequentialist theories assert that outcomes should guide choices. For example, according to utilitarianism, the morally superior choice is the one that creates the greatest good for the greatest number of people. Deontological theories hold that certain rules of behavior determine what is right and wrong: according to Kant's categorical imperatives one should always treat oneself and others as ends in themselves, never as means to other ends. Virtue theory requires that personal development of proper characteristics, such as honesty, technical and intellectual competence, and compassion, will lead to good choices among competing options [2].

A commonly applied framework in health care is a combination of those approaches, the principlism approach advocated by Beauchamp and Childress [3] shown in Table 3.1. Certain structures or aids to ethics analysis have been

Table 3.1 The principlism approach [3]

Autonomy	**Beneficence**
The patient has the right to select a treatment from among several options after understanding the risks, benefits, and consequences of each	When caring for patients, the physician's paramount obligation is to the best interest of the patient. To best serve that interest, the physician must maintain competence, good clinical judgment, life-long education, and accountability
Non-maleficence	**Justice**
A physician must not cause more harm than good, which includes recognizing one's limitations as well as appropriate disclosure and discussion of complications, among many other means of avoiding harm	A physician should ensure equal treatment of similarly situated patients, without any medically unjustified discrimination

recommended. Jonsen et al. have described a four-topics model approach [4], which includes examining the medical indications, patient preferences, quality of life, and contextual features of a case to select the best course of action (see Fig. 3.1).

The Four Topics Chart	
Medical Indications	**Preferences of Patients**
The Principles of Beneficence and Nonmaleficence 1. What is the patient's medical problem? Is the problem acute? chronic? critical? reversible? emergent? terminal? 2. What are the goals of treatment? 3. In what circumstances are medical treatements not are the probabilities of success of various treatment options? 5. In sum, how can this patient be benefited by medical and nursing care, and how can harm be avoided?	The Principle of Respect for Autonomy 1. Has the patient been informed of benefits and risk of diagnostic and treateement recommendations, understood this information, and given consent? 2. Is the patient mentally capable and legally competent or is there evidence of incapacity? 3. If mentally capable, what preferences about treatment is the patient stating? 4. If incapacitated, has the patient expressed prior preferences? 5. Who is the appropriate surrogate to make decisions for an incapacitated patient? What standards should govern the surrogate's decisions? 6. Is the patient unwilling or unable to cooperate with medical treatment? It so, why?
Quality of Life.	**Contextual Features**
The Principles of Beneficence and Nonmaleficence and Respect for Autonomy 1. What are the prospect, with or without treatment, for a return to normal life and what physical, mental, and social deficits might the patient experience even if treatment succeeds? 2. On what grounds can anyone judge that some quality of life would be undesirable for a patient who cannot make or express such a judgement? 3. Are there biases that might prejudice the provider's evaluation of the patient's quality of life? 4. What ethical issues arise concerning improving or enhancing a patient's quality of life? 5. Do quality-of-life assessment raise any questions that might contribute to a change of treatment plan, such as forgoing life-sustaining treatment? 6. Are there plans to provide pain relief and provide comfort after a decision has been made to forgo life-sustaining interventions? 7. Is medically assisted dying ethically or legally permissible? 8. What is the legal and ethical status of suicide?	The Principles of Justic and Fairness 1. Are there professional, interprofessional, or business interests that might create conflicts of interest in the clinical treatment of patients? 2. Are there parties other than clinician and patient, such as family members, who have a legitimate interest in clinical decisions? 3. What are the limits imposed on patient confidentiality by the legitimate interests of third parties? 4. Are there financial factors that create conflicts of interest in clinical decisions? 5. Are there problems of allocation of resouces that effect clinical decisions? 6. Are there religious factors that might influence clinical decisions? 7. What are the legal issues that might effect clinical decisions? 8. Are there considerations of clinical research and medical education that affect clinical decisions? 9. Are there considerations of public health and safety that influence clinical decisions? 10. Does institutional affiliation create conflicts of interest that might influence clinical decisions?

Fig. 3.1 The four-topics matrix of Jonsen, Siegler, and Winslade, which is based on the Ethical Principlism approach of Beauchamp and Childress [4]. With permission, from Jonsen AR, Siegler M, Winslade WJ. Clinical ethics. 8th ed. McGraw-Hill; 2015

3.3   Why Do Surgical Ethics Matter?

> Surgery is a moral practice, and every surgeon is a moral agent—Pellegrini [5]

Surgical ethics is a subcategory of medical ethics that focuses on issues concerning issues related to the care of surgical patients. It encompasses, but is not limited to, providing a framework to address dilemmas surgeons face in the daily care of patients, research, education, leadership, and management. Surgery is inherently a technical skill, but it is also, in more general terms, a healing art. A technically excellent outcome that fails to regard the relevant ethical principles in an encounter with a patient falls short of surgical excellence. A truly optimal outcome can result only when the technical and the ethical elements are in concordance. The ethical question in patient care is not "what *can* be done for this patient?" but rather, "what *should* be done for this patient?"

Surgical ethics is not a static system; it is dynamically informed by evolving technologies, value systems—both personal and societal—and worldviews. Ethical issues should be revisited periodically, and underlying assumptions may need to be overturned. Principles do not change, but their application may have to be tailored to changing needs or values of a specific community to best serve its members. The role of surgeons, too, may evolve. At various career stages, surgeons function as health care providers, teachers, learners, innovators, researchers, administrators, and leaders. Ethical principles that surgeons apply conform to a varied hierarchy of importance based on the roles and responsibilities they embody [1]. Pellegrini [5] proposed characteristics of excellence of a modern competent surgeon that include: (1) clinical skills and surgical judgment; (2) technical skills; (3) knowledge and practice of humanism, ethics, and moral values.

3.4   What Makes Surgical Ethics Different?

1. *Training and education*

By definition and function of the specialty, surgeons necessarily inflict harm by performing an operation to heal—i.e., anatomical correction or removal of disease. The benefits of surgery, however, overbalance the harm. Surgery as a discipline requires technical performance as well as decisions based on appropriateness, acceptability, and standards of care, all of which are mastered during education and training, and refined through professional practice.

According to Chap. 9 of the American Medical Association (AMA) Code of Ethics [6], physicians have a responsibility to teach and mentor those who follow, for they are the future of our caring profession. The process of training the future generation of physicians, however, must be balanced with a physician's obligation to the patient, and the patients' freedom to choose from whom they received their medical treatment. The obligation to educate trainees is especially challenging in surgical specialties, because the acquisition of technical skills and judgment comes with a learning curve that is uniquely consequential in surgery—errors made during operations can lead to immediate and grave consequences. To ensure patient safety and quality of care, appropriate faculty supervision is an absolute ethical requirement. Trainees gain competence through graduated responsibility that is linked to their level of training and expertise, as determined by their instructing surgeons. Trainees must be aware of their own limitations, and educators are obligated to evaluate and understand their trainees' abilities and readiness before advancing their responsibilities. Patients should be informed about modifications to standard procedures, if there are any, for educational purposes and be given the opportunity, without coercion, to agree or refuse.

In providing education for technical knowledge and skills, physicians have not only an ethical responsibility to accurately evaluate trainees for the welfare of future patients, but because no formal objective test for technical performance or proficiency is usually available upon completion of surgical training, educators have the vital role to constantly evaluate each trainee's technical performance throughout residency. This ensures the trainee has an environment to allow for successful achievement of competency and provides pathways for self-improvement should deficiencies be identified. Concurrently, educators must be aware of their own biases, both implicit and explicit, in their assessment of trainees' surgical competence and autonomous functioning to ensure that all receive equitable opportunities to succeed in their professional careers [7].

A major objective of surgical training is to provide trainees the tools and motivation to practice lifelong learning and self-improvement throughout their careers, ensuring that their future patients will continue to receive excellent care.

2. *Patient care*

The surgeon's mantle bestows many roles, but the role of caring for patients engenders the most distinctive and demanding ethical circumstances. Those unique ethical demands arise from the special relationship between surgeon and patient, a relationship that is characterized by professional intimacy and mutual reliance. No other professional relationship requires the same degree of trust, as is required when patients undergo anesthesia, rendering them completely helpless while allowing their surgeon to cut into their body. The profession therefore carries a heavy weight of responsibility for patients' well-being. They can never treat that responsibility lightly.

The process of informed consent is ethically necessary to respect the patient's autonomy in clinical and research settings. This process can be particularly challenging and nuanced in surgery for several reasons. Contrary to the paternalistic decision-making paradigm of the past, the current ethically best practice in planning a patient's treatment is shared decision making, in which the surgeon and patient together choose a treatment option that is best for the patient. It is an amalgamation of medical-surgical facts, which are provided by the surgeon, and the patient's value system. Together they decide on the best course to take. No matter the agreement or disagreement, the patient makes the final decision, thereby exercising the right of personal autonomous decision making [8].

In the shared decision-making framework, the patient's autonomy is balanced with the surgeon's clinical experience, knowledge, and recommendation [8]. Transferring to the patient the medical knowledge required to understand the rationale and alternatives to treatment is not always possible, particularly when the time before surgery is limited. The stakes may be high, however, when the procedure at hand is highly invasive and carries life-threatening or life-altering risks while the patient is incapacitated under general anesthesia. If the need for treatment is time-sensitive, all of the necessary decision-making information is unlikely to be available [8]. Moreover, decision making is often complicated by factors such as varying degrees of capacity, minor status, language barriers, educational status, or religious factors that limit therapeutic options.

Despite these barriers, the profound depth of trust that characterizes the surgeon-patient relationship requires for its sustenance surgeons' uncompromising adherence to ethical principles. Many examples illustrate the importance of ethical principles that help to cultivate trust. Surgeons bear the responsibility of preserving the patient's physical and informational privacy, as well as maintaining strict confidentiality of all patient-related interactions. They must hold their patients' best interests above all potentially conflicting motives (e.g., promoting their own financial interests, rejecting high-risk patients because of public reporting, increasing productivity, enhancing a positive reputation, and burnishing relationships with industry). If errors have occurred, surgeons must fully disclose them to patients and families with honesty and humility. In return for surgeons' full dedication to patients' best interests, patients trust surgeons to take them safely through the surgical experience, navigating expected and unexpected intra- and post-operative events, which often require that decisions be made under conditions of uncertainty.

3. *Physician wellness and professional conduct*

Physicians are responsible for maintaining their own health and wellness to ensure that they are capable of continuing to provide safe and effective medical and surgical care for their patients according to Chaps. 8 and 9 of the AMA Code of Ethics [6]. Surgeons and surgical trainees are particularly at risk for burnout due to the length of working hours, delayed career gratification, and high-stakes operative outcomes [9]. The negative effects of emotional and physical fatigue, stress, burnout, and illness can prevent physicians from being able to perform at their best. When physicians' health or wellness is compromised, they are obligated to take measures to mitigate the problem, seek appropriate help, and take appropriate measures to protect patients. Physicians and their colleagues have a collective obligation to create communities and environments that foster their own wellness and that of others. A corollary obligation is to assist, intervene, and report impaired colleagues according to Chaps. 8 and 9 of the AMA Code of Ethics [6].

The way physicians and surgeons conduct themselves, in person and online, must uphold the values and standards of the medical profession. Surgeons take on various roles beyond being a physician, such as advocate, scholar, collaborator, leader, and educator of not only trainees, but also of patients, colleagues, and the public. They have an obligation to communicate truth and information, and to counter misinformation. Best practices for surgeons' social media have been published by the Cardiothoracic Ethics Forum [10] and are consistent with the Codes of Ethics of Society of Thoracic Surgeons (STS) [11] and the American Association for Thoracic Surgery (AATS) [12]. In brief, as with in-person relations, online interactions must preserve patient confidentiality and privacy, uphold professionalism, maintain boundaries, appropriately disclose conflicts of interest, portray oneself and content accurately, understand the permanence of all online activity, and recognize that great responsibility accompanies the influence arising from respect and authority.

4. *Surgical research*

The common purpose of all operations, which are inherently invasive and are often costly, is to maximize healing and reduce harm. This purpose can be undermined if the rationale for a treatment is not objectively rooted in empirical facts, in which case standard therapies would then remain in general use without demonstrable efficacy. Surgical research provides the means to evaluate, improve, and disseminate facts about the science and art of surgery.

The nature of innovation is such that some treatments in early stages of development may be without benefit or may appear to be harmful, futile, or unethical. Historical texts contain many examples of declarations that certain treatments or operations are beyond the realm of possible. Theodor Billroth, possibly the greatest of all nineteenth century surgeons, famously exclaimed, "A surgeon who tries to suture a heart wound deserves to lose the esteem of his colleagues" [13]. Progress has often arisen, however, from courageous innovation and has erased doubt, such as Ludwig Rehn's suture repair of a heart laceration that challenged Billroth's declaration just a few years later. Innovation and research have been the processes by which new approaches are realized and hypotheses are proven and generalized into surgical practice.

The methodology of surgical research is different from most medical research for several reasons (see Chap. 48). Randomized controlled trials (RCTs) are more difficult to carry out for surgical procedures than, for example, for pharmaceutical trials. A 50 mg pill is the same no matter who prescribes it or where it is administered. Surgical procedures, however, are highly variable, depending on who the surgeons are, how many such procedures they have performed, what innovative technical variations they have introduced, and the local surgical culture at the institution in which it is done. The surgical learning curve of individual surgeons is more or less steep, depending on their experience and skill. Because of the need for substantial numbers of patient-subjects in order to achieve sufficient statistical power for valid conclusions, an increasing number of studies in surgery are multi-institutional. Unlike the standard dose of a medication, the standard techniques for a particular surgical procedure are highly variable, so comparison of one procedure with another when multiple surgeons are involved, is subject to important consistency errors [14].

Another challenge for surgical RCT studies is the unavailability of blinding for both the patients and investigators—surgeons always know what they are doing to their patients, so double-blinded RCTs are difficult, often impossible, to carry out. Although sham surgery, in which some subjects receive the true operation and the control group receive only an incision and a scar, has been ethically criticized, some have been successful in defining the efficacy or ineffectiveness of a procedure. In addition, the culture of surgery often encourages projecting confidence (e.g., "sometimes in error but never in doubt") [15], combined with the cognitive bias that doing something is more beneficial than withholding action, may not be conducive to careful, and at times tedious, adherence to protocols.

Overcoming these challenges requires anticipating pitfalls in ethical conduct of surgical research and establishing policies or structures to protect patients. The Belmont Report of 1979 established ethical principles for protection of research subjects and defined what constitutes research in distinction from practice [16]. Its principles—respect for persons, or autonomy, beneficence, and justice—were codified in 1984 in federal regulations that became known as the Common Rule [17], which established enforceable guidelines for research, including research oversight committees that the regulations termed Institutional Review Boards. Those regulations are intended to protect surgical research subjects, as all clinical research subjects, from potential exploitation, undue risks, or false or misleading information about a research protocol. Seven requirements for the ethical conduct of clinical research have been described: (1) socially valuable health-related knowledge, (2) rigorous methods that produce scientifically valid data, (3) fair selection of participants, (4) favorable risk-benefit ratio, (5) independent committee review and oversight, (6) thorough informed consent and (7) respectful treatment of patients during the course of research [14]. Together, these tenets ensure that clinical research is carried out within an ethical framework.

5. *Administration*

Surgeons' roles extend beyond clinical care and the operating theater, to include ethical obligations in the administrative, societal, and leadership realms. In administrative roles such as committee members and department and division leaders, surgeons wield substantial influence over the conduct of department, hospital, or university functions, including operating room culture, research directions and facilities, and education of students and trainees. Surgeons also face various pressures to meet the needs of their multispecialty teams, their employers, government regulations, a complex web of referral patterns, and national societies. This requires them to remain cognizant of the terrain of potential ethical problems and navigate them with thoughtful analysis and honest communication.

Surgeons may also contribute to developing and administering ethical standards at a local and national level through participation in groups such as the ACS Committee on Ethics and the STS Committee on Standards and Ethics [18]. Such committees and their members infuse ethical conversations into the surgical literature and conferences in various ways: publishing textbooks or manuscripts in specialty journals, hosting salient ethical presentations and debates at national conferences, and performing regulatory roles such as peer-review functions. Surgeons can also be directly involved in writing and implementing policies regarding the standards of the profession on topics such as engaging with social media, industry, and other entities that may be fraught with ethical dilemmas.

At a societal level, surgeons may exercise an ethical obligation to advocate for their patients through political activism, such as fundraising, lobbying, and testifying before congressional committees. Some have argued for an ethical obligation to testify in medically related court proceedings [19] (See Chap. 18). These activities can ultimately influence health policymaking at all levels of government.

3.5 How to Teach Surgical Ethics

1. *Teaching ethics*

Teaching surgical ethics (See Chap. 11) can provide an opportunity for surgeons and those in training to develop a proper framework and vocabulary for moral reasoning and deliberation. As they attempt to make sense of ethical problems as they arise, they can continue to refine their understanding [20]. Furthermore, teaching surgical ethics would meet most components of professionalism as required by the Accreditation Council for Graduate Medical Education (See Chap. 16). The Council's professionalism standard states:

> Residents must demonstrate a commitment to carrying out professional responsibilities and an adherence to ethical principles. Residents are expected to demonstrate:
>
> - Compassion, integrity, and respect for others
> - Responsiveness to patient needs that supersedes self-interest
> - Respect for patient privacy and autonomy
> - Accountability to patients, society and the profession; and,
> - Sensitivity and responsiveness to a diverse patient population, including but not limited to diversity in gender, age, culture, race, religion, disabilities, and sexual orientation. [21]

2. *Perspectives on an ethics curriculum*

A taxonomy of ethics curricula describes three overlapping spheres: (1) a formal curriculum taught in the classroom; (2) an informal curriculum consisting of ad hoc lessons, values, and attitudes learned through interactions with others; and (3) a "hidden curriculum", which includes all socialized influences embedded in task-specific experiences [22]. A qualitative study of surgical faculty and trainees demonstrated unanimous agreement on the importance of ethics education as a component of surgical training [22]; however, despite clinical exposure to ethical topics, residents' knowledge base was poor [23]. Furthermore, participants indicated that although some ethical issues can be conveyed in a formal curriculum, informal curricular teaching is also highly valued through real case discussion and varied teaching methods including but not limited to role-playing, debates, objective structured clinical examinations, and small group discussions, to bridge the divide between knowledge and application [22]. Furthermore, feedback on how one handles ethically difficult situations in informal curricula teaching or clinical practice was valued by participants in order to help identify areas for improvement, much like the process to refine and cultivate one's surgical skills.

3. *Challenges in teaching surgical ethics*

Trainees have identified challenges in teaching surgical ethics [22]: (1) providing trainees with an ethical framework; (2) providing practical insight into the issues they face within their particular specialties; and (3) demonstrating real-life perspectives using case-based examples to learn to apply their knowledge to clinical practice. Trainee respondents also identified challenges when facing and navigating situations involving unethical faculty behavior or ill-conceived administrative decisions.

In the field of cardiothoracic surgery, surgical ethics has been taught and fostered by the Cardiothoracic Ethics Forum, which provides ethics education for cardiothoracic surgeons through presentations and debates on ethical issues at national meetings of cardiothoracic surgical societies. In addition to their ethics committees, the STS and the AATS also have established the position of ethics editors of their respective journals, *The Annals of Thoracic Surgery (ATS)* and the *Journal of Thoracic and Cardiovascular Surgery (JTCVS)*, through which publication of articles on ethical issues in surgery can be facilitated. In a survey of 578 cardiothoracic surgeons [24], 83% of respondents believed that cardiothoracic surgeons would benefit from ethics education to improve their understanding of complex ethical issues in cardiothoracic surgery; 64% agreed or strongly agreed that ethics sessions at national meetings improved their understanding. In addition to the aforementioned efforts, the Cardiothoracic Surgery Ethics Forum supports opportunities for intellectual development and preparation for leadership roles in surgical ethics through scholarships for surgeons and trainees to obtain formal education and training in biomedical ethics.

3.6   Future Directions

Surgical ethics is not a static discipline, but is dynamic and constantly evolving, shaped by scientific advances, administrative demands, national and world events, and shifting societal values. The practice of surgery requires a deep fund of knowledge and sound judgment about ethical challenges encountered in daily practice. Educators should seek to continually evaluate and refine education in surgical ethics to ensure it remains relevant and able to meet the needs of trainees and faculty. Surgeon teachers can capitalize on their past experiences to provide case-based examples and discuss with learners the options, decision-making process, potential solutions and outcomes. A specific program to accomplish this through morbidity and mortality rounds has been described recently [25] and should be adopted by surgical training programs more widely. Trainees should make every effort to be present during faculty discussions with patients and their families regarding the risks, benefits, and uncertainties of a proposed surgical treatment, and should seek guidance when faced with ethical dilemmas. Furthermore, just as surgical simulation laboratories help trainees improve technique and self-confidence in technical skills, proficiency at managing ethical problems can be strengthened through demonstration and varied active learning methods with trainee engagement.

3.7   Concluding Remarks

Over 20 years ago, we studied a previously described disparity in the rate of discussion of ethical issues between the medical and the surgical literatures [1, 24]—such discussions had been found to be four times more frequent in the medical than in the surgical literature. In the two decades since that publication, efforts to address the gap by increasing discussion of ethical issues in surgical meetings and publications and to introduce ethics education in surgical training programs have flourished. In cardiothoracic surgery alone in the last two decades, members of the Cardiothoracic Ethics Forum have published nearly 500 papers on ethical issues in the surgical and related literature, have presented over 50 hour-long ethics discussions and debates at national cardiothoracic surgical society meetings, and have developed numerous ethics-related policies for surgical societies.

Methods and programs for formal ethics education in surgical training programs have been developed and disseminated by such institutions as the MacLean Center for Clinical Medical Ethics of the University of Chicago, and the Joint Centre for Bioethics, Dalla Lana School of Public Health of the University of Toronto.

The depth of trust demanded between patients and surgeons in clinical surgery place the surgeon in unique ethical circumstances, and ethical practice has been deeply ingrained in surgeons for well over a century; that embedded ethical tradition was not recognized as such, however, nor were ethical issues often explicitly discussed in formal settings until recently. Our thoracic surgeon colleague and ethicist, Martin McKneally, has said, "Surgeons are practicing ethicists throughout their career" [26]. To that idea we could add that surgeons *have always been* practicing ethicists. Now, ethics discussions and education has been made a permanent and explicit part of surgical meetings, conferences, and rounds, as well as of surgical training—we believe this will redound to the ultimate betterment of surgical practice.

3.8   Selected References

- Sade RM. The Ethics of Surgery: Conflicts and Controversies. Oxford University Press; 2015. p. 1–13.

  - The author begins with an overview of the ethics gap in surgery and then delves into case examples of cardiothoracic surgical ethics related to issues of professional integrity, relationships with patients in terms of autonomy and consent, innovation and use of technology as well as organ donation and transplantation. In addition, conflicts of interest in surgery as well as ethical issues in health-care policy are also explored.

- Devon K, Sade R. Surgical ethics: How I teach it. Ann Thorac Surg. 2020;110(6):1805–1808. https://doi.org/10.1016/j.athoracsurg.2020.07.010

  - A step-by-step of how to teach surgical ethics to trainees from the perspective of a surgeon-ethicist. Emphasis is placed on the importance of utilizing every interaction as an opportunity to discuss ethical issues, integrating ethics into clinical training, as well as academic events and activities. Ethics "teaching moments" are emphasized throughout all aspects of clinical training, including morbidity and mortality rounds, journal clubs, and patient interactions.

- Brewster LP, Hall DE, Joehl RJ. Assessing residents in surgical ethics: We do it a lot; We only know a little. J Surg Res. 2011;171(2):395–398. https://doi.org/10.1016/j.jss.2011.04.008

  - Surgical residents' exposure to ethical scenarios and their confidence level and understanding of ethical principles are explored. Despite clinical exposure to and self-perceived confidence of ethical topics, surgical residents' knowledge was low, highlighting the need for a formal ethics curriculum.

References

1. Sade RM. The ethics of surgery: conflicts and controversies. Oxford University Press; 2015. p. 1–13.
2. Bonde S, Firenze P. A framework for making ethical decisions. Science and technology studies. Brown University; 2013. https://www.brown.edu/academics/science-and-technology-studies/framework-making-ethical-decisions. Accessed 15 Dec 2020.
3. Beauchamp TL, Childress JF. Principles of biomedical ethics. 8th ed. Oxford University Press; 2019.
4. Jonsen A, Siegler M, Winslade W. Clinical ethics: a practical approach to ethical decisions in clinical medicine. 8th ed. McGraw-Hill; 2015. p. 9.
5. Pellegrini CA. Presidential address: the surgeon of the future: anchoring innovation and science with moral values. Bull Am Coll Surg. 2013;98(12):8–14.
6. American Medical Association. Opinion 9.2.2. Code of medical ethics. American Medical Association; 2017. p. 142–143.
7. Kim GJ, Clark MJ, Meyerson SL, et al. Mind the gap: the autonomy perception gap in the operating room by surgical residents and faculty. J Surg Educ. 2020;77:1522–7. https://doi.org/10.1016/j.surg.2020.05.023.
8. Kon AA. The shared decision-making continuum. JAMA. 2010;309:903–4. https://doi.org/10.1001/jama.2010.1208.
9. Swain JD, Soegaard Ballester JM, Luc JGY, Han JJ. Burning the candle at both ends: Mitigating surgeon burnout at the training stages. [Published online ahead of print June 21, 2020]. J Thorac Cardiovasc Surg. https://doi.org/10.1016/j.jtcvs.2020.06.122.

10. Varghese TKJ, Entwistle JW, Mayer JE, Moffatt-Bruce SD, Sade RM, for the Cardiothoracic Ethics Forum. Ethical standards for cardiothoracic surgeons' participation in social media. Ann Thorac Surg. 2019;108:666–70. https://doi.org/10.1016/j.athoracsurg.2019.04.003.
11. Code of Ethics. Society of thoracic surgeons. https://sts.org/about-sts/policies/code-ethics. Accessed 15 Dec 2020.
12. Code of Ethics. American association for thoracic surgery. https://www.aats.org/aatsimis/AATSWeb/Association/About/Governance/By-Laws_and_Policies/Code_of_Ethics.aspx. Accessed 15 Dec 2020.
13. Mueller U. Medizingeschichte: Herznaht wider ethische Bedenken. Dtsch Arztebl. 2007;104(1–2):A26–8.
14. Guiding Principles for Ethical Research. National Institutes of Health (NIH). https://www.nih.gov/health-information/nih-clinical-research-trials-you/guiding-principles-ethical-research. Accessed 15 Dec 2020.
15. Gawande A. Complications. Metropolitan Books; 2002:15.
16. The Belmont report. Ethical principles and guidelines for the protection of human subjects of research. National Commission for the Protection of Human Subjects of Biomedical and Behavioral Research; 1979. https://www.hhs.gov/ohrp/regulations-and-policy/belmont-report/read-the-belmont-report/index.html. Accessed 15 Dec 2020.
17. Federal Policy for the Protection of Human Subjects ('Common Rule'). https://www.hhs.gov/ohrp/regulations-and-policy/regulations/common-rule/index.html. Accessed 15 Dec 2020.
18. Sade RM, McKneally MF. Evolution of STS ethical standards: adjudication, policy making, and education. Ann Thorac Surg. 2014;97:S44–7. https://doi.org/10.1016/j.athoracsurg.2013.10.007.
19. Watson DC, Robicsek F, Sade RM. Are thoracic surgeons ethically obligated to serve as expert witnesses for the plaintiff? Ann Thorac Surg. 2004;78(4):1137–41. https://doi.org/10.1016/J.athoracsurg.2004.07.001.
20. Devon K, Sade R. Surgical ethics: how I teach it. Ann Thorac Surg. 2020;110(6):1805–8. https://doi.org/10.1016/j.athoracsurg.2020.07.010.
21. ACGME Common Program Requirements. Accreditation Council for Graduate Medical Education; 2017. p. 11. https://www.acgme.org/Portals/0/PFAssets/ProgramRequirements/CPRs_2017-07-01.pdf. Accessed 15 Dec 2020.
22. Howard F, McKneally MF, Upshur REG, Levin AV. The formal and informal surgical ethics curriculum: views of resident and staff surgeons in Toronto. Am J Surg. 2012;203(2):258–65. https://doi.org/10.1016/j.amjsurg.2011.02.008.
23. Brewster LP, Hall DE, Joehl RJ. Assessing residents in surgical ethics: we do it a lot; we only know a little. J Surg Res. 2011;171(2):395–8. https://doi.org/10.1016/j.jss.2011.04.008.
24. D'Amico TA, McKneally MF, Sade RM. Ethics in cardiothoracic surgery: a survey of surgeons' views. Ann Thorac Surg. 2010;90(1):11–13.e1–4. https://doi.org/10.1016/j.athoracsurg.2010.03.061.
25. Snelgrove R, Ng SL, Devon K. Reconceptualizing ethics through morbidity and mortality rounds. J Am Coll Surg. 2020;231:233–48. https://doi.org/10.1016/j.jamcollsurg.2020.04.038.
26. Devon K. Turning the spotlight on the Editor. The Surgical Spotlight. University of Toronto. Fall-Winter; 2015–2016. p. 15. http://www.surgicalspotlight.ca/Shared/PDF/SS_Winter-Spring_16.pdf. Accessed 13 Dec 2020.

Chapter 4
Notable Ethical Surgeons

Vassyl A. Lonchyna (iD), **Peggy Kelley** (iD), **and Peter Angelos** (iD)

Abstract As the three co-editors of this volume considered our own experiences as surgeons, we realized that each of us were dramatically influenced by many surgeons and other physicians who have been role models of the ethical care of patients. While not wanting to be too self-indulgent, we thought it valuable to discuss the influences of some notable ethical physicians and surgeons on our own careers and practices. In an acknowledgement of the impact of the pandemic that has raged as we worked on this volume, Vassyl Lonchyna has written about healthcare workers who have selflessly cared for patients. Peggy Kelley cites the influences of two distinguished otolaryngologists, Dr. John J. Conley and Dr. Sylvan Stool, who transcended their specific practices to become role models for all surgeons. Peter Angelos explores the impact of Sir William Stokes who may have been the first to use the term "surgical ethics" in print and Dr. C. Rollins Hanlon who led the American College of Surgeons for many years and also influenced the growing acceptance of surgical ethics in American surgery. Vassyl Lonchyna concludes the chapter by considering the personal sacrifice of Dr. Ostap Selianski, a Ukrainian country doctor, who heroically served patients until his death in World War II.

Keywords Healthcare workers · COVID-19 · John J. Conley · Sylvan S stool · Sir William Stokes · C. Rollins Hanlon · Ostap Selianski

V. A. Lonchyna (✉)
MacLean Center for Clinical Medical Ethics, University of Chicago, Chicago, IL, USA

Institute for Bioethics, Ukrainian Catholic University, Lviv, Ukraine
e-mail: vassyl@aol.com

P. Kelley
Providence Children's Surgical Services, St. Vincent Hospital, Portland, OR, USA
e-mail: peggy.kelley@providence.org

P. Angelos
Department of Surgery and MacLean Center for Clinical Medical Ethics,
The University of Chicago, Chicago, IL, USA
e-mail: pangelos@surgery.bsd.uchicago.edu

© The Author(s), under exclusive license to Springer Nature
Switzerland AG 2022
V. A. Lonchyna et al. (eds.), *Difficult Decisions in Surgical Ethics*, Difficult
Decisions in Surgery: An Evidence-Based Approach,
https://doi.org/10.1007/978-3-030-84625-1_4

4.1 The Healthcare Worker in the Time of COVID

The twentieth century is bookended by two deadly pandemics …

> It was the best of times, it was the worst of times …. Charles Dickens, *A Tale of Two Cities* (1859)

We begin this chapter, neigh book, in acknowledging our utmost respect, thankfulness and gratitude to all of the healthcare workers of the world. They ran into the face of the enemy without hesitation, fought bravely and tirelessly to vanquish this enemy virus. Despite potential grave danger to themselves and their families, they worked long hours as the onslaught mounted and seemed never to abate.

Who are these heroes? They are your neighbors. Every day, ordinary people who chose the vocation of helping others. At the beginning of the pandemic, they could not have imagined how our world would be turned upside down and inside out and badly shaken with the ravages of an unseen disease. The disease that did not discriminate, that attacked young and old, and especially our most vulnerable, the elderly, those with chronic diseases, those facing disparities of healthcare access due to their socio-economic status, and unwittingly the healthcare workers themselves. These are the heroes of the frontline: paramedics, clerks, nurses, laboratory technicians, phlebotomists, doctors. They are joined in brother/sisterhood with those that help the system work to keep an everyday, but highly strained, infrastructure purring at an overtaxed speed: the maintenance workers, transporters, cooks, bio-technical support, drivers, and morgue workers.

Every day we see images of the frontline caregivers, decked out in space age protective gear, working exhaustive hours to care for critically ill patients. (see Fig. 4.1). We see the tears on the faces of workers dealing with death on, not a daily, but hourly basis. We see the strain in the eyes and faces of workers, who care for patients who are not able to have family with them, who become the last human touch the patients feel before leaving this life. We see long lines of people waiting for COVID testing, enabled by healthcare volunteers placing their health and lives on the line to be part of the nationwide/worldwide response to controlling this pandemic.

This has resulted in a myriad of victims. Firstly, those HC workers, who themselves became infected, with a high mortality rate. Secondly, the families of the HC workers, who despite a myriad of complicated safety measures, including self-quarantine, could not escape being infected and suffering the wrath of this disease. Thirdly, the extreme fatigue and emotional toll on the HC workers, who see no end to this war, who suffer from PTSD and even have succumbed to suicide.

Next, but not lastly, the everyday anticipation of relief, in the form of vaccination. The HC workers are the first to receive it, as they are our frontline soldiers. But the eradication of this enemy will depend on herd immunity, achievable only by having 80–90% of the entire population immunized with one of the many effective and safe vaccines brought into service within a year by the immense efforts and cooperation of scientists, physicians, industry and government. The HC worker will be spearheading this massive relief for our population, without which we will not see an end to this pandemic.

Fig. 4.1 Self-portrait: working with COVID patients. By Nurse Maribel Huerta, a surgical ICU nurse at Advocate Christ Medical Center in Oak Lawn, IL [1]

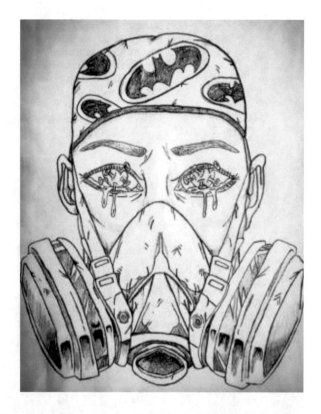

The years 2020–2021 have been incredible for mankind. Our healthcare workers, whom we often take for granted, have stepped up to the challenge, and without hesitation, have fought for each of us. To each and every healthcare worker, we owe our gratitude, and we acknowledge them as our heroes.

Complaint

They call and I go,
It is a frozen road
past midnight, a dust
of snow caught
in the rigid wheeltracks.
The door opens.
I smile, enter and
shake off the cold.
Here is a great woman
on her side in the bed.
She is sick,
perhaps vomiting,
perhaps laboring
to give birth to
a tenth child. Joy! Joy!
Night is a room

darkened for lovers,
through the jalousies the sun
has sent one golden needle!
I pick the hair from her eyes
and watch her misery
with compassion.

William Carlos Williams 1921 [2]
—Vassyl A Lonchyna

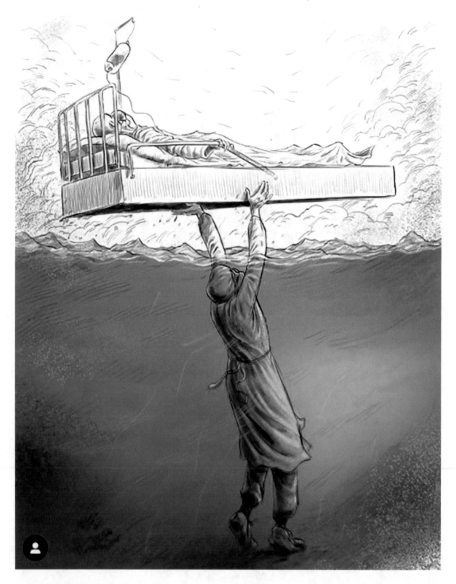

Fig. 4.2 "The Sacrifice" (2020), dedicated to all the doctors of the world, by Iranian artist Bozorgmehr Hosseinpour

4.2 John J. Conley MD (1912–1999)

Dr. Conley, a native Pennsylvanian and graduate of the University of Pittsburgh School of Medicine, became a New York City otolaryngologist who specialized in treating patients with head and neck cancer (see Fig. 4.3). And, for many surgeons, his name is synonymous with surgical ethics. As a surgeon, he had a long career that encompassed the development of head and neck cancer extirpation and reconstructive surgery. He innovated operations for speech following laryngectomy and one step myocutaneous flaps for reconstruction following ablative cancer surgery of the face and neck as well as made contributions leading to successful nerve grafting.

As a Clinical Professor of Otolaryngology at Columbia University College of Physicians and Surgeons, he published nearly 300 surgical papers and eight books. He was willing to share both his excellent [4] and catastrophic [5] surgical results for the advancement of the nascent field. **He was known for being a master surgical technician with deliberate, delicate precision when indicated and rapid, utilitarian and courageous cuts where needed. His passion for both performing and teaching surgery was well known.** Among his clinical accolades, he was named the first president of the American Society of Head and Neck Surgery. He also served as president of the American Academy of Ophthalmology and Otolaryngology and later the American Academy of Facial Plastic and Reconstructive Surgery.

Fig. 4.3 Dr. John J. Conley. With permission from John Wiley and Sons [3]

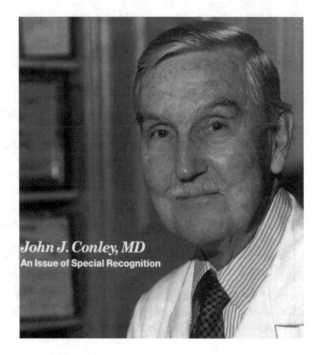

John J. Conley, MD
An Issue of Special Recognition

As an ethicist, Dr. Conley wrote thoughtfully about the difficult decisions that surgeons face. Beginning in the 1980's his papers started reflecting his ideas on ethics but as early as the mid 1970's he was writing about justice issues [6]. After retiring from performing surgery at 80 years of age, he founded the John Conley Foundation for Ethics and Philosophy in Medicine. Difficult decisions that surgeons face was addressed in his essay *Have I performed the right operation?* [7] Here Conley outlines the difficulty of acknowledging that there is no one right operation and that even the right operation, performed well, may result in a treatment failure. For him, the important thing in finding the right operation was to have a working relationship with each patient to understand how various surgical options would affect them and in taking the time to review the outcome of each operation a surgeon completes so that there is no hiding behind a mask of "well I tried".

We are in unprecedented times: a theme also addressed by this sage. In *Concepts of ethics in medicine*, [8] Conley writes that the ideal laws of Moses (laws for social behavior) and Hippocrates (laws for doctors) set us up to deal with incomprehensible progress and change in science and technology. He states, "we are better prepared to meet these challenges as we are compelled to mutate in another direction." A prophetic call to rely on the stabilizing forces and intrinsic good of the Hippocratic oath he summarizes as:

1. Be humble and proud you are a doctor.
2. Be grateful to your teachers.
3. Honor your colleagues and your patients with natural and honest respect.
4. Defend the rights and dignity of the patient.
5. Accept and help all patients, without exclusion to the best of your ability.
6. Do not perform unnecessary surgery.
7. Inform the patient and his or her family about the disease process, the possible complications of treatment, answer questions, and recognize options and alternatives.
8. Do not give guarantees but tell the truth as you see it.
9. Never hesitate to advise a second opinion, seek help, or refer a patient to another doctor.
10. Be fair in your charges and be generous to those who cannot pay. The professionality of medicine should be higher than business. Recognize the essentiality of business in all aspects of medicine and use it to improve medical elegance and service.
11. Respect confidentiality.
12. Appreciate the complexities of illness, the hazards of treatment, and the sanctity of life.
13. Recognize that not all problems can be solved, and that there is often an association with religion, politics, ethics, and society [8].

Reading Conley's summary of the Hippocratic oath reminds me that even in the midst of change and pandemic, basic principles of treating others how I would like to be treated is a sound foundation from which to practice medicine and surgery.

Dr. Conley's contributions to the field of surgical ethics have been recognized as the surgeon ethicist for whom both the American College of Surgeons and the American Academy of Otolaryngology-Head and Neck Surgery have named their national ethics lectureships.

From the American College of Surgeons:

> The Conley Ethics and Philosophy Lecture is sponsored by the Committee on Ethics and has been generously supported since 1991 by John J. Conley, MD, FACS, New York, NY, to explore ethical issues in surgery. Dr. Conley died in 1999, but his legacy continues, and his memory is honored at this annual lecture [9].

From the American Academy of Otolaryngology Head & Neck Surgery:

> The John Conley, MD Lecture on Medical Ethics has been given annually since 1986. It is based on Dr. John Conley's passion for head and neck surgery and belief in the professionalism of the practice of medicine. He was dedicated to the highest standard of moral and ethical behavior from physicians [10].

From the John Conley Foundation of Surgical Philosophy and Ethics:

> This lectureship was established by a well-known surgeon, John J Conley, an otolaryngologist who dedicated most of his professional life to the treatment of head and neck cancer. Dr. Conley was primarily a surgeon, not a philosopher or an ethicist. Yet, he believed that to provide the best care to patients with cancer, the surgeon should be trained in other areas, in addition to the traditional technical aspects of surgery. To that end, in the early 1990s, he founded the John J Conley Foundation for Ethics and Philosophy in Medicine, through which he established this lectureship to provide a forum within the American College of Surgeons where ethical questions facing surgeons could be discussed. He once said, "I consider ethics and philosophy to be in one sense, the essence of the medical profession … I am particularly interested in maintaining the highest ethical principles as a frontline for the practicing surgeon."

Dr. Conley embodied the idea that the practice of surgical ethics is part of the very fabric of who we, as surgeons, are and it is the philosophy that gave birth to this book. The study, the basic science of ethics, is rooted in philosophy. Whereas in the past, surgeons studied the Morbidity & Mortality of what went wrong, we now are teaching the science of how to make the right decision and what principles we can use to bolster our decision making. The four principles of clinical ethics: autonomy, beneficence, non-maleficence and justice are analogous to basic tenets of surgical practice: gentle handling of tissue, meticulous hemostasis, preservation of blood supply, and strict aseptic technique (Halstedian tenets). The surgeons chosen in this chapter are highlighted not because they didactically taught ethical principles out loud but because they demonstrated them day in and day out. They lived them.

Today, as we bring together various chapters in difficult decisions in surgical ethics, it is amazing to see the breadth of surgical specialty representation—all turning around the four principles of ethics. I find it interesting that the practice of surgical ethics is so much just a part of how we do surgery well and for the right reasons that this is the tenth book in the series *Difficult Decisions in Surgery: An Evidence Based Approach*. If ethics in surgery were so foreign and difficult, wouldn't it have been called out much earlier? Instead, the practice of surgery as an artform, as a service to mankind, is only able to be performed ethically. We are taught by our mentors and those whom we hold sacred, to trust our gut feelings, and embrace the mantle of "always gracious, always courteous, and always considerate." [11] The chapters that follow use cases to demonstrate how difficult life can be for our patients and families who may require us to perform heroic surgery or to choose not to.

—Peggy Kelley

4.3 Sylvan S. Stool MD (1925–2004)

When I think of an ethical person or someone who works ethically, I conjure up a person who always has the "ought" at the forefront of their approach to the patient in front of them, the colleague alongside of them, or the system that looms over them. For me the wise face that accompanies the *ought* principles of our ethical teachings is Sylvan Stool (see Fig. 4.4a).

Dr. Stool was one of the founders of pediatric otolaryngology [12]. Born and raised in Texas, he had a circuitous course through a year of pediatric surgery training in Seattle, WA, then pediatric training in Salt Lake City, UT and a pediatric residency at Boston Children's hospital. He set up a pediatric practice in Denver, CO where he lived in the flat above his medical office and was an Instructor in the Department of Pediatrics at the University of Colorado (CU).

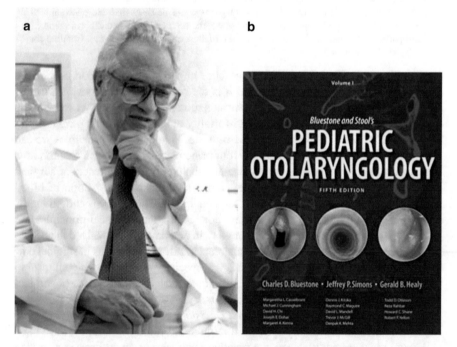

Fig. 4.4 (a) Dr. Sylvan S. Stool. With permission from Elsevier [12]. (b) Two-volume fifth edition of *Bluestone and Stool's Pediatric Otolaryngology* (2014). With permission from PMPH-USA [13]

He became fascinated with children's hearing, and he was seeing many children with fluid in the middle ear. He figured if he could get the fluid out of the child's ear, they would hear better. He went to the Chairman of Otolaryngology at CU and asked to be taught how to remove the middle ear fluid. He was told he needed training in ENT, so he secured funding as well as his first research grant from the NIH—Division of Neurological Diseases and Blindness in 1960 and became the first otolaryngology resident at CU (while teaching pediatrics at the same institution). The act of not being stopped because there was no program previously, brings us to the first *ought* I learned from Sylvan: **One ought to advance one's capabilities as they become available**.

His first Otolaryngology faculty appointment was at the University of Pennsylvania. At Children's Hospital of Philadelphia (CHOP) he honed his second *ought:* **You ought to do your best for the child in the era you find yourself now.** At CHOP, he became known for being an innovator in the pediatric airway. Dr. Stool was first to use and describe stay sutures placed at the edge of the trachea at the time of tracheostomy to minimize difficulty in replacing a tracheostomy tube if the child accidentally decannulated while healing (a significant cause of tracheostomy associated mortality). He brought the Hopkins rod telescope to the US and changed forever the field of bronchoscopy and laryngoscopy with the use of direct light and magnification and was instrumental in developing the first plastic tracheotomy tubes which were much more comfortable than the metal Jackson tracheostomy tubes.

He continued work on ear fluid and during this time had research funding for basic science work on an Animal Model for Serous Otitis. Throughout his career, otitis media was a consistent area of interest both in research and in treating children to restore their hearing. Later in his career he would be asked to speak about what he had learned over the years. Several times I heard his address on "There are no Golden Eras, just Golden days." When others bemoaned the passing of THE GOLDEN ERA OF MEDICINE, he would point out that when he started as a house officer in pediatrics, children died of Acute Lymphocytic Leukemia (ALL)—sometimes more than a handful every night and now ALL carries a 90% cure rate [14]. O'Dwyer tubes to hold open a constricting airway have been replaced by antibiotics, intubation and endoscopic management. He would note that while the issues at hand would always be present, ever changing but present, if we focused on the child who lived, the child who breathed because of our help, we would have the energy and the wherewithal to continue being a physician called to care for our patients.

While we may have the goal to CURE, with advances and innovation and success in business, it is our responsibility always to CARE. We cannot guarantee to always know what to do or when to do it or not, but we CAN guarantee our patients that we will be thoughtful and caring in our approach to their problems, to their concerns. He would ask, "What ought to be your priority today?" Just writing about his way of thinking about problems makes my pulse slow, my shoulders relax. When we are focused on the "ought" so much of the "what ifs" fall away.

With the dream of practicing otolaryngology only for children, this otolaryngologist nee pediatrician joined Dr. Charles Bluestone in Pittsburgh and there established the first pediatric otolaryngology fellowship at Children's Hospital of Pittsburgh—again securing the first NIH training funding for the field, as well as writing the first and still preeminent text on pediatric otolaryngology, now in its fifth edition (see Fig. 4.4b) [13].

This brings me to the final *ought*: **You ought to multiply your care by sharing your expertise with others.** By others, he did not mean just other pediatric otolaryngologists. The fellowship was certainly one of the most prolific in the US but as a pediatrician he knew that it was necessary to involve all those that treat the whole child, so he established the first multidisciplinary group, The Society for Ear Nose and Throat Advancement in Children (SENTAC). SENTAC is a collective group of like-minded health care professionals involved in the care of children with otolaryngology, hearing, speech and swallowing disorders. Uniquely composed of physicians and allied health care professionals, SENTAC's members include otolaryngologists, pediatricians, basic scientists, audiologists, speech therapists, occupational therapists, nurse practitioners, and physician assistants [15].

Dr. Stool was not satisfied in treating only the children of the US, he felt called to serve internationally. He developed a Pneumatic Otoscopy Workshop which allowed him to have a mobile educational platform. He traveled several times to the remote islands of the South Pacific where he and colleagues taught and trained health care workers to do simple surgical procedures. He took the Otoscopy Workshop to 31 central and South American Countries. He was a founding father and first president of the Interamerican Association of Pediatric Otolaryngologists (IAPO). The IAPO organization benefited from his guidance in those embryonic days and owes much current success to his soft-styled guidance. Both U.S. and Latin colleagues gave testimony to his role as teacher, mentor, friend, and "father." (see Fig. 4.5) [16].

Currently, IAPO) has translated its publications into more than 10 languages and the main website is available in English, Spanish and Portuguese. He also co-founded the Latin America Otitis Media Research and Training Program. He traveled to Geneva to counsel the World Health Organization about ear programs in less economically advantaged countries. He also supported the newly forming global groups of pediatric otolaryngologists such as ESPO (European Society of Pediatric Otolaryngology).

Back home, he cared for the disadvantaged and "coveted" the privilege of treating that group of patients that needed the most help. Sylvan's patient impact sometimes was less visible yet even more profound than daily office visits or surgery. In a masterstroke of prevention, Sylvan and his son, Daniel, approached the McDonald's Corporation to decrease the hazards of foreign body aspiration from the famous "Happy Meals." Sylvan felt that giving a small child a colorful meal with food to eat, plus a colorful toy that was not meant for consumption, too often resulted in an ingested toy. The concept he proposed was to redesign the small toys. Now there are age-appropriate labeled toys which have saved many lives.

The Laryngoscope
Lippincott Williams & Wilkins, Inc.
© 2005 The American Laryngological,
Rhinological and Otological Society, Inc.

Sylvan Stool

Peggy Kelley, MD; James Reilly, MD; Roland D. Eavey, MD, SM

Sylvan Stool will be remembered fondly as a unique, fascinating, and comfortable friend by his numerous colleagues. Tragically, earlier this year, Sylvan died suddenly. Yet, in many ways, he survives.

Sylvan accomplished much for the field of otolaryngology; perhaps most well known is the signature textbook *Pediatric Otolaryngology*, along with many other pioneering educational and research contributions at the Children's Hospital of Pittsburgh. Among his many accomplishments, perhaps lesser known in the United States, was being named the first President of the Interamerican Association of Pediatric Otolaryngology (IAPO), and organization that recently held a meeting at which Sylvan was honored. IAPO has grown in the past decade to convene several successful Congresses, has published three books, and has been joined by about 5000 mostly Latin pediatri-

corpus and created the first and most prolific Pediatric Otolaryngology Fellowship training program. Sylvan capt ured National Institutes of Health (NIH) resources to fund the fellowship. Sylvan initiated the group SENTAC (Society of ENT Advances in Children). He was a charter member of ASPO (American Society of Pediatric Otolaryngology). Before those accomplishments, as a solo Chief of Otolaryngology at the Children's Hospital of Philadelphia, he pioneered surgical airway management advances, such as the use of the Hopkins rod telescope for bronchoscopy and the plastic tracheotomy tube with stay sutures for safety.

Few people know that Sylvan did not start out his medical career as an otolaryngologist. Sylvan was a practicing pediatrician in Denver, and he and June already

Fig. 4.5 In memorium for Sylvan Stool by his Fellows. (With permission from John Wiley and Sons [16])

The lessons of how I ought to consider the patients before me, my colleagues around me and systems that I work in and through, travel with me daily. I was fortunate to be Dr. Stool's medical student and later pediatric otolaryngology colleague. I ought to take advantage of opportunities, I ought to treat the child before me the best way I know now, and I ought to be willing to learn from and teach others so that children's lives are better everywhere.

This is the lesson that Dr. Sylvan Stool, the son of a Jewish storekeeper in West Texas and father of the field of pediatric otolaryngology taught. It is a lesson I try to carry with me each day. Thank you for the opportunity to remind myself.

—Peggy Kelley

4.4   Growth of Surgical Ethics

In recent decades, there has been a growth of interest in surgical ethics. This burgeoning interest in surgical ethics can be tracked through the table of contents of surgical journals or the programs from many surgical societies over recent years. This focus on the ethical dimension of the care of surgical patients has had several important results. First of all, patients have gotten higher quality care because their surgeons have attended to the importance of communication, disclosure, and developing trust in the informed consent process. Secondly, surgeons have also found that by acknowledging the importance of their relationships with patients, the work of surgery becomes even more enjoyable. In recent years, surgeons have seen significant focus on the central question, "What should be done for this patient?" This question has added importance when there is often so much than can be done to keep patients alive even when their quality of life may be very poor. For contemporary surgeons, it may seem as though the growth of interest in surgical ethics has happened over the last 5–10 years. However, careful scrutiny of our remote and more recent history in surgery suggests a longer history of attention to ethical questions.

4.5 Sir William Stokes, M.Ch. Univ. Dubl., F.R.C.S.I. (1838–1900)

The late 1800s was a time when much of surgical treatment involved draining pus and setting fractures. Antisepsis had just recently been accepted and the central question for surgeons was always, "What can be done for this patient?" In that historical setting, consider the radical ideas of Sir William Stokes (see Fig. 4.6a). We do not know as much about him as we would like, but Mr. Stokes (as surgeons in Great Britain and Ireland are known) was a prominent individual. He was described as "Surgeon-in-Ordinary" to her Majesty Queen Victoria and was also past President of the Royal College of Surgeons and of the Pathological Society of Ireland. In November of 1894, the Dublin Journal of Medical Sciences published a copy of an address Mr. Stokes gave to medical students of the Meath Hospital and County Dublin Infirmary on October 8, 1894, entitled "The Ethics of Operative Surgery." (see Fig. 4.6b).

In that address [17], Mr. Stokes stated:

> A consideration of surgical ethics that frequently exercises the mind of the operating surgeon is the question of the principles that should guide him in dealing with cancerous growths. The question as to what constitutes justification in dealing with them in an operative way is ever present and surrounded with difficulty, as the result of such interference must end in weal or woe, satisfaction or regret to the patient as to the operator.

Several important points are valuable to consider about this statement. First of all, this may have been the very first use of the term "surgical ethics" in the literature. For that reason alone, it would be notable and something for which we should acknowledge Mr. Stokes' forward thinking in the use of the term. Perhaps more importantly though, in this quotation, we see the same central question that remains in the care of every patient with cancer or other surgical problems even today—"Do the risks of the operation outweigh the potential benefits to the patient?" This question of whether a surgeon *should* do something that he or she *could* do is a very modern question and truly the most important question in surgical ethics. We would do well to reflect on the importance of Mr. Stokes noting this central question in 1894.

—Peter Angelos

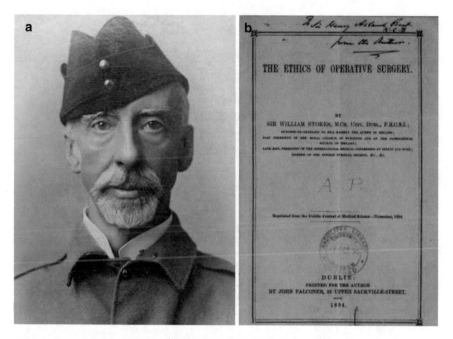

Fig. 4.6 (a) Sir William Stokes (surgeon). (b) "The Ethics of Operative Surgery" 1894 [17]

4.6 C. Rollins Hanlon, MD, FACS (1915–2011)

Dr. Hanlon, known by his friends as Rollo, was a surgical hero for many as both chair of surgery at St. Louis University and then as Executive Director of the American College of Surgeons (ACS) for 17 years (see Fig. 4.7a). He not only was a pioneering cardiac surgeon and a thoughtful leader of the ACS, but he was also a visionary who helped shift the ACS to a greater focus on the ethical dimension of surgical care in the annual Clinical Congress.

In 1987, Dr. Hanlon pioneered the teaching of humanism to surgeons with the annual Science and Humanism Seminar at the ACS Clinical Congress [18]. This early focus on humanism in surgery flew in the face of the more common focus on the techniques and technology of surgery that was so appealing in the late 1980s when laparoscopic surgery was beginning to gain traction.

The Science and Humanism Seminar at the Clinical Congress was organized each year by Dr. Hanlon and gained in popularity over the years. After the 2000 program that addressed creativity and disease, Dr. Hanlon transitioned the program into the College's Committee on Ethics that had begun regular ethics educational programs at the Clinical Congress (see Fig. 4.7b). The early attention to humanism in surgery and his efforts at bringing the ethical dimension of surgical care to the forefront would be reason enough for most surgeons to consider Dr. Hanlon to be among the notable ethical surgeons. However, I consider Dr. Hanlon to be a surgical

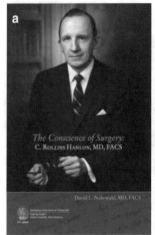

Fig. 4.7 (**a**) "The Conscience of Surgery: C. Rollins Hanlon" by David L Nahrwold sums up the life of Dr. Hanlon (Image courtesy of the Archives of the American College of Surgeons [18]). (**b**) Ethics in Surgery (Reprinted from the Journal of the American College of Surgeons, 1998 [19], with permission from Elsevier)

ethics hero also because of the friendship that he extended to me when I was a young surgical faculty member.

In 1995, when I first joined the faculty in the Department of Surgery at Northwestern University, Dr. Hanlon had long since "retired" as Executive Director of the ACS. However, he continued to work as Executive Consultant. In that role he served on the Regents Committee on Ethics. I am not certain how I was first introduced to Dr. Hanlon, but since the ACS was in a building just a block away from my office at Northwestern, I was able to make appointments to speak with Dr. Hanlon about issues in ethics intermittently during my early years on the faculty. I found his willingness to spend time with me to be amazing. He treated me, and everyone else, with absolute professionalism.

Through Dr. Hanlon's efforts, I was given the task of creating an "Annotated Bibliography of Ethics in Surgery," for the Regents Committee on Ethics. I shudder to think now at how ill-prepared I was for the task. However, Dr. Hanlon fortunately offered to advise me on the project. Without his encouragement and wise assistance, I would have never completed the job. However, I did eventually complete the project and got the bibliography published in the Journal of the American College of Surgeons (see Fig. 4.8) [20].

Despite my wanting Dr. Hanlon to be a co-author with me, he insisted that it was my work and would only allow me to acknowledge his assistance in a footnote. I was fortunate to have the opportunity to interact with Dr. Hanlon for several more years until his death in 2011. He will always be remembered by me as an ethical surgeon and a personal hero.

—Peter Angelos

Annotated Bibliography of Ethics in Surgery

Peter Angelos, MD, PhD

The ethical issues faced by physicians have never been more challenging than they are today. New technologies and techniques, increased financial pressures, and greater acknowledgment of treatment limits have put increased ethical pressure on practicing physicians. For surgeons, the need to be aware of ethical questions is perhaps even greater than for other physicians. Surgeons are often those who introduce new techniques or technologies. They are often consulted as the last option for the treatment of critically ill patients. Surgeons are the primary physicians involved in emergency procedures for critically injured trauma patients. A certain familiarity with the current literature on medical ethics can help surgeons to deal effectively with many contemporary ethical dilemmas.

This annotated bibliography of readings in ethics has been selected specifically for a surgical audience. First, major ethics books are presented. Second, a small sample of videotapes on ethics is listed. The third and largest section is a list of publications on ethics topics that are particularly relevant to surgeons. The list provides a taxonomy of ethical problems in surgical practice. Although the list is not meant to be exhaustive, it is designed to provide surgeons with an understanding of fundamental issues and to assist them in reaching sound clinical ethical decisions.

ethics can be analyzed usefully in terms of the principles of benef-icence, nonmaleficence, autonomy, and justice.

2. Jonsen AR, Siegler M, Winslade WJ. Clinical Ethics: A Practical Approach to Ethical Decisions in Clinical Medicine. 4th ed. New York: McGraw-Hill; 1998.

   This book uses a simple four-part approach and is designed as a practical handbook for physicians, residents, and medical students. Case presentations address most of the ethical issues faced in medical and surgical practice. References for each chapter are particularly complete.

3. LaPuma J. Managed Care Ethics: Essays on the Impact of Managed Care on Traditional Medical Ethics. New York: Hatherleigh Press; 1998.

   This collection of published essays examines how the contemporary managed care environment affects many of the traditional ethical issues that physicians encounter.

4. McCullough LB, Jones JW, Brody BA, eds. Surgical Ethics. New York: Oxford University Press; 1998.

   This recent authoritative text focuses on topics of particular concern to surgeons. The editors have covered issues at the end of life, issues in surgical education, and problems in surgical research. Joint authorship of chapters by a surgeon and an ethicist adds to the practicality of the presentations. An outstanding work.

5. Reich WT, ed. Encyclopedia of Bioethics. Rev ed. New York: Macmillan; 1995.

   This multivolume encyclopedia provides well-written entries on a broad list of topics in bioethics. It is a useful place to start when exploring most major issues in medical ethics.

6. Reiser SR, Dyck AJ, Curran WJ, eds. Ethics in Medicine: Historical Perspectives and Contemporary Concerns. Cambridge, MA: MIT Press; 1977.

   This book collects the major primary sources from which contem-

Fig. 4.8 Annotated Bibliography of Ethics in Surgery. (Reprinted from the Journal of the American College of Surgeons, 1999 [20], with permission from Elsevier)

4.7   Ostap Selianski, MD (1898–1945)

> The purpose of human life is to serve, and to show compassion and the will to help others.
> (Albert Schweitzer (1875–1965))

During my Fulbright year in Ukraine, on May 31, 2017, I was invited by my physician colleagues to a memorial service in the underground crypt of St. George's Cathedral in Lviv (see Fig. 4.9a). The occasion was the entombment of an urn containing an aliquot of soil from the common grave of the victims of the firebombing of Dresden on February 13 and 14, 1945 (see Fig. 4.9b and c). Over 25,000 civilians died in the carpet-bombing destruction of this centuries-old city by the Allied forces. Among the victims of this fire-bombing was a little-known surgeon Ostap Selianski, from Western Ukraine (Galicia).

Who was Ostap Selianski? (see Fig. 4.10) I had not heard of him, and he is not known in regional or world literature. He was not a Nobel Laureate nor a director of a large clinic. I had the privilege of meeting his 90-year-old daughter, Vera Vovk,

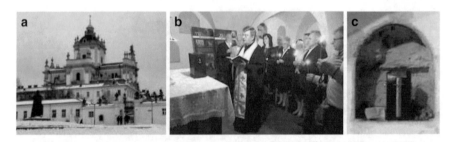

Fig. 4.9 (**a**) St. George's Cathedral in Lviv, Ukraine. (**b**) Entombment of remains in crypt. (**c**) Urn containing soil from the common graves of the victims of the Dresden bombing. (Photos by author)

Fig. 4.10 Ostap Selianski, MD. (Family photo)

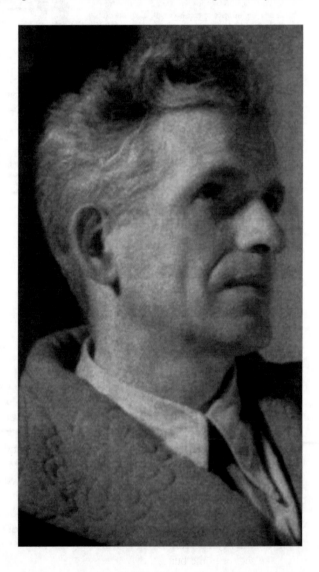

and learned about him [21]. He was a country physician raised in a family who valued service to mankind, to country and to God, and whose religious upbringing saw value in every living creature.

Ostap Selianski was born in 1898 in a large family. His father was a village priest. Interestingly, the family name for generations was Vovk (meaning wolf in Ukrainian). Knowing that he was going to be assigned to a village in the Carpathian Mountains, and knowing how superstitious village folk are in assigning temperament and characteristics to names, he could not risk coming to his flock with the name Vovk. He changed it to Selianski (meaning villager). Ostap's secondary school education in the neighboring towns was interrupted at the age of 16 when he quit school, ran away from home and joined the forces of the Ukrainian Sich Riflemen (Ukrainski Sichovi Striltsi) [22], a unit of the Austrian army, where he quickly rose to the rank of a junior lieutenant. He was wounded in battle and ended up a POW in the Polish camp in Tuchola [23].

After the war he began the study of medicine in Poznan and completed his degree requirements in Prague. During these years he married Stephania Vonok, and their daughter Vera was born. After his internship in Poznan he returned to Galicia, to the city of Lviv and served as the personal physician to the Metropolitan of the Greek Catholic Church in Ukraine, Andrey Sheptytsky. He lived on the grounds of the Metropolitan's residence. When the Metropolitan became seriously ill and required more specialized care by a hospital physician, Ostap took his family and moved to the village of Kuty to serve the poor people in the Carpathian Mountains.

Despite the prevalent climate of tribalism and nationalism, factors which helped to ignite the two World Wars, Dr. Selianski maintained a non-discriminating attitude towards his patients. He looked at each patient as a human being who needed his help and gave himself fully to their care, often to the point of exhaustion. He often did not take payment from the villagers who could not afford to pay and even helped them out with free medications. He took care of a variety of problems from dental to deliveries to trauma. Despite being a village doctor, he was well ahead of his times. He purchased a portable X-ray machine in Germany, as this helped him to be precise in diagnosing disease and fractures. It was the only such machine in all of Western Ukraine. Ironically, he paid his last installment for the loan just before the start of the war.

With Hitler's invasion, he was on the wrong side of the front line, under Russian occupation. He was serendipitously warned by a Russian military officer that he might be executed (part of the genocidal program of the Soviets towards Ukrainian leaders and intelligentsias). He immediately decided to flee with his family westward. He ended up in Dresden. As there was a lack of doctors due to the call up of the German doctors into the armed forces, he easily found work, first at the Frederiksted Pathological Institute and subsequently as a surgeon at the Gerhardt Wagner Hospital. He was extremely busy, often operating into the night. He gave every patient the same attention and care, regardless of their nationality, race or religion, often to the consternation of the nationalistic German support staff.

Air raids were a common occurrence. The medical personnel had to evacuate the patients into the bunker. Dr. Seliansky himself was seen to personally carry the sickest of the children into the bunker during these raids. One evening, he was about to embark on an emergency operation when the air sirens went off. He was encouraged to leave and take shelter in the bunker. He refused to leave his patient, who he felt would not

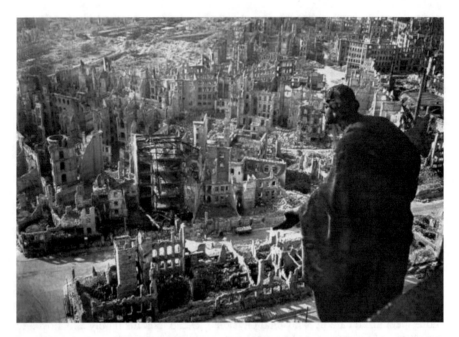

Fig. 4.11 The Bombing of Dresden: "Operation Thunderclap" 13–15 February 1945 [24] (Cassowary Colorizations, CC BY 2.0, via Wikimedia Commons)

survive until morning without the operation. He stayed with only a skeleton crew as the Allies began bombing the city on the night of February 13, 1945. (See Fig. 4.11) [24].

The roof caved in on the operating theater … there were no survivors [25]. The bodies could not be recovered as they were blown up or incinerated. The ashes of the victims of this inferno throughout Dresden were buried in a common grave.

He was a renaissance man with interests in music, theater and literature, especially poetry. This gave him great solace to withstand the stresses of his professional duties in the midst of those of surrounding world events. His life's guide was to be merciful and maintain respect for all creatures. He was not famous, he was everyman, but his life serves as an example of how to live.

—Vassyl A Lonchyna

Acknowledgements Copyright permission for Fig. 4.2 is kindly granted by Iranian artist Bozorgmehr Hosseinpour as his gift to the doctors of the world.

References

1. Bowen A. Creative Process. *Chicago Tribune*. May 5, 2021. Sec 6, pg 4.
2. Williams WC. *Complaint*. Poet.org. https://poets.org/poem/complaint-0. Accessed 14 May 2021.

3. Bailey BJ, Blaugrund SM, Biller H, et al. John J. Conley, MD an issue of special recognition. Laryngoscope. 1996;106(4):385–95. https://doi.org/10.1097/00005537-199604000-00001.
4. Conley JJ, Donovan DT. A new technique for total reconstruction of the lower lip in a patient with malignant melanoma. Otolaryngol Head Neck Surg. 1986;94(3):393–7. https://doi.org/10.1177/019459988609400328.
5. Conley JJ, Baker DC. Catastrophic necrosis of the neck. Otolaryngol Head Neck Surg. 1979;87(5):610–3. https://doi.org/10.1177/019459987908700513.
6. Conley JJ. Symposium: health science liability. The medical-legal problem. Trans Am Acad Ophthalmol Otolaryngol. 1972;76(3):718–20.
7. Conley JJ, Have I. Performed the right operation? Arch Otolaryngol Head Neck Surg. 1986;112:385–7. https://doi.org/10.1001/archotol.1986.03780040025006.
8. Conley JJ. Concepts of ethics in medicine. Otolaryngol Head Neck Surg. 1993;109(6):973–4. https://doi.org/10.1177/019459989310900601.
9. American College of Surgeons. John J. Conley Ethics and Philosophy Lecture. Virtual Clinical Congress 2020. Bull Brief. September 8, 2020. https://bulletin.facs.org/2021/01/clinical-con-gress-2020-highlights/. Accessed 12 June 2021.
10. American Academy of Otolaryngology. John Conley, MD Lecture on Medical Ethics. Annual Meeting 2020. https://www.entnet.org/about-us/awards-lectures/john-conley-md-lecture-on-medical-ethics/. Accessed 12 June 2021.
11. McCabe BF, Blaugrund SM, Harrison DFN, et al. John J. Conley, MD, 1912–1999. Ann Otol Rhinol Laryngol. 2000;109(1):1–8. https://doi.org/10.1177/000348940010900101.
12. Chan KH. Sylvan stool, MD. November 7, 1925—April 11, 2004. Inter J Pediatr Otolaryngol. 2004;68:1221–2. https://doi.org/10.1018/j.ijporl.2004.07.001.
13. Bluestone CD, Simmons JP, Healy GB, editors. Bluestone and Stool's Pediatric otolaryngology. 5th ed. People's Medical Publishing House; 2014.
14. American Cancer Society. Survival rates for childhood leukemia. https://www.cancer.org/cancer/leukemia-in-children/detection-diagnosis-staging/survival-rates.html. Accessed 11 May 2021.
15. The Society for Ear, Nose, and Throat Advancement in Children (SENTAC). Homepage. http://sentac.org. Accessed 15 May 2021.
16. Kelley P, Reilly J, Eavey RD. Sylvan Stool. Laryngoscope. 2005;115(1):2–3. https://doi.org/10.1097/01.mlg.0000152158.25710.4d.
17. Stokes, W. The ethics of operative surgery. Reprinted from the Dublin Journal of Medical Science, November 1894.
18. Nahrwold DL. *The conscience of surgery: C. Rollins Hanlon, MD, FACS*. American College of Surgeons; 2018.
19. Hanlon CR. Ethics in surgery. J Am Coll Surg. 1998;186(1):41–9. https://doi.org/10.1016/s1072-7515(97)00157-9.
20. Angelos P. Annotated bibliography of ethics in surgery. J Amer Coll Surg. 1999;188(5):538–44.
21. Hryhoruk A. Vera Vovk: 'I will always be a Ukrainian.' January 25, 2021. National Writer's Union of Ukraine. https://nspu.com.ua/novini/vira-vovk-ya-zavzhdi-zalishalasya-ukrainkoju/. Accessed 12 June 2021.
22. Sodol P. Ukrainian Sich Riflemen. Internet Encyclopedia of Ukraine. http://www.encyclope-diaofukraine.com/display.asp?linkpath=pages%5CU%5CK%5CUkrainianSichRiflemen.htm. Accessed 15 May 2021.
23. Tuchola prisoner of war camp. Wikipedia. https://en.wikipedia.org/wiki/Tuchola_prisoner_of_war_camp. Accessed 15 May 2021.
24. Chodacki A. Doktor Selianski. Lublin: Liber Duo; 2015.
25. McKay S. The fire and the darkness: the bombing of Dresden, 1945. St. Matthew's Press; 2020.

Part II
Communication

Chapter 5
Transparency in Surgery

Alan T. Makhoul ⓘ**, Brian C. Drolet** ⓘ**, and Alexander Langerman** ⓘ

Abstract For most patients, surgery is an unknown experience laden with unfamiliar terms and complex considerations. Inevitably, this foreign environment creates uncertainty, which can give rise to fear and anxiety. For patients to make informed decisions, surgical teams must work to help patients understand the peri-operative process. These discussions should disclose relevant information a patient would need to make decisions, while avoiding unnecessary details. This delicate balance has become even more challenging with the advent of audiovisual recording capabilities that can offer an objective account of operating room proceedings while the patient is under anesthesia. Does the potential for "total transparency" require more thorough disclosures from the surgeon? Should patients have access to audio and/or video recordings? What should surgeons discuss with patients regarding the logistics and proceedings of a routine operating room? These questions fall under the purview of surgical transparency research and will be explored in this chapter.

Keywords Transparency · Disclosure · Audiovisual recording · Surgical literacy
Informed consent · Patient autonomy

A. T. Makhoul
Vanderbilt University School of Medicine, Nashville, TN, USA
e-mail: alan.t.makhoul@vanderbilt.edu

B. C. Drolet
Department of Plastic Surgery, Department of Biomedical Informatics and Center for Biomedical Ethics and Society, Vanderbilt University Medical Center, Nashville, TN, USA
e-mail: Brian.c.drolet@vumc.org

A. Langerman (✉)
Department of Otolaryngology—Head and Neck Surgery, Department of Radiology and Radiological Sciences, Center for Biomedical Ethics and Society, Vanderbilt University Medical Center, Nashville, TN, USA
e-mail: Alexander.Langerman@vumc.org

© The Author(s), under exclusive license to Springer Nature
Switzerland AG 2022
V. A. Lonchyna et al. (eds.), *Difficult Decisions in Surgical Ethics*, Difficult
Decisions in Surgery: An Evidence-Based Approach,
https://doi.org/10.1007/978-3-030-84625-1_5

Case

A 58-year-old man with a history of squamous cell carcinoma of the tongue presents to a head and neck surgeon who determines that a lymph node dissection is medically indicated. The surgeon explains to the patient why she believes the procedure is necessary, the risks of the procedure, and the alternatives. The surgeon answers the patient's questions, and the patient consents to the procedure. The surgeon then asks the patient if he would be willing to have the procedure recorded for training purposes, and he agrees.

During the operation, the internal jugular vein is injured by a chief resident while he is gaining exposure of the lymph node packet. The surgeon is not present at the time of the injury, as she is involved in an "overlapping" case in a nearby room. Approximately 300 mL of blood are lost from the internal jugular vein while it is repaired. The repair is successful, but the case is prolonged by 30 min.

Afterwards, the surgeon is apprehensive about disclosing the error. In her mind, the error did not result in significant clinical harm, and disclosure might put her at risk for litigation, not to mention psychological distress to both her and the patient. In addition, she is unsure how the patient will react to her absence during the error. She ultimately discloses the error to the patient but does not reveal that it was made by the chief resident while she was in another room. The patient is upset and requests a copy of the audiovisual recording that was created.

5.1 Introduction

Every patient presents with a unique history that shapes their understanding of surgical care. Some patients have undergone dozens of procedures; others have never been inside a hospital. Some patients have very little formal education; others are surgeons themselves. Yet, all must be counseled so that they are able to make informed decisions about their health care. The surgeon directs this conversation and therefore must appreciate the patient's level of understanding and tailor the conversation to meet the patient's needs.

Low healthcare literacy is present in up to a third of surgical patients [1]. This not only hinders discussion of the details of a procedure but may also affect medication adherence and compliance with discharge instructions [1, 2]. In addition, differences in healthcare literacy magnify existing disparities in healthcare access, such as those resulting from socio-economic status, educational attainment, and English fluency [1]. Furthermore, few patients fully understand the nuances of surgical practice, such as the role of trainees, overlapping scheduling practices, and surgeon learning curves (see Chap. 49) [3, 4]. Online medical literature may narrow this literacy gap, but information gathered online must be distilled by the surgeon to ensure patient-centered care [5].

Table 5.1 Elements of ethics relating to transparency in surgery

Elements of ethics relating to transparency in surgery
Beneficence: A surgeon's chief objective is to provide beneficial care for the patient. Trust is established when surgeons communicate what good is expected to come from a procedure (to justify the risk), as well as what good ultimately resulted. By giving a patient comprehensive information about the proceedings of their treatment, they are put in the best position to make future healthcare decisions, which further improves their care
Nonmaleficence: Surgeons must minimize harm to the patient. Potential harms can be of commission or omission of physical acts or communication. When harm occurs, the surgeon has a duty to be fully transparent and clarify whether an error may have contributed. Doing so helps protect the surgeon-patient alliance, maintains trust, and enables the patient to make the best possible decisions about future care
Respect for autonomy: Surgeons must disclose certain minimum information about the procedure for patients to act intentionally and with understanding (i.e., informed consent). Furthermore, patients need to know what occurred during the procedure in order to make informed decisions about future care and actions (e.g., self-care, future medical interventions, litigation). Informing patients of their role in training future surgeons acknowledges their contribution to medical education and ensures they are not unwilling participants. Beyond minimum disclosure, the degree of understanding is determined by the patient's goals and values
Justice: Transparency must be practiced equitably with all surgical patients. Surgeons must identify their implicit biases and seek to counteract them in their conversations with patients

In addition, surgery under general anesthesia presents a unique circumstance with regard to patient understanding. Unlike most medical interventions, general anesthesia requires a complete transfer of autonomy from patient to surgeon. For a period of time, patients are unaware of—and unable to participate in—what is being done to their bodies [6]. As a result, they cannot witness their procedure in real-time; rather, they must be informed of the events beforehand and debriefed afterwards. This necessitates special considerations with regards to transparency, disclosure, and informed consent (see Table 5.1).

Because the surgeon's post-operative disclosure and operative note are a patient's only window into the operating room, it would be impossible for patients to know all the activities and interactions of the surgical team during their surgeries. Our profession, however, is on the verge of a paradigm shift where objective recordings of surgery are increasingly being used for performance assessment, patient safety, efficiency improvement, and documentation. Theoretically, this same technology could offer patients an unedited account of everything that happened in the OR, including a first-person perspective of the surgery, ambient video of the operating room, and audio of the team's conversation during the procedure. Legislation has even been proposed to permit or require patient access to such recordings [7, 8]. The capability to implement such technology creates a new upper limit for 'total transparency' against which lesser forms of disclosure can be compared.

While total transparency is attractive from patient autonomy, documentation, and quality improvement perspectives, it also presents potential challenges for both the patient and surgical team. These challenges stem in part from the healthcare literacy gap preventing most patients from interpreting the events of a complex procedure, risking anxiety and misunderstanding for the patient and placing an obligation on the surgeon to explain the recording. Patients may also find the graphic images of their surgery disturbing, and the mere existence of recordings might threaten their sense of privacy. From a provider perspective, OR staff may find ambient recordings intrusive, distracting, and threatening to workplace privacy.

These potential harms, plus the medical-legal challenges, make it unlikely that 'total transparency' through audiovisual recording would become routine without federal or state mandate [8]. But even as a theoretical exercise, the concept of total transparency forces us to differentiate between what *can* be shared with a patient and what *should* be shared. Optimal transparency balances meaningful disclosure and unnecessary harm. In practice, this requires identifying the information that should be discussed with a particular patient, using suitable language, and navigating the obstacles inherent to such conversations.

5.2 Search Strategy

Published studies discussing surgical transparency, surgical informed consent, surgical disclosure, and operating room recording were searched using the National Library of Medicine's PubMed database between January 1, 1970 and June 1, 2020. "All field" terms 'transparency,' 'surgical literacy,' 'surgical trainee involvement,' 'video recording,' 'operating room privacy,' 'surgical informed consent,' 'surgical disclosure,' 'consent training,' and 'surgery error litigation,' were used. No language restrictions were applied. This search yielded 40 relevant studies.

5.3 Discussion

5.3.1 A Spectrum of Understanding

The appropriate degree of transparency for a surgical patient exists along a spectrum, from minimal to total disclosure (see Fig. 5.1). To respect autonomy, a surgeon must work to identify where a patient's desired disclosure best fits on this

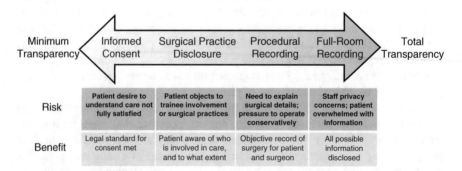

Fig. 5.1 Spectrum of transparency

spectrum and tailor the communication of information accordingly. No degree of disclosure is 'superior'—trade-offs exist at all levels, and the compromise that best aligns with a patient's goals should be pursued.

Certain minimum disclosures must occur before and after surgery for all patients. This duty to disclose arises from the need to protect autonomous decision-making and align care with patient values. Therefore, minimum disclosure must occur regardless of patient preference. Pre-operatively, the surgeon must provide the information necessary for informed patient consent, including a description of the procedure, its risks, anticipated benefits, potential side effects, as well as alternative treatment options [9]. Legal standards for informed consent vary by jurisdiction, with some using a reasonable patient standard and others a reasonable physician standard, but all require disclosure of certain information to help protect patients [5, 10]. Likewise, post-operative disclosure should, at a minimum, complete the pre-operative conversation. For example: Did any risks manifest during surgery? Were the objectives of the procedure met entirely? Post-operative disclosure not only enables autonomous decision-making regarding follow-up care, but also upholds beneficence and non-maleficence by allowing patients to direct additional care and avoid complications.

Many patients, however, desire to know more than the minimum. For instance, it is now common to disclose aspects of routine surgical practice, such as whether the attending surgeon will be present for an entire procedure or if a portion will be per-formed independently by an assistant or trainee. This came into the mainstream most notably through the practice of "double booking" procedures, which was not well known to the public or routinely discussed with patients until a 2015 Boston Globe exposé shed light on this unseen practice and spurred demand for increased transparency [4, 11]. In response, the American College of Surgeons provided clarification on what constituted acceptable forms of this practice ("overlapping" rather than "concurrent" surgery) and highlighted the need for disclosure [12].

One concern patients have about "double-booking" surgery is that they would be operated on by a trainee in the absence of an attending surgeon [13]. However, the attending surgeon may intentionally leave a room to allow their trainee graduated autonomy, even if they are not needed elsewhere. The need for graduated trainee autonomy is well-recognized and may require the attending to step away from the table or even leave the operating room as a trainee becomes more advanced [14]. Furthermore, patients are frequently unaware of the differences between medical students, residents, and fellows [15], and are therefore less attuned to the fact that trainees are allowed graduated independence over the course of their training. Patients may not like this; in a field that relies heavily on technical skill, many patients naturally prefer the most experienced set of hands [16]. Taken a step further, the preference for expertise also extends to the experience and ability of the attending surgeon (see Chap. 50).

It is therefore incumbent upon the attending surgeon to discuss the realities of surgical practice with patients and demonstrate that the proposed care is not inferior. Yet, such conversations are often difficult. Surgeons in competitive markets may worry that disclosing these realities will divert business to surgeons that minimize the role of assistants or trainees. Some research suggests, however, that objections to trainees are not fixed and might be allayed by explaining the benefit of improved quality of care and the need to train the next generation of surgeons [17]. Patients may also benefit from knowing that trainees provide key assistance to the surgeon and have been shown to improve patient outcomes [18]. Development of scripts and methods for discussing these topics truthfully *and* reassuringly is an important area of surgical transparency research.

Audiovisual recordings have been proposed as a means of bridging the information gap between surgeon disclosure and the actual proceedings of the operating room. Unlike surgeon disclosure, audiovisual recordings provide an objective, portable account of operating room events.

Modern recording technology could allow surgeons to offer an unparalleled degree of transparency. Patients could be given a "full-room" multi-feed continuous audiovisual recording of their procedure, verbally annotated in real-time by the surgeon. A 2010 survey of colonoscopy patients suggested patients may be interested in procedural recordings, and some patients have taken to intentionally (and even surreptitiously) audio-recording their procedures [19, 20].

Although the desire for total transparency through full-room audiovisual recording may stem from a legitimate desire of some patients to understand their care, making such recordings widely available to patients may be prohibitively impractical. For one, the volume and complexity of information contained in an operating room recording would be too much for almost any patient to adequately interpret, with many opportunities for misunderstanding. To avoid this, transparency would likely require an extensive debriefing of the recording with the surgeon; such debriefings are unrealistic due to limitations in time and healthcare literacy. While full-room recordings may help prevent hidden practices or inappropriate behavior, it is unlikely they would convey a deeper understanding of a patient's care. Full-room recordings may also serve as a stressor for the surgical team and stifle operating room conversation. These potential downsides make it unlikely that full room recording would be made available to patients in the near future. Rather, the notion of 'total transparency' functions best as a theoretical upper limit to which other lesser degrees of transparency can be compared.

A more focused approach, "*procedural* transparency," involves capture of first-person video of the procedure for the medical record [20]. First-person video could be captured using operating room cameras or wearable recording devices and uploaded directly into the medical record, similar to medical photography. Recordings of the procedure itself are more reasonably considered "medical data" than the movements or conversations of the team members and would offer an objective record of how a patient's anatomy has been altered and manipulated. However, making even these videos available to patients will create new responsibilities for the surgeon to explain the details captured on the recording. This may include explaining the roles of trainees (whose hands may be visible) or recorded errors, even if they did not cause harm. Debriefing strategies regarding surgical videos are therefore in need of further investigation.

The creation of any recording also raises privacy concerns that must be discussed. Before a recording is made, the patient and surgeon must agree to its purpose, audience, how it will be stored, and for how long. Whether the recording will be integrated into the medical record, used for training purposes, or given to the patient for personal use has implications for ownership and legal status. A recording may need to be edited to protect the privacy of other patients discussed during the procedure or the privacy of the OR staff. Furthermore, some staff may not consent to being recorded if given the choice and may need to be edited out of the recording through voice alteration or facial blurring. Such audiovisual processing would likely come at a cost. Whether patients should pay a fee to obtain a recording raises equity concerns, as disadvantaged patients may not be able to afford such charges [7].

Furthermore, procedural recording may have consequences on surgeon performance. Surgeons may consciously or subconsciously operate more "defensively" knowing that the recording may someday be shown in a court room. They may be less eager to involve trainees when the "cameras are rolling" for fear of litigation, as some surgeons do when they have awake patients [20, 21], or be reluctant to depart from standard protocol, even if innovation is warranted (Chap. 49). On the other hand, recording may promote attentiveness and meticulousness if surgeons know they might later be evaluated by their peers. It would also allow surgeons to analyze, and potentially improve, their technique [22]. These advantages and disadvantages are being weighed as this technology matures.

Ultimately, each patient will seek a different degree of understanding. Where a patient exists on the transparency spectrum depends not only on their goals and values, but also on the procedure itself. A patient may feel comfortable with the minimum disclosure for a simple, routine procedure such as a lipoma excision, but may desire a greater degree of understanding for cardiac bypass surgery (or the contrary may be true). Thus, the surgeon must determine the degree of disclosure on an individual basis through patient-centered conversation. A reasonable discussion about transparency might begin with an explanation of the spectrum of options and the compromises that exist at each level. If a video of the surgical procedure is going to be made, the patient should know its purpose and whether they would have access to it. Out of respect for autonomy, patients should be allowed sufficient time to fully consider all options and should be able to change their chosen degree of transparency at any point. In fact, some patients may not know what degree of transparency is suitable for them—they may simply want to be reassured that more information is available, if desired.

Offering patients the information that best suits their needs builds trust, strengthens the patient-surgeon relationship, and upholds autonomy. Challenges exist, however, that can impede effective transparency. Barriers range from surgeon inexperience to complex team dynamics to fears of litigation. Fortunately, multiple strategies have been shown to improve transparency and assist surgeons with navigating these sometimes-difficult conversations. These challenges and opportunities for improvement will be discussed in the next two sections.

5.3.2   Challenges to Transparency

Disclosure of an adverse surgical event is among the most difficult conversations a surgeon can have. Fear of a negative patient reaction, professional embarrassment, personal feelings of guilt, and the possibility of malpractice litigation have all contributed to a culture of blame and silence regarding mistake-making in surgery [23]. In 2000, the publication of "To Err is Human" by the U.S. Institute of Medicine paved the way for the healthcare community to rethink this flawed mentality [24]. Today, the principles of beneficence and non-maleficence guide open discussions regarding adverse events, as stakeholders seek to understand how similar mistakes can be prevented. At the center of these conversations is an acknowledgement of the adverse event and disclosure to the patient.

Yet, problems exist with adverse event transparency. A 2012 interview study revealed that relatively few disclosures met patient expectations for basic information and apology [25]. In addition, ambiguity persists regarding which events require disclosure and by whom. A 2006 survey found that only 66% of surgeons would disclose an error involving a bile duct injury, while 97% would disclose an error associated with a retained sponge [26]. "System-related" errors further complicate transparency conversations. In a 2006 interview study, surgeons were more likely to provide partial disclosure in the event of a system-related error [27].

A scarcity of surgeon education further hinders the provision of appropriate transparency. Trainees have indicated a need for additional disclosure preparation, and those who have received it have reported greater confidence in their abilities [28]. The social skills required to have difficult conversations—such as empathy and humility—are difficult to teach and have not been a focus of medical education [29]. Moreover, a central conclusion of "To Err is Human" was that most adverse events are born out of poorly designed systems, not negligence [30]. Yet, undergraduate and graduate education rarely offers substantial human factor and patient safety education [30].

Likewise, surgeons are infrequently taught the skills—or provided the resources—needed to cope with the psychological distress that accompanies an adverse event and its disclosure. A culture of perfectionism permeates medicine and is especially common in the operating room, where a single error can cause serious harm. While a perfectionist mindset can promote self-improvement and attentiveness, it can devastate a surgeon when harm occurs, decreasing confidence and promoting anxiety [31]. In a 2010 survey, surgeons who reported a recent error were significantly more likely to report feelings of emotional exhaustion and depersonalization, both of which contribute to the epidemic of surgeon burnout [32]. An absence of support often accompanies the negative emotions felt by surgeons following an error. In a 2007 survey, over 80% of physicians expressed interest in counseling following an adverse event, yet only 10% agreed that healthcare organizations provided adequate help [33]. This unmanaged emotional burden may deter some surgeons from acknowledging and being transparent about all adverse events.

The dynamics of an interdisciplinary surgical team can also obscure the provision of surgical transparency. Before and after surgery, "ownership" of the various aspects of the surgery must be clarified. Should the surgeon explain the risks associated with anesthesia? Should the surgeon take responsibility and apologize for a counting error made by the surgical technician? What role does the anesthesiologist have in disclosing errors? Left unaddressed, ambiguity encourages a diffusion of responsibility that interferes with transparency. Additionally, adverse events due to "system irregularities"—which may not be the fault of any individual—should be handled through a consistent framework. While the surgeon has traditionally been considered the "captain of the ship" in the OR and represents the surgical endeavor to the patient, the surgeon cannot control all aspects of the perioperative process and explicitly acknowledging this to patients may elevate the roles of other team members.

Medical-legal issues intersect directly with transparency concerns. Because full disclosure does not guarantee protection in most U.S. malpractice cases, fear of litigation may deter surgeons from acknowledging mistakes and taking responsibility [27]. Fear that an apology will be construed as an admission of guilt may even prevent some surgeons from being emotionally vulnerable with patients, despite a genuine interest from patients and surgeons. To combat this reluctance, some states have enacted 'apology laws' that prohibit a physician's apology from being used as admissible evidence in a legal proceeding [34]. However, each law has specific nuances, such as the timeframe during which an apology is considered inadmissible and to whom it may be delivered (see Chap. 16) [34].

Audiovisual recording adds another layer of legal complexity. Massachusetts and Wisconsin have introduced bills under which patients can request a recording of their surgery [7, 8]. Because it is unclear what constitutes "normal practice" for a given procedure, it is unknown what degree of variance will constitute "malpractice" to a court viewing a recording [20]. Consequently, surgeons may be hesitant to adopt recording technology in the operating room until it is understood how recordings will be used in the legal system. Furthermore, ownership of the recording would have implications for the admissibility of a recording in a legal proceeding.

Current evidence, however, suggests that objective recordings can be protective or harmful. Video recordings have been used as evidence of *good* practice by documenting that all surgical steps occurred correctly and verifying that no surgical equipment was retained [35]. On the other hand, surreptitious audio recordings have been used to establish malpractice based on what was spoken by the provider during a procedure [36]. The role audiovisual recordings would have in malpractice cases if they were available to patients is a critical area of research.

While much of the work on error disclosure has focused on errors that result in clinically significant harm, minor errors are much more common. Surgeons are often unsure whether to disclose an adverse event if they are able to repair the injury. Surgeons may worry that disclosure of clinically insignificant adverse events (or other nuances of surgical practice, such as trainee involvement) may cause psychological distress for the patient. Similar arguments were used as recently as the 1980s to claim that surgical risks should not be disclosed during the informed consent process, since disclosure may "frighten the patient" [37]. Just as non-disclosure of risks seems unthinkable in our current practice, non-disclosure of adverse events, trainee roles, and other "difficult topics" may eventually become unimaginable. Routine operative video recording would require surgeons to hone their skills for discussing these topics with patients.

5.3.3   Improving Transparency

Simplifying documents, demystifying medical jargon, and using multimedia formats all improve patient-surgeon communication [38]. In a 2012 review, nine randomized controlled trials of multimedia interventions, including computerized programs, graphic animations, and videos, were effective in improving understanding among surgical patients [39]. Communication techniques, such as "repeat back" have also demonstrated efficacy [39]. Such tools become even more relevant when the desired degree of transparency increases. In the case of a recording, viewing a de-identified "stock" recording of the procedure beforehand may allow patients to judge if they wish to see that graphic content on their bodies. If they elect to receive a recording of their surgery, a graphic animation tailored to that procedure type may facilitate patient understanding. Multimedia interventions may ultimately allow for patients to better interpret the information conveyed through a high degree of transparency.

Surgical team dynamics and responsibilities should be established before patient care has begun. Each team member must understand the scope of their responsibilities and should be prepared to have open conversations with the patient before and after surgery. This requires that all team members develop a level of rapport suitable to their role. While the surgeon will likely have the strongest relationship with the patient, transparency should not, and cannot, be solely their responsibility. Anesthesiologists, surgical staff, and trainees must all feel comfortable communicating openly with the patient. In the case of an adverse event, a "disclosure time-out" can allow the surgical team to plan accurate communication of all relevant information and to identify the most appropriate individual to have the conversation with the patient [27].

Although surgeons often fear litigation following an adverse event, many studies suggest these fears are overdone. The overwhelming majority of adverse events do not result in litigation, and surgeons routinely overestimate this risk [27]. Some U.S. states now offer protection against the use of apologies (e.g., "I'm sorry") as an admission of guilt in malpractice litigation [34]. Furthermore, multiple studies suggest that transparency decreases the likelihood of litigation in the case of an adverse event [27]. Moreover, while transparency does not fully safeguard against litigation, intentionally withholding information can have far greater consequences for the surgeon and the surgical profession.

Transparency training must begin during medical education. A 2013 review found that disclosure curricula develop knowledge, skills, and competencies that are valued by trainees [28]. However, educational interventions are usually brief, stand-alone events that occur within a patient safety course or simulation exercise [28]. To be most successful, transparency education should be integrated longitudinally in undergraduate and graduate medical education. Trainees should be afforded the benefit of multiple exercises throughout their training so that they may grow incrementally in their understanding. Standardized patient feedback, in particular, has been shown to be helpful to surgical residents [40]. For example, including trainees in pre-operative and post-operative conversations not only promotes transparency for patients, but also provides the trainee with exposure to transparency conversations.

Lastly, equity studies are needed. Little is known about how unconscious biases affect transparency conversations with patients. To support justice, surgeons must provide all patients the appropriate level of understanding, and this may require recognizing and counteracting implicit biases. Likewise, the ideal language of transparency remains uncharacterized. Surgeons must individualize their language to communicate effectively and optimize understanding. The appropriate terminology, when to use it, and with whom should be studied further.

Returning to our case at the start of the chapter, transparency could have been improved by beginning the encounter with a discussion of the patient's goals for understanding. If desired, the surgeon should have explained the involvement of trainees and overlapping case scheduling in her practice. Being transparent about these topics from the beginning would likely have prevented a more challenging situation after the error occurred. In addition, the surgeon should have clarified the ownership of the recording and whether the patient may request a copy; recordings are often conducted as part of research studies that have explicit directives about video access. The surgeon was correct to disclose the error even though it did not result in significant clinical harm but should have also been fully transparent about the circumstances under which the error took place.

5.4 Concluding Remarks

Offering all patients the degree of transparency that aligns with their goals and values is just, is patient-centered, and contributes to high-quality patient care. Doing so requires identification of the information that a patient desires, use of language that is suitable for the patient, and navigation of the obstacles inherent to such conversations. We believe that promoting a culture of surgical transparency will allow surgeons to continue to be leaders in the ethical provision of health care. To accomplish this, further research is needed to develop a "language of transparency" that is truthful and reassuring.

In our practice as academic surgeons, we discuss the role of trainees and the setting of an academic medical center with all patients to promote trust and allow trainees to develop as independent surgeons. We value transparency in adverse event and error disclosure, including trainees whenever possible in those discussions. Lastly, we individualize our approach to transparency using a patient-centered informed consent process.

5.5   Selected References

- Spatz ES, Krumholz HM, and Moulton BW. The New Era of Informed Consent: Getting to a Reasonable-Patient Standard Through Shared Decision Making. JAMA. 2016;315(19):2063–2064. https://doi.org/10.1001/jama.2016.3070

  – This article focuses on the importance of a patient-centered informed consent process, especially as U.S. and U.K. governments shift from a "reasonable-physician standard" to a "reasonable-patient standard." Transparent, bias-free communication with a provider is integral to the informed consent process, but should also include decision aids and written information at a basic reading level.

- van Dalen ASHM, Legemaate J, Schlack WS, Legemate DA, Schijven MP. Legal perspectives on black box recording devices in the operating environment. Br J Surg. 2019;106(11):1433–1441. https://doi.org/10.1002/bjs.11198

  – Using parallels to the aviation industry and the successful use of "black box" recording devices, the authors examine the medical-legal concerns surrounding operative recordings, including privacy issues, data usage, and existing litigation. They provide examples of how recordings have been used to demonstrate both good and bad surgical practice.

- Mulsow JJ, Feeley TM, Tierney S. Beyond consent--improving understanding in surgical patients. Am J Surg. 2012;203(1):112–120. https://doi.org/10.1016/j.amjsurg.2010.12.010

  – The authors review the literature on the efficacy of patient understanding interventions: informational leaflets, multimedia, patient decision aids, and the internet. They characterize the gap in patient understanding among various surgical populations and common barriers, such as low health literacy and patient-surgeon discrepancies regarding what information is important.

References

1. Chang ME, Baker SJ, Dos Santos Marques IS, et al. Health literacy in surgery. Health Lit Res Pract. 2020;4(1):e46–65. https://doi.org/10.3928/24748307-20191121-01.
2. De Oliveira GS Jr, McCarthy RJ, Wolf MS, Holl J. The impact of health literacy in the care of surgical patients: a qualitative systematic review. BMC Surg. 2015;15:86. https://doi.org/10.1186/s12893-015-0073-6.

3. Wojcik BM, Phitayakorn R, Lillemoe KD, Chang DC, Mullen JT. Preoperative disclosure of surgical trainee involvement: Pandora's box or an opportunity for enlightenment? Ann Surg. 2017;265(5):869–70. https://doi.org/10.1097/sla.0000000000002136.
4. Langerman A. Concurrent surgery and informed consent. JAMA Surg. 2016;151(7):601–2. https://doi.org/10.1001/jamasurg.2016.0511.
5. Spatz ES, Krumholz HM, Moulton BW. The new era of informed consent: getting to a reasonable-patient standard through shared decision making. JAMA. 2016;315(19):2063–4. https://doi.org/10.1001/jama.2016.3070.
6. Langerman A, Siegler M, Angelos P. Intraoperative decision making: the decision to perform additional, unplanned procedures on anesthetized patients. J Am Coll Surg. 2016;222(5):956–60. https://doi.org/10.1016/j.jamcollsurg.2016.02.011.
7. H.R. 633, 2011 Leg., Reg. Sess. (Mass. 2011). https://malegislature.gov/Bills/187/H633/CoSponsor. Accessed 23 Sept 2020.
8. Assemb. B. 255, 2015 Leg., (Wis. 2015). https://docs.legis.wisconsin.gov/2015/related/proposals/ab255.pdf. Accessed 23 Sept 2020.
9. Bagnall NM, Pucher OH, Johnston MJ, et al. Informing the process of consent for surgery: identification of key constructs and quality factors. J Surg Res. 2017;209:86–92. https://doi.org/10.1016/j.jss.2016.09.051.
10. Hall DE, Prochazka AV, Fink AS. Informed consent for clinical treatment. CMAJ. 2012;184(5):533–40. https://doi.org/10.1503/cmaj.112120.
11. Abelson J, Saltzman J, Kowalczyk L, Allen S. Clash in the Name of Care. *Boston Globe*. October 25, 2015. http://apps.bostonglobe.com/spotlight/clash-in-the-name-of-care/story/. Accessed 23 Sept 2020.
12. American College of Surgeons. Statements on principles. April 12, 2016. https://www.facs.org/about-acs/statements/stonprin. Accessed 23 Sept 2020.
13. Langerman A, Arambula A, Bonnet K, Schlundt DG, Brelsford KM. Patient values regarding overlapping surgery: identification of distinct patient subgroups. Laryngoscope. 2020;130(12):2779–84. https://doi.org/10.1002/lary.28405.
14. Kovatch KJ, Prince MEP, Sandhu G. Weighing entrustment decisions with patient care during residency training. Otolaryngol Head Neck Surg. 2018;158(6):1024–7. https://doi.org/10.1177/0194599818764652.
15. Unruh KP, Dhulipala SC, Holt GE. Patient understanding of the role of the orthopedic resident. J Surg Educ. 2013;70(3):345–9. https://doi.org/10.1016/j.jsurg.2013.01.004.
16. Porta CR, Sebesta JA, Brown TA, Steele SR, Martin MJ. Training surgeons and the informed consent process: routine disclosure of trainee participation and its effect on patient willingness and consent rates. Arch Surg. 2012;147(1):57–62. https://doi.org/10.1001/archsurg.2011.235.
17. Counihan TC, Nye D, Wu JJ. Surgeons' experiences with Patients' concerns regarding trainees. J Surg Educ. 2015;72(5):974–8. https://doi.org/10.1016/j.jsurg.2015.03.007.
18. Hutter MM, Glasgow RE, Mulvihill SJ. Does the participation of a surgical trainee adversely impact patient outcomes? A study of major pancreatic resections in California. Surgery. 2000;128(2):286–92. https://doi.org/10.1067/msy.2000.107416.
19. Raghavendra M, Rex DK. Patient interest in video recording of colonoscopy: a survey. World J Gastroenterol. 2010;16(4):458–61. https://doi.org/10.3748/wjg.v16.i4.458.
20. Langerman A, Grantcharov TP. Are we ready for our close-up?: why and how we must embrace video in the OR. Ann Surg. 2017;266(6):934–6. https://doi.org/10.1097/sla.0000000000002232.
21. Smith CS, Guyton K, Pariser JJ, Siegler M, Schindler N, Langerman A. Surgeon-patient communication during awake procedures. Am J Surg. 2017;213(6):996–1002 e1. https://doi.org/10.1016/j.amjsurg.2016.06.017.
22. Langerman A. Using surgical video to classify intraoperative events. Ann Surg. 2020;272(2):227–8. https://doi.org/10.1097/SLA.0000000000003934.
23. Kaldjian LC, Jones EW, Rosenthal GE. Facilitating and impeding factors for physicians' error disclosure: a structured literature review. Jt Comm J Qual Patient Saf. 2006;32(4):188–98. https://doi.org/10.1016/s1553-7250(06)32024-7.

24. Kohn LT, Corrigan JM, Donaldson MS, editors. For the Institute of Medicine (US) committee on quality of health Care in America. In To err is human: building a safer health system. National Academies Press; 2000.
25. Iedema R, Allen S, Britton K, Gallagher TH. What do patients and relatives know about problems and failures in care? BMJ Qual Saf. 2012;21(3):198–205. https://doi.org/10.1136/bmjqs-2011-000100.
26. Gallagher TH, Garbutt JM, Waterman AD, et al. Choosing your words carefully: how physicians would disclose harmful medical errors to patients. Arch Intern Med. 2006;166(15):1585–93.
27. Lipira LE, Gallagher TH. Disclosure of adverse events and errors in surgical care: challenges and strategies for improvement. World J Surg. 2014;38(7):1614–21. https://doi.org/10.1007/s00268-014-2564-5.
28. Stroud L, Wong BM, Hollenberg E, Levinson W. Teaching medical error disclosure to physicians-in-training: a scoping review. Acad Med. 2013;88(6):884–92. https://doi.org/10.1097/acm.0b013e31828f898f.
29. Falcone JL, Claxton RN, Marshall GT. Communication skills training in surgical residency: a needs assessment and metacognition analysis of a difficult conversation objective structured clinical examination. J Surg Educ. 2014;71(3):309–15. https://doi.org/10.1016/j.jsurg.2013.09.020.
30. Tevlin R, Doherty E, Traynor O. Improving disclosure and management of medical error—an opportunity to transform the surgeons of tomorrow. Surgeon. 2013;11(6):338–43. https://doi.org/10.1016/j.surge.2013.07.008.
31. Robertson JJ, Long B. Suffering in silence: medical error and its impact on health care providers. J Emerg Med. 2018;54(4):402–9. https://doi.org/10.1016/j.jemermed.2017.12.001.
32. Shanafelt TD, Balch CM, Bechamps G, et al. Burnout and medical errors among American surgeons. Ann Surg. 2010;251(6):995–1000. https://doi.org/10.1097/sla.0b013e3181bfdab3.
33. Waterman AD, Garbut J, Hazel E, et al. The emotional impact of medical errors on practicing physicians in the United States and Canada. Jt Comm J Qual Patient Saf. 2007;33(8):467–76.
34. Saitta N, Hodge SD Jr. Efficacy of a physician's words of empathy: an overview of state apology laws. J Am Osteopath Assoc. 2012;112(5):302–6.
35. van Dalen ASHM, Legemaate J, Schlack WS, Legemate DA, Schijven MP. Legal perspectives on black box recording devices in the operating environment. Br J Surg. 2019;106(11):1433–41. https://doi.org/10.1002/bjs.11198.
36. Jackman T. Anesthesiologist trashes sedated patient—And it ends up costing her. *The Washington Post*. June 23, 2015. https://www.washingtonpost.com/local/anesthesiologist-trashes-sedated-patient-jury-orders-her-to-pay-500000/2015/06/23/cae05c00-18f3-11e5-ab92-c75ae6ab94b5_story.html. Accessed 23 Sept 2020.
37. Morton WJ. The doctrine of informed consent. Med Law. 1987;6(2):117–25.
38. Perrenoud B, Velonaki VS, Bodenmann P, Ramelet AS. The effectiveness of health literacy interventions on the informed consent process of health care users: a systematic review protocol. JBI Database System Rev Implement Rep. 2015;13(10):82–94. https://doi.org/10.11124/jbisrir-2015-2304.
39. Mulsow JJ, Feeley TM, Tierney S. Beyond consent--improving understanding in surgical patients. Am J Surg. 2012;203(1):112–20. https://doi.org/10.1016/j.amjsurg.2010.12.010.
40. Leeper-Majors K, Veale JR, Westbrook TS, Reed K. The effect of standardized patient feedback in teaching surgical residents informed consent: results of a pilot study. Curr Surg. 2003;60(6):615–22. https://doi.org/10.1016/s0149-7944(03)00157-0.

Chapter 6
Is Informed Consent Ever Truly Informed?

T. Johelen Carleton (iD) **and Pringl Miller** (iD)

Abstract The clinical ethical imperative to provide patients or their surrogate decision makers with relevant and tailored information is a serious endeavor that has challenged many generations of surgeons. The surgical informed consent process (SIC) is a critical aspect of surgical practice that is especially complex because patients are diverse individuals who do not automatically fit into algorithms. The sensitivity and specificity with which the SIC process must be embraced should be seen through the lens of each autonomous person. During SIC it is vital to understand what matters most to the patient. Only then can a surgeon facilitate a meaningful discussion that will honor a patient's rights, dignity, preferences, goals and values. This chapter will address the evolution of the medicolegal and ethical aspects of the surgical informed consent process and how to optimally satisfy the communication needs. Additionally, this chapter will explore the adaptations to the surgical informed consent process during the COVID-19 pandemic.

Keywords Surgical ethics · Surgery · Surgical informed consent · Shared-decision making · Patient–surgeon relationship

T. J. Carleton
Hospice & Palliative Medicine, Phoenix, AZ, USA

P. Miller (✉)
Physician Just Equity, San Francisco, CA, USA

© The Author(s), under exclusive license to Springer Nature
Switzerland AG 2022
V. A. Lonchyna et al. (eds.), *Difficult Decisions in Surgical Ethics*, Difficult
Decisions in Surgery: An Evidence-Based Approach,
https://doi.org/10.1007/978-3-030-84625-1_6

77

Case

Mr. Y is a morbidly obese 75-year-old man with full decision-making capacity who presents in septic shock secondary to a strangulated ventral hernia. He consents to an emergent ventral hernia repair and is apprised of the risks including, but not limited to: bleeding, infection, bowel resection, ostomy, myocardial infarction, pneumonia, thromboembolic events, recurrent ventral hernia, and death. He undergoes emergent ventral hernia repair with a small bowel resection. Mr. Y steadily improves postoperatively though with significant debility due to sepsis and postoperative ileus. Mr. Y eventually discharges to a rehabilitation facility where he unfortunately contracts SARS-CoV-2. He is readmitted to the medical intensive care unit (MICU) and requires intubation. Mr. Y no longer has decision making capacity and his sister becomes his surrogate. They never discussed his wishes regarding life sustaining medical treatment or end of life (EOL) care. His FiO2 requirement increases and tracheostomy is performed for prolonged mechanical ventilation. Mr. Y is transferred to a long-term acute care facility (LTAC) for ventilator weaning and wound care. After a week at the LTAC he requires less ventilatory support, but he develops a mucus plug that causes cardiopulmonary arrest. Although successfully resuscitated, he suffers a catastrophic anoxic brain injury resulting in a minimally conscious state. He becomes medically stable and returns to the LTAC where his sister considers transitioning care to comfort.

6.1 Introduction

The single biggest problem in communication is the illusion that it has taken place. (George Bernard Shaw)

Elements of the SIC process include the exchange of information between surgeon and patient, ethical standards, legal standards, and practice patterns. The SIC process is an underestimated part of surgery and neither surgeons nor patients sufficiently realize its importance [1].

From an ethical standpoint, it is well established that surgical interventions should confer more benefit than harm. We approach operations every day that may offer benefit if we are skilled enough, and fortunate enough, that harm is minimized or does not enter into the equation. We can predict what might happen, but we don't know for sure what will happen. Although there is movement toward precision medicine, many of our best objective predictors of outcomes give us odds based on a population, not certainty for an individual.

One of the most enduring questions confronting practicing surgeons regarding the SIC process is "can informed consent *truly* be informed?" A patient with

Table 6.1 Ethical principles of surgical informed consent

Autonomy	Effective SIC requires that each patient have as much information as possible for a treatment decision free of coercion. The information should be delivered with sensitivity and sophisticated communication tailored to each patient's needs.
Beneficence	The SIC process for operative intervention should start with why the procedure is beneficial. This requires knowledge of a patient's preferences, goals, and values in order to meet the patient's definition of beneficial.
Non-Maleficence	Patients should be informed of the potential harm and complications of operative intervention and to the best of our ability the benefit of surgery should outweigh the risk. Surgeons must be transparent about the expected outcomes of treatment and the impact of this treatment on a patient's quality of life.
Justice	All patients deserve equitable treatment which means that consistent efforts must be extended during the SIC process that also conform to the unique needs of each individual patient.

decision making capacity or their surrogate should not be expected to understand what a trained surgical specialist knows about risks, benefits, complications, and alternatives. Conversely, surgeons will not understand what matters most to their patients unless they ask and respect the answers. A dialogue, not a physician monologue, is crucial to the SIC process and honors patient autonomy. This dialogue often elicits differing perspectives about what constitutes risk, what constitutes benefit, and what ratio of risk and benefit is acceptable for each patient. For example, from the surgeon's point of view the greatest risk may be operative mortality but from the patient's point of view the greatest risk may be loss of function and independence. Physicians can outline the potential complications of treatment but only the patient can speak to what the consequences of treatment mean for their quality of life and whether the trade-offs are worth it (See Table 6.1).

The SIC process has evolved over time, and more recently has been anchored by the ethical principle of autonomy and a patient's right to self-determination. Jonsen et al. have stated that informed consent is a practical application of respect for the patient's autonomy [2]. The purpose of this chapter is to improve the understanding and application of the SIC process.

6.2   Search Strategy

The literature search was initiated in PubMed using keywords "informed consent" and "surgery" and MeSH terms "informed consent" and "surgical procedures, operative". Separate searches were performed for MeSH terms "informed consent, history" and "informed consent, standards" and "shared decision making". The initial search yielded 2645 references. Preference was given to articles published within the last two decades in major English language journals.

6.3 Discussion

6.3.1 History

The concept of informed consent was mentioned as early as Hippocrates' writings [3, 4]. In medieval times doctors asked for a "hold harmless document" aimed at releasing them from future responsibility to the patient or family in the event anything adverse happened following therapy [3, 4]. This concept was called *pro corpore mortuoto* and can be found in Italian, French, and Middle Eastern archives as early as the fourteenth century and is considered a precursor to IC, although its purpose at that time was to protect the doctor and not the patient [5–7].

Respect for patient autonomy and the right to self-determination changed the informed consent process. The first lawsuit showcasing the failure to obtain IC prior to a surgical procedure was the English case *Slater vs Baker & Stapleton* that occurred in 1767. Slater sued his physician for re-fracturing his leg, as an experimental application of external fixation [8]. Following this case, the concept of assault and battery surfaced in English Common Law, establishing that a surgeon is liable for breach of duty if [he] failed to receive authorization from a patient before performing surgery [9].

The Slater case also illustrates the overlap between informed consent for surgery and informed consent for human subjects research. Both processes share the obligation to inform, to confirm the understanding of the person participating, and to assure the consent is given freely, without coercion. The goal for both is an informed choice to participate. Following the Second World War, the unethical medical experiments conducted by the Nazi party on involuntary subjects in concentration camps led to the Nuremberg trials (*USA v. Karl Brandt et al.*) and the Nuremberg Code [10]. The Code speaks directly to the absolutely essential voluntary consent of the human subject. The Nuremberg Code protects human research subjects and influenced the modern concept of informed consent for individual treatment. Modern work that is pertinent to consent for human subject's research and extends to operative consent includes the work of Flory et al. in "Interventions to Improve Research Participants Understandings in Informed Consent for Research: A Systemic Review". They find that the time spent for a given amount of information is important and that the best way to increase patients' comprehension is to simply spend more time talking one-on-one with them [11]. Patients want verbal information from a healthcare professional, which presents yet another challenge because surgeons are paid far more to operate than they are to talk.

Case-based litigation provided a contemporary legal framework for SIC as a result of the development of anesthesia and more invasive surgery. In the 1905 case *Mohr v. Williams*, the patient sued the surgeon for hearing loss after he performed a procedure on the right ear when the proposed operation was for the left ear. The suit was successful and the patient's informed consent for the precise procedure and site was deemed necessary. This case has since been used as an example in Torts classes and solidified informed consent as a binding contract between the patient and the surgeon [12]. In 1914, Mary Schloendorff was admitted to New York Hospital with a uterine fibroid. She declined the recommended surgery but consented to an exam under ether anesthesia during which the fibroid was removed. Following surgery, she suffered postoperative complications and sued in the case Schloendorff v. Society of New York Hospital [13]. Justice Benjamin Cardozo of the New York Court of Appeals ruled that involuntary removal of the fibroid constituted medical battery and wrote in the Court's opinion:

> Every human being of adult years and sound mind has a right to determine what shall be done with his own body; and a surgeon who performs an operation without [his] patient's consent commits an assault for which [he] is liable in damages. This is true except in cases of emergency where the patient is unconscious and where it is necessary to operate before consent can be obtained [13].

In 1957 Martin Salgo sued a physician and the trustees of Stanford University for malpractice, *Salgo vs. Leland Stanford, Jr. University Board of Trustees*, when his lower extremities were paralyzed after an aortogram. He claimed he was not informed of the risks associated with the procedure. The Salgo lawsuit was successful and the decision not only introduced the term "informed consent" for the first time but also established standards for the informed consent process in modern medical practice. In the lawsuit, the involved physicians admitted that they had failed to warn Salgo about his risks [14]. The Court judgment read:

> A physician violates [his]duty to[his] patient … if [he] withholds any facts which are neces-sary to form the basis of an intelligent consent by the patient to the proposed treatment [14].

6.3.2   Standards

The concept of a professional practice standard in negligence cases was introduced in the United Kingdom by *Bolam v FHMC* in 1957. Bolam sued after he was injured during electroconvulsive therapy when he was not given a muscle relaxant or restrained and did not understand the risks. Bolum lost the case because these ele-ments were not a part of the standard of care at that time. However, the ruling estab-lished the concept of a reasonable body of medical opinion to which a physician's practice should adhere. Assessing whether a physician practices in accordance with other reasonable physicians, which is without negligence, became known as the Bolam Test [15]. The Bolam test focuses on the one-sided delivery of information from the doctor and became the standard of care defining negligence. A paradigm shift to a more patient centered view was established in 1972 by the *Canterbury v. Spence* case which focused on information pertinent to a reasonable patient, estab-lishing a new precedent for informed consent [16, 17]. In the interim, patient-centered surgery has gained traction as the new standard of care. The more paternalistic "reasonable doctor standard" that focuses on surgeon practice patterns has become secondary to the "reasonable patient standard" that focuses on pertinent information for patient decision making in most countries [18].

As surgeons, we have a professional ethical responsibility to disclose information that informs patients about anticipated risks of surgery. The *reasonable person standard* characterizes the risks to disclose as those that a reasonable person would want to know under the given circumstances in order to make an informed decision. The *subjective standard* is contingent on a patient's decision to accept therapy, whereas the *community practice standard* is reliant on what other local clinicians consider appropriate [19]. Thus, the obligation faced by surgeons to disclose risk and provide comprehensive SIC when caring for a diverse patient population with individualized needs is challenging to say the least.

Based on historical cases and legislation, modern SIC is supported by three concepts: "preconditions," "information," and "consent" [20].

Preconditions include the ability of a patient to exercise their right to self-determination without coercion. The Patient Self Determination Act (PSDA) of 1990 encourages all people to make decisions now about the extent of medical care they would choose to accept or refuse in the event of a future serious illness [20]. Advance directives provide a blueprint of patient preferences for the care if decision making capacity is lost. These documented preferences for care may avert and or transform a SIC process for life saving procedures if such intervention is not desired.

Information includes disclosure of medical facts about conditions, proposed procedures, the potential risks, benefits, complications, and alternatives of proposed procedures, including the effect of nontreatment. All this information must be disclosed by the surgeon to honor the patient's right to self-determination and to make an informed choice.

Consent is the written registration of the patient's decision on a consent form. Documentation of the SIC process that leads to the consent usually exists in a separate, distinct location within the patient's electronic health record.

6.3.3   Legal

According to West's Encyclopedia of American Law, informed consent, is "an agreement to do something or to allow something to happen only after the relevant facts are known" [21]. Full disclosure must be completed by each party entering the agreement. Informed consent is also defined as "voluntary authorization, by a patient or research subject, with full comprehension of the risks involved, for diagnostic or investigative procedures, and for medical and surgical treatment" [22]. The clinical/ethical and legal aspects of IC are intertwined because medical expertise is necessary for the physician to inform and satisfy the legal burden of full disclosure to the patient. The first definition is a reminder that disclosure is not unidirectional, and both patient and physician are responsible for communicating relevant information. The second definition is a reminder that the ICP is often viewed as offering protection for patients who must know the risks to be in full agreement to proceed with surgery. Ideally, informed consent protects both providers and patients in litigation. The optimally informed patient will have more realistic expectations regarding a surgical procedure and its associated risks. Well-informed patients will be more satisfied and file fewer legal claims [4, 23]. Therefore, surgeons have incentive to be facile with the legal aspects of the informed consent process, which is enhanced by clear communication and shared decision-making.

6.3.4   Communication

A surgeon has the ethical obligation to communicate the therapeutic options to patients or surrogates and selflessly guide the therapeutic choices aligned with the patient's preferences, goals and values according to the best available evidence. The 2005 American College of Surgeons Statement on Principles of Palliative Care the fourth principle states,

> Identify the primary goals of care from the patient's perspective, and address how the surgeon's care can achieve the patient's objectives [24].

Sindhu wrote about the ethical complexities and inherent limitations of the informed consent process. Posing the question: "Can Consent Ever Truly Be Informed?" he describes the consent process between himself and his patient. Mr. J. has advanced cancer and is consulting him about radiation therapy. The patient is portrayed as a highly educated and fully resourced patient. After Sindhu has relayed information as part of the informed consent process which includes a recommendation for radiation therapy, Mr. J nods in agreement with the proposed plan without uttering a single word. Dr. Sindhu asks if he has questions and Mr. J does not. When he specifically elicits Mr. J's thoughts about treatment, his response is, "Whatever you think. You're the doctor" [25].

Dr. Sindhu's case illustrates the challenges of how the intention of shared decision making may not be realized depending on patient willingness and capability of engagement. It is understandable why some patients might be inclined to defer to the surgeon's judgement. The surgeon has dedicated years of study to render an opinion and each patient will process the exchange of information with varying degrees of comfort and comprehension. Clinicians must assess where patients fall on that spectrum and, to the best of their ability, satisfy the patient's particular communication needs.

Brezis found that half of patients did not remember receiving explanations about risks and two-thirds did not remember having a discussion about alternatives to proposed procedures. Their work revealed that expectations about decisions varied: about 20% of the study patients desired physicians to make decisions as opposed to 20% who favored autonomous decision making and 60% who preferred shared decision making [26].

Regardless of a patient's ability or willingness to take in information, the amount of material shared matters and varies with individuals. Silvia and Sorrel found that patients who perceived that the amount of information given to them was "just right" score significantly higher on comprehension tests than patients who said that the amount of information they received was either too much or too little [27].

Volpe has written about the amount of information delivered to patient's… She highlights the existence of expressed and unexpressed needs for information. Expressed needs are related to the quantity and source of information and unexpressed needs are the emotional tone and rank order of the information. Volpe's work suggests that patient autonomy is best served by meeting expressed and unexpressed information needs in tandem. It is especially important that providers are careful not to overwhelm patients with too much material. This communication skill set is subtle and enters the realm of cognitive psychology to support patients in the process of informed consent [28].

Another variable influencing the demand for communication in an informed consent process is the operation itself. Consent to remove a skin tag is not the same as the same as consent to repair an abdominal aortic aneurysm because the associated risks are very different for any given patient. In a uniquely logical approach to shared decision making, Whitney describes a model based upon risk and certainty that stratifies simple consent and informed consent accordingly. This work proposes that shared decision making is more complicated and more important when there is more than one reasonable treatment option. Informed consent does not require more than one clinical option but does require an exchange of information that includes risk, certainty, and patient preference [29].

Objective risk calculation is becoming an expected standard for modern surgery. Weisen et al. explore how the Surgical Risk Preoperative Assessment System (SURPAS) improves the informed consent process. Their study compares usual informed consent with a SURPAS guided informed consent that includes printed risk information for the patient. Eighty-two percent of the SURPAS patient cohort were very satisfied with the risk discussion versus 16% of the usual patient cohort. In addition, 75.3% of the SURPAS cohort reported that the modified risk discussion made them feel more comfortable with having surgery versus 19% of the usual SIC process cohort. The introduction of SURPAS also significantly reduced anxiety when compared to the control group [30].

A number of publications have proposed tools to improve the informed consent process, however literature on the quality of SIC is generally scarce [31, 32]. Surgical training has significant opportunity to encourage the communication skills integral to the process of informed consent. Although interpersonal skills and communication are a core competency for the Accreditation Council for Graduate Medical Education, development of curricula specific to informed consent could help standardize the skill set necessary to maximize patient understanding about risk and benefit. Kruser proposes and evaluates a framework for informed consent utilizing a novel communication tool of "best case/worst case (BC/WC) scenario" for difficult in-the-moment surgical decisions. Training surgeons to use this novel communication tool for high-risk acute surgical problems, they found that 79% of surgeons reported best case/worst case (BC/WC) was better than their usual approach and 71% endorsed active use of BC/WC in clinical practice. Patients and families found that BC/WC established expectations, provided clarity and facilitated deliberation [33, 34].

6.4 COVID Considerations—SIC has been Challenged by So Many Uncertainties

This SIC chapter is being drafted during the COVID-19 pandemic and in the perils of this new practice environment, surgeons are confronted by unprecedented unknowns that have complicated the SIC process. By practicing as surgeons we are consenting to exposure but don't know what that exposure might actually mean personally, professionally, and for those we love. The prospect of being exposed to SARS-CoV-2 and contracting the virus during this pandemic, is an inherent challenge to the informed consent process for surgeons and patients alike. COVID-19 is new to our world leaving our statistically rich fund of knowledge with limited data about the risks to surgical patients. We don't know how often COVID negative patients will contract the virus from operating room staff. We don't know how often a COVID positive patient will transmit the virus to staff during an operation. The pandemic changes everyone's risk, creates an entirely different scope and functional ability to engage in the SIC process raising a number of ethical questions including, "should there be elective operations in a pandemic?", "what constitutes an elective operation?", and how do we address COVID-19 positive patients who need emergent surgery?" Prachand described a departmental development of a quantitative, rational system for scoring medically necessary, time-sensitive procedures (MeNTS), based on current resource availability, patient risk factors, degree of resource utilization presented by a proposed procedure, and the medical and surgical feasibility of postponing an intervention [35]. Additionally, communication practices have been adapted by the constraints imposed by COVID-19. Many academic medical centers have reinforced the role of attending surgeons to maintain full responsibility for the SIC process. This practice is a result of recognition that significant scientific, ethical, and moral uncertainties surround the care of patients and families during the COVID-19 pandemic and how they might be reflected in informed consent discussions [36]. For example, routine use of personal protective equipment (PPE) such as masks that cover the mouth have limited the ability for some to read lips and interpret facial expressions. For multi-lingual patients or patients with disabilities and their families it may be that shared decision making is disrupted by visitor restrictions and the absence of advocates and surrogates present at the bedside. These new COVID-19 related barriers to usual communication might be preventing our best attempt to honor patient autonomy in the SIC process.

As the case of Mr. Y illustrates, we can't know for sure who will have what complications and how many different elements must be considered during the informed consent process. That is why transparency about potential but unknown risks and honest admission of how little we currently understand about the surgical outcomes of COVID-19 positive patients and patients with unknown COVID-19 status is especially important. In the case presented, the surgeon performs much of what is expected for the informed consent process. The risks, benefits, and alternatives are well communicated even under the pressure of an emergent operation. And yet, as is frequently the case, what should be an essential component of informed consent is omitted. Throughout the trajectory of Mr. Y's clinical course nobody asks how he defines quality of life or his thoughts on prolonged life support. Physicians can outline the potential consequences of treatment but only the patient can speak to what they mean to their quality of life. If their physician doesn't listen, they could be performing an operation for the wrong indications.

6.5   Conclusion

The Surgical Informed Consent process is complex because there are so many disparate elements that must be fused into a coherent decision for an individual who may not fit homogeneous algorithms. SIC requires medical expertise and sophisticated communication skill to satisfy the ethical, legal, and rapidly evolving, shared decision-making standards for a diverse patient population. When examining the process of SIC in today's clinical landscape, it can only be *reasonably* achieved by effectively providing the *right* amount of information, delivered in the right way, to enable an informed treatment decision for each individual patient.

We have challenges to achieve a meaningful SIC. The process is often perfunctory and adequate only to satisfy minimum standards of ethical, legal, and institutional requirements. Optimal SIC is not the surgeon's presentation of a menu of options outlining the risks, benefits, complications, and alternatives, but rather starts with getting to know our patients. Instead of revering SIC as an opportunity to really understand our patients and their goals of care, or counsel them in depth about post intervention scenarios, we are willing to consider SIC a task suitable for the junior resident, who has limited experience with the consequences of surgery [37]. We do not train surgeons how to communicate in general, much less specifically about SIC. Meredyth at al explore these challenges, calling it "(Under)Valuing" Surgical Informed Consent. The authors advocate for changes in surgical culture and propose standardized training. They also point out that all of health care culture has accountability for better informed consent, including hospital administrators and insurers [1].

Perhaps the way forward is to consider the SIC process a valuable interaction during which the *surgeon* is informed about the patient's preferences, goals and values, after which they can present a patient centered recommendation. Only by engaging with, and listening to, our patients can we deliver optimal care. If we initiate this type of discussion, chances are our patients will rise and openly participate in the shared decision-making process thereby making SIC the best that it can be.

6.6   Selected References

- Leclercq WKG, Keulers BJ, Scheltinga MRM, Spauwen PHM, van der Wilt G. A review of surgical informed consent: past, present, and future. A quest to help patients make better decisions. World J Surg. 2010;34:1406–14. https://doi.org/10.1007/s00268-010-0542-0

    – A most comprehensive review of surgical informed consent cited by many authors in the current literature.

- Meredyth NA, de Melo-Martin I. (Under)valuing surgical informed consent. J Am Coll Surg. 2020;230(2):257262. https://doi.org/10.1016/j.jamcollsurg.2019.10.001

    – The authors review the challenges and potential solutions to modern surgical informed consent framed by the context of surgical and health care culture.

- Prachand VN, Milner R, Angelos P, et al. Medically necessary, time-sensitive procedures: scoring system to ethically and efficiently manage resource scarcity and provider risk during the COVID-19 pandemic. J Am Coll Surg. 2020;231(2):281–8. https://doi.org/10.1016/j.jamcollsurg.2020.04.011

    – The authors outline the relationship between the COVID pandemic and surgical ethics which has profound implications for surgical informed consent.

Acknowledgements Yuk Ming Liu, MD for her assistance with the original literature search.

References

1. Meredyth NA, de Melo-Martin I. (Under)valuing surgical informed consent. J Am Coll Surg. 2020;230(2):257–62. https://doi.org/10.1016/j.jamcollsurg.2019.10.001.
2. Jonsen A, Siegler M, Winslade WJ. Clinic ethics: a practical approach to ethical decisions in clinical medicine. McGraw Hill Education; 2015. p. 54.
3. Chotai PN, Tubbs RS, Huang EY. History and philosophy of surgical informed consent in children. Int J Philos Med. 2016;6:10601. https://doi.org/10.18550/ijhpm.0116.0601.
4. Leclercq WKG, Keulers BJ, Scheltinga MRM, Spauwen PHM, van der Wilt G. A review of surgical informed consent: past, present, and future. A quest to help patients make better decisions. World J Surg. 2010;34:1406–14. https://doi.org/10.1007/s00268-010-0542-0.
5. Ajlouni KM. History of informed medical consent [letter]. Lancet. 1995;346(8980):980. https://doi.org/10.1016/s0140-6736(95)91608-3.
6. Vollmann J, Winau R, Baron JH. History of informed medical consent [letter]. Lancet. 1997;347(8998):410. https://doi.org/10.1016/s0140-6736(96)90597-8.
7. Rothman DJ. History of informed medical consent [letter]. Lancet. 1995;346(8990):1633. https://doi.org/10.1016/s0140-6736((5)91970-8.
8. *Slater v. Baker & Stapleton*, 95 Eng. Rep. 860 (K.B. 1767).
9. Murray PM. The history of informed consent. Iowa Orthop J. 1990;10:104–9.

10. Records of the United States Nuerenberg war crimes trials. *United States of America v. Karl Brandt et al.* (Case I). November 21, 1946–August 20, 1947. National Archives and Records Service, General Services Administration; 1974. https://www.archives.gov/files/research/captured-german-records/microfilm/m887.pdf. Accessed 16 Mar 2021.

11. Flory J, Emanuel E. Interventions to improve research participants' understanding in informed consent for research: a systemic review. JAMA. 2004;292(13):1593–601. https://doi.org/10.1001/jama.292.13.1593.

12. *Mohr v. Williams*, 104 N.W. 12 (SC Minn 1905).

13. *Scholendorff v. Society of New York Hospital*, 211 N.Y. 215, 105 N.E. 92 (1914).

14. *Salgo v. Leland Stanford Jr. Univ. Bd. Trustees*, 317 P.2d 170 (1957).

15. *Bolam v Friern Hospital Management Committee*, 1957 1 WLR 582, 587.

16. *Canterbury v. Spence*, 464 F.2d 772 (D.C. Cir. 1972).

17. Robert S. Jerry Canterbury, whose paralysis led to informed consent laws, is dead at 78. *New York Times*. May 16, 2017. https://www.nytimes.com/2017/05/16/us/jerry-canterbury-medical-consent-paralysis.html. Accessed 17 Feb 2021.

18. Kastelein WR. Informed consent and medical liability: jurisprudence 1994–1998. [in Dutch]. Tijdschr Gezondhd. 1998;22:134–46. https://doi.org/10.1007/bf03055782.

19. Ganai S. Informed consent and disclosure of surgeon experience. In: Ferreres AR, editor. Surgical ethics. Principles and practice. Springer; 2019. p. 219.

20. *Patient Self-Determination Act of 1990*, Omnibus Budget Reconciliation Act of 1990. Omnibus Budget Reconciliation Act of 1990, 42 U.S.C., §§ 1395cc, 1396a (1990). https://www.congress.gov/bill/101st-congress/house-bill/4449. Accessed 2 Mar 2021.

21. West's encyclopedia of American law: Fri to Jam. Thomson/Gale; 2005.

22. Wortz G. Reducing liability risk through informed consent. J Med Pract Manage. 2011;26(4):203–8.

23. MeSH Database. Informed consent. Term introduced 1973. https://www.ncbi.nlm.nih.gov/mesh/68007258?ordinalpos=1&itool=EntrezSystem2.PEntrez.Mesh.Mesh_ResultsPanel.Mesh_RVDoc%20Sum. Accessed 12 Oct 2020.

24. Statement on principles of palliative care. American College of Surgeons. August 1, 2005. https://www.facs.org/about-acs/statements/50-palliative-care. Accessed 12 Oct 2020.

25. Sindhu K. Can consent ever truly be informed? November 2, 2018. Doximity Op-Med. https://www.doximity.com/articles/57ea0c6b-1439-437d-95c0-ad2864579c94?utm_campaign=identified_redirect&utm_source=opmed. Accessed 12 Oct 2020.

26. Brezis M, Israel S, Weinstein-Birenshtock A, Pogoda P, Sharon A, Tauber R. Quality of informed consent for invasive procedures. Int J Qual Health Care. 2008;20(5):352–7. https://doi.org/10.1093/intqhc/mzn025.

27. Silvia MC, Sorrell JM. Enhancing comprehension of information for informed consent: a review of empirical research. IRB: Ethics Hum Res. 1988;10(1):1–5. https://doi.org/10.2307/3564101.

28. Volpe RL. Patient's expressed and unexpressed needs for information for informed consent. J Clin Ethics. 2010;21(1):45–57. 20465076.

29. Whitney SN, McGuire AL, McCullough LB. A typology of shared decision making, informed consent, and simple consent. Ann Intern Med. 2004;140(1):54–9. https://doi.org/10.7326/0003-4819-140-1-200401060-00012.

30. Wiesen BM, Bronsert MR, Aasen DM, et al. Use of Surgical Risk Preoperative Assessment System (SURPAS) and patient satisfaction during informed consent for surgery. J Am Coll Surg. 2020;230(6):1025–33.e1. https://doi.org/10.1016/j.jamcollsurg.2020.02.049.

31. Kinnersley P, Phillips K, Savage K, et al. Interventions to promote informed consent for patients undergoing surgical and other invasive healthcare procedures. Cochrane Database Syst Rev. 2013;7:CD009445. https://doi.org/10.1002/14651858.CD009445.pub2.

32. Loftus TJ, Tighe PJ, Filiberto AC, et al. Artificial intelligence and surgical decision-making. JAMA Surg. 2020;155(2):148–58. https://doi.org/10.1001/jamasurg.2019.4917.

33. Kruser JM, Nabozny MJ, Steffens NM, et al. "Best case/worst case": qualitative evaluation of a novel communication tool for difficult in-the-moment surgical decisions. J Am Geriatr Soc. 2015;63(9):1805–11. https://doi.org/10.1111/jgs.13615.
34. Schwarze ML, Kehler JM, Campbell TC. Navigating high-risk procedures with more than just a street map [letter]. J Palliat Med. 2013;16:1169–71. https://doi.org/10.1089/jprn.2013.0221.
35. Prachand VN, Milner R, Angelos P, et al. Medically necessary, time-sensitive procedures: scoring system to ethically and efficiently manage resource scarcity and provider risk during the COVID-19 pandemic. J Am Coll Surg. 2020;231(2):281–8. https://doi.org/10.1016/j.jamcollsurg.2020.04.011.
36. Bryan AF, Milner R, Roggin KK, Angelos P, Matthews JB. Unknown unknowns: surgical consent during the COVID-19 pandemic. Ann Surg. 2020;272(2):e161–2. https://doi.org/10.1097/SLA.0000000000003995.
37. Angelos P, DaRosa DA, Bentram D, Sherman H. Residents seeking informed consent: are they adequately knowledgeable? Curr Surg. 2002;59(1):115–8. https://doi.org/10.1016/s0149-7944(01)00591-8.

Chapter 7
Goals of Care Discussions in High-Risk Surgery

Eric M. Curto, Robert P. Sticca, and Sabha Ganai ⓘ

Abstract In patients with complex surgical problems, goals of care discussions can be challenging. These discussions are paramount and are often a multi-layered process that should include two-way communication in developing a plan of action centered around the patient's wishes. We should start our surgeon-patient discussions in the preoperative period and span the entirety of the patient's care timeline. Risks, goals, uncertainty, prognostication, and expectations should all be addressed. There are a multitude of clinical tools that we can use to help augment the goals of care discussions. Surgical "buy-in" and "best case/worst case" clinical scenarios can provide an agreed upon treatment pathway and clarity to both the patient and the surgeon. We can utilize these discussions and tools to address the ethical principles of respect for autonomy and beneficence. With these tools and knowledge available, we can strive towards providing our patients with full disclosure even in the setting of complex surgical situations.

Keywords High-risk surgery · Goals of care · Informed consent
Decision-making · Ethics · Surgical "buy-in"

E. M. Curto
University of North Dakota School of Medicine and Health Sciences, Grand Forks, ND, USA
e-mail: eric.curto@und.edu

R. P. Sticca · S. Ganai (✉)
University of North Dakota School of Medicine and Health Sciences, Grand Forks, ND, USA

Sanford Clinic, Fargo, ND, USA
e-mail: robert.sticca@und.edu; sabha.ganai@und.edu

© The Author(s), under exclusive license to Springer Nature
Switzerland AG 2022
V. A. Lonchyna et al. (eds.), *Difficult Decisions in Surgical Ethics*, Difficult
Decisions in Surgery: An Evidence-Based Approach,
https://doi.org/10.1007/978-3-030-84625-1_7

Case

Our patient is a 64-year-old Caucasian gentleman who was a retired music teacher. He battled chronic pain for many years due to spinal stenosis causing severe radiculopathy to both lower extremities requiring a lumbosacral fusion. As a consequence of his lifestyle and debilitated status, the patient was morbidly obese. After talking with his neurosurgeon, it was considered prudent to lose weight to help improve his ability to recover from a repeat spinal fusion.

He was referred to a bariatric surgeon for this, and after a year-long informed consent process, he was scheduled for a sleeve gastrectomy. He underwent the laparoscopic surgery without complication and lost approximately 80 pounds. This was followed by a repeat spinal fusion with improvement to his neurologic symptoms. Unfortunately, the patient had return of his radicular pain and gained back most of the weight he had lost.

During a follow-up visit with bariatric surgery clinic, our patient reported symptoms of odynophagia and dysphagia. Work up for these symptoms led to findings of locally advanced distal esophageal adenocarcinoma. He was seen by a multidisciplinary team, including medical, surgical, and radiation oncologists, and plans were made to start neoadjuvant chemoradiation.

Due to the patient's history of a sleeve gastrectomy, the altered blood supply to his stomach would make it insufficient as a conduit, an unintended consequence of his prior bariatric surgery. After the patient had completed chemoradiation, he underwent a transhiatal esophagectomy with colonic interposition.

Before surgery, we spent time discussing and progressing through the informed consent process. We discussed the risks, goals, expectations of surgery, and touched on prognosis of his disease. These were not easy discussions to have, touching on the uncertainty ahead and the real possibility of morbidity, altered quality of life, and death. Goals of care discussions in high-risk situations, while daunting, have been shown to be feasible and able to align a patient's goals in relation to surgery [1]. It is an ongoing process, one that started well before his day of surgery, and stretched long beyond it to his final days.

7.1 Introduction

In patients with complex surgical problems, goals of care discussions can be challenging. While these situations call for a high level of diagnostic skills, decision-making, and surgical acumen, they also bring on the need for proficient and sufficient

Table 7.1 Ethical principles to help guide difficult decisions in surgery

Respect for Persons	The basis of all discussions when it comes to goals of cares in high-risk surgery should be rooted in *shared decision-making*. It is with this principle that we continue to strive towards *patient autonomy*. In this chapter, most clinical tools mentioned are significantly promoting and assisting the patient and their ability to making a fully disclosed decision. Through utilization of these tools and centering decision making around the patient's wishes, we can progress towards succeeding with respect for persons and patient autonomy.
Nonmaleficence	We arrive upon this discussion when it comes to providing a treatment pathway for a patient. It is paramount to ascertain a pathway that first *respects their autonomy* and their wishes. With that, we can avoid actions or behaviors (even if unintentional or in good will) that could cause harm to patient if it were against their wishes. Additionally, we address perioperative judgment and the ability to balance competing priorities to place the patient's best interest of "*first, do no harm*" at the center of the decision making.

The most significant ethical principles influenced in this chapter: *respect for persons* and *nonmaleficence*
Source: Authors own work

informed consent for the patient. Goals of care should be addressed in the first conversation with the patient and should continue throughout their course of care with shared decision-making at the forefront. It is a multi-layered process that should include two-way communication in developing a plan of action centered around the patient's wishes. In many instances, we unfortunately provide inadequate informed consent for our patients [2]. It is the goal of this chapter to provide our readers with the knowledge and tools to provide patients with a competent discussion in goals of care and a complete informed consent process (see Table 7.1).

7.2 Search Strategy

The topic of goals of care discussion in high-risk surgery was the center of our search strategy. The following keywords were used in general search engines Google Scholar and PubMed through August 2020: high-risk surgery; goals of care; informed consent; decision-making. These general keywords along with the idea of having tools for discussing high-risk surgery goals brought us to 27 key papers included in the references. Additional searches were used to refine our discussion and centered around risk, uncertainty, prognostication, palliative care and end of life discussions, perioperative decision-making and differences on outcomes in high-risk surgeries, as well as more general reviews on shared decision making and the informed consent process.

7.3 Discussion

7.3.1 Preoperative Period and Informed Consent

The first patient encounter is the entry into the surgical realm and informed consent process, which can be integrated into discussion on goals of care. In its most basic form, informed consent should include a discussion of diagnosis (or potential diagnoses); the proposed and alternative treatments with its risks, benefits, and goals; and the overall prognosis for each proposed pathway [3]. While these elements are vital, the picture can look increasingly different with any number of clinical situations.

For example, the patient in our illustrative case underwent at least three "elective" surgeries. The first was a lumbosacral fusion for chronic symptoms of back pain and radiculopathy. The potential benefits of the surgery included improvement of his symptoms and quality of life. His second surgery, a sleeve gastrectomy, had more abstract potential benefits, which included weight loss, metabolic and physiologic improvements, as well as psychological and social effects. Finally, his esophagectomy for cancer and subsequent emergent revision surgery had the potential benefit of curing him of cancer and saving his life, respectively.

To provide ethically correct consent, we must provide disclosure of the treatment pathway(s) with proper patient understanding and decision-making [4]. We must use a language that can be understood, which can be a challenge when discussing complex anatomical and medical terminology. It is important to provide enough contextual information for the patient but to also not overwhelm them with minutia and details. Understanding the level of information to convey to the patient and their family is a critical one and something seldom achieved from a single encounter.

To assist with informing the patient in a manner where full disclosure can be ascertained, three models have been constructed:

- **Professional**: disclosure and discussion by physicians in similar circumstances.
- **Reasonable**: disclosure and discussion based on what a reasonable patient would want to know.
- **Subjective**: disclosure and discussion based on patient's specific interests, values, and life plans.

A professional standard for disclosure can bear risk of medical paternalism and is not compatible within the framework of shared decision-making. Childers et al. discussed the utility of combining the reasonable and subjective models in the disclosure process [4]. While the reasonable person standard is considered legally valid in most states, there are ethical considerations to consider elements of both the reasonable and subjective standards, particularly in respect of shared decision-making. It is with this hybrid method that we can move past some of the pitfalls of the two individually. The reasonable standard can ignore individual patient preferences while attempting to maintain justice for all patients. On the other hand, the subjective standard focuses more on respecting patient autonomy, but cannot always be feasible due to time constraints and limitations in ability to ensure patient comprehension and understanding of complex scenarios. A reasonable and subjective standard, however, can provide patients and physicians the ability to identify what values and interests take precedence and make certain of their inclusion in disclosure and discussion. For example, a professional musician may require additional discussion of material risks relevant to their career prior to considering options of carpal tunnel surgery versus continued splinting for median neuropathy, even if those foreseen risks are low.

7.3.2   Discussing Risk

In high-risk surgeries, the discussion of risk becomes paramount. There is evidence that despite poor patient comprehension of the risks involved with surgery, it is not necessarily associated with feelings of being poorly informed or reservations on the decision for surgery [5]. Nonetheless, it is our ethical obligation to provide patients with a thorough understanding of the potential risks that coincide with surgery. Discussing complex surgical problems with patients and their families can be challenging as a true understanding of the diagnosis, treatment, and risks involved may never be achieved across all circumstances. Appropriately, there is qualitative evidence that demonstrates despite the aptitude of surgeons communicating risk and their personal commitment to a patient's survival, the topics of life-supporting postoperative treatments and patient preferences are rarely discussed [6]. Although these topics can be delicate and challenging to approach, they should be considered to promote shared decision-making.

Maneuvering discussions on the level of detail to provide in regard to a complex and high-risk surgery can be daunting. One technique that can be used as conduit for further deliberation on risks is the "fix-it" strategy first introduced in 1991 by Lynn and Degrazia, a model of medical decision-making where the identified problem is a medical deviation from normalcy [7]. With this model, a surgery can be described in layman's terms or analogously as the "fix," for the medical disease—the "it." This has been described as a reliable technique which surgeons often employ in an attempt to describe the details and goals for a proposed operation. However, it must be done with caution to avoid creating an environment that culminates with normalcy and the patient returning to their baseline status before surgery was undertaken. Additionally, this tool can create an environment of oversimplification in terms of expectations and possible outcomes. It can be used as a bridge along with other tools in further discussion on goals of care and risks involved [8].

It is important to start the conversation of potential risks and complications in the very first patient encounter. Much can be learned from the patient regarding their beliefs, interests, and goals. You can allow for natural growth in your relationship with the patient, which can propel discussions of complicated topics. Although this may be difficult to complete in an acute care setting where time may be short, there should be time in the clinic and in telephone encounters to create a clear clinical picture and plan with the patient. Regarding the illustrative case at the beginning of the chapter, these may include short-term risks like postoperative bleeding and long-term risks including internal hernias and weight regain with respect to bariatric surgery, as well as risks of anastomotic leak, recurrent laryngeal nerve injury, or postoperative stricture and dysphagia when considering an esophagectomy. The patient needs to know that this operation could lead to more procedures or operations if things do not go precisely as the patient and the surgeon plan.

With these discussions, you and your patient can be prepared for the treatment that comes after. In these high-risk surgeries where morbidity is more frequently encountered, it is important to discuss the possibility of postoperative intubation, need for placement of a feeding tube for nutrition, or dialysis. Knowing these risks of a surgery can assist a patient in deciding if these treatment modalities align with their interests and goals. This benefits the patient two-fold: it provides them with a more thorough understanding about the potential complications and sequalae of treatments, and it allows them to have these decisions made beforehand in a controlled environment. In situations when urgent or emergent surgery is needed, patients are not always of full mind and body. Having these discussions preoperatively allows them to utilize the provider, friends, family, and others as needed to make these vital decisions about their future healthcare.

Dr. Schwarze described this process of commitment as surgical "buy-in." [9] It allows surgeons to negotiate a postoperative commitment from the patient before undergoing these high-risk surgeries. As a result, the surgeon and the patient understand leading into surgery the patient's commitment as well as their limitations on postoperative interventions. Additionally, this allows for negotiations of time restrictions for postoperative cares, can shift a share of the responsibility to the patient, and can even allow the surgeon to refuse surgery if he or she felt proceeding was unsafe or unreasonable given patient requested limitations. If these measures are taken preoperatively, there can be significant reduction of emotional stress for the patient as well as the surgeon [9].

Nabozny et al. specified that surgical "buy-in" cannot be presumed and must be explicitly discussed otherwise patient preferences on treatment options postoperatively may be incongruent to the surgeon's expectations [10]. Advanced directives should be addressed if already present or newly constructed to provide the patient and surgeon with full disclosure. It is important that these complex discussions include the patient's spouse, close relatives, and/or legal healthcare power of attorney as it is difficult and frustrating for everyone when a predictable postoperative complication occurs, such as reintubation and the need for short-term ventilator support, which obviate the patient's ability to make rational healthcare decisions during that time. If the patient's healthcare proxy does not understand the commitment made preoperatively to manage short-term complications in the postoperative period, they may apply general statements made by the patient in sometimes distant past conversations ("I do not want to be on life support"). This may lead to a decision to withdraw critical support and let the patient expire even though the surgical team feels the complications are correctable and the patient has a reasonable chance of meaningful survival. Although the family may feel they are complying with the patients previously stated wishes ("he/she would not want to live like that"), this may be framed out of context of their current intentions. The surgical team may also feel betrayed as they have invested much time, work, and energy into performing a major surgery, and in their opinion the patient is not given a reasonable chance to get through the surgery and postoperative period.

7.3.3   Managing Expectations, Uncertainty, and Prognostication

Providing a detailed description of potential complications in the surgical "buy-in" process can provoke a cascade of questions about expectations. Patients and their families may ask what is expected as the most likely outcome? Will their grandparent, parent, sibling, or child survive surgery? If they survive, what would you expect their quality of life to be? What is the chance of the most severe of complications happening? These questions delve into the reality of uncertainty when it comes to biologic results even when technical execution of the surgery is exemplary. These expectations can be extremely challenging to convey and ensure comprehension from a patient perspective when there is a high level of uncertainty and unknown, which is often the case in high-risk surgeries. Surgeons frequently spend ample time describing surgical details and associated risks, but they often come up short from the patient's perspective when it comes to terms of recovery, quality of life afterwards, and survival [11].

There are many strategies and techniques when it comes to providing a patient or their family with expectations and in discussion of uncertainty. One technique that has classically been described, especially in the intensive care setting, is "hanging the crepe." In brief, this phrase characterized a "no-lose" situation where the patient is portrayed to be on the precipice of death and will almost certainly die unless a miraculous turn of events occurs, which may be remedied surgical intervention. This scenario can provide the physician with two outcomes as seen by the patient or their family: (1) the patient passes on as was predicted by the physician due disease progression, or (2) the patient survives and the physician is regarded as their savior [12]. This strategy entails painting an overly dire and pessimistic picture, and although straightforward and possibly necessary when actual outcomes in certain situations are hard to predict, bypasses the in-depth discussion and disclosure of information that can lead to a more educated decision by the patient or their decision-maker.

Thankfully, there are other strategies that we can use to support the decision-making process. One such strategy was introduced by Kruser et al. who presented "best case/worst case" scenarios to patients and used a novel communication tool to assist in coming to a decision on a difficult surgical situation [13]. With this tool, a graphic is constructed by the physician that displays a confined range of treatment options that may include different surgical options or supportive care. Best- and worst-case scenarios are then listed and described under each treatment option, and the most likely outcomes are identified. The advantages of this support tool were that it establishes a choice for the patient, provides clarity on their situation, encourages deliberation with family and the physician, and can be individualized to the patient's goals. This methodology also puts context to the esoteric discussion of complications by conveying how likely they may impact their long-term quality of life. For a previously independent person, this technique opens up discussions of the implications of discharge to a nursing facility versus home, as well as the extreme scenarios of requiring prolonged intensive care unit care leading to death.

Just as surgeons use objective data to guide their clinical decision-making, it can be beneficial to provide our patients with the same. The techniques based on "best case/worst case" scenarios are great at comparing different treatment options and their expected outcomes but can lack a discussion on objective data points when comparing their clinical picture to the general populations. There are multiple prognostic tools available that can also be utilized in discussions, but they can be time intensive, difficult to locate, or difficult to know their reliability. The American Society of Anesthesiologists physical status classification can be used to risk-stratify but lacks individual association of patients' comorbidities and their relation to the specific surgery and can have less than optimal inter-rater reliability [14]. A tool that can be specified to general surgical procedures, the National Surgery Quality Improvement (NSQIP) calculator from the American College of Surgeons, has been shown to be relatively easy to use with good predictive ability as well as the capability to make adjustments based on the surgeon's clinical experience and judgement. Additionally, the use of a frailty index can help better inform outcomes [15]. Overall, it is important to use a clinical tool that can be used with the surgeon's comfort, is understandable for the patient and family, and has been shown to demonstrate reliability and validity.

When using objective numbers and data, we should avoid manipulation of the information provided to prevent framing bias and effect. It has been shown that both physicians and patients are susceptible to framing bias, and a comprehensive presentation of absolute mortality, absolute survival, and relative risk reduction can lead to the least biased scenario when included in the informed process [16]. This should be done delicately and other aspects that can include risks of serious and any complications, discharge to a rehab or nursing facility, and readmission rate should be discussed as well. Importantly, degree of uncertainty specific to data given and context to the patient's situation, for example the impact on quality of life, should be disclosed when using data in the goals of care discussions.

While it is important to include the topic of prognostication, it should not be used in isolation and can be intertwined into larger discussions (i.e., the best-case/worst-case scenarios). Additionally, relying on too many numbers and percentages can be troublesome and overwhelming to the patient. There is a fine line of giving too much information and too little. Some patients want a wide range of information and details while others only want selected information [17]. Knowing this, it is important to follow the patient's cues and learn their preferences which can shape discussions in a more productive manner.

7.3.4   Shared Decision-Making

Over the years, physicians have moved away from the paternalistic model for decision-making where selected information is conveyed to the patient, and the choice for treatment is made by the physician. In the extreme situation, the physician makes the decision on an intervention and "informs the patient when the intervention will be initiated" [18]. As consequence to this often-criticized model, the informed model was proposed where information is explained in full, but no advice or recommendations are made [19]. This leaves the patient having to shoulder the load on preference for treatment, which can be expectantly overwhelming. The concept of shared decision-making looks to rectify these previous models and provides a mode of two-way communication. This process was first clarified by Charles where four key characteristics were suggested [20]:

- There are at least *two* participants (the physician and the patient),
- Both parties share information,
- Both parties work together to create the preferred treatment, and
- Agreement on a treatment to implement.

One difficulty some surgeons may have is engagement of the patient and their families in the discussion of care. To help remedy these findings, Schwarze et al. had performed a randomized clinical trial introducing a question prompt list to be given to patients before their first clinic visit who were to undergo surgery deemed as being high risk [21]. Unfortunately, this study did not find statistically significant effect on patient engagement and well-being compared to the control group; however, the surgeons who participated in the study believed it empowered patients to ask questions and desired its continued use in their practices.

Creating an environment that can provide the patient and the surgeon with a shared platform for decision-making can be difficult. We should provide the patient with an empathetic and encouraging presence while avoiding coddling or providing false hope. We need to use the tools we have discussed thus far to educate the patient fairly without overloading them with information. We face the challenge of oftentimes feeling we know what is best for the patient, while patients may feel that we are not always hearing their concerns. With the patient's autonomy at the center of care, shared decisions can be made that align with the patient's culture, interests, beliefs, and goals.

7.3.5   Perioperative Judgment and Outcomes

Often, decisions in high-risk surgeries are considered a decision between "life and death." These surgical situations can lead to several emotions from all parties involved and can lead to a buildup of clinical momentum that can be hard to stop once it has started and push into action potentially unnecessary and unwanted interventions [10]. It can be difficult to undo this momentum with a single discussion with the patient or their family; however, it is important to take the steps to provide the most accurate picture for goals, risks, and expectations of what surgery entails. With this approach the outcome that is most aligned with the patient's goals can be pursued.

While things often can move fast perioperatively, it is important to slow things down as necessary. Intraoperatively, Moulton et al. demonstrated a type of attentive automaticity that surgeons exhibit in the operating room that can be "slowed down" in times where effortful attention and judgement is required [22]. This can be a spectrum of actions that range from fine tuning technique, removing distractions, or even stopping completely [22]. It is in these times experienced and expert surgeons can perform life-saving maneuvers where less experienced surgeons may not succeed. Accordingly, this may be indicative of findings that support better outcomes when high-risk surgeries such as pancreatectomy, gastrectomy, and esophagectomy are performed by high-volume surgeons [23].

It is important when considering high-risk surgeries that competing priorities be explicit. The outcome of surgical intervention is paramount, but the path leading to the outcome is not always clear. As described by Leung et al., surgeons must balance priorities such as reputation, hierarchal culture, ego, time, monetary gain, and trainee teaching when making decisions with consideration of the patient's best interest of "first, do no harm."[24] They postulate that creating a more transparent discussion on these processes may create a full disclosure situation that can reduce errors and resultingly improve outcomes [24].

7.4 Case Conclusion

In our illustrative case, the patient ultimately succumbed to his disease after many days in the hospital postoperatively.

7.4.1 Goals of Care in End-of-Life Discussions

There is often a tremendous strain on patients and their families at the end of life. As surgeons, the emotional strain experienced is not insignificant and can be present when their patients have complications that subsequently lead to poor outcomes. What can often be more intrusive is the ongoing distress from possible complications arising, regardless of whether they occur [25]. These experiences may certainly act as stressors that impact future interactions with patients.

While there is no perfect formula to approaching end-of-life discussions, multiple strategies have been developed that can aid in a productive conversation. These conversations should start at the first clinical encounter or shortly thereafter but before surgical intervention is performed when possible. The patient's family should ideally be present, and a surrogate decision maker should be appointed in cases where the patient loses their decision-making capacity. Every patient will be different and cues on the path of discussion should be gathered and performed with empathy and compassion. Studies demonstrate patients at both ends of the spectrum where the details are wanted in their entirety, while on the other hand, other participants felt that the information was too blunt and wanted a softer discussion about death and dying [8].

Strong consideration should be made to include palliative care consultation before high risk surgery. Such consultation has demonstrated efficacy in improvement to ratings of overall end of life care, communication, and support as rated by families of deceased patients [26]. Palliative care consultations should not replace the surgeon-patient discussion about end-of-life issues but can augment it. End of life discussions, like other surgical skills, take practice and continued medical training on palliative topics as well as integrating these topics into core resident curricula is critical to producing surgeons that are prepared, knowledgeable, and skilled in navigating in these difficult situations [27, 28].

7.5 Conclusion

The goals of care discussions prior to high-risk surgery are of paramount importance but are nevertheless challenging. The discussion starts in the first encounter with the patient and their family and must include a thorough informed consent process such as the one described by Abaunza [3] and be rooted in shared decision-making. A well-established patient-surgeon relationship can nurture the tough discussions on risks and aid in negotiations with the surgical "buy-in" [9, 10] established that "buy-in" cannot be presumed and must be explicitly discussed and advanced directives should be constructed to provide the surgeon and patient full disclosure.

With high-risk surgery, there will be a level of uncertainty for what the future holds. We can use the tools provided by Kruser et al. [13] and present the "best case/worst case" scenarios to our patients and their families to address the multitude of possible outcomes. Additionally, we should look to utilize the clinical tools that are available to us such as the NSQIP calculator and the frailty index to potentiate reduction of uncertainty and assist with prognostication. By using these tools and refining our perioperative judgement within the basis of "first, do no harm"; we can create a situation that provides the patient with full disclosure while reducing errors and improving outcomes [24].

7.6   Selected References

- Schwarze ML, Bradley CT, Brasel KJ. Surgical "buy-in": the contractual relationship between surgeons and patients that influences decisions regarding life-supporting therapy. Crit Care Med. 2010;38(3):843–848. https://doi.org/10.1097/ccm.0b013e3181cc466b.

    - A great tool for surgeons discussing high-risk surgeries and the plan of action. It allows the surgeon and the patient to create a situation that can be agreed upon. It gives the patient AND the surgeon the ability to set parameters to the care. Using explicit discussion provides full disclosure and the patient and surgeon can come to a shared decision on the treatment options. It highlights what is and is not expected by the surgeon and the patient.

- Kruser JM, Nabozny MJ, Steffens NM, et al. "Best Case/Worst Case": qualitative evaluation of a novel communication tool for difficult in-the-moment surgical decisions. J Am Geriatr Soc. 2015;63(9):1805–1811. https://doi.org/10.1111/jgs.13615.

    - A description of the "best case/worst case" communication tool for surgical decision making at difficult in-the-moment periods in a patient's care timeline. The tool was praised by both surgeons and patients as providing clarity on challenging topics in an easy-to-understand manner. Additionally, it also promoted further discussions on goals of care and coming to a decision based on the patient's wishes.

References

1. McGreevy C, Kunac A, Chokshi R, Smith JH, Mazza D, Mosenthal AC. Discussing goals of care preoperatively in high-risk oncologic surgery [ASCO Abstract]. J Clin Oncol. 2015;33(29):38. https://doi.org/10.1200/jco.2015.33.29_suppl.38.
2. Lomas DJ, Ziegelmann MJ, Elliott DS. How informed is our consent? Patient awareness of radiation and radical prostatectomy complications. Turk J Urol. 2018;45(3):191–5. https://doi.org/10.5152/tud.2018.81522.
3. Abaunza H, Romero K. Elements for adequate informed consent in the surgical context. World J Surg. 2014;38(7):1594–604. https://doi.org/10.1007/s00268-014-2588-x.
4. Childers R, Lipsett PA, Pawlik TM. Informed consent and the surgeon. J Am Coll Surg. 2009;208(4):627–34. https://doi.org/10.1016/j.jamcollsurg.2008.12.012.
5. Ruske J, Sharma G, Makie K, et al. Patient comprehension necessary for informed consent for vascular procedures is poor and related to frailty [SAVS Abstract 15]. J Vasc Surg. 2020;71(1):23–4. https://doi.org/10.1016/j.jvs.2020.06.131.
6. Pecanac KE, Kehler JM, Brasel KJ, et al. It's big surgery: preoperative expressions of risk, responsibility, and commitment to treatment after high-risk operations. Ann Surg. 2014;259(3):458–63. https://doi.org/10.1097/sla.0000000000000314.
7. Lynn J, DeGrazia D. An outcomes model of medical decision making. Theor Med. 1991;12(4):325–43. https://doi.org/10.1007/bf00489892.

8. Kruser JM, Pecanac KE, Brasel KJ, et al. "And I think that we can fix it": mental models used in high-risk surgical decision making. Ann Surg. 2015;261(4):678–84. https://doi.org/10.1097/sla.0000000000000714.

9. Schwarze ML, Bradley CT, Brasel KJ. Surgical "buy-in": the contractual relationship between surgeons and patients that influences decisions regarding life-supporting therapy. Crit Care Med. 2010;38(3):843–8. https://doi.org/10.1097/ccm.0b013e3181cc466b.

10. Nabozny MJ, Kruser JM, Steffens NM, et al. Patient-reported limitations to surgical buy-in: a qualitative study of patients facing high-risk surgery. Ann Surg. 2017;265(1):97–102. https://doi.org/10.1097/sla.0000000000001645.

11. McNair AGK, MacKichan F, Donovan JL, et al. What surgeons tell patients and what patients want to know before major cancer surgery: a qualitative study. BMC Cancer. 2016;16:258. https://doi.org/10.1186/s12885=016-2292-3.

12. Siegler M. Pascal's wager and the hanging of the crepe. N Engl J Med. 1975;293(17):853–7. https://doi.org/10.1056/nejm197510232931705.

13. Kruser JM, Nabozny MJ, Steffens NM, et al. "Best Case/Worst Case": qualitative evaluation of a novel communication tool for difficult in-the-moment surgical decisions. J Am Geriatr Soc. 2015;63(9):1805–11. https://doi.org/10.1111/jgs.13615.

14. Fitz-Henry J. The ASA classification and peri-operative risk. Ann R Coll Surg Engl. 2011;93(3):185–7. https://doi.org/10.1308/rcsann.2011.93.3.185a.

15. Eamer G, Al-Amoodi MJH, Holroyd-Leduc J, Rolfson DB, Warkentin LM, Khadaroo RG. Review of risk assessment tools to predict morbidity and mortality in elderly surgical patients. Am J Surg. 2018;216(3):585–94. https://doi.org/10.1016/j.amjsurg.2018.04.006.

16. Perneger TV, Agoritsas T. Doctors and patients' susceptibility to framing bias: a randomized trial. J Gen Intern Med. 2011;26(12):1411–7. https://doi.org/10.1007/s11606-011-1810-x.

17. Elkin EB, Kim SHM, Casper ES, Kissane DW, Schrag D. Desire for information and involvement in treatment decisions: elderly cancer patients' preferences and their physicians' perceptions. J Clin Oncol. 2007;25(33):275–5280. https://doi.org/10.1200/jco.2007.11.1922.

18. Emanuel EJ, Emanuel LL. Four models of the physician-patient relationship. JAMA. 1992;267(16):2221–6. https://doi.org/10.1001/jama.1992.03480160079038.

19. Levine MN, Gafni A, Markham B, MacFarlane D. A bedside decision instrument to elicit a patient's preference concerning adjuvant chemotherapy for breast cancer. Ann Intern Med. 1992;117(1):53–8. https://doi.org/10.7326/0003-4819-117-1-53.

20. Charles C, Gafni A, Whelan T. Shared decision-making in the medical encounter: what does it mean? (or it takes at least two to tango). Soc Sci Med. 1997;44(5):681–92. https://doi.org/10.1016/s0277-9536(96)00221-3.

21. Schwarze ML, Buffington A, Tucholka JL, et al. Effectiveness of a question prompt list intervention for older patients considering major surgery: a multisite randomized clinical trial. JAMA Surg. 2019;155(1):6–13. https://doi.org/10.1001/jamasurg.2019.3778.

22. Moulton CA, Regehr G, Lingard L, Merritt C, Macrae H. 'Slowing down when you should': initiators and influences of the transition from the routine to the effortful. J Gastrointest Surg. 2010;14(6):1019–26. https://doi.org/10.1007/s11605-010-1178-y.

23. Mamidanna R, Ni Z, Anderson O, et al. Surgeon volume and cancer esophagectomy, gastrectomy, and pancreatectomy: a population-based study in England. Ann Surg. 2016;263(4):727–32. https://doi.org/10.1097/sla.0000000000001490.

24. Leung A, Luu S, Regehr G, Murnaghan L, Gallinger S, Moulton CA. "First, do no harm": balancing competing priorities in surgical practice. Acad Med. 2012;87(10):1368–74. https://doi.org/10.1097/acm.0b013e3182677587.

25. Orri M, Revah-Lévy A, Farges O. Surgeons' emotional experience of their everyday practice – a qualitative study. PLoS One. 2015;10(11):e0143763. https://doi.org/10.1371/journal.pone.0143763.

26. Yefimova M, Aslakson RA, Yang L, et al. Palliative care and end-of-life outcomes following high-risk surgery. JAMA Surg. 2020;155(2):138–46. https://doi.org/10.1001/jamasurg.2019.5083.

27. Raoof M, O'Neill L, Neumayer L, Fain M, Krouse R. Prospective evaluation of surgical palliative care immersion training for general surgery residents. Am J Surg. 2017;214(2):378–83. https://doi.org/10.1016/j.amjsurg.2016.11.032.
28. Wancata LM, Hinshaw DB, Suwanabol PA. Palliative care and surgical training: are we being trained to be unprepared? Ann Surg. 2017;265(1):32–3. https://doi.org/10.1097/sla.0000000000001779.

Chapter 8
The Ethics of Telehealth in Surgery

Karishma B. Mistry, Karen Devon ⓘD, **and Sabha Ganai** ⓘD

Abstract The global pandemic of COVID-19 has brought telehealth services into rapid full implementation after decades of incremental advances. In this chapter we explore ethical principles of justice, autonomy, and nonmaleficence, duties towards professionalism and continuing education, and how the practice of surgery is impacted by virtual care.

Keywords Telehealth · Telemedicine · Virtual care · Ethics · Surgery

Case

Our patient is a 67-year-old male farmer who presents with a dark, irregular, ulcerated mole on his back. His wife had initially noticed it because of staining on the bedsheets and requested further evaluation. Their local primary care provider performed a punch biopsy which confirmed a 1.8-mm Breslow thickness, ulcerated melanoma. They are referred to a surgical oncologist at a facility with capacity to perform lymphoscintigraphy, wide excision, and sentinel node biopsy, but it is 4 hours away by car. The surgeon arranges a

K. B. Mistry
Sanford Clinic, Fargo, ND, USA
e-mail: kmistry@sgu.edu

K. Devon
Women's College Hospital, University Health Network, Toronto, ON, Canada

Department of Surgery, University of Toronto, Toronto, ON, Canada
e-mail: karen.devon@wchospital.ca

S. Ganai (✉)
Sanford Clinic, Fargo, ND, USA

University of North Dakota School of Medicine and Health Sciences, Grand Forks, ND, USA
e-mail: sabha.ganai@und.edu

© The Author(s), under exclusive license to Springer Nature
Switzerland AG 2022
V. A. Lonchyna et al. (eds.), *Difficult Decisions in Surgical Ethics*, Difficult
Decisions in Surgery: An Evidence-Based Approach,
https://doi.org/10.1007/978-3-030-84625-1_8

telehealth consultation and performs a limited physical examination, visualizing the lesion as his wife holds the smart-phone camera towards the patient's back. The surgeon is required to take their word on not being able to self-palpate any "lumps or bumps" in various nodal stations described around the neck, collar bone, armpits, and groins. Their surgeon is still able to establish trust and rapport with the couple and discuss risks, benefits, and alternatives as part of informed consent.

A few weeks later, the couple travel to have ambulatory surgery. Their primary care physician asynchronously has provided documentation of a complete physical examination, which is transmitted securely into the electronic medical record. A few hours after arrival, their surgeon performs a focused physical exam in the preoperative holding area after the lymphoscintigraphy is completed by nuclear medicine in order to confirm the absence of clinically palpable lymph nodes. Due to nodal drainage patterns present on lymphoscintigraphy to both axillae, a bilateral sentinel lymph node biopsy is recommended and performed, along with the wide margin excision of the melanoma.

Questions that arise prior to the telehealth visit:

- What if the couple are not digitally literate?
- What if they live in a rural area without access to high-speed internet connection leading to a grainy distortion of the video image, or no image at all?

Questions that arise during the process of the telehealth visit:

- What if there were discussion points not understood about material risks during the process of informed consent due to technical issues or asynchronous conversation?
- What if the patient would like to record the visit to share with other family members?

Questions that arise during the process of management:

- What if there was a clinically palpable axillary lymph node present discovered when the surgeon saw the patient in the preoperative holding area?
- Should the surgeon postpone the procedure, to order a PET/CT, possibly a week later, to complete staging and potentially change the timing and plan for the procedure to accommodate neoadjuvant therapy? Should the surgeon modify consent and proceed with definitive surgery at the originally scheduled time, sparing the patient an additional 8-hour round trip?

Questions that arise during the plan for future surveillance:

- In order to plan recommended survivorship care, do we require the patient to travel for care to have a physical exam by the original surgeon, rely on the patient's local primary care provider for surveillance, or perform synchronous telehealth visits paired with asynchronous local axillary ultrasound reports?

8.1 Introduction

The World Health Organization (WHO) defines telehealth as "the delivery of health care services, where patients and providers are separated by distance." [1] Circumstances amid a global pandemic have brought the world of telehealth from an emerging practice to a rapid standard of care given the need for such distancing. In addition, in the context of the United States, guidelines for telehealth reimbursement were previously limited to patients physically present at specific telehealth capable facilities in rural locales, whereas now, reimbursement has become available for most patients who have access to a smartphone or the internet [2]. In this chapter we explore the ethics of telehealth in surgical practice with an understanding that technology and capacity to advance has been in a state of incremental change but variable implementation.

Technology advancements have made the benefits of health care widely accessible from a distance for years, and nearly two decades ago, telesurgery was conducted using robot assistance, allowing for a cholecystectomy to be performed in New York City, USA with instrument manipulation directed synchronously by a surgeon located in Strasbourg, France [3]. The electronic ICU, also called tele-ICU, has been a successful advancement in the field of critical care for the past 20 years. It was put in place to support high volume areas and high acuity patients; it has allowed 24-hour care, care in times of staff shortages, and better monitoring of ill patients [4]. Advancements in the field of artificial intelligence (AI) have also allowed for improved performance of medicine. With greater accuracy of diagnosis in a variety of fields such as identifying images of cancer in dermatology, x-rays in radiology, and digitized pathology slides AI has proven its potential in the future of technology in medicine [5]. In the context of the COVID-19 pandemic, AI technology can be used to minimize the human interaction while continuing to diagnose and treat patients efficiently.

While many of these advancements have now rapidly become implemented, telehealth has created ethical concerns for both the patient and physician in the conduct of care from a distance. Due to rapid uptake of synchronous clinic visits during the COVID-19 pandemic, this novel way of providing healthcare has revealed some uncertainty and ethical challenges that may not have been considered or addressed (see Table 8.1). These include whether telehealth is as effective for quality patient diagnosis, treatment, and care, and whether there are significant harms, direct or indirect, to patient care or the patient-physician relationship.

Table 8.1 Ethical concerns that can arise during a telehealth visit

• Justice: access to digital technology and ensuring digital literacy for the population
• Autonomy: obtaining consent from the patient and upholding patient privacy
• Nonmaleficence: ensuring there is either no change in standard care or reconciling the shortcomings of telehealth and providing ways to mitigate risk
• Professionalism: ensuring the doctor-patient relationship is valued and fiduciary duties toward the patient are respected
• Continuous Education: ensuring the health system learns and improves to provide better care for future generations

8.2   Search Strategy

A literature review was conducted through February 2021 utilizing PubMed. MESH Search terms included: Telemedicine, Physician Patient relations, social justice, Digital technology, Privacy, Informed Consent, Social Responsibility, Beneficence, Patient Care, Health Services Accessibility, Medically Underserved Area, Reference Standards, Risk Assessment, Standard of Care, Medical Education, COVID-19, Rural Population, Literacy, Curriculum, Clinical Medicine, Policy. Keywords used included ethics in telemedicine, telemedicine, standard of care in telemedicine, and telemedicine education. From available literature, 16 articles were selected for their contribution to the topic of ethics and telemedicine in the context of delivery of surgical care. Additional references were added during the editorial peer review process.

8.3   Justice

While telemedicine has been recently recognized as an advantageous new way of healthcare delivery that comes with benefits, it also has risks (see Table 8.2). Some issues that providers may have with telemedicine are user-based, such as interacting with patients who are hard-of-hearing or who do not own a computer, smartphone, or tablet. Even if they do have access to technology, questions arise such as: is the

Table 8.2 Analysis of risks and benefits in delivering care via telehealth modalities

Risks	Benefits
Digital literacy of patients (justice)	Reduced transmission and exposure for patient/provider in time of pandemic (nonmaleficience)
Loss of traditional doctor-patient relationship (professionalism)	Reduced travel burdens (justice)
Limited physical exam capability (nonmaleficence)	Improved compliance by optimizing the ease, frequency, and consistency of care (autonomy, beneficence)
Overuse of Telehealth due to ease and convenience (nonmaleficence)	Broadened access to care for rural communities (justice)
Reduced physician accountability (professionalism)	Improving patient's sense of autonomy over their care (autonomy)
Uncertain reliability of virtual diagnosis (nonmaleficence)	Decreased missed appointments (autonomy)

Source: Authors own work

connection stable, is the video clear enough to properly assess the melanoma, and also, was it critically important to see the lesion at all given that it was already biopsied? In addition, what if his wife was not available to hold the camera to allow the surgeon to visualize the patient's back? Would patients with family support be at an advantage compared to those who live alone?

Older generations may not be as familiar with technology and use of applications, and those in rural locales may not have a stable internet connection to do so even if they have a device with video capabilities [6]. How do we as surgeons, or the health system overall, adjust for technological capacity and not further disadvantage those with socioeconomic disparities? Furthermore, by conducting virtual visits, we may lose aspects of the overall visit such as the opportunity to take vital signs and conduct auscultation of the thorax. While it can be debated if these are essential pieces of a focused physical examination, it forces several questions: are patients getting equal care by opting-in for the virtual visit? Are vital signs and other clinical findings something patients can provide if they have access to technology at home, or access to a primary care provider, and if so, can the clinician trust that information?

The advancement of technology is expanding in the healthcare field, including integrated applications with various personal devices that can track your heart rate, temperature, blood pressure, blood glucose, menstrual cycle, and physical activity at home. Teledermatology using mobile phones has been shown to be a cost-effective way of improving access to care and facilitating specialist consultations [7]. In addition, we have witnessed the performance of telehealth in surgical practice, including a successful transatlantic robotic surgery, video-based instruction of techniques using remotely performed live surgery, as well as increasing capacity to hold large-scale international medical conferences through virtual means, all with minimal need to travel. Small incremental advances will also provide valuable gains in efficiency, ease of care, and satisfaction through the use of these technologies.

Justice concerns remain present and disparities in care may be accentuated by cost, reimbursement, and access to these technologies. In fact, with the advantages of obtaining surgical consultation via telehealth means, one can envision that a patient with wealth or the right kind of insurance can obtain a virtual visit with an expert surgeon located in a different state, as long as the surgeon has appropriate licensure in the state where the patient is located at the visit. What is still uncertain is whether this improved access to care can equitably be promoted to individuals without means.

8.4   Autonomy

During the COVID-19 pandemic, telehealth became an industry necessity, aiming to minimize disease transmission, but this implementation has also provided opportunities to address challenges faced in clinical practice on a regular basis [8]. Patient preference and need are important reasons telehealth has been implemented, but we must remember this was also tied to improved reimbursement after March 2020, with reimbursement previously focused on patients in isolated rural areas with poor access to medical care [2]. In this context, reimbursement potential has introduced telehealth in the clinical encounter as a reasonable option that still favors patient autonomy. Telehealth has allowed the travel and time burden for patients to be diminished with the potential for more frequent management via virtual checkups, including postoperative wound checks [8]. Frequent and consistent follow-up by physicians may be beneficial in ensuring compliance with a treatment plan [8]. Through the asynchronous use of external technologies such as "wrist-watch" heart rate monitors and smartphone tracking systems, patients are able to provide updated information more frequently per visit [9, 10]. Telehealth services of the future may also enhance the care of non-English speaking patients or those that converse with American Sign Language through the ability to obtain a virtual interpreter in a matter of seconds.

The inner workings of telemedicine go beyond the role of the physician-patient relationship and relies on factors such as obtaining proper informed consent and upholding patient privacy. At the annual American Medical Association (AMA) meeting in 2016, the downside of using technology discussed security breaches and unauthorized access as a concern in maintaining patient confidentiality [6]. In regard to these obligations of privacy and confidentiality, there is a difference between legal and ethical implications. For example, if you are initiating a conversation with a patient who is physically located in an unknown location and you have private information to share with them, doubts may be raised if you should disclose information to them using telehealth capacities. From a legal context, it may be considered safe if a patient is the one putting themselves at risk of potential disclosure to family or public during a conversation.

Uncertainty remains whether it is ethically appropriate for the physician to disclose private information knowing that it may not be via a secure method. Even if the patient is located alone behind a closed door, cybersecurity and protection of shared information may not be perfect using standard platforms. While hospital and clinic-based medical informatics teams exist to protect and maintain the security of asynchronously transmitted medical information in accordance with the Security Rule of the Health Insurance Portability and Accountability Act of 1996 (HIPAA; 45 CFR Part 160 and Part 164, Subparts A and C) [11], there is currently no optimal method of synchronous telehealth communication between providers and patients. Communication via telehealth has been flexible between using a combination of secure patient portals, proprietary HIPAA-compliant telehealth applications, and telephone as a flexible back-up, as system failures are not uncommon in clinical practice, particularly when access disparities exist. In the context of the COVID pandemic, the Department of Health and Human Services recognized a need for greater HIPAA security flexibilities and allow video chat applications and various text-based applications in clinical practice, with preference for HIPAA-compliant technologies [12]. In addition, while telephone calls can be performed via a hospital or clinic office landline, they can also be performed using dialer applications on smart phones that can mimic a clinic telephone number, maintaining the privacy of the physician's mobile phone number.

This leads to the question if there is a responsibility to obtain consent from the patient prior to a conversation as a risk of loss of privacy may be present before sharing of information. However, this also creates uncertainty whether conduct needs to be different via video versus phone, and if so, why? To provide clarity, the Agency for Healthcare Research and Quality (AHRQ) has created a three-step outline to follow when obtaining informed consent from a patient specific to the use of telehealth [13]. It starts prior to the discussion where the provider gives the patient the opportunity to ask questions in order to provide them with relevant information necessary to make an informed decision about using telehealth. Next, during the discussion about telehealth, the teach-back method is recommended in order to appreciate comprehension by the patient about relevant risks and benefits. Finally, after the discussion, documentation of the encounter is recommended to ensure the information is clearly communicated [13].

Furthermore, in regard to conducting an exam virtually, there are sensitive areas of examination, including genitalia, the perineum, and female breasts, that should raise caution on video transmission out of respect for patient privacy and dignity, but may be important to examine in a non-virtual setting. If elements of a visit are recorded, even momentarily for image capture, should examinations or discussions of sensitive issues be entirely avoided, or should consent for recording be obtained? This has professional liability implications for medical professionalism, where in-person standards may need to be re-evaluated to accommodate telehealth visits. Addressing these questions will be important moving forward in order to define the privacy and confidentiality concerns of both patient and provider. From an autonomy standpoint, there are competing risks to virtual care which may supersede the choice to have a virtual visit as opposed to an in-person visit.

8.5   Non-maleficence

In telehealth, there are tradeoffs where access to care may be perceived as more important than perfect care. In weighing risks and benefits of what some may consider "gold-standard" guideline-concordant care compared to performing "silver- or bronze-level" care, we have to reconcile that no physician is perfect, and even an expert can miss a subtle clinical finding. The physical encounter with a patient is a key element of the role of a physician in establishing a diagnosis and capitalizes on sensory input including vision, touch, temperature, kinesthesia, sound, and even smell. While symptoms can be discussed on a telephone or virtual visit, signs that are derived from a constellation of physical exam findings may be necessary to efficiently and cost-effectively focus an otherwise broad differential diagnosis [14]. Virtual care does not and cannot replace this physical and human element of medicine and could in fact negatively impact the relationship between the physician and patient. Conversation, emotion, body language, and overall comfort can potentially get lost through the barrier of a screen.

However, as the physical exam is an art, there are certainly trained subspecialists and experts who have better acumen at clinical detection than others. With our case, conducting the initial physical exam and even surveillance follow-up appointments virtually may have posed challenges to delivering a reasonable standard of care. While our patient had an obvious melanoma primary, what if the patient also had in-transit metastases, clinically palpable nodes, or a disease process that was more subtle or nuanced requiring physical exam skills or techniques not available locally? Do we require the patient to travel for care to have their physical exam by the original surgeon prior to decision making, or do we accommodate the possibility that surgical decision making may occur on the day of surgery? In regard to follow-up, do we rely on the patient's local primary care provider for surveillance, or do we learn to perform telehealth visits paired with local axillary ultrasound reports? The options to mitigate the shortcomings that can arise with a telehealth consultation are many and ought to be considered in maintaining a standard level of care for all patients. There is great potential that the use of additional (albeit initially costly) technology to supplement or replace clinical exams may ultimately improve and add value to clinical care for all patients [5].

While we have suggested a minimal distinction between "gold"-standard care and second-best, "silver- or bronze- level" care, it is uncertain whether substandard delivery of services should be accepted, as this can decrease trust and cause harm, indirectly to the doctor-patient relationship, and possibly directly to patients themselves if problems are missed. Physicians must provide the same standard of care for all patients in order to uphold equity, therefore, some patients may require in-person visits and some patients may receive telehealth visits to achieve favorable outcomes. It is unclear that a breast exam can be appropriately performed using telemedicine, but it is possible that patients with a new breast lesion or cancer could be scheduled for an initial consultation to discuss surgical options and timing of therapies with plans to have an in-person exam performed at a later time, including the day of surgery. This may not be perceived as time efficient, but the approach may ultimately respect a patient's autonomy by providing more time and discussion for the process of informed consent, as well as satisfying their secondary need for convenience. Thus far, all information on the benefits of telehealth have solely been focused on psychosocial factors and have not been able to directly quantify if telehealth is providing better health outcomes, a more accurate diagnosis, or increased survival rates [15]. Such issues should be further investigated as the advancement of telehealth proves to be transformative in the time of the COVID-19 pandemic with its expansions helping physicians in maintaining care and decreasing exposure for both sides.

8.6   Professionalism

The "Ethics of Telemedicine" were discussed at the AMA annual meeting in 2016 [6], and also codified in the 2017 AMA Code of Medical Ethics [16], bringing up valid ethical concerns for implementation of telemedicine, including physician accountability to uphold their duty to provide adequate care from the comfort of a screen. There may be additional barriers to development of the doctor-patient relationship in regard to establishing a connection that leads to trust and being able to deliver on that trust by providing a similar level of care as would be received in-person. These barriers can be divided into two categories: verbal and non-verbal. Verbal issues can be reduced by engaging in "small talk" at the beginning of each appointment and educating the physician on important factors like tone of voice and style of questions asked. Nonverbal cues such as body language that are lost via telehealth can be made up for by camera placement and paying attention to facial expressions and body posture [17]. Empathy and respect may be facilitated by appropriate use of facial expressions, nodding, gestures, and providing space to pause, actively listen, and answer questions [18]. Pellegrini described trust as the keystone of the patient-physician relationship, providing integrity and stability to the relationship, and defined good communication as "not necessarily about what we say, but it is more about how we say what we say, and how another mind interprets what we say" [19]. The process of creating trust must be fostered through development of an unforced relationship between the physician and the patient.

A conflict of commitment to note is the possibility that physicians may lose sight of their duty to each individual patient and focus more on productivity and the convenience of the extrinsic rewards of medical practice, as more tele-visits now equate to more billable hours at the touch of a button. This could inevitably change the future of healthcare as physicians become more reliant on technology for diagnosis and lose their own expertise and clinical acumen. The expectations of physicians for how to achieve their productivity goals may differ in telemedicine, but they must still be equipped to effectively interact and communicate with the individual patient, including confirmation of patient comprehension and adequately answering their questions.

Telemedicine visits for patients prior to March 2020, before being spurred by the COVID-19 pandemic, were determined by state-specific coverage rules [2, 20]. Prior to COVID-19 coverage expansions, all states could provide some reimbursement for qualified live video appointments via Medicaid, but as of November 2019, only 8 states fully covered their Medicaid patients for all telehealth services. The Centers for Medicare and Medicaid Services (CMS) could only reimburse payment for telehealth if certain criteria were met, including patient location at Federally Qualified Health Centers (FQHCs) and/or Rural Health Clinics (RHCs). This favored use by patients with diminished access to healthcare, but facility requirements did not allow a patient to have a telehealth visit from home, and likely limited implementation by limiting to access to providers with established relationships with these facilities.

When non-essential in-person activity was abruptly halted in the United States due to the COVID-19 pandemic, the CMS issued a press release on March 6, 2020, as President Trump signed a section 1135 waiver of the Social Security Act, extending CMS capacity to temporarily allow clinicians to provide telehealth services [20]. Subsequently, the Coronavirus Aid, Relief, and Economic Security Act of 2020 (CARES Act) broadened the waiver authority under section 1135 of the Social Security Act [21]. This provided CMS additional authority to waive requirements which specified the types of practitioners that could bill for professional services using telehealth, and also allowed for audio-only telehealth reimbursement. In order to allow for flexibility, CMS has permitted these emergency declaration blanket waivers to allow for greater flexibility in scope of practice and in reimbursement for telehealth services retroactive from March 1, 2020, until the end of the emergency declaration [22]. As a consequence of these waivers, patients could be located at home during a telehealth encounter, and providers could also provide services when at home, paid with a fee-for-service rate rather than a separate telehealth rate. Since coverage had thus increased and expanded for all patients in all states, uncertainty remains whether telehealth visits will continue to be fully covered once the pandemic is over, and whether access to telehealth services will be equitable depending on the terms of eligibility for these services.

There are limitations to implementation of telemedicine based on licensing regulations for physicians, which are generally determined by each state's medical practice act, requiring a physician to hold a medical license in the specific state where the patient is physically present during virtual visits [23]. There are a few areas where federal law overrides state laws. The National Defense Authorization Act (2012) allows physicians to only require a license in the state they are physically located in when providing care under Tri-Care, a military health plan, "regardless of where such health-care professional or the patient are located so long as the practice is within the scope of the authorized Federal duties" [24]. In addition, within the Veterans Affairs (VA) system, the VA MISSION Act of 2018 allows out-of-state clinicians to provide care for veterans as long as they have an active, unrestricted medical license [25]. States have different requirements for physicians to be licensed to conduct virtual visits, including telehealth-limited licenses, and many of these processes were relaxed during the coronavirus pandemic, as the need to be able to provide virtual care exploded. Further exploration of expansion of licensure, either creation of a national licensing system, or by broader implementation of the 2017 Interstate Medical Licensure Compact, a voluntary expedited pathway to obtain licensure between participating states [26], would be invaluable for permitting the practice of medicine across state lines [23]. Further research and adoption of changes in health care policy will be necessary to ensure that telehealth provides benefits for all parties, is being properly conducted, covered, and billed, and delivers care in a fair, efficient, and equitable fashion.

8.7   Continuous Education

Clinical medicine is an art that medical students strive to achieve and master from the moment they obtain their white coat. Throughout the four years of medical education, students are required to complete certain clinical hours per semester to ensure a proper foundation and acquired skills for effective in-person education. Students are graded on all aspects of human interaction from greetings and small talk to verbal cues, body language, and facial expressions, all with an aim to build a successful patient relationship. By the end of the formal medical education, clinical service and physical examination instruction constitutes more than half of the student's time. With the current advancement of telehealth and online medical education, this brings up the following questions: Should medical schools integrate telehealth courses to ensure competency in this new form of communication? As telehealth is prioritized, will the art of medicine get lost behind a screen? School curriculums and further training of physicians who use telehealth services are a work in progress as the ethical considerations are being uncovered with time.

For those in practice, we foresee that distance learning will become more important for continuing medical education and the process of certification. While a relative isolation of non-academic physicians during clinical practice has been described for over a century [27], one can envision improved access to education through the ability to not only maintain education as medicine evolves, but also socialize with other practitioners in a professional context without needing to travel. The scope of telehealth overlaps with distance learning, as while patients can seek access to consultation at a distance, so can physicians. The opportunities for a primary surgeon to seek consultation with an expert at a tertiary center during an operation have already been in progress, and technology may allow further expansion of the capacity of consultants to provide assistance. Such efforts may pose conflicts with current state licensure requirements but may be ethically valid as potentially improving delivery of safe and effective patient care.

8.8   Case Conclusion

In our case, the patient's oncologic and surgical care was facilitated by the use of a telehealth appointment via expediting access to an initial clinic visit, establishing the patient-surgeon relationship, and improving the efficiency of being able to schedule their procedure. The patient was able to successfully conduct the appointment via video, and while some ethics concerns and areas of uncertainty exist, these could potentially be mitigated by strategic use of telehealth. For example, a telehealth conversation with a patient who is not fluent in English could be addressed by preparation prior to the visit and using technology that allows for having a translator added to the video call in real time. In the event that there are concerns about technical issues that could impair conversation, the AHRQ three-step process to obtaining informed consent for telehealth use would be beneficial prior to the clinician visit and could be done with a medical assistant as an initial screen prior to "rooming the patient". This would help ensure the patient is able to comprehend the information being communicated both prior to the encounter, during the encounter, and post encounter with the teach back method to clear up any missed information. Patients who are homeless or resource constrained may still benefit from using FQHCs and RHCs as an access point for the telehealth encounter, especially if there is an intersection of constraints due to travel distance, internet access, and technology.

In terms of starting the conversation, the limitations of telehealth as previously outlined can be mitigated by good communication strategies summarizing areas of uncertainty using the telehealth platform and by letting the patient know that all preliminary diagnosis or suspicions will be confirmed with an in-person visit in case of further action. Finally, with the plan of continuing care and oncologic survivorship care, follow up via telehealth services can provide more up to date and frequent check-ins as it may facilitate patients to make their appointments. In particular, patients located in rural areas may be better able to achieve postoperative follow up visits via a combination of telehealth and seeing their local primary care provider, mitigating the factors that come with travel distance, low energy from recovery, and the time inconvenience of travel.

Finally, through development of collaborative relationships with rural surgeons, surgical oncologic sub-specialists can use telehealth strategically to optimize care for their rural patients. With esophageal cancer patients, for example, telehealth can be used for the initial encounter at diagnosis, and the care of the patient can be co-managed with the local rural surgeon who performed initial endoscopic diagnosis and biopsy. The patient can travel for their PET/CT and endoscopic ultrasound and have an in-person or telehealth visit with the oncologic surgeon at the high-volume center. If the patient requires pre-therapy nutritional support, for example, the local rural surgeon can place a jejunostomy tube laparoscopically if that is within their skill set. The patient can then receive neoadjuvant therapy by medical and radiation oncologists closer to home, and then after an additional telehealth visit to complete the process of informed consent, the patient can travel for their esophagectomy at the high-volume center. If the patient has a wound infection or requires a postoperative dilation, the patient can elect to travel, or stay within their locale for care according to patient preferences, surgeon preferences, and the quality of the collaborative relationship between the surgeons.

8.9 Conclusion

The breadth of use of telehealth services has expanded in a short amount of a time, and with this forward momentum comes areas of uncertainty and considerations on both the surgeon and patient side that need to be addressed. Health care providers must ensure they are delivering a standard of care and upholding the ethical principles of justice, autonomy, beneficence, and nonmaleficence as part of fiduciary duties to the patient. Modality of delivery is not always equal for all, especially in terms of digital literacy of the populations. Obtaining informed consent over a screen or telephone potentially involves a different protocol of communication and engagement than an in-person visit. While telehealth may provide ease for some people and has advantages in times of a pandemic, it is important to note potential vulnerabilities towards maintaining a standard of care and losing the art of the physical exam. Finally, there are issues including licensing pathways, reimbursement methods, and professional standards that are changing with time and will need to be further discussed to ensure that both equity in service and respect to patients is delivered by surgeons who provide telehealth towards those patients who are eligible to receive this service. Telehealth is an extremely useful tool that has been shown to have benefits for both physician and patient, however with those benefits comes risks and areas of vulnerability that should be mitigated in order to add value to and improve delivery of healthcare in an ethical fashion.

8.10 Selected References

- American Medical Association. AMA telehealth implementation playbook. American Medical Association; 2020.

  - Created as a response to the COVID-19 pandemic, this is a guide for physicians how to set up and use telemedicine in their practice. It defines telemedicine, its components, how to set up your team and how to implement it. There is also information about vendors, cybersecurity and coding.

- Chaet D, Clearfield R, Sabin JE, Skimming K; for the Council on Ethical and Judicial Affairs, American Medical Association. Ethical practice in telehealth and telemedicine. J Gen Intern Med. 2017;32(10);1136–1140. https://doi.org/10.1007/s11606-017-4082-2.

  - A pre-pandemic report of the AMA Council on Ethics about this new field of telemedicine. In utilizing this new technology, among a myriad of known and unknown problems, privacy, confidentiality, transparency and informed consent need to be maintained.

- Dixon RF, Rao L. Asynchronous virtual visits for the follow-up of chronic conditions. Telemed e-Health. 2014;20(7):669–672. https://doi.org/10.1089/tmj.2013.0211.

  - An early study of how telemedicine can help in the management of chronic diseases.

- Kruse CS, Krowski N, Rodriguez B, Tran L, Vela J, Brooks M. Telehealth and patient satisfaction: A systematic review and narrative analysis. BMJ Open. 2017;7(8):e016242. https://doi.org/10.1136/bmjopen-2017-016242.

  - A systematic review of the effects of telemedicine from the viewpoint of the patient.

Such positive factors as improved outcomes, ease of use, improved communication and decreased travel time warrants the continued incorporation of telemedicine in daily medical practice.

References

1. World Health Organization. Global diffusion of eHealth: making universal health coverage achievable. Report of the third global survey on eHealth. World Health Organization; 2016.
2. Centers for Medicare and Medicaid Services. List of Telehealth Services for Calender Year 2021. Updated on April 7, 2021. https://cms.gov/Medicare/Medicare-General-Information/Telehealth/Telehealth-Codes. Accessed 9 May 2021.
3. Marescaux J, Leroy J, Rubino F, et al. Transcontinental robot-assisted remote telesurgery: feasibility and potential applications. Ann Surg. 2002;235(4):487–92. https://doi.org/10.1097/00000658-200204000-00005.
4. Essay P, Shahin TB, Balkan B, Mosier J, Subbian V. The connected intensive care unit patient: exploratory analyses and cohort discovery from a critical care telemedicine database. JMIR Med Inform. 2019;7(1):e13006. https://doi.org/10.2196/13006.
5. Topol EJ. High-performance medicine: the convergence of human and artificial intelligence. Nat Med. 2019;25:44–56. https://doi.org/10.1038/s41591-018-0300-7.
6. Chaet D, Clearfield R, Sabin JE, Skimming K, the Council on Ethical and Judicial Affairs, American Medical Association. Ethical practice in telehealth and telemedicine. J Gen Intern Med. 2017;32(10):1136–40. https://doi.org/10.1007/s11606-017-4082-2.
7. Zuo KJ, Guo D, Rao J. Mobile teledermatology: a promising future in clinical practice. J Cutan Med Surg. 2013;17(6):387–91. https://doi.org/10.2310/7750.2013.13030.
8. American Medical Association. AMA telehealth implementation playbook. American Medical Association; 2020.
9. Dixon RF, Rao L. Asynchronous virtual visits for the follow-up of chronic conditions. Telemed e-Health. 2014;20(7):669–72. https://doi.org/10.1089/tmj.2013.0211.
10. Tuckson RV, Edmunds M, Hodgkins ML. Telehealth. N Engl J Med. 2017;377(16):1585–92. https://doi.org/10.1056/nejmsr1503323.
11. US Department of Health & Human Services. Summary of the HIPAA security rule. https://www.hhs.gov/hipaa/for-professionals/security/laws-regulations/index.html. Accessed 9 May 2021.
12. US Department of Health & Human Services. HIPAA flexibility for telehealth technology. https://telehealth.hhs.gov/providers/policy-changes-during-the-covid-19-public-health-emergency/hipaa-flexibility-for-telehealth-technology/. Accessed 5 May 2021.
13. Agency for Healthcare Research and Quality. How to obtain consent for telehealth. Content last reviewed September 2020. https://www.ahrq.gov/health-literacy/obtain-consent-telehealth.html. Accessed 2 Dec 2020.
14. Kruse CS, Krowski N, Rodriguez B, Tran L, Vela J, Brooks M. Telehealth and patient satisfaction: a systematic review and narrative analysis. BMJ Open. 2017;7(8):e016242. https://doi.org/10.1136/bmjopen-2017-016242.
15. Rising KL, Ward MM, Goldwater JC, Bhagianadh D, Hollander JE. Framework to advance oncology-related telehealth. JCO Clin Cancer Inform. 2018;2:1–11. https://doi.org/10.1200/cci.17.00156.
16. American Medical Association. Code of medical ethics. American Medical Association; 2017.
17. Bulik R. Human factors in primary care telemedicine encounters. J Telemed Telecare. 2008;14:169–72. https://doi.org/10.1258/jtt.2007.007041.
18. Nemetz ET, Urbach DR, Devon KM. The art of surgery: balancing compassionate with virtual care. J Med Internet Res. 2020;22(8):e22417. https://doi.org/10.2196/22417.

19. Pellegrini CA. Trust: the keystone of the patient-physician relationship. J Am Coll Surg. 2017;224(2):95–102. https://doi.org/10.1016/j.jamcollsurg.2016.10.032.
20. Centers for Medicare & Medicaid Services. Medicare telemedicine health care provider fact sheet. March 17, 2020. https://www.cms.gov/newsroom/fact-sheets/medicare-telemedicine-health-care-provider-fact-sheet. Accessed May 2021.
21. Coronavirus Aid, Relief, and Economic Security Act (CARES Act), Pub L No. 116-136, §§3701, 3703–3707, 134 Stat 285 (2020). https://www.congress.gov/116/plaws/publ136/PLAW-116publ136.pdf. Accessed 5 May 2021.
22. Centers for Medicare & Medicaid Services. COVID-19 emergency declaration blanket waivers for health care providers. April 8, 2021. https://www.cms.gov/files/document/summary-covid-19-emergency-declaration-waivers.pdf. Accessed 5 May 2021.
23. Mehrotra A, Nimgaonkar A, Richman B. Telemedicine and medical licensure – potential paths for reform. N Engl J Med. 2021;384(8):687–90. https://doi.org/10.1056/nejmp2031608.
24. National Defense Authorization Act for Fiscal Year 2012, Pub L No. 112-81, §713, 125 Stat 1298 (2011). https://www.congress.gov/112/plaws/publ81/PLAW-112publ81.pdf. Accessed 5 May 2021.
25. VA MISSION Act of 2018, S. 2372, Pub L No. 115-182, 132 Stat 1393 (2018). https://www.congress.gov/115/plaws/publ182/PLAW-115publ182.pdf. Accessed 5 May 2021.
26. Interstate Medical Licensure Compact. A faster pathway to physician licensure. https://www.imlcc.org/a-faster-pathway-to-physician-licensure/#WhoDevelopedTheCompact. Accessed 5 May 2021.
27. Starr P. The social transformation of American medicine: the rise of a sovereign profession & the making of a vast industry. 2nd ed. Basic Books; 2017.

Chapter 9
How to Deliver Bad News: A Family Postmortem

Jaishankar Raman (iD)

Abstract Conveying bad news after complications occur following surgical intervention is always emotionally fraught. We use a case study to highlight possible mechanisms of communicating with patient's families after they have suffered a major setback. The importance of prompt feedback is highlighted. The detrimental effects of bad outcomes on surgeons and medical practitioners are under-recognized and not handled well. In this chapter, recommendations are made about an ethical framework that could be adapted for use in dealing with critically ill patients. This could then be used as curriculum for teaching residents and medical students.

Keywords End-of-life care · Adverse outcomes · Communication · Conveying bad news · Feedback · Complications

Case
He looked vaguely familiar. A solitary figure in the waiting area of the consulting room, leafing through a magazine rather desultorily. My patient list just had him itemized by his name with no referring physician and no inkling of his clinical problem. I shall call him Mr. Twiddle, partly because it appeared that he just sat there twiddling his fingers and thumbs.

J. Raman (✉)
University of Melbourne, Fitzroy North, VIC, Australia

Deakin University, Melbourne, VIC, Australia

Deakin University, Geelong, VIC, Australia

University of Illinois at Urbana-Champaign, Champaign, IL, USA

Oregon Health & Science University, Portland, OR, USA

James Cook University, Townsville, Queensland, Australia

St Vincent's Hospital, Melbourne, VIC, Australia
e-mail: jraman@unimelb.edu.au

© The Author(s), under exclusive license to Springer Nature
Switzerland AG 2022
V. A. Lonchyna et al. (eds.), *Difficult Decisions in Surgical Ethics*, Difficult
Decisions in Surgery: An Evidence-Based Approach,
https://doi.org/10.1007/978-3-030-84625-1_9

When I finally got him into my consulting room and started enquiring about his health, something in his manner and demeanor alerted me to the reason behind his visit. He had an air of despondency and started mentioning his wife. Mrs. Twiddle had been a patient of mine who underwent emergency coronary artery bypass surgery along with reconstruction of a large scar that occupied the anterior aspect or front of the left ventricle. She had been very sick and unstable going into the procedure—she was supported with a balloon pump and inotropic drugs to keep her alive. The operation went well, and she made it off the operating table in a reasonable state, with a stable circulation and improved cardiac function. After a long day of surgery, I was happy to inform her husband that we had managed to salvage her from cardiogenic shock but emphasized to him that she was still critically ill. About 15 hours post-operatively, in the wee hours of the morning, an inappropriate adjustment of a crucial inotrope led to a rapid downward spiral, a lethal arrhythmia & cardiac arrest. I raced in with members of the surgical team and managed to resuscitate her. We placed her on a temporary cardiac assist device in the hope of resting her heart and allowing her organ systems to recover. Despite her cardiac stabilization, the combination of advanced age, pre-existing shock and the post-operative arrest conspired to cause a syndrome of severe liver injury or "shock liver". The liver is one of the few organs that we cannot support; in contrast to supporting the failing kidneys with dialysis, failing lungs with the ventilator, failing heart with an extra-corporeal pump, etc. Liver failure progresses quickly and even with treatment, is associated with a high mortality rate over 80%. Needless to say, she passed away a few hours later.

9.1   Introduction

How does one convey the devastating news about the death of a loved one, after a seemingly promising initial course after surgery? Indeed, how do we convey bad news? Is it enough just to call the relative over the phone and just allow the profound intake of breath, sobbing, or stunned silence, at the other end be ignored? Do we call them and ask them to come into the hospital right away? Or as I have seen some surgeons do, just let the fellow/trainee call the relatives, because they are usually very busy attending to the next lot of patients? This is a case-based exposition of how bad news can be communicated. We also try to make a strong argument for a delayed communication strategy well after the event, to provide closure and clear up misconceptions. The benefits are provided to patient's families as well as the healthcare workers involved.

9.2 Search Strategy

We used PubMed for articles with over 20 citations as a means of searching for relevant articles on important aspect of communication.

9.3 Discussion

This most important foundation in communication with patients' relatives is not dealt with consistently in medical schools [1]. This maybe a casualty of the teaching system and lack of emphasis on clinical medicine in the US and many western medical systems. Interestingly, an early "How to do it" article was published in the BMJ in 1990 by a senior registrar in the Emergency department, who had to deal with a lot of distressed relatives of trauma victims [2]. Despite a lot of descriptions, publications of experiences, meta-analyses of publications [3], there is no consistent teaching centered around Conveying Bad News.

There are reports in the medical literature of how these events can affect medical students and doctors [4]. The existing guidelines or published methods have been predominantly in the realm of cancer and deal with patients in outpatient settings. In high-risk specialties such as trauma surgery and high acuity settings such as critical care, the need is even more evident [5]. There are some interesting insights and publications that try to provide guidelines in these circumstances [6].

Regardless, I had no formal training in any of this as a medical student or as a surgical trainee. I tried to develop a protocol or technique, that incorporated the practices of my surgical mentors and some of the needs of the relatives that I perceived were important. I must say I am old-fashioned and maybe a trite masochistic—in insisting on conveying the bad news in person. As I found out later, this follows the SPIKES principles which seemed to have been developed for cancer patients [7] and are grounded in common sensical approaches to communication. SPIKES represents a stepwise approach incorporating the pillars outlined in Table 9.1. The conversation is tailored to the particular family dynamics and the clinical situation.

My version of the SPIKES principles are as follows and it sort of evolved over time and happened almost by accident:

> If a complication or an untoward bad outcome occurs, I ask the bedside nurse or resident to invite the family to come in. I then go in to meet them in a quiet room with my resident and a nurse to convey the bad news. I spend as much time as possible with them. There are many variations on the theme and there is no specific method that is taught us as trainees. This is despite the fact that most clinicians are confronted with this situation of conveying bad news many times during their careers [8].

Table 9.1 SPIKES system of communication with patients

S—Setting up the interview or encounter. Preferably done in a quiet area, with others in attendance, with no major time constraints and preferably with everyone sitting down.
P—Perception of the patient and the family of the situation. Of course, if the patient is critically ill and unable to participate, all of this perspective falls on the family members and/or next of kin.
I—Invitation of the patient or the family in this instance to ask for information. Essentially this is a request for information.
K—Knowledge being provided to the patient and the family. This provides an opportunity to fill them in on the clinical situation and the details of sequence of events.
E—Emotions with empathetic response. The communication is based on empathy and works with establishment of an emotional connection.
S—Strategy of the intervention and summary of the situation. This provides an overview or summary of the patient's condition, complications and clinical course.

Adapted from Baile [7]

In this instance, I went into the ICU waiting room, met with Mr Twiddle and ushered him into an adjoining room. I sat down with him and explained the unfortunate course of events. There was a surgical resident and an ICU nurse with me. He looked shell shocked and could barely say anything. After he had been counseled in this manner, I offered him the opportunity of a debriefing session in my consulting offices a few weeks later. For want of a better term, I shall call this the Family Postmortem. We then embarked on this technique that I have termed the "Family Post-mortem". It harks back to the days when all deaths in a hospital underwent a post-mortem examination to identify causes of death. We adapted this technique as a method of assessing the causes and sequence of events leading to the adverse outcomes. This then served as a basis for debriefing the family—and providing data, more information and the possibility of closure.

The appointment was scheduled, and I got back to the daily grind of operating in multiple hospitals. I did not have luxury of time to fully get over the trauma of losing that patient. To illustrate the mechanism I follow, we return to Mr Twiddle in the consulting rooms. This was the deceased patient's husband waiting patiently in the lobby of the consulting rooms. As I ushered him in to his chair, the unpleasant chain of events of that night resurfaced through the fog of repressed memory. I explained the circumstances of her clinical presentation, the surgery, her early post-operative stability and the cause of her post-operative decline. It is very easy for us to lapse into medicalese and jargon-filled talk. I tried hard to keep the language as "lay" and simple as possible. He appeared to get a much better grasp of those fateful sequence of events. He then reminisced about his long and happy marriage. Touchingly, he thanked me and the team for all our efforts. He said he particularly appreciated the opportunity to talk about her death and "now could understand what had happened". We drank some tea, talked about his early days as an engineer in Northeast England. I felt a sense of relief and felt like a weight had been lifted off my shoulders.

This technique of talking to families of patients that have had unexpectedly bad outcomes a few weeks after the event was a technique of communication that I learnt from my mentor Dr. Brian Buxton. A supremely gifted and energetic cardiac surgeon in Melbourne, who pioneered arterial grafting in CABG surgery, Dr. Buxton combined academia and a very busy practice. In keeping with the traditional cardiac surgeon mold, his economy of movement also extended to patient communication. However, he had this unwritten rule of offering to meet with families of patients who had bad outcomes or death a few days to weeks after the incident.

My first experience of this unique method of communication was when I was a fellow or senior registrar (as they are called in Australia) in adult cardiac surgery. It involved a stroke that proved fatal in a lady who had undergone emergency coronary artery surgery in the setting of cardiogenic shock. Dr. Buxton called the patient's family after they withdrew support and spent some time discussing the clinical cascade that led to the unfortunate sequence of events. He then managed to convince the husband of the recently deceased patient to give us permission for an autopsy. Based on the autopsy findings, we were able to work out a mechanism behind the unexpected stroke. We then met with the family for a debriefing session that proved therapeutic to both the family and to us the surgical team. Notwithstanding the family's gratitude, I found the whole experience strangely settling after the funk and depression I had sunk into following that patient's decline.

There is a significant body of literature documenting the importance of feedback to the family and to the team members, after a major adverse event [9]. This aspect of following up when bad news is disclosed is mentioned in a 9-step guide set out to help young ophthalmologists deal with these situations (Table 9.2) [10]. In addition, these mechanisms also allow communication in times of stress for the patient's relatives [11].

I have taken the liberty of suggesting a mnemonic for the use of the 9-step guide set out by the ophthalmologists, since it seems so pragmatic and easy to adapt to a variety of clinical circumstances. These guidelines may not necessarily be applicable in the setting of a catastrophic outcome but serve as a simple set of guiding principles for communication.

Table 9.2 9-Step method of communicating news of adverse effects with patients and families

Suggested acronym for Mnemonic BuilDemPerL TAViSH	Action
Buil	Build a relationship
Dem	Demonstrate empathy
Per	Understand the patient's perspective
L	Speak in plain language
T	Schedule enough time
A	Remain available for more interaction
Vi	Optimize the next visit
S	Encourage second opinions
H	Allow for hope

Adapted from Smith [10]

In all of these bad news scenarios and communications around them, the ethical principles of patient autonomy, beneficence, non-maleficence, and justice have to be kept foremost. Patient autonomy is reflected in the need for full disclosure of the events and the consequences. This is especially important after adverse events; more so when the family needs to be informed. Beneficence and non-maleficence are implied in the consent for the procedure or the interventions prior to the acute decompensation. However, these aspects may need to be re-visited when the communication occurs with the family after the event. The justice component usually pertains to the fact that the procedure, the outcome and response are uniformly applied to all patients.

When I went into practice, I used this system of a *family post-mortem* to help families deal with grief and achieve closure. Invariably, I found it a valuable mechanism of coping, debriefing, learning, and a valuable mechanism of getting feedback on all aspects of care. It has also helped other members of the team to come to terms with a loss especially after heroic attempts at salvage of life. We often neglect the stress suffered by the surgeon and the members of the caring team at losing a patient [12]. There is a significant body of literature talking about supports provided to nurses who have suffered the loss of a patient [13]. There are specific resources offered in terms of support groups and work experience being limited by shift work. Nurses also tend to be able to talk among themselves, have debriefing sessions and undergo specific education programs that help them cope with loss. Surgical specialties seem to do this in a haphazard manner or not at all.

Interestingly, institutions also vary in the way bad news is handled and messaged to families. There is now a trend in some Intensive Care Units to invite families to participate in their rounds and there is data that this may help with communication [14]. The other important change is in culture of accountability and transparency. The Just Culture initiative moves from a blame culture to a more open method of evaluation of organizational issues and contributing factors to adverse events [15]. The Just Culture strategies incorporating non-blame-based analyses of adverse outcomes and providing feedback to patients' families have implications in reduction of errors and minimizing legal ramifications of adverse events [16].

Initially, I held these family post-mortem meetings just by myself, often meeting with one close bereaved family member. Over the years this has morphed into a multidisciplinary group that often includes the social workers, pastoral care/chaplaincy personnel, the resident staff, the nurse/nurses who cared for the deceased patient and sporadically a patient advocate from among the nursing staff. So that when we finally sit down for that "dreaded" meeting, the presence of people of different perspectives helps bring closure to the family as well the house staff. Participation is entirely voluntary, and all the caregivers are invited.

In roughly half these cases, the family may not turn up. In which case, the social worker often follows up twice with phone calls to reschedule the meeting. At the very least, I try to have a telephonic conversation. We have found the families that do attend these meetings sometimes have valid complaints or concerns about the care of their loved one. The meeting often helps clarify matters, sort out problems or identify errors if they were made and address lapses in communication. We try to be forthright and honest about the sequence of events. Occasionally, a relative has pointed out a glaring act of omission that might have precipitated a catastrophic chain of events. I try to use these as teaching exercises for nurses and residents—reinforcing the need to respond to concerned family members promptly. They are often the best judges of a patient's clinical condition, in the absence of objective criteria of physiological dysfunction.

What are the advantages of this approach? [17] It helps families come to terms with their grief. The nursing staff members often learn from the experience and feel that their efforts have been worthwhile. The surgical team uses it to debrief, and the episode often acts as a focus for quality improvement. We should not forget that as surgeons, we feel depressed when we have complications, and this process helps us come to terms with a mortal complication.

The disadvantages of this approach are theoretical and have been mentioned by clinicians. Some feel it stirs the pot of emotions in the bereaved family. Others feel it may worsen the grief reaction and make the family ask "searching questions". In this litigious society there is always the potential risk of malpractice claims. Even though the opposite is actually true [18], only a few institutions adopt this approach. There is also a perception that the surgeon's time is often too valuable for the "touchy-feely" interaction that accompanies this kind of family post-mortem.

Finally, when one looks at the field of the doctor-patient relationship in high-tech medicine, the casualty most often is direct communication between the two. Conflicting information, messages conveyed after complications have occurred and miscommunication are quite common. More importantly, there is a small body of literature suggesting that bereaved family rarely get to talk to the doctors after the loss of their loved one, often causing depression [19]. This concept of the *family post-mortem* tries to rectify some of that, albeit after the fact. It has proved satisfactory and satisfying in my practice which specializes in complex and high-risk cardiothoracic surgery.

How do we use these anecdotal, experiential and narrative instances to transform the nature of communication provided to patients and families who are at the end of life? By extension, what can we do to make the family's grieving process easier after the death of a loved one or a major setback in their clinical course? Many critical care units, especially in North America tend to turf the responsibilities of detailed communication about bad news to palliative care teams.

9.4   Conclusions

Communication about prognosis and possible outcomes should be a fundamental aspect of the treating physician's message to the patient and their relatives. Expectations need to be managed, especially in critically ill patients. Frequent, if not daily updates are essential. Moreover, prompt communication when complications occur is common sensical. Families should be kept in the loop when the clinical course takes an expected or unexpected turn for the worse. We as doctors should be at the forefront of handling the information. As most of us have experienced, all it takes is one miscommunication or a muddled message to make the families lose trust in the process of care. Educational initiatives as part of medical school curricula would serve as a first step. This should be further reinforced when doctors emerge from the cocoon of training and the communication skills honed over the course of their training. The fundamentals and principles of communication maybe facets of Clinical Ethics training as the specialty evolves. My hope and recommendation would be that every medical student and doctor be provided the skills to deal with these end-of-life communications.

9.5   Selected References

- Baile WF, Buckman R, Lenzi R, Glober G, Beale EA, Kudelka AP. SPIKES-A six-step protocol for delivering bad news: application to the patient with cancer. Oncologist. 2000;5(4):302–311. https://doi.org/10.1634/theoncologist5-4-302

  - This article was one of the first to provide a simple step by step protocol to oncologists for delivery of bad news. While this is aimed at oncologists, it has wide applicability.

- Smith D, Braga-Mele R, Day SH, Schwab IR. 9 Tips for delivering bad news. A guide for the young ophthalmologist. Eyenet Suppl. 2016:17–18.

  - This collection of thoughts from a dynamic group of ophthalmologists was set out as a guide to young ophthalmologists early in their practice to help them navigate the demands of dealing with adverse events.

- Khatri N, Brown GD, Hicks LL. From a blame culture to a just culture in health care. Health Care Manage Rev. 2009;34(4):312–322. https://doi.org/10.1097/hmr.0b013e3181a3b709
- Kachalia A, Mello MM, Nallomuthu BK, Studdert DM. Legal and Policy Interventions to Improve Patient Safety. Circ. 2016;133:661–671. https://doi.org/10.1161/CIRCULATIONAHA.115.015880

  - This publication is a corner stone of the patient safety movement and seeks to codify the elements of just culture. This moves away from assigning and casting blame, transitioning to looking at systemic issues.

References

1. Kiluk JV, Dessurealt S, Quinn G. Teaching medical students on how to break bad news to standardized patients. J Cancer Educ. 2012;27(2):277–80. https://doi.org/10.1007/s13187-012-0312-9.
2. MacLaughlan CAJ. ABC of major traum. Handling distressed relatives and breaking bad news. BMJ. 1990;301:1145–9. https://doi.org/10.1136/bmj.301.6761.1145.

3. Johnson J, Panagioti M. Interventions to improve the breaking of bad or difficult news by physicians, medical students, and interns/residents: a systematic review and meta-analysis. Acad Med. 2018;93:1400–12. https://doi.org/10.1097/acm.0000000000002308.
4. Rhodes-Kropf J, Carmody SS, Seltzer D, et al. "This is just too awful; I just can't believe I experienced that …": medical students' reactions to their "most memorable" patient death. Acad Med. 2005;80:634–40.
5. Jackson VA, Sullivan AM, Gadmer NM, et al. "It was haunting …": physicians' descriptions of emotionally powerful patient deaths. Acad Med. 2005;80:648–56.
6. Buckman R. How to break bad news: a guide for health care professionals. Baltimore: Johns Hopkins University Press; 1992.
7. Baile WF, Buckman R, Lenzi R, Glober G, Beale EA, Kudelka AP. SPIKES-A six-step protocol for delivering bad news: application to the patient with cancer. Oncologist. 2000;5(4):302–11. https://doi.org/10.1634/theoncologist5-4-302.
8. Fallowfield L, Lipkin L, Hall A. Teaching senior oncologists communication skills: results from phase I of a comprehensive longitudinal program in the United Kingdom. J Clin Oncol. 1998;16:1961–8.
9. Kearney MK, Weininger RB, Vachon MLS, Harrison RL, Mount BM. Self-care of physicians caring for patients at the end of life: "being connected … a key to my survival.". JAMA. 2009;301:1155–64. https://doi.org/10.1001/jama.2009.352.
10. Smith D, Braga-Mele R, Day SH, Schwab IR. 9 Tips for delivering bad news. A guide for the young ophthalmologist. Eyenet Suppl. 2016:17–8.
11. Premi JN. Communicating bad news to patients. In: Division of Mental Health, World Health Organization, editor. Communicating bad news. Geneva: Division of Mental Health, World Health Organization; 1993. p. 15–21.
12. Whitehead PR. The lived experience of physicians dealing with patient death. BMJ Support Palliat Care. 2014;4:271–6. https://doi.org/10.1136/bmjspcare-2012-000326.
13. Zheng R, Lee SF, Bloomer MJ. How nurses cope with patient death: a systematic review and qualitative meta-synthesis. J Clin Nurs. 2018;27(1–2):e39–49. https://doi.org/10.1111/jocn.13975.
14. Au SS, des Ordons AR, Soo A, Guienguere S, Stelfox HT. Family participation in intensive care unit rounds: comparing family and provider perspectives. J Crit Care. 2017;38(4):132–6. https://doi.org/10.1016/j.jcrc.2016.10.020.
15. Khatri N, Brown GD, Hicks LL. From a blame culture to a just culture in health care. Health Care Manag Rev. 2009;34(4):312–22. https://doi.org/10.1097/hmr.0b013e3181a3b709.
16. Kachalia A, Mello MM, Nallomuthu BK, Studdert DM. Legal and policy interventions to improve patient safety. Circulation. 2016;133:661–71. https://doi.org/10.1161/CIRCULATIONAHA.115.015880.
17. Donovan K. Breaking bad news. In: Division of Mental Health, World Health Organization, editor. Communicating bad news. Geneva: Division of Mental Health, World Health Organization; 1993. p. 3–14.
18. Kraman SS, Cranfill L, Hamm G, Woodard T. Advocacy: the Lexington Veterans Affairs Medical Center. John M Eisenberg patient safety awards. Jt Comm J Qual Patient Saf. 2002;28(12):646–50. https://doi.org/10.1016/s1070-3241(02)28069-4.
19. Tolle SW, Bascom PB, Hickam DH, Benson JA Jr. Communication between physicians and surviving spouses following patient deaths. J Gen Intern Med. 1986;1(5):309–14. https://doi.org/10.1007/bf02596210.

Chapter 10
Surgical Empathy

Erin Fennern ⓘ and Malini D. Sur ⓘ

Abstract Empathy is critical to developing and maintaining a surgeon-patient relationship built on trust. Vulnerable patients rely on this connection to move forward with their care. Emotional empathy entails sharing in the experience of another's emotions. Clinical empathy, however, takes a cognitive approach aimed at predicting patient emotions as a means of guiding empathic communication. While emotional empathy, which is linked to physician burnout, may risk inaccuracy and heterogeneity in clinical judgment across patient groups, *clinical empathy* can lead to improved patient outcomes and can enhance the meaning of the surgeon's work. Fortunately, there are several strategies for fostering clinical empathy skills.

Keywords Empathy · Empathic communication · Emotional labor · Implicit Bias Burnout

10.1 Introduction

The concept of empathy has always been central to explorations of the doctor-patient relationship. At a time of great vulnerability, patients and families look to their surgeon for support and reassurance to go forward with or without treatment. Trusting that their surgeon understands the particular difficulty of their situation naturally influences the willingness of patients to engage in their care, and that trust—much like technical skill—contributes to positive clinical outcomes. When time is of the essence, such as in a high-acuity perioperative setting, relaying

E. Fennern
Department of Surgery, The Mount Sinai Hospital, New York, NY, USA

M. D. Sur (✉)
Northside Hospital Cancer Institute, Atlanta, GA, USA
e-mail: Malini.Sur@northside.com

© The Author(s), under exclusive license to Springer Nature Switzerland AG 2022

V. A. Lonchyna et al. (eds.), *Difficult Decisions in Surgical Ethics*, Difficult Decisions in Surgery: An Evidence-Based Approach,
https://doi.org/10.1007/978-3-030-84625-1_10

Table 10.1 Surgical empathy is an important element of all four pillars of medical ethics

Beneficence	• Surgical empathy is linked to improved clinical outcomes and greater patient satisfaction
Non-maleficence	• With knowledge of empathy's benefit, surgeons have a duty to cultivate this skill • Without empathy, they risk violating the principle of non-maleficence or doing no harm, as patient may be alienated and left vulnerable at a time of distress
Respect for autonomy	• While respecting patients' abilities to make decisions for themselves, surgical empathy can foster a trusting relationship • Trust is what enables the surgeon to guide patient decisions based on their expert knowledge and insight into the patient's values
Justice	• Surgical empathy can foster a trusting relationship that enables the surgeon to guide their patient's self-determined decision-making in a manner that is based on expert knowledge and insight • Surgeons must be mindful of checking personal feelings and implicit biases that may lead to inequitable emotional responses and resulting care to maintain justice in health care delivery

surgical empathy may be even more challenging and more critical than in a more paced, outpatient medical setting (see Table 10.1).

10.2 Search Strategy

A PubMed search was performed using the search terms ["ethics" + "empathy"], ["empathy" + "surgery"], ["empathy" + "burnout"], ["empathy" + "surgeon"] between 2010 and 2020. Embedded references to historical papers were also explored, with the goal of focusing our discussion on the following: the concept of empathy, the benefits and risks to surgeons in exhibiting and practicing empathy in their practice, and the ethical challenges of demonstrating empathy in the surgical setting, as well as future directions for the cultivation and preservation of empathy in surgeons. This search yielded 231 papers, of which 55 were utilized for this chapter. Following a brief introduction, we incorporate a series of short case vignettes as a starting point for subsequent discussion.

10.3 What Is Empathy and How Can It Be Measured?

From a nonmedical perspective, empathy is commonly defined as the action of vicariously *experiencing* the situation and emotions of another person without having them explicitly communicated [1]. In the medical literature, however, empathy often takes on a more cognitive and more detached role, with an emphasis on the ability of the physician to neutrally evaluate and treat a patient while *predicting* the patient's emotions without necessarily experiencing them [2, 3]. While based in compassion, this clinical empathy isn't merely supportive; it is fueled by a purpose-driven desire to help the person in need [4].

Demonstrating empathy is considered a critical component of a physician's "emotional labor," a term introduced by sociologist Arlie Hochschild in 1983 to describe workers' demonstration of emotions to meet job requirements [5]. Emotional labor can be achieved through deep-acting, when the physician's reactions are based on an actual experience of the patient's emotions, consistent with the typical understanding of empathy [3]. This requires the physician to change their emotional state and respond to the patient accordingly [6]. Emotional labor can also be achieved through surface-acting, when the physician does not actually feel the patient's feelings, but is able to display empathy through voice, facial expressions, posture, and supportive comments [3, 5]. In this way, the physician does not alter their true emotional state. Surface-acting may be considered more consistent with the neutral medicalized approach to empathy. While there continues to be a great deal of overlap among specific definitions used in the medical literature, all are based on a combination of thinking, feeling, and acting to connect with and predict the patient's emotional state [4, 7].

Regardless of the precise definition used, it is clear that medical education programs have long embraced the cultivation of empathy as a critical element in the development of independent practitioners [8]. The Jefferson Scale of Physician Empathy, a self-administered 20-item assessment of empathy in patient-care situations, has been adapted to a student version which is the most commonly utilized in studies aiming to measure, understand, and intervene on empathy among medical students from their pre-clinical years to clerkships [9–12]. This instrument enables students to identify their level of agreement with statements relating to the value of empathy, such as "My patients feel better when I understand their feelings" and "It is difficult for me to view things from my patients' perspectives." One can imagine that medical students' abilities to respond to the desperation of a terminally ill patient as in Case 1 may vary tremendously based on personality, background, personal experience, and training.

Case 1

A third-year medical student was asked to see an inpatient consult on the neurosurgery service. The clerkship requirements include documentation of a complete neurology exam. The patient was a 68-year-old man who was post-operative day 10 from a resection of a glioblastoma multiforme tumor. His post-surgical course was complicated by a stroke. After asking the patient a few questions, while nervously trying to remember and perform the steps of a comprehensive neurology exam, the patient interrupted the student and abruptly stated, "I don't want to do this. I just want to die." Not certain as to how to respond, the student did not know whether to continue or end the assessment.

Given the perceived importance of empathy in student doctors, it is not surprising that many investigations have also explored the continued development and maintenance of empathy in residency. In the preamble to the common core requirements of the Accreditation Council for Graduate Medical Education (ACGME), training programs are specifically asked to allow residents not only to gain the knowledge, skills, and attitudes for autonomous practice, but also the empathy to do so. While surgical subspecialty trainees are often perceived as merely technically-oriented and prone to a reduced ability or interest in patient communication, the preservation of empathy throughout surgical training has been of particular interest in recent years [6, 13–15].

10.4 Why Is Empathy Important for the Surgeon?

Empathy is a fundamental trait of a morally upright surgeon. Upon completion of surgical residency and initiation into practice, surgeons inducted into the American College of Surgeons recite a fellowship pledge to prioritize the welfare of the patient above all, and to treat the patient as though they were in the patient's position [16]. Such an oath arises from the timeless model of the surgeon as the patient's moral fiduciary [6, 17]. The surgeon-patient relationship is unique because of the surgeon's need to weigh imposing bodily harm and the attendant risk of complications against the anticipated health benefits of surgery, and the patient's trust in the surgeon to do so in a thoughtful and safe manner on their behalf. For a patient to provide informed consent, they must develop such trust not only in the surgeon's technical ability and intelligence, but also in the surgeon's desire to do what is right for the patient [18]. Whether through feeling or surface-acting, the surgeon must connect with the patient and gain that trust in order to proceed with the operation. Empathy, then, is central to the delivery of beneficence—the ethical obligation of surgeons to help their patients achieve the best health possible [6].

As demonstrated in Case 2, validation of empathy through effective communication leads to patient engagement in the plan of care (see Table 10.2). In this way, empathy can be valued through a utilitarian lens, as it helps to generate the desired consequence of good patient health. The idea that providing emotional support fosters physical healing is not simply a theoretical or philosophical one. Numerous studies have demonstrated that physician empathy is correlated with better health outcomes [4], including improved information-gathering and diagnostics [3, 19–25], greater patient buy-in and adherence to a plan of treatment [26–28], and improved patient quality of life and outcomes [18, 29].

Case 2

A surgical resident working in the emergency room evaluated a 34-year-old woman who was 25 weeks pregnant and had clinical findings consistent with acute appendicitis. The attending surgeon oncall was notified and recommended emergency appendectomy. As they prepared the operating room, the patient refused to sign the consent form as presented by the resident. The attending surgeon came in to see her, held her hand and said calmly: "You must be so worried about your baby's safety. I completely understand your concerns and appreciate that this all must be very overwhelming. You have done the right thing by coming to the hospital this evening. While there are risks to surgery, there are also risks to leaving your infected appendix in. It's a difficult decision, but I strongly recommend that we operate, and I am hopeful that you and your baby will do well. What other concerns do you have that I can address?" Assured that her surgeon understood her feelings and cared for her interests, the patient consented to the procedure.

Table 10.2 Statements that facilitate empathy

Queries
"Would you (or could you) tell me a little more about that?"
"What has this been like for you?"
"Is there anything else?"
"Are you OK with that?"
Clarifications
"Let me see if I have this right."
"I want to make sure I really understand what you're telling me. I am hearing that …"
"I don't want us to go further until I'm sure I've gotten it right."
"When I'm done, if I've gone astray, I'd appreciate it if you would correct me. OK?"
Responses
"That sounds very difficult."
"Sounds like …"
"That's great! I bet you're feeling pretty good about that."
"I can imagine that this might feel …"
"Anyone in your situation would feel that way …"
"I can see that you are …"

Note: Reprinted from *Let Me See If I Have This Right …": Words That Help Build Empathy*, by Coulehan JL, Platt FW, Egener B, et al. [19]. Copyright 2001 by Annals of Internal Medicine

Surgeons' demonstration of empathy might also help patients feel respected as individuals at a time when they may feel they have lost control over their lives. In this way, patients' perceptions of their care can be influenced by empathy. For example, nearly three decades ago, detailed reviews of plaintiff depositions from medical malpractice cases showed that failing to understand or devaluing the patient or family perspective, or delivering information poorly, were central to patients' complaints about physicians [24, 30]. Moreover, surgeon empathy is known to be linked to overall patient satisfaction [18]. While technical skill and medical knowledge are certainly fundamental, the role of the surgeon is still to provide a human service. By affecting patients' desire for information about their condition and their motivation to heal, the subjective perception of health can be positively impacted—even when technical and medical tools fall short, and patients do not fully recover [31, 32].

10.5 What Are the Costs of Surgical Empathy?

Whereas empathy in a traditional, nonmedical context has purely favorable connotations, it has been long recognized as a double-edged sword in the health care setting. In their daily work, physicians are required to regulate their emotional responses to patients in order to formulate an assessment and plan of care based on the objective facts at hand. Tens of thousands of hours of training establish accurate symptomatology, laboratory results, and imaging findings as the foundations of diagnosis and treatment based on evidence in the literature. Being overly connected with one's feelings might lead to straying from standard of care and resulting errors in surgical management and decision making. Physicians who have emotional responses to critically ill patients have been shown to perform more life-prolonging procedures compared to those with more cognitive responses [33]. In Case 3, a surgeon who strongly connects with the emotion of the surrogate might be convinced to proceed to emergency surgery despite an almost certain risk of perioperative mortality, while one who stays more emotionally neutral might be able to remain steadfast in the medical recommendation to avoid operative intervention.

Case 3

The on-call surgeon was asked to see an 83-year-old woman with a history of metastatic ovarian cancer on third line chemotherapy, signs and symptoms of abdominal sepsis, and radiographic findings of pneumoperitoneum. As the patient had altered mental status, the surgeon engaged her surrogate decision makers in a conversation regarding the expected outcomes of emergency laparotomy and whether this would be in line with the patient's wishes. The patient's son interjected, "Please, Doc, you just gotta do everything to save my mom—she's everything to us." The surgeon is troubled, knowing that even with a technically successful surgery, the patient is at very high risk of perioperative death.

In addition to potentially clouding surgical judgment, emotional empathy is problematic because it introduces room for tremendous heterogeneity in the treatment of patients based on the strength of the surgeon-patient connection. Empathy requires an ability to relate to another human being, and therefore is susceptible to influence from social factors [34]. Traits such as race, gender, education level, and physical appearance can impact perceptions of empathy [35]. A pro-White empathy bias has been demonstrated among college students viewing a patient's pained facial expressions and linked to pain treatment bias [36, 37]. Extensive research, outside the scope of this chapter, demonstrates the unfortunate role of implicit biases among surgeons in contributing to disparate health outcomes among minority groups [38, 39]. Excessive reliance on an empathic physician response might also cloud the ability of the physician to recognize critical differences between themselves and their patients, seeing their patients through their own, prejudiced lens of experience [40, 41]. Consequently, the ability of socially learned bias to influence physician empathy threatens the very principle of justice in our health care system. Surgeons who are overly reliant on traditional forms of empathy may unconsciously be inequitable in their treatment decisions across patient groups, perhaps responding to the patient in Case 3 with more or less willingness to intervene based on their level of identification with the patient's personal characteristics.

In addition to precluding fair treatment of patients, reliance on physician empathy as a basis for delivery of good medical care has another practical challenge in the surgical setting. Empathy is often felt to require time and patience, whereas the modern surgical care paradigm relies on speed and efficiency. There is a noticeable decline in measures of empathy during the clinical years of medical school, and both resident and attending surgeons demonstrate missing up to 70% of opportunities for empathic responses during patient encounters [13, 23, 42]. The reasons for this are likely manifold, however perceived time constraints in today's practice settings undoubtedly play a part [10, 31]. Furthermore, a strong practice emphasis on surgeon productivity as measured by relative value units does not incentivize the physician to take the opportunity to elicit and respond to patient emotions.

Finally, there is clearly a close and complicated relationship between the decline of empathy and physician burnout during training. Whether one factor causes the other, or both are rooted in other changes during the transition to independent practice, is unclear. Specialties such as general surgery and urology have been identified as having higher rates of burnout, defined commonly as a state of mental, physical, and emotional exhaustion induced by prolonged stress [43]. Empathy appears to have a bidirectional impact—for some, it decreases the propensity for burnout [44]; for others, it enhances it [45]. Several studies have shown that medical students who demonstrate higher empathy in school are observed to have lower burnout rates in residency [45, 46]. However, taking on emotional distress from patients by *experiencing* their suffering can increase the risk of emotional burnout and compassion fatigue [43, 47–49]. But this "risky strength" of heightened empathy, in turn, may also lead to enhanced meaning for the work of the surgeon [13]. This is why we emphasize the importance of a clinical empathy that emphasizes the surgeon's ability to connect with the patient through communication strategies and deep-acting, with the aim of predicting the patient's emotions without necessarily experiencing them [4]. The ability to conceptualize the patient's perspective and use their perceived values to motivate and guide the plan of care, while also showing oneself compassion and protecting against emotional exhaustion—this is the goal of surgical empathy.

10.6   How Can We Train Surgeons to Develop and Maintain Clinical Empathy?

In procedural specialties, the act of healing is often intertwined with trauma and pain. Surgery itself is a type of calculated violence with a long-term goal of inducing healing. It makes sense then, that there would be an increased risk of dehumanization in surgical care. Thus far, we have examined the potential benefits and challenges of empathy in the context of ethical surgical practice. Can empathy be cultivated and maintained in an ethically conscious yet healthy manner among resident and attending surgeons? Fortunately, there is a developing body of literature that answers in the affirmative. Well-designed studies show that measures of physician empathy can be improved through education and training [13, 45, 50, 51].

In surgery, several targeted interventions to foster empathy have shown promise. Interactive workshops focused on fundamental aspects of empathetic communication with standardized patients and small-group learning have been shown to be effective at improving perceived empathy among medical students and surgical trainees [51, 52]. Interestingly, research suggests that longer visits may not necessarily be required for adequate delivery of empathy—rather, physicians need assistance in recognizing and responding to empathic opportunities [19, 42].

To this end, surgical trainees would benefit from a curriculum for the development of communication skills and surface acting. Clinical empathy entails both the formation of insights as well as acts of compassionate communication [22, 51, 52]. In this sense, it is both innate and also teachable. Perhaps the greatest tool for the development of clinical empathy skills is role modeling by empathic faculty (See Table 10.2) [19, 50, 53]. Programs could develop mentorship or preceptorship opportunities where residents directly learn empathic skills from selected faculty. Additionally, didactics, patient simulations, and role-playing have also been shown to positively impact residents' subjective sense of their own clinical empathy skillset [4, 50, 51]. Demonstration of clinical empathy skills should be a required ACGME competency for which residents should be evaluated, provided feedback with individualized learning plans, and remediated when gaps in skills are found.

Additional training programs centered specifically around mindfulness and well-being have also been associated with decreased burnout [14, 40, 54]. This skillset training ought not end when residency is completed. Continued education through immersion physician communication programs like VitalTalk (www.vitaltalk.org) should be encouraged, and elements of these could be included in credentialing and maintenance of certification. Implicit bias training, common in business settings, could also be adjusted to raise awareness of subconscious discrimination in health care settings that can influence health outcomes.

Finally, a prerequisite for physicians to be able to display empathy may be that they themselves are in an emotionally stable state [55]. Given this, organizations that prioritize physicians' mental and physical well-being may find a valuable return on investment. Work hours should be humane, with adequate coverage for rest and self-care, and the clinical pace must allow for thoughtful patient care, utilizing physician extenders, when possible, to provide relief and buffer against unsafe work volume. The workplace should be free from bullying and discrimination, whether by other staff or by patients. Although not well-studied, we believe these factors to be intuitively associated with the ability to connect with and provide emotional support for others.

10.7 Conclusion

Surgeons have much to gain by considering the expression of emotion through *clinical empathy* part of their work role. Neither purely emotional nor purely cognitive, clinical surgical empathy can help patients overcome a challenging period in their health while allowing for accurate and ethical clinical decision-making. As there are vast differences in personalities among surgeons and among patients, it is understood that each surgeon-patient relationship will be unique and require a tailored approach. Just as recognition of common patterns of disease guide surgeons in their patient-specific treatment recommendations and operative planning as indicated, an appreciation of shared human emotional needs can serve to inform the surgeon's armamentarium of patient-specific empathic communication strategies.

10.8 Selected References

- Han JL, Pappas TN. A Review of Empathy, Its Importance, and Its Teaching in Surgical Training. J Surg Educ. 2018;75(1):88–94. https://doi.org/10.1016/j.jsurg.2017.06.035

    - This paper highlights the importance of empathy in the surgeon-patient relationship, its relationship to patient outcomes, and its value in surgical education.

- Hochschild AR. *The Managed Heart: Commercialization of Human Feeling.* University of California Press; 1983.

    - A seminal work in sociology for its recognition of the value and cost of emotional labor, this book won the American Sociological Association's Charles Cooley Award in 1984.

- Khan S, Jung F, Kirubarajan A, Karim K, Scheer A, Simpson J. A Systematic Review of Interventions to Improve Humanism in Surgical Practice. J Surg Educ. 2020;78(2):548–560. https://doi.org/10.1016/j.surg.2020.07.032

  - This is a comprehensive summary of strategies for improving empathic communication in surgical trainees.

- Larson EB, Yao X. Clinical empathy as emotional labor in the patient-physician relationship. JAMA. 2005;293(9):1100–1106. https://doi.org/10.1001/jama.293.9.1100

  - The authors propose that physicians are emotional laborers, and that engagement in the process of empathy leads to more effective clinical care and professional satisfaction.

References

1. "Empathy". *Merriam-Webster Dictionary*. Merriam-Webster. Accessed February 20, 2021. https://www.merriam-webster.com/dictionary/empathy.
2. Aring CD. Sympathy and empathy. JAMA. 1958;167(4):448–52. https://doi.org/10.1001/jama.1958.02990210034008.
3. Halpern J. From idealized clinical empathy to empathic communication in medical care. Med Health Care Philos. 2014;17(2):301–11. https://doi.org/10.1007/s11019-013-9510-4.
4. Neumann M, Bensing J, Mercer S, Ernstmann N, Ommen O, Pfaff H. Analyzing the "nature" and "specific effectiveness" of clinical empathy: a theoretical overview and contribution towards a theory-based research agenda. Patient Educ Couns. 2009;74(3):339–46. https://doi.org/10.1016/j.pec.2008.11.013.
5. Hochschild AR. The managed heart: commercialization of human feeling. University of California Press; 1983.
6. Larson EB, Yao X. Clinical empathy as emotional labor in the patient-physician relationship. JAMA. 2005;293(9):1100–6. https://doi.org/10.1001/jama.293.9.1100.
7. Sulzer SH, Feinstein NW, Wendland C. Assessing empathy development in medical education: a systematic review. Med Educ. 2016;50(3):300–10. https://doi.org/10.1111/medu.12806.
8. Rafaeli A, Sutton RI. Expression of emotion as part of the work role. Acad Manag Rev. 1987;12(1):23–37. https://doi.org/10.5465/amr.1987.4306444.
9. Hojat M, Mangione S, Nasca TJ, et al. The Jefferson scale of physician empathy: development and preliminary psychometric data. Educ Psychol Meas. 2001;61(2) https://doi.org/10.1177/00131640121971158.
10. Chen DCR, Pahilan ME, Orlander JD. Comparing a self-administered measure of empathy with observed behavior among medical students. J Gen Intern Med. 2010;25(3):200–2. https://doi.org/10.1007/s11606-009-1193-4.
11. Chen D, Lew R, Hershman W, Orlander J. A cross-sectional measurement of medical student empathy. J Gen Intern Med. 2007;22(10):1434–8. https://doi.org/10.1007/s11606-007-0298-x.
12. Brazeau CMLR, Schroeder R, Rovi S, Boyd L. Relationships between medical student burnout, empathy, and professionalism climate. Acad Med. 2010;85:S33–6. https://doi.org/10.1097/acm.0b013e3181ed4c47.
13. Han JL, Pappas TN. A review of empathy, its importance, and its teaching in surgical training. J Surg Educ. 2018;75(1):88–94. https://doi.org/10.1016/j.jsurg.2017.06.035.

14. Stephen AE, Mehta DH. Mindfulness in Surgery. Am J Lifestyle Med. 2019;13(6):552–5. https://doi.org/10.1177/1559827619870474.

15. Branson CF, Chipman JG. Improving surgical residents' communication in disclosing complications: a qualitative analysis of simulated physician and patient surrogate conversations. Am J Surg. 2018;215(2):331–5. https://doi.org/10.1016/j.amjsurg.2017.10.041.

16. American College of Surgeons. ACS Fellowship pledge. Accessed February 19, 2021. https://www.facs.org/member-services/join/fellows/fellowreq.

17. Jones JW, McCullough LB, Richman BW. The ethics of surgical practice: cases, dilemmas, and resolutions. Oxford University Press; 2008.

18. Weng H-C, Steed JF, Yu S-W, et al. The effect of surgeon empathy and emotional intelligence on patient satisfaction. Adv Health Sci Educ. 2011;16(5):591–600. https://doi.org/10.1007/s10459-011-9278-3.

19. Coulehan JL, Platt FW, Egener B, et al. "Let me see if I have this right …": words that help build empathy. Ann Intern Med. 2001;135(3):221–7. https://doi.org/10.7326/0003-4819-135-3-200108070-00022.

20. Squier RW. A model of empathic understanding and adherence to treatment regimens in practitioner-patient relationships. Soc Sci Med. 1990;30(3):325–39. https://doi.org/10.1016/0277-9536(90)90188-x.

21. Maguire P, Faulkner A, Booth K, Elliott C, Hillier V. Helping cancer patients disclose their concerns. Eur J Cancer. 1996;32(1):78–81. https://doi.org/10.1016/0959-8049(95)00527-7.

22. Beckman HB, Frankel RM. Training practitioners to communicate effectively in cancer care: it is the relationship that counts. Patient Educ Couns. 2003;50(1):85–9. https://doi.org/10.1016/s0738-3991(03)00086-7.

23. Levinson W, Chaumeton N. Communication between surgeons and patients in routine office visits. Surgery. 1999;125(2):127–34. https://doi.org/10.1016/s0039-6060(99)70255-2.

24. Levinson W, Roter DL, Mullooly JP, Dull VT, Frankel RM. Physician-patient communication: the relationship with malpractice claims among primary care physicians and surgeons. JAMA. 1997;277(7):553–9. https://doi.org/10.1001/jama.1997.03540310051034.

25. Levinson W, Hudak P, Tricco AC. A systematic review of surgeon–patient communication: strengths and opportunities for improvement. Patient Educ Couns. 2013;93(1):3–17. https://doi.org/10.1016/j.pec.2013.03.023.

26. Mercer SW, Reynolds WJ. Empathy and quality of care. Br J Gen Pract 2002;52(Suppl): S9–S12. PMID:12389763.

27. Howie JGR, Heaney DJ, Maxwell M, Walker JJ, Freeman GK, Rai H. Quality at general practice consultations: cross sectional survey. BMJ. 1999;319(7212):738–43. https://doi.org/10.1136/bmj.319.7212.738.

28. Di Blasi Z, Harkness E, Ernst E, Georgiou A, Kleijnen J. Influence of context effects on health outcomes: a systematic review. Lancet. 2001;357(9258):757–62. https://doi.org/10.1016/s0140-6736(00)04169-6.

29. Rakel DP, Hoeft TJ, Barrett BP, Chewning BA, Craig BM, Niu M. Practitioner empathy and the duration of the common cold. Fam Med 2009;41(7):494–501. PMID:19582635.

30. Beckman HB. The doctor-patient relationship and malpractice. Arch Intern Med. 1994;154(12):1365–70. https://doi.org/10.1001/archinte.1994.0040120093010.

31. Steinhausen S, Ommen O, Antoine S-L, Koehler T, Pfaff H, Neugebauer E. Short- and long-term subjective medical treatment outcome of trauma surgery patients: the importance of physician empathy. Patient Prefer Adherence 2014; 8:1239–1253. PMID:25258518.

32. Pollak KI, Alexander SC, Tulsky JA, et al. Physician empathy and listening: associations with patient satisfaction and autonomy. J Am Board Fam Med. 2011;24(6):665–72. https://doi.org/10.3122/jabfm.2011.06.110025.

33. Nightingale SD, Yarnold PR, Greenberg MS. Sympathy, empathy, and physician resource utilization. J Gen Intern Med. 1991;6(5):420–3. https://doi.org/10.1007/bf02598163.

34. Humbyrd CJ. Virtue ethics in a value-driven world. Clin Orthop Relat Res. 2019;477(5): 2639–41. https://doi.org/10.1097/corr.0000000000000908.
35. Riess H. The science of empathy. J Patient Exp. 2017;4(2):74–7. https://doi.org/10.1177/2374373517699267.
36. Kaseweter KA, Drwecki BB, Prkachin KM. Racial differences in pain treatment and empathy in a Canadian sample. Pain Res Manag. 2012;17(6):381–4. https://doi.org/10.1155/2012/803474.
37. Drwecki BB, Moore CF, Ward SE, Prkachin KM. Reducing racial disparities in pain treatment: the role of empathy and perspective-taking. Pain. 2011;152(5):1001–6. https://doi.org/10.1016/j.pain.2010.12.005.
38. Santry HP, Wren SM. The role of unconscious Bias in surgical safety and outcomes. Surg Clin North Am. 2012;92(1):137–51. https://doi.org/10.1016/j.suc.2011.11.006.
39. Forgiarini M, Gallucci M, Maravita A. Racism and the empathy for pain on our skin. Front Psychol. 2011;2:108. https://doi.org/10.3389/fpsyg.2011.00108.
40. Carmel S, Glick SM. Compassionate-empathic physicians: personality traits and social-organizational factors that enhance or inhibit this behavior pattern. Soc Sci Med. 1996;43(8):1253–61. https://doi.org/10.1016/0277-9536(95)00445-9.
41. Wilmer HA. The doctor-patient relationship and the issues of pity, sympathy and empathy. Br J Med Psychol. 1968;41(3):243–8. https://doi.org/10.1111/j.2044-8341.1968.tb02029.x.
42. Morse DS, Edwardsen EA, Gordon HS. Missed opportunities for interval empathy in lung Cancer communication. Arch Intern Med. 2008;168(17):1853–8. https://doi.org/10.1001/archinte.168.17.1853.
43. Dyrbye LN, Burke SE, Hardeman RR, et al. Association of Clinical Specialty with Symptoms of burnout and career choice regret among US resident physicians. JAMA. 2018;320(11):1114–30. https://doi.org/10.1001/jama.2018.12615.
44. Thirioux B, Birault F, Jaafari N. Empathy is a protective factor of burnout in physicians: new neuro-phenomenological hypotheses regarding empathy and sympathy in care relationship. Front Psychol. 2016;7:763. https://doi.org/10.3389/fpsyg.2016.00763.
45. Wilkinson H, Whittington R, Perry L, Eames C. Examining the relationship between burnout and empathy in healthcare professionals: a systematic review. Burn Res. 2017;7:18–29. https://doi.org/10.1016/j.bern.2017.06.003.
46. Neumann M, Edelhäuser F, Tauschel D, et al. Empathy decline and its reasons: a systematic review of studies with medical students and residents. Acad Med. 2011;86(8):996–1009. https://doi.org/10.1097/acm.0b013e318221e615.
47. Manczak EM, DeLongis A, Chen E. Does empathy have a cost? Diverging psychological and physiological effects within families. Health Psychol. 2016;35(3):211–8. https://doi.org/10.1037/hea0000281.
48. Buffone AEK, Poulin M, DeLury S, Ministero L, Morrisson C, Scalco M. Don't walk in her shoes! Different forms of perspective taking affect stress physiology. J Exp Soc Psychol. 2017;72:161–8. https://doi.org/10.1016/j.jesp.2017.04.001.
49. van Mol MMC, Kompanje EJO, Benoit DD, Bakker J, Nijkamp MD, Seedat S. The prevalence of compassion fatigue and burnout among healthcare professionals in intensive care units: a systematic review. PLoS One. 2015;10(8):e0136955. https://doi.org/10.1371/journal.pone.0136955.
50. Kelm Z, Womer J, Walter JK, Feudtner C. Interventions to cultivate physician empathy: a systematic review. BMC Med Educ. 2014;14:219. https://doi.org/10.1186/1472-6920-14-219.
51. Khan S, Jung F, Kirubarajan A, Karim K, Scheer A, Simpson J. A systematic review of interventions to improve humanism in surgical practice. J Surg Educ. 2020;78(2):548–60. https://doi.org/10.1016/j.surg.2020.07.032.
52. Shapiro J, Youm J, Kheriaty A, Pham T, Chen Y, Clayma R. The human kindness curriculum: an innovative preclinical initiative to highlight kindness and empathy in medicine. Educ Health. 2019;32(2):53–61. https://doi.org/10.4103/efh.efh_133_18.

53. Silvester J, Patterson F, Koczwara A, Ferguson E. "Trust me…": psychological and behavioral predictors of perceived physician empathy. J Appl Psychol. 2007;92(2):519–27. https://doi.org/10.1037/0021-9010.92.2.519.
54. Yuguero O, Marsal J, Esquerda M, Galvan L, Soler-González J. Cross-sectional study of the association between empathy and burnout and drug prescribing quality in primary care. Prim Health Care Res Dev. 2019;20:e145. https://doi.org/10.1017/s1463423619000793.
55. Martín-Brufau R, Martin-Gorgojo A, Suso-Ribera C, Estrada E, Capriles-Ovalles ME, Romero-Brufau S. Emotion regulation strategies, workload conditions, and burnout in healthcare residents. Int J Environ Res Public Health. 2020;17(21):7816. https://doi.org/10.3390/ijerph17217816.

Part III
Surgical Education

Chapter 11
Teaching Surgical Ethics

Elisheva T. A. Nemetz ⓘ, Sabha Ganai ⓘ, and Karen Devon ⓘ

Abstract Surgical ethics education is essential to the practice of surgery and has an evolving small body of literature. Teaching surgical ethics occurs informally as well as formally. Informal surgical ethics education includes role-modelling, bedside teaching, and the hidden curriculum. Formal surgical ethics education includes modalities such as: lectures, case-based learning, small-group learning, role-play, standardized patients, and ethics morbidity and mortality rounds. In this chapter we identify challenges to implementing ethics education and discuss assessment in surgical ethics education.

Keywords Teaching surgical ethics · Informal ethics education · Formal ethics education · Resident ethics education · Teaching surgical trainees · Surgical resident ethics

E. T. A. Nemetz
Faculty of Medicine, University of Toronto, Toronto, ON, Canada
e-mail: elisheva.nemetz@mail.utoronto.ca

S. Ganai
Department of Surgery, University of North Dakota School of Medicine and Health Sciences, Grand Forks, ND, USA
e-mail: sabha.ganai@und.edu

K. Devon (✉)
Department of Surgery, Women's College Hospital and University Health Network, University of Toronto, Toronto, ON, Canada
e-mail: karen.devon@wchospital.ca

© The Author(s), under exclusive license to Springer Nature Switzerland AG 2022
V. A. Lonchyna et al. (eds.), *Difficult Decisions in Surgical Ethics*, Difficult Decisions in Surgery: An Evidence-Based Approach,
https://doi.org/10.1007/978-3-030-84625-1_11

Case

A senior surgery resident sees a patient in the emergency department with acute appendicitis. She goes through the informed consent process and books the patient for the operating room. The attending surgeon greets the patient just prior to the patient going to sleep and says, "Don't worry, the team will take great care of you." The attending then says to the resident, "Go ahead, and call me if you need me. I'll be upstairs in my office." The resident tells the attending that she did not specifically mention to the patient that she would be doing the case, wondering if it is okay. The attending tells her that given that this is an emergency, "You needn't worry."

11.1   Introduction

Good clinical medicine relies upon the practice of moral and ethical medicine. Surgery, an act with the potential to harm, is performed with the intention of providing the patient with a good outcome, and thus requires a balance of risks and benefits. An education in clinical ethics assists surgeons in confronting emerging issues, ensures care is delivered in a responsible manner, prepares residents for leadership positions, and permits trainees to identify and resolve ethics problems as they arise [1, 2]. Ethics education may also be of personal benefit during surgical training, as trainees may encounter significant moral angst from moral dilemmas [3]. Ethical dilemmas not only affect the patient-physician relationship but also impact the interactions between multidisciplinary healthcare providers and the team-based provision of care [4]. Surgical practice is fertile ground for ethical dilemmas and improper handling of ethical quandaries results in significant costs, including the breakdown of public trust in the healthcare professions [4]. Deficiencies have been noted in the provision of ethics education, including limited faculty possessing expertise, time constraints of surgical training programs, and the view that an education in ethics is peripheral to the learning agenda [5–7].

Ethics should be incorporated into surgical curriculum in a purposeful and practical way (see Table 11.1) [8]. This chapter explores various components of ethics education including informal and formal educational methods, challenges to surgical ethics education, and assessments of ethics knowledge.

11.2   Search Strategy

A literature review was conducted between 1976 and 2020 utilizing MEDLINE and OVID. Search terms included: surgical ethics AND training, surgical ethics, core competency, professionalism, surgical bioethics, ethics AND training, ethics AND

Table 11.1 Principles of ethics as incorporated into a surgical ethics education curricula

Principles or duties explored	Methods of exploration
Autonomy and respect for persons	• Communication and management of an unforeseen outcome to a standardized family: "delivery of bad news" • Discussion of privacy, confidentiality, and posting of photographs on social media
Nonmaleficence and beneficence	• Discussion of process of informed consent prior to a central line placement technical simulation • Teaching best case/worst case framework for complex surgical decision-making • Exploring the ACS NSQIP surgical risk calculator estimates and alternative options during M&M case discussion
Justice	• Informal discussion of disparities in patient outcome by race/ethnicity during bedside rounds and working to address social determinants of health • Didactic discussion of system of allocation of organs for transplantation • Discussion of approaches to gender-related differences in salary during formal leadership and negotiation workshop for chief residents
Professionalism	• Articulating elements of the hidden curriculum that should be avoided during bedside rounds • Demonstrating respectful and educational discourse focused on quality improvement during M&M conference • Discussion of proper expectations for documentation during a billing and coding workshop

residency, moral culture, bioethics AND residency, bioethics AND surgical residents, curricula, education, bioethics AND medical school, moral deliberation, teaching AND surgical ethics, teaching AND medical ethics, professional competence, virtues, and surgical ethics AND education. From available literature, twenty-nine articles were chosen for their contribution to the topic of teaching surgical ethics.

11.3 Informal Ethics Education

Many surgical residents learn how to deal with ethical challenges through what is known as the hidden curriculum [2, 9–13]. The hidden curriculum is more than the unintentional transfer of knowledge and skills but rather, includes the values, norms, and beliefs taught to medical trainees, such as maintaining medical hierarchy and assuming emotional neutralization in patient care along the way [14]. Although there are textbooks on the subject matter of surgical ethics, surgical trainees often learn through the actions and decisions of their surgical faculty [6]. Brewster et al. determined that surgical residents advance through their training and mitigate ethical dilemmas in the ways that were modeled to them by faculty.

However, the disadvantage of informal surgical ethics education is that the ethical reasoning is often not explicit, nor is it openly discussed, making it difficult to acknowledge and understand [9]. The calculus that a surgeon grapples with mentally and the framework utilized to reach a conclusion are often not explained, especially as the surgeon advances in his/her field and engages in these determinations frequently [9]. Nonetheless, if performed explicitly and openly, modeling can be a good opportunity to elucidate an ethical quandary and its resolution as applied to the practice of medicine [9].

Teaching at the bedside is a legacy of the Oslerian revolution in education, which focuses upon the convergence of formal and informal education [15], "*Ethicists might issue their principles from their proverbial ivory tower. Physicians, immersed in the immediacy of wards, clinics, and surgical suites may find them of little value in alleviating the pain of decisions.*" [16] Clinical interactions at the 'bedside' lead to personal accountability for the ethical decisions being made with consequences that are tangible for surgical trainees [15]. In order to be successful in real-time ethical decision-making, surgical trainees require formal ethics education as a foundation, concurrent with 'bedside' ethics education [6].

Academic exploration may be another way for interested learners to pursue ethics education. Grossman et al. encouraged residents to analyze and publish their own experiences formally, in order to improve ethics education and engage surgical trainees effectively [7].

11.4 Formal Ethics Education

Many pedagogical methods have been utilized to add ethics into surgical education, with varying degrees of success, and with such success being difficult to measure. The goals of ethics curricula include teaching students to identify and manage ethical issues in practice, ensuring trainees develop core knowledge, skills, and competencies in bioethics, improving confidence in surgical ethics and shared decision-making, enabling the practice of moral and ethical medicine, and providing space for moral reasoning. [1, 15, 17–19]. As many trainees enter medicine with a science background, formal ethics education often first begins in medical school [9].

Thirunavukarasu et al. demonstrated that surgical trainees deal with the same ethical issues repeatedly on specific rotations, and an ethics education can address gaps in knowledge and improve trainees' confidence in ethical decision-making [19]. Additionally, both the Royal College of Physicians and Surgeons of Canada (RCPSC) and the American College of Surgeons (ACS) in the United States recognize competency in ethics as an essential component of being a good surgeon [2]. Both Colleges have constructed their curriculums to cover areas they view as critical.

The RCPSC includes ten modules that focus on the following: truth telling, consent and capacity, disclosure, substitute decision-making, confidentiality, conflict of interest, surgical competence, end of life issues, resource allocation, and research ethics [2]. Similarly, the ACS Ethics Curriculum for Surgical Residents consists of six chapters which cover: conflict of interest, professional obligations of surgeons, substitute decision-making, truth telling and communication, end of life issues, and confidentiality [2]. In a 2010 survey of 113 surgical program directors, most had an established surgical ethics curriculum [7]. A mixed modality of educational methods is often used when designing and implementing ethics curricula in surgical programs [7].

11.5   Lectures

Lectures are beneficial when background information or frameworks lend themselves to be taught in a topic specific manner, for example teaching the principles of the consent process or how to make a capacity determination [20]. There is a heavy reliance on lecture series for ethics education due to its ease of knowledge exchange in an organized manner, but mixed modalities promote active learning and is more appealing for learners [7].

11.6   Case-Based Learning

Case based learning moves surgical ethics from the abstract principles to the concrete and applicable, thus is a popular modality within ethics education through lectures or small-group work [21]. A positive aspect of live case-based ethics discussions is the promotion of participation and inclusivity of those in attendance [6]. For instance, Snelgrove et al. noted in their study on Ethics Morbidity and Mortality rounds, that an open discussion of cases minimized the surgical hierarchy that often makes trainees reluctant to speak up in a group forum [8]. When done temporally with real scenarios, a case-based format also allows for diversity of voices in a multidisciplinary team, some of which may include lawyers, chaplains, and ethics consult teams [22]. Cases can be chosen based on specific ethical principles demonstrated and relevant facts of the case, which may aid and elucidate lecture topics [6]. An important study demonstrated that a case-based ethics program with a primary focus on end of life care resulted in an increase in documented discussions regarding care and a decreased duration of hospitalization among dying patients in the intensive-care unit [23].

11.7   Small-Group Learning

Small-group learning has numerous advantages, as it is a method that sparks discussion and opinions, encouraging the exchange of various values and beliefs [24]. Small group learning employs vignettes and open-ended questions, which can either be broad or specific such as, *"Has anyone encountered a situation like this before?"* to *"What do we think about undertaking a treatment not detailed on the consent form?"* [24] For maximum efficacy, small group learning should incorporate facilitators who correct factual errors gently, who do not interrupt contributors, and who encourage a diversity of opinions [24].

11.8   Role-Play/Standardized Patients

Another valuable approach to ethics education is role-play. Trainees are presented with instructions about priorities, responsibilities, or roles and learn through scenarios, such as a preoperative interview or office visit [24]. It is beneficial for trainees to assume the roles of others such as patients, caregivers, nursing staff, etc. in order to gain an understanding of complex circumstances from different points-of-view [24].

A similar strategy to role-play is integrating standardized patients for trainees to engage with. These are trained actors that provide trainees with an experience that closely mimics issues in surgical practice [25] and the opportunity to discuss and resolve ethical issues in a low-stakes environment. If done in the audience of peers, trainees might also learn from others and provide with feedback [25]. Incorporating video review for feedback so that trainees can discern what they executed well and what areas they need to improve on, is also helpful [20]. However, the use of standardized patients is not always superior to more traditional formats, as shown by Robb et al., and ought to be used selectively depending on the goal and content of the educational session [26].

11.9   Ethics Morbidity and Mortality Rounds

Ethics morbidity and mortality (M&M) rounds refers to devoting time during surgical M&M rounds to discuss a case with a moral dilemma. Ethics M&M rounds utilize real cases, adding an aspect of reality and complexity seen with ethical quandaries in the practice of surgery, reflecting the "complex and value-laden world of clinical ward medicine." [27] An opportunity to work through the case with a preceptor is presented in advance, potentially guided by a template and supported by literature search. When contrasted with traditional methods of ethics education, in one academic center, traditional methods were perceived by participants as disconnected from surgical practice, with surgeons' uncertain about applying their knowledge of ethics [27]. Conversely, it was determined that ethics morbidity and mortality rounds made ethics education engaging, integral to surgical practice, valuable, and relevant [27]. Ethics morbidity and mortality rounds encourages participants to elucidate ethical issues and learn frameworks, allowing them to learn the "language" of ethics, promoting dialogue and critical reflection among the participants [4].

11.10 Challenges to Surgical Ethics Education

There are challenges inherent to implementing ethics curricula, including the time, perceived faculty ethics expertise, and lack of faculty interest [5, 9, 28]. Further, in a survey 94% of U.S. program directors (44% response rate) believed the current level of ethics education to be adequate in preparing residents to handle ethically challenging situations [7]. Being connected with a bioethics center can assist in overcoming some of these barriers. Bioethics centers may be able to support specific curriculum development and assist physician-ethicist faculty interested in ethics education, acting as a centralized support [7, 18]. Effective bioethics centers offer mixed modalities of ethics education. For instance, the Johns Hopkins Berman Institute of Bioethics integrates small group learning, residents' own experiences aided by discussion, provision of frameworks, practice through the utilization of standardized patients, and constructive feedback from faculty and peers [9].

Another challenge to ethics education is that ethical issues are ever present and constantly evolving thus resulting ethics education needs to be relevant and applicable; with delivery at various time-points throughout a surgeon's career i.e. from medical students to practicing surgeons-in-chief [2]. Different levels of experience and responsibility must be taken into consideration when determining appropriate ethics education [2]. Notwithstanding which phase of their career a surgeon is in, mixed methods of ethics education are beneficial as they provide overarching ethical values, principles, and frameworks relevant to everyone [27]. For example, ethics morbidity and mortality rounds presented in the same format as the already occurring surgical morbidity and mortality rounds format can provide an educational opportunity applicable to all attendees from various disciplines and levels of experience [21]. Challenges to surgical ethics education must be recognized and addressed.

Finally, the culture of surgery includes ethics issues not often addressed within non-surgical ethics training [3, 10]. In addition to the anticipated ethics issues that surgical trainees face such as consent and end of life decisions, surgical trainees may encounter ethical dilemmas related to the nature of surgical education in general, such as disagreement with faculty about clinical decisions or questions about surgical innovation or research [3, 10]. Formal surgical education needs to encompass not only the ethics issues affecting patients, but also those that surgical trainees face in their learning environments.

11.11   Assessment of Learning

Whether or not ethics education can or should be assessed is a matter of debate. Surgical training programs vary in their employment of tests to assess trainees' ethics knowledge often utilizing traditional testing, such written examinations. Brewster et al. compared ethics knowledge between post-graduate year 1 (PGY-1) residents and more senior residents. While the confidence levels of both groups were comparable, both groups showed low test scores, with the PGY-1 students outperforming senior residents. Similarly, a couple of studies tested residents before and after implementing an ethics curriculum [20, 29]. In one, through post-test evaluations, confidence levels of residents increased, but given post-test scores ranging from 42% to 90%, the authors acknowledged the challenges of utilizing a survey to test ethics knowledge [20].

In a study of orthopedic residents, knowledge about ethics improved in the group that had a curriculum specific to orthopedics [29]. Moreover, some programs appreciate the complexity of testing ethics education and may not test students in a formal manner [1]. Helft aptly discusses the difficulty of measuring virtue and suggests that the focus should be on developing a student's ability to handle ethical dilemmas rather than obtaining good results on standardized testing [17]. Holloran e.t al.'s study on case-based teaching in the ICU is poignant as it evaluates the central goal of ethics education improvements to everyday patient care-rather than simply improvement via in assessments [23]. Qualitative approaches to evaluation may yield evidence of transformative changes in learners that may not be exclusively related to "knowledge", but rather a maturity that occurs through critical reflection.

11.12   Case Resolution

The case we present is a common occurrence in academic surgery, where moral distress may be present in the resident because of a conflict of obligations to the patient and to the attending. There are a multitude of ethics issues that could be explored through the case, including: was the process of informed consent adequate, and how do we manage the conflict of obligation between duty to teach and duty to provide patient care? There are many different methods one could use to accomplish some of the learning points.

Informally, it may appear that the unintended dominant message of the hidden curriculum is that expectations for a patient receiving emergency care are different from the expectations of patients receiving elective surgery. Ideally, this attending physician may have confidence in their chief resident and wishes to foster autonomy in the learning process, recognizing that future patients will benefit from resident entrustment towards independent surgery during their training; however, the attending has not made this explicit.

There are concerns about respect for patient autonomy in the case as described, and the attending in this case might have used this opportunity to explore the resident's concern further. However, depending on the duties and values created by a hierarchical system, the resident may not have wished to contradict the attending, leading to the issue of moral distress for the resident. Formally, a group learning or lecture format regarding the process of informed consent and resident supervision could provide definitions and standards that could help reconcile future management of these conflicts. Using the M&M format to delve deeper into ethics issues surrounding surgical education would likely prove useful.

11.13   Conclusion

The field of surgery demands moral awareness in addition to technical excellence [7]. Ethics education is a complex yet important task and can take many forms. Despite challenges, great strides have recently been made to explicitly define surgical ethics education and evaluation, with the ultimate goal of improving surgical care.

11.14   Selected References

- Brewster LP, Hall DE, Joehl RJ. Assessing residents in surgical ethics: we do it a lot; we only know a little. J Surg Res. 2011;171(2):395–8. https://doi.org/10.1016/j.jss.2011.04.008.

  - Despite clinical experience, ethics knowledge can be poor, thus ethics education is essential for surgical residents.
- Helft PR, Eckles RE, Torbeck L. Ethics education in surgical residency programs: a review of the literature. J Surg Educ. 2009;66(1):35–42. https://doi.org/10.1016/j.jsurg.2008.10.001.

  - A review of the literature on ethics education in postgraduate surgical training programs.
- Keune JD, Kodner IJ. The importance of an ethics curriculum in surgical education. World J Surg. 2014;38(7): 1581–6. https://doi.org/10.1007/s00268-014-2569-0.

  - This paper discusses the benefits of ethics curriculum in surgical education.
- Klingensmith ME. Teaching ethics in surgical training programs using a case-based format. J Surg Educ. 2008;65(2):126–8. https://doi.org/10.1016/j.jsurg.2007.12.001.

  - This paper discusses the use of a monthly, case-based learning as a method of teaching ethics including aspects instrumental for success.

- Snelgrove R, Ng SL, Devon K. Reconceptualizing ethics through morbidity and mortality rounds. J Am Coll Surg. 2020;231(2):244–248.e3. https://doi.org/10.1016/j.jamcollsurg.2020.04.038.

  – Morbidity and Mortality rounds makes ethics education engaging and relevant to participants, allowing for transformative learning to occur.

References

1. Keune JD, Kodner IJ. The importance of an ethics curriculum in surgical education. World J Surg. 2014;38(7):1581–6. https://doi.org/10.1007/s00268-014-2569-0.
2. Kodner IJ. Ethics curricula in surgery: needs and approaches. World J Surg. 2003;27(8):952–6. https://doi.org/10.1007/s00268-003-7173-7.
3. Knifed E, Goyal A, Bernstein M. Moral angst for surgical residents: a qualitative study. Am J Surg. 2010;199(4):571–6. https://doi.org/10.1016/j.amjsurg.2009.04.007.
4. Ganai S, Devon KM. Teaching surgical ethics. In: Kohler TS, Schwartz B, editors. Surgeons as educators. A guide for academic development and teaching excellence. Springer; 2018. p. 377–85.
5. Downing MT, Way DP, Caniano DA. Results of a national survey on ethics education in general surgery residency programs. Am J Surg. 1997;174(3):364–8. https://doi.org/10.1016/s0002-9610(97)00112-8.
6. Scott KK, Chesire DJ, Burns JB Jr, Nussbaum MS. Proficiency of surgical faculty and residents with ethical dilemmas: is modeling enough? J Surg Educ. 2012;69(6):780–4. https://doi.org/10.1016/j.jsurg.2012.04.014.
7. Grossman E, Posner MC, Angelos P. Ethics education in surgical residency: past, present, and future. Surgery. 2010;147(1):114–9. https://doi.org/10.1016/j.surg.2009.04.011.
8. Snelgrove R, Ng S, Devon K. Ethics M&Ms: toward a recognition of ethics in everyday practice. J Grad Med Educ. 2016;8(3):462–4. https://doi.org/10.4300/JGME-D-15-00645.1.
9. Brewster LP, Hall DE, Joehl RJ. Assessing residents in surgical ethics: we do it a lot; we only know a little. J Surg Res. 2011;171(2):395–8. https://doi.org/10.1016/j.jss.2011.04.008.
10. Howard F, McKneally MF, Upshur RE, Levin AV. The formal and informal surgical ethics curriculum: views of resident and staff surgeons in Toronto. Am J Surg. 2012;203(2):258–65. https://doi.org/10.1016/j.amjsurg.2011.02.008.
11. Hafferty FW, Franks R. The hidden curriculum, ethics teaching, and the structure of medical education. Acad Med. 1994;69(11):861–71. https://doi.org/10.1097/00001888-199411000-00001.
12. Hafferty F, Castellani B. The hidden curriculum: a theory of medical education. In: Brosnan C, Turner BS, editors. Handbook of the sociology of medical education. Routledge; 2009. p. 15–35.
13. Mahajan R, Aruldhas BW, Sharma M, Badyal DK, Singh T. Professionalism and ethics: a proposed curriculum for undergraduates. Int J Appl Basic Med Res. 2016;6(3):157–63. https://doi.org/10.4103/2229-516X.186963.
14. Mahood SC. Medical education: beware the hidden curriculum. Can Fam Physician. 2011;57(9):983–5. PMID: 21918135
15. Siegler M. A legacy of Osler. Teaching clinical ethics at the bedside. JAMA. 1978;239(10):951–6. https://doi.org/10.1001/jama.239.10.951.
16. Jonsen AR. Ethicist's heyday. Am Rev Respir Dis. 1976;113:5–6.
17. Helft PR, Eckles RE, Torbeck L. Ethics education in surgical residency programs: a review of the literature. J Surg Educ. 2009;66(1):35–42. https://doi.org/10.1016/j.jsurg.2008.10.001.
18. Howard F, McKneally MF, Levin AV. Integrating bioethics into postgraduate medical education: the University of Toronto model. Acad Med. 2010;85(6):1035–40. https://doi.org/10.1097/ACM.0b013e3181dbebb8.

19. Thirunavukarasu P, Brewster LP, Pecora SM, Hall DE. Educational intervention is effective in improving knowledge and confidence in surgical ethics-a prospective study. Am J Surg. 2010;200(5):665–9. https://doi.org/10.1016/j.amjsurg.2010.08.002.
20. Angelos P, Da Rosa DA, Derossis AM, Kim B. Medical ethics curriculum for surgical residents: results of a pilot project. Surgery. 1999;126:701–7. https://doi.org/10.1016/s0039-6060(99)70125-x.
21. Devon K, Sade RM. Surgical ethics: how I teach it. Ann Thorac Surg. 2020;110:1805–8. https://doi.org/10.1016/j.athoracsur.2020.07.010.
22. Klingensmith ME. Teaching ethics in surgical training programs using a case-based format. J Surg Educ. 2008;65(2):126–8. https://doi.org/10.1016/j.jsurg.2007.12.001.
23. Holloran SD, Starkey GW, Burke PA, Steele G, Forse RA. An educational intervention in the surgical intensive care unit to improve ethical decisions. Surgery. 1995;118(2):294–9. https://doi.org/10.1016/s0039-6060(05)80337-x.
24. Johnston C. Teaching ethics in the operating theatre by small group teaching. Clin Teach. 2010;7(4):240–3. https://doi.org/10.1111/j.1743-498X.2010.00397.x.
25. Moon MR, Hughes MT, Chen JY, Khaira K, Lipsett P, Carrese JA. Ethics skills laboratory experience for surgery interns. J Surg Educ. 2014;71(6):829–38. https://doi.org/10.1016/j.jsurg.2014.03.010.
26. Robb A, Etchells E, Cusimano MD, Cohen R, Singer PA, McKneally M. A randomized trial of teaching bioethics to surgical residents. Am J Surg. 2005;189:453–7. https://doi.org/10.1016/j.amsurg.2004.08.066.
27. Snelgrove R, Ng SL, Devon K. Reconceptualizing ethics through morbidity and mortality rounds. J Am Coll Surg. 2020;231(2):244–248.e3. https://doi.org/10.1016/j.jamcollsurg.2020.04.038.
28. Levin AV, Berry S, Kassardjian CD, Howard F, McKneally M. "Ethics teaching is as important as my clinical education": a survey of participants in residency education at a single university. UTMJ. 2006;84(1):60–3.
29. Wenger NS, Liu H, Lieberman JR. Teaching medical ethics to orthopaedic surgery residents. J Bone Joint Surg Am. 1998;80:1125–31.

Chapter 12
Communication During Awake Surgery: Training Residents and Disclosure to Patients

Kristina Guyton ⓘ

Abstract As local anesthetic techniques have improved, awake procedures are increasingly utilized. During awake surgical procedures the patient has real-time awareness of the operative process. Surgeon communication with the patient, management of the patient's emotional reactions, and patient trust in the provider all contribute to the success of the awake surgery. Involvement of surgical trainees in operative procedures—including awake procedures—is an integral part of surgical training. Disclosure and discussion of trainee involvement increasingly is recognized as important in respecting patient autonomy. Awake surgical procedures present unique ethical challenges in surgeon-patient communication and in trainee involvement.

Keywords Surgical resident/trainee · Surgeon-patient communication · Awake surgery · Trainee involvement · Patient disclosure · Resident role

12.1 Clinical Scenario

Mr. Smith is a 67-year-old man with carpal tunnel syndrome. He undergoes a right carpal tunnel release under local anesthetic. He follows up in clinic two weeks later and demonstrates symptomatic improvement and appropriate healing; yet he seems withdrawn. He does not say anything to the surgeon but mentions to the nurse that during the surgery he heard the surgeon teaching someone else how to do the procedure and whispering corrections. He doesn't know who did his surgery and he doesn't feel that the surgery was done well. Mr. Smith leaves poor reviews and does not recommend the surgeon or institution to family or friends.

K. Guyton (✉)
Department of Surgery, University of Iowa, Iowa City, IA, USA
e-mail: kristina-guyton@uiowa.edu

© The Author(s), under exclusive license to Springer Nature
Switzerland AG 2022
V. A. Lonchyna et al. (eds.), *Difficult Decisions in Surgical Ethics*, Difficult
Decisions in Surgery: An Evidence-Based Approach,
https://doi.org/10.1007/978-3-030-84625-1_12

12.2 Ethical Problem

Despite appropriate medical care and a good outcome, the patient does not feel that he was adequately cared for. This impacts his impression of the care he received, and he is ultimately dissatisfied.

12.3 Introduction

Surgeons often attribute patient satisfaction to technical success of the surgery. However, many aspects of the patient's experience influence their assessment of their overall care; thereby impacting their perception of the surgical outcome and their likeliness to recommend their surgeon to other people. Patient experience is an increasingly utilized marker of quality. Interventions to enhance the perioperative experience improve overall patient satisfaction [1]. This effect has been demonstrated in situations where patients have little to no awareness or memory of the procedure itself. In contrast, during awake surgery the patient directly experiences and participates in the performance of surgery. The patient is fully alert, often scared, and listening intently. Surgeons who perform and teach awake procedures develop distinct skills and techniques to manage the patient's intraprocedural experience and incorporate trainees.

12.4 Search Strategy

The search terms utilized: Awake surgical/procedural communication, awake surgery, surgeon patient communication, ethics, local anesthesia, anxiety, resident, resident participation, teaching, consent. Search of the PubMed database was conducted using combinations of these search terms. 8058 articles were identified in the search results. Some additional articles were identified from the references of the articles encountered. 24 of the articles reviewed contributed unique perspectives in the development of this chapter.

12.5 Awake Procedures

Awake procedures constitute a wide range of practices in many different fields of medicine (see Table 12.1). While in this chapter the word 'surgeon' is utilized, the techniques described are not limited to use only within the surgical field. These communication techniques may be useful for any proceduralist or assistant involved in awake procedures. Table 12.1 lists many specialties which utilize awake surgical procedures. The list grows larger when including more formal procedures where

Table 12.1 Examples of frequently performed awake or semi-awake procedures by specialty

Medical Specialty	Procedure
Anesthesiology	Epidural placement, nerve block
Cardiology	Pacemaker placement, cardiac catheterization
Dermatology	Cyst excision, Mohs excision, punch biopsy, skin lesion excision
Gastroenterology/ Colorectal surgery	Upper endoscopy, colonoscopy, flexible sigmoidoscopy
General Surgery	Abscess drainage, central line placement, port placement
Interventional Radiology	Imaging guided biopsy or drain placement, port placement
Neurosurgery	Lumbar puncture, craniotomy
Obstetrics and Gynecology	IUD placement, colposcopy, uterine biopsies, vaginal delivery, cesarean section with epidural, D&Cs, early abortions
Orthopedics	Extremity surgery with nerve block
Ophthalmology	Cataract surgery, eyelid blepharoplasty
Otolaryngology	Laryngoscopy
Plastic Surgery	Skin lesion removal
Urology	Vasectomy, prostate biopsy, cystoscopy
Vascular	Vein ablation, dialysis access, angiogram

patients are given some degree of anxiolysis or sedation and less formal procedures done at the bedside in the hospital and clinic (e.g., placement of intravenous catheters, nasogastric tubes or foley catheters). A procedure with little or no sedation offers the advantages of lower cost, shorter patient recovery time, greater flexibility in location of procedure, and a shorter hospital visit. However, awake procedures can be quite anxiety provoking for the patient [2, 3].

The foundation of the doctor-patient relationship is establishment of trust. Trust is a necessary component of every surgeon-patient relationship as performance of any procedure requires patient relinquishment of situational control. For awake procedures, the patient will directly experience and participate in the procedure, amplifying patient vulnerability. Successful completion depends on the awake patient continuously deciding to cooperate to allow the procedure to continue. Unlike under general anesthesia, the awake patient retains capacity to revoke consent for the procedure at any time even in the middle of a complex surgery [4]. During awake procedures, surgeon-patient trust must be actively maintained with communication and management of pain and anxiety.

Development of trust prior to an awake surgical procedure can be challenging. The patient must be convinced of the necessity of the procedure and must develop a confidence that it will be performed well. Preexisting factors that contribute to trust include institutional reputation, surgeon reputation, and the patient's prior experiences with medical care. Potentially modifiable factors include the development of surgeon-patient rapport and the explanation of the disease process and the proposed intervention. Patients need to feel confident that the provider will effectively perform the procedure as well as manage their pain and anxiety during an awake procedure. Ultimately, a proceduralist must develop patient trust and create an environment in which the patient is willing to be vulnerable. While we cannot make patients completely comfortable there are many techniques that can be utilized to increase comfort and decrease anxiety.

12.6 Awake Procedure Communication

Awake surgical procedures pose unique challenges for both the physician-directed care team and the patient. Successful management of patient anxiety during awake procedures requires constant patient reassurance while minimizing pain and anxiety-provoking stimuli. Pain management is frequently achieved with local anesthetic, whether injected or topical; it but can also be achieved with regional nerve blocks. Even with adequate pain control, many factors contribute to patient anxiety. Anxiety-provoking stimuli include seeing aspects of the surgery or surgical instruments, feeling tugging or pressure, hearing sounds associated with the procedure like the buzz of the cautery device or clicks of instruments, and smelling odors of antiseptics or cauterized tissue. Perhaps the most influential facet of awake surgery are the words, phrases, and tones of voice that the surgeon and staff use to communicate with each other and with the patient [5].

Surgeons who frequently perform awake procedures describe various techniques for communication with the alert patient. Management of patient expectations begins in the office when discussing the procedure; this continues into the periprocedural and intraprocedural settings with explanation of the steps of the procedure; and on-going instructions prepare the patient for any anticipated change in stimulation or sensation. Surgeons frequently check in with the patient during the procedure regarding their physical and emotional comfort. This allows modification of the local anesthetic or reassurance to help the patient through the procedure. The surgeon can bring attention to the procedure through explaining and teaching the patient or they can distract the patient from the experience by talking about unrelated topics. Surgeons frequently cite discussing the patient's job, family, pets, vacations, sports, etc.—tailoring the conversation to their patient. Depending on the procedure, it may work best for another team member to be the one communicating with the patient [5]. Some providers advocate for inclusion of a family member in the procedure room [6]. For some procedures, less interactive communication may be necessary to avoid patient movement and methods of distraction may include playing music, hypnosis or utilizing a virtual reality headset [7].

Whether they are actively included in the conversation, the awake patient is listening carefully. Surgeons who perform awake procedures recognize that words, phrases, and tone of voice contribute to patient anxiety. Many avoid certain words like 'knife' or 'blade' and utilize a number, code word or hand motion instead: 'please pass me a 15.' During awake procedures surgeons try to avoid any verbal indication of error or intonation of alarm or anxiety in their voice. It is very helpful for the surgeon to have the assistance of experienced staff who are familiar with the procedure as this decreases the required technical communication [5].

Unique to awake procedures is the intraprocedural or intraoperative experience of the patient. With standard anesthesia—whether general or monitored anesthesia or even proceduralist directed sedation (e.g., colonoscopies)—there is a component of periprocedural amnesia for the patient. With the patient sedated or asleep, the surgical team is more at liberty to discuss the technical aspects of the case, to hold conversations about unrelated topics, or to teach without considering or needing to involve a listening patient. With an awake patient, some of that typical conversation does not occur or is intentionally hidden from the patient. Here the surgeon must balance respect for patient autonomy and nonmaleficence, not causing unnecessary anxiety or distress as a result of conversation overheard from the surgical team. Table 12.2 outlines the interplay between ethical principles during awake surgical procedures.

12.7   Ethical Challenges of Awake Surgical Communication

Much of the communication during awake surgery falls into the realm of what Dr. Komesaroff termed 'microethics': the ethics of everyday clinical practice [8, 9]. As Dr. Truog describes it, microethics "is unique to each situation, arises spontaneously at a particular moment in time, and is created in the relational space between the participants [see Table 12.2]. It is inextricably connected to the verbal and

Table 12.2 Ethical principles involved in communication with patients during awake procedures

Patient autonomy
• Respect for the patient as an independent decision maker
• Right to know and understand what is happening with their medical care
• Right to decide if they are comfortable proceeding with an awake procedure
• Disclosure of trainee involvement in their care
Nonmaleficence
• Minimize undue worry or distress prior to the procedure
• Minimize discomfort both physically and emotionally during the procedure
• Ensure no harm to the patient by including a trainee
Beneficence
• Facilitating early return to normal activities
• Efficient care of the medical condition
• Reassurance and education during the procedure
• Opportunity to strengthen the physician-patient relationship
Justice
• Minimizing resource utilization
• Facilitating early return of the patient to normal activities
• Training the next generation of physicians in specialized surgical techniques and communication
• Ensure trainees are not involved only in the setting of more vulnerable populations

nonverbal ways in which we communicate." [9]. He gives the example of a clinician choosing between the words "fetus" and "baby" when counseling a young woman after finding out about an unplanned pregnancy. These choices include "the most appropriate way to approach the patient, to talk with him, to allay his fears and to establish the common ground on which mutual decisions can be taken" [8]. Microethics considers the impact that these small choices can have on the patient's emotions and decisions. Word choice, tone of voice, and the environment of the conversation can impact a patient's perception of their choices and options.

12.8   Trainees in Awake Surgical Procedures

Few surgeons learn their awake surgical communication techniques through formal teaching. Most develop their methods through participation in awake procedures during training and through observation of attendings' techniques and styles; they subsequently trial these different approaches with their own patients. These procedures are frequently performed, many providers express insecurity about their communication methods and wish to improve upon their awake procedure communication. Each of these physicians learned communication techniques by working in training with other surgeons. Adding a trainee to the team in awake surgery adds additional ethical and communication challenges for the surgeon to manage [5].

12.9   Surgical Training

Surgical training has evolved over time from an individual apprenticeship to a model of graduated responsibility assisting in caring for patients of numerous attending surgeons. Training transitions from the clinic and inpatient wards to operative procedures, starting with lower complexity, increasing in technical difficulty over time. Integral to this process is participation in procedures with gradual acquisition and mastery of technical skills. Trainee involvement in and education during operative procedures is an essential part of surgical training.

The medical profession has a responsibility to train the next generation of physicians in both technical and professional skills required to successfully practice independently. Trainees make up the primary workforce at teaching hospitals. Historically, the medical field has not been transparent about the level of independence of trainees in surgical procedures. Articles and lawsuits exposing concerns regarding trainee oversight have undermined the general public's confidence in this process. While all recognize that it is necessary to train the next generation of surgeons, no patient wants to feel that they are potentially receiving inferior care. Patients have legitimate concerns about the involvement of trainees. The historical adage of "see one, do one, teach one" does not emphasize an evaluation of competence or technical mastery. In response to public concern the pendulum of resident oversight has swung back. Modern training has increased oversight of trainees. Less frequently are trainees performing surgeries or procedures completely independently without the involvement or oversight of an attending surgeon [10, 11].

12.10   Disclosure of Resident Involvement

Increasingly, disclosure and discussion of trainee involvement is recognized as critical in respecting patient autonomy. While there is a responsibility to society to train the next generation of physicians and surgeons in the art and craft of awake surgery, this must be balanced with respect for patient autonomy. Disclosure of trainee participation, discussion of roles, and consent for resident involvement differs widely by institution and physician practice. When discussed preoperatively in a scripted manner, patients are typically very accepting of trainee involvement in their care [12, 13]. More resistance is encountered if the patient feels the teaching is hidden. Discussion of trainee participation is most well accepted by patients when disclosed by the attending surgeon in advance of the day of surgery [14, 15]. Often this is incorporated into the preoperative consent discussion. Understandably, patients who may not understand the training structure can be quite frustrated when not informed of resident involvement until right before the procedure and are surprised by the information when it is "too late" to object. Willingness to have residents involved with their care improves with education on roles and setting expectations [16–18]. Conversely, more detail could adversely impact willingness to have residents involved [12].

A frequently cited patient concern about involvement of surgical trainees is that the surgical trainee is not the surgeon with whom the patient consented to have the surgery. Only meeting the trainee the day of surgery or after surgery, patients don't have the same opportunity to build a trusting relationship with the trainee. Their trust must be built within a few moments before surgery or it must form as an extension of the trusting relationship built with the attending surgeon. Often their concern is for inadequate or suboptimal surgery in the hands of a trainee. Interestingly, studies demonstrate that while procedures with residents may not be as fast, there is no evidence of lower quality or higher rates of complications [19–21]. Rather, in the setting of colonoscopy, adenoma detection rate (a marker for quality) tends to be a reflection of the instructing surgeon rather than the trainee [22, 23].

12.11   Modifying Communication with the Awake Patient

The level of anesthesia a patient receives alters the quantity, type, and content of communication the surgeon has with both the patient and the trainee. In the setting where deeper anesthesia is induced—resulting in less patient awareness and involvement—the surgeon may focus more on the technical aspects of the case, teaching aloud without intentional patient inclusion. When patients are awake and listening during procedures, surgeons can modify communication with their staff and assistants—operating, communicating, and teaching while patients are awake to positively influence the patient experience.

Striking the appropriate balance between open communication and hiding potentially distressing aspects of awake procedures from the patient can be challenging. While we strive for transparency, there are certain words or phrases that will distress even the most understanding patient, such as 'oops' and 'oh no'. There is clear benefit to the patient's emotional wellbeing to hide these emotions and reactions while performing a procedure. Remaining calm and using neutral language is important for the surgeon, the trainee, and any assistants. Trainees add an additional degree of unpredictability to an awake procedure which may make verbal slips like this more likely. Whispering and nonverbal communication may also be interpreted by patients as an attempt to conceal information and cause unnecessary distress [5].

12.12 Communication with the Trainee during Awake Procedures

While communication during an awake procedure typically revolves around patient comfort and completion of the procedure, involvement of a trainee may alter intraoperative communication content and techniques. Teaching during awake procedures must account for the real-time patient awareness of the teaching process. Preoperative discussion of teaching is critical to make this a comfortable experience for the patient. If there is honest disclosure of trainee involvement, the teaching discussion does not have to be hidden; rather it can be used as an opportunity to educate both the trainee and the patient. Some surgeons specifically involve the patient in the teaching discussion, teaching both the student and the patient [5].

Not all teaching about the procedure needs to take place in front of the patient. Some surgeons use preoperative discussion and postoperative debriefing with the trainee to make the intraoperative teaching more succinct. This preoperative time can also be used to set trainee expectations and ground rules as to what they should expect to experience, say, and do during the procedure. While, in one light, this may be seen as hiding the teaching or the level of the trainee, it could also be reasoned that this is adequate preparation prior to and appropriate debriefing after the procedure. These adjustments work to balance transparent communication respecting patient autonomy and the responsibility to teach these skills to the next generation [5].

It is also important to consider resident responses to their experiences with awake procedures. This is a challenging position to be in for a trainee; they report hesitating to ask questions and feeling frustrated when the attending takes over the procedure. Interviews with residents emphasized the benefit of preprocedural preparation of both the patient and the trainee: disclosure of trainee involvement to the patient; antecedent preparation of the trainee on the steps of the procedure; how to communicate during the procedure; and what parts of the procedure they should expect to be involved in. Interestingly, whispering and nonverbal communication could be both effective techniques when helping to guide the trainee in the next step and potential sources of discomfort to the patient if they were felt to be deceptive regarding who was performing the procedure. Residents noted that if they were involved in the consent process more details about the steps of the procedure were included to adequately prepare the patient for the experience of an awake procedure including management of discomfort and anxiety [24].

12.13   Clinical Scenario Revisited

During Mr. Smith's preoperative clinic visit, the initial history and physical is performed by a trainee. This is followed by examination and discussion with the attending surgeon, Dr. Jones. The surgeon discusses the recommended procedure and what to expect on the day of surgery and for recovery. Dr. Jones says, "Mr. Smith, thank you for talking with our resident today. Teaching the next generation of surgeons is an important part of what I do. Residents will be involved in multiple parts of your care, but please understand that I will be responsible for and directing every aspect of your care. What questions or concerns can I address for you?"

The morning of surgery the resident introduces herself to Mr. Smith. Prior to entering the operating room, Dr. Jones and the resident discuss the technical aspects of the case and set ground rules for their communication during the procedure. During the procedure, Dr. Jones utilizes techniques to distract Mr. Smith, talking about his work, but also teaches the surgical resident about important aspects of the case, including Mr. Smith in the discussion. At his follow up visit, Mr. Smith asks Dr. Jones about the resident who participated in the case, stating "I was so impressed with her. Doc, she can be my doctor after you retire. I've been telling everyone I know what a great experience I had."

12.14   Clinical Scenario Review

Discussion of trainee involvement at the preoperative visit gives the patient advance notice of the interaction, allowing him to have time to consider the arrangement and withdraw consent if desired. The surgeon outlines his/her assumption of responsibility for the patient's care and dedication to surgical education. Then the surgeon asks about questions in a manner which indicates that she expects him to have questions, decreasing the barrier to asking a question. Finally, Dr. Jones utilizes intraprocedural communication techniques to minimize distressing components of the procedure and maximize the comfort of the patient. Ultimately, this results in a positive perceived outcome for the patient.

12.15   Conclusion

Awake surgical procedures are efficient and cost effective for both the patient and the surgeon. Success of the procedure depends on the surgeon's ability to keep the patient calm and relaxed. Management of the patient experience during awake procedures can be multifactorial: modify the environment, alter methods of communication, and distract the patient from the details of the procedure. These techniques are primarily taught indirectly as trainees participate in awake surgeries with the attending surgeon. During awake surgical procedures the patient has real-time awareness of the teaching process. This poses unique ethical challenges in surgeon-patient communication and trainee involvement. With advanced disclosure to the patient and preemptive teaching to the trainee, teaching during awake surgical procedures can be a valuable and rewarding experience for both the patient and the trainee.

12.16   Selected References

- Smith CS, Guyton K, Pariser JJ, Siegler M, Schindler N, Langerman A. Surgeon-patient communication during awake procedures. Am J Surg. 2017;213(6):996–1002.e1. https://doi.org/10.1016/j.amjsurg.2016.06.017

  – This is a thematic analysis of focused surgeon interviews regarding communication techniques utilized during awake procedures. Surgeons were also questioned regarding any prior training that they had received for these procedures and methods they utilized to manage trainee involvement.

- Truog RD, Brown SD, Browning D, et al. Microethics: The ethics of everyday clinical practice. Hastings Cent Rep. 2015;45(1):11–17. https://doi.org/10.1002/hast.413

  – This essay is a compelling argument to include discussion of microethics within medical ethics education. Microethics are the small choices made from moment to moment in clinical encounters which influence the patient ethical decisions. This perspective helps students understand the impact a small thing like word choice can have on a patient's emotional reactions and decisions.

- Gamboa J, Cameron MC, Fathi R, Alkousakis T. A review of non-pharmacologic approaches to enhance the patient experience in dermatologic surgery. Dermatol. Online J. 2020;26(3). Accessed March 15, 2021. https://escholarship.org/uc/item/7mp372nd

- This review is a thorough discussion of non-pharmacologic approaches to optimize the patient experience during awake procedures. Adjuncts discussed include mechanoanesthesia, cold therapy, verbal and audiovisual distraction, music, optimal needle insertion methods, hypnosis and guided-imagery, perioperative communication and educational strategies

References

1. Chow A, Mayer EK, Darzi AW, Athanasiou T. Patient-reported outcome measures: the importance of patient satisfaction in surgery. Surgery. 2009;146:435–43. https://doi.org/10.1016/j.surg.2009.03.019.
2. Caddick J, Jawad S, Southern S, Majumder S. The power of words: sources of anxiety in patients undergoing local anaesthetic plastic surgery. Ann R Coll Surg Engl. 2012;94(2):94–8. https://doi.org/10.1309/003588412x13171221501267.
3. Mitchell M. Conscious surgery: influence of the environment on patient anxiety. J Adv Nurs. 2008;64(3):261–71. https://doi.org/10.1111/j.1365-2648.2008.04769.x.
4. Ford PJ, Boulis NM, Montgomery EB, Rezai AR. A patient revoking consent during awake craniotomy: an ethical challenge. Neuromodulation. 2007;10(4):329–32. https://doi.org/10.1111/j.1525-1403.2007.00119.x.
5. Smith CS, Guyton K, Pariser JJ, Siegler M, Schindler N, Langerman A. Surgeon-patient communication during awake procedures. Am J Surg. 2017;213(6):996–1002.e1. https://doi.org/10.1016/j.amjsurg.2016.06.017.
6. Coffey MJ. Patient-centered communication during procedures [letter]. Am J Surg. 2017;213(6):1188. https://doi.org/10.1016/j.amjsurg.2016.08.004.
7. Gamboa J, Cameron MC, Fathi R, Alkousakis T. A review of non-pharmacologic approaches to enhance the patient experience in dermatologic surgery. Dermatol Online J. 2020;26(3). Accessed March 15, 2021. https://escholarship.org/uc/item/7mp372nd
8. Komesaroff PA, editor. Troubled bodies: critical perspectives on postmodernism, medical ethics, and the body. Duke University Press; 1995.
9. Truog RD, Brown SD, Browning D, et al. Microethics: the ethics of everyday clinical practice. Hast Cent Rep. 2015;45(1):11–7. https://doi.org/10.1002/hast.413.
10. Potts JR. Shifting Sands of surgical education. J Am Coll Surg. 2018;227(2):151–62. https://doi.org/10.1016/j.jamcollsurg.2018.02.012.
11. Dickinson KJ, Bass BL, Nguyen DT, Graviss EA, Pei KY. Public perception of general surgery resident autonomy and supervision. IJ Am Coll Surg. 2021;232(1):8–15.e1. https://doi.org/10.1016/j.jamcollsurg.2020.08.764.
12. Porta CR, Sebesta JA, Brown TA, Steele SR, Martin MJ. Training surgeons and the informed consent process: routine disclosure of trainee participation and its effect on patient willingness and consent rates. Arch Surg. 2012;147:57–62. https://doi.org/10.1001/archsurg.2011.235.
13. Gan KD, Rudnisky CJ, Weis E. Discussing resident participation in cataract surgery. Can J Ophthalmol. 2009;44(6):651–4. https://doi.org/10.3129/i09-075.
14. Kirsch MJ, Kasten SJ. What about learners' roles in the operating room should be disclosed to patients? AMA J Ethics. 2018;20(4):336–41. https://doi.org/10.1001/journalofethics.2018.20.4.ecas2-1804.
15. Vallance JH, Ahmed M, Dhillon B. Cataract surgery and consent: recall, anxiety, and attitude toward trainee surgeons preoperatively and postoperatively. J Cataract Refract Surg. 2004;30(7):1479–85. https://doi.org/10.1016/j.jcrs.2003.11.050.
16. Kempenich JW, Willis RE, Al Fayyadh MA, et al. Video-based patient education improves patient attitudes toward resident participation in outpatient surgical care. J Surg Educ. 2018;75(6):e61–7. https://doi.org/10.1016/j.jsurg.2018.07.024.

17. Beale KG, Kempenich JW, Willis RE, et al. Surgical Inpatient's attitudes toward resident participation: all about expectations. J Surg Educ. 2020;77(6):e28–33. https://doi.org/10.1016/j.jsurg.2020.02.025.
18. Kempenich JW, Willis RE, Blue RJ, et al. The effect of patient education on the perceptions of resident participation in surgical care. J Surg Educ. 2016;73(6):e111–7. https://doi.org/10.1016/j.jsurg.2016.05.005.
19. Uecker J, Luftman K, Ali S, Brown C. Comparable operative times with and without surgery resident participation. J Surg Educ. 2013;70(6):696–9. https://doi.org/10.1016/j.surg.2013.06.011.
20. Davis SS, Husain FA, Lin E, Nandipati KC, Perez S, Sweeney JF. Resident participation in index laparoscopic general surgical cases: impact of the learning environment on surgical outcomes. J Am Coll Surg. 2013;216(1):96–104. https://doi.org/10.1016/j.amcollsurg.2012.08.014.
21. Papandria D, Rhee D, Ortega G, et al. Assessing trainee impact on operative time for common general surgical procedures in ACS-NSQIP. J Surg Educ. 2012;69(2):149–55. https://doi.org/10.1016/j.surg.2011.08.003.
22. Turner JS, Henry D, Chase A, Kpodzo D, Flood MC, Clark CE. Adenoma detection rate in colonoscopy: does the participation of a resident matter? Am Surg 2018;84(6):1064–1068. PMID: 29981650.
23. Sapci I, Aiello A, Hassab TH, et al. Colorectal surgery resident participation in screening colonoscopies: how does it impact quality? Dis Colon Rectum. 2019;62(12):1528–32. https://doi.org/10.1097/dcr.0000000000001503.
24. Smith CS, Nolan R, Guyton K, Siegler M, Langerman A, Schindler N. Resident perspectives on teaching during awake surgical procedures. J Surg Educ. 2019;76(6):1492–9. https://doi.org/10.1016/j.surg.2019.04.007.

Chapter 13
Trainee Involvement in Surgical Care

Darren S. Bryan ⓘ **and Peter Angelos** ⓘ

Abstract In the modern practice of surgery, the process of informed consent provides the framework for patients to make knowledgeable decisions about how their care will proceed. Surgical trainees are intimately involved in care that occurs at teaching hospitals, which have dual missions to provide patient care, and train the next generation of surgeons. Here, we review the ethical principles surrounding trainee involvement, and the literature delving into the ways in which that involvement is communicated with patients. Available evidence suggests that when included as part of a discussion, patients are in large part accepting and supportive of resident and fellow participation in operations. Patients should be aware that trainees are involved in their treatment and the surgical community should reject a "don't ask, don't tell" policy that relies on an unstated but understood lack of transparency.

Keywords Surgical education · Ethics · Surgical ethics · Trainee involvement
Educational ethics · Surgical transparency · Operative ethics

> **Case**
> A 47-year-old woman is admitted from the Emergency Department at an academic medical center with three days of nausea, emesis, and obstipation. She has no medical problems. Her surgical history, however, is significant for an exploratory laparotomy and small bowel resection five years ago following a

D. S. Bryan (✉)
Department of Surgery, Brigham and Women's Hospital, Boston, MA, USA
e-mail: DSBryan@partners.org

P. Angelos
Department of Surgery and MacLean Center for Clinical Medical Ethics,
The University of Chicago, Chicago, IL, USA
e-mail: pangelos@surgery.bsd.uchicago.edu

© The Author(s), under exclusive license to Springer Nature
Switzerland AG 2022
V. A. Lonchyna et al. (eds.), *Difficult Decisions in Surgical Ethics*, Difficult
Decisions in Surgery: An Evidence-Based Approach,
https://doi.org/10.1007/978-3-030-84625-1_13

gunshot wound. On examination, she is distended and uncomfortable, but has no peritoneal signs. An upright x-ray of her abdomen demonstrates multiple air fluid levels. A complete blood count and basic metabolic panel show no notable abnormalities. The surgical team on call is consulted and, following nasogastric decompression, admits the patient for management of a suspected adhesive bowel obstruction.

After four days of nil-per-os (NPO) status, the patient has failed to improve. Computed tomography (CT) demonstrates dilated small bowel transitioning acutely to decompressed bowel in the pelvis, and the patient is booked for operative exploration the following morning. The attending surgeon, chief surgical resident, and junior surgical resident visit the patient in her room the night before surgery, where they discuss her failure to improve with a non-operative approach, as well as the risks and benefits of the recommended exploration. The patient is agreeable, asking several clarifying questions, including, directed at the attending surgeon with raised eyebrows, "you're the one doing this, right?" The attending smiles and responds "Of course. I'm your surgeon. They'll [gestures to the residents] be helping me, though."

In the operating room the following day, following induction of general anesthesia, the attending surgeon participates in the pre-surgical safety pause ("time-out") before instructing the chief resident to gain access to the abdomen and evaluate the bowel. The attending observes, un-scrubbed, as the chief and junior resident safely perform a midline laparotomy through the patient's prior incision. On exploration, an adhesive band of tissue is discovered. The attending surgeon, before leaving the room, tells the resident team to lyse the adhesion, evaluate the bowel once more, and close the abdomen. As she begins to do so, the chief resident's thoughts briefly move to the conversation with the patient the day prior, and the brief verbal exchange between attending and patient. The patient had clearly expressed some degree of concern over *who* was performing the operation, and the attending surgeon had clearly assuaged any fears of the patient through his assurance that *he* was the "surgeon" and would be "assisted" by the residents. But what lay within this statement? What was the meaning of being one's surgeon? Did it require physical handling of instruments and performance of the operation, or in an academic care model, were the residents themselves the instruments, and the attending still the acting surgeon? Though the current situation was under control and felt safe, would the patient be comfortable with what was unfolding in the OR? These questions would have to wait.

13.1   Introduction

A fundamental tenant of the ethical practice of medicine is the patient's right to self-determination. Almost by definition, for a patient to make decisions about his or her care, they must be well informed. While the concept of an informed patient able to participate in care is seemingly uncomplicated, the flow of patients through the modern healthcare delivery apparatus, and the complexity of that delivery, is anything but straightforward. In academic medical centers as well as in many hospital systems, graduate medical education (GME) and the training of the next generation of physicians are considered to be part of a multifaceted mission including direct patient care, and often, research. Thus, medical education must be balanced with and occur within the context of direct patient care.

While teaching hospitals must balance these sometimes-competing missions of education and patient care, the relationship between the two is symbiotic. Multiple studies have demonstrated that care provided in academic centers is safe and clinically effective, with some even demonstrating that outcome measures, including overall survival, are improved in large teaching hospitals [1–4]. Furthermore, studies have demonstrated that resident involvement in care is safe and does not lead to worse outcomes [5–7]. Alternatively, the "ends" (namely, of equivalent, if not improved, patient outcomes) do not necessarily justify the means through which a patient arrives at them. Those receiving healthcare, particularly in vulnerable settings such as an anesthetized state, have a right to self-determination—that is, a right to declare *how* they receive their care. To make such a determination, transparency in care delivery, and care as it relates to resident involvement, is necessary.

When faced with periods of uncertainty or vulnerability, patients look to practitioners for reassurance and hope, often relying heavily on the experience and honesty of the care team. In the same encounter, the team must truthfully inform the patient, often while feeling the obligation to provide much desired reassurance and comfort. The navigation of conversations, that result in the patient becoming comfortable with resident involvement, is both necessary, and potentially uncomfortable. We performed a review of literature examining patient perceptions of trainee involvement in care, aiming to make recommendations for communication strategies in such situations.

13.2   Search Strategy

We utilized the PubMed database to conduct a literature review. We searched for publications indexed with MeSH terms and subheadings falling under: Disclosure/ethics, Informed Consent/ethics, Internship and Residency/ethics, Surgical Procedures, Operative/ethics, and Specialties, Surgical/education. Results were limited to English language, human clinical trials and perspectives pieces published in the last 20 years. Articles were hand screened for relevancy. We further examined references and crosschecked for relevant articles not identified by the original search criteria. We included 16 studies focusing on communication of information as it relates to resident, medical student, or fellow involvement in care.

13.3 Discussion

13.3.1 Ethical Principles for Consideration

Resident involvement in care is necessary for surgical training. The bioethical principles of beneficence and non-maleficence, or, diagnosing and treating illness with the greatest possible efficacy and lowest associated risk, are central to clinical medical ethics [8, 9]. Through training, largely performed while working side by side with practicing surgeons, trainees become capable in the discipline of surgery. Practical experience within graduate medical education and the need for exposure to the operating room with graduated responsibility are both necessary to educate capable surgeons. The beneficence and non-maleficence experienced by future patients when treated by a well-trained workforce must be balanced with the rights of autonomy and self-determination of present patients who are actively receiving care (Table 13.1).

In the modern era, free and informed consent by the patient is widely recognized to be necessary for the legal and ethical practice of medicine and surgery. Modern day understanding of morality, that which is right, and which is wrong, is heavily influenced by the Kantian concept of respect for persons, in which individuals are seen as free, rational beings with dignity, who are owed respect simply by virtue of being persons [10]. An extension of this respect for persons is the bioethical principle of "respect for autonomy", recognizing a moral right for the individual to determine their own choices and life trajectory [8, 9]. Clinically, respect for patient autonomy is born out through the practice of informed consent, the phrase given to the forging of a mutually agreed upon plan of care recommended by a physician and consented to by a patient who understands the proposed treatment, along with associated risks, benefits, and alternatives. As such, transparency as it relates to resident involvement in care, is necessary.

Table 13.1 Ethical principles for consideration

Ethical principle	Consideration
Autonomy	• Patients have a right to choose (or not) to receive care that is provided in part by trainees • The ability to dictate one's own care and who is involved when in a vulnerable (i.e., anesthetized) state, speaks to a fundamental right to self-determination
Beneficence	• The involvement of trainees in patient care is *necessary* in order to "do good" and be effective future independent clinicians • Research suggests improved outcomes at teaching hospitals
Non-maleficence	• Trainees, in order to avoid doing harm, must learn good practice while in training. Best accomplished through active participation
Justice	• Adequate training and education is necessary to ensure a well-staffed future workforce, capable of needs and ensuring access to care for populations in need

Many argue that in practice, *truly* informed consent is a fallacy (see Chap. 6). Can any patient, no matter the depth of education or prior conversation with their treating physician, completely understand a proposed treatment and the associated risks? Nevertheless, the practice acts as a safeguard that protects against deceit or coercion and further helps to form a therapeutic alliance between physician and patient [11]. Recognizing this, the extent and the scope of patient education for a patient to be considered "informed" is a topic of debate among medical ethicists. Few believe in a "more is better" approach, instead advocating for the content of such conversations to include what a "reasonable patient" would want to know (the reasonable patient standard), or more recently, for individually tailoring such conversations to the patient and their beliefs and values [8]. Therefore, the necessity of pre-operative discussion of resident involvement in care depends on whether or not a reasonable patient would want to know. We explore this, below.

13.3.1.1   Patient Perceptions of Trainee Involvement in Care

Some argue that by virtue of receiving care at an academic medical center, patients are aware of and thus consent to trainee involvement, obviating the need for further discussion. Such opinions have not been supported by data, with multiple studies showing that academic hierarchy, trainee designations, and even the nomenclature (i.e., "attending", "intern", "resident") commonly used in graduate medical education is a virtual black box for patients [12]. Patients do, in fact, seem to have opinions about their interactions with trainees. A Canadian study performed in 2008 by Knifed and colleagues sought to examine a patient's baseline knowledge of and comfort with resident involvement in their intra-operative care [13]. They performed a hypothesis-generating qualitative study, interviewing 30 patients who were scheduled to undergo elective neurosurgical operations. Consistently, patients showed a low level of understanding of resident roles and responsibilities. However, once described, their anxiety level diminished. Furthermore, patients recognized the need for education, and exhibited trust in the medical system (in this case, in Canada). Interestingly and importantly, patients expressed a desire to meet the resident physicians prior to the operation in which they would take part, underlining their consideration as members of the treatment team.

In another study designed to evaluate patient willingness to be cared for by residents, Porta and colleagues administered surveys to more than 300 patients scheduled for elective general surgery [14]. Patients additionally were overwhelmingly in support of more detailed information as to resident roles and participation in care. They further found that patients at baseline were highly supportive of resident education (more than 90% consented to having a resident participate in their operation), however when given specific scenarios with increasing rates of resident participation, the patients' willingness to consent to the operation fell. This correlates with other published reports, generally finding that patients appreciate and desire more information [15, 16].

13.3.2   Interventions Directed at Information Communication

Several groups have examined the ways in which resident involvement in care is communicated. Sharda and colleagues evaluated three different methods of directly obtaining consent for resident involvement in cataract surgery [17]. One method involved delivering a pre-scripted statement explaining the role of a resident, introducing the resident (if present), and assuring the patient of adequate supervision before asking for consent. Another method supplied a written statement explaining resident roles and participation, allowing the patient to indicate their choice for resident participation (or not). In a third method, surgeons simply stated that residents would be involved in care in the operating room, observing or performing the operation under supervision. The authors observed starkly contrasting rates of consent. Patients exposed to the first method, in which surgeons took time to explain the role of a resident, introduce them if present, and to ensure adequate supervision, yielded a consent rate of 86%, compared to just 21% for those patients given a written statement asking for consent. In another study, Bryan et al. randomized pre-operative general surgery patients to standard informed consent practices (in which discussion of trainee involvement in care was not mandated) or enhanced informed consent, which included a standardized statement describing the roles and involvement of trainees [18]. Similar to Sharda's group, a significant increase in consent rates was observed when patients were exposed to the standardized script. Both studies highlight the importance of conversation and openness when discussing resident participation and underline the value of surgeon advocacy for trainee involvement in care.

13.4   Case Resolution

The chief resident pressed on in the operation, lysing the band of adhesive tissue as instructed by her attending surgeon. As she began to trace the small intestine, looking for other causes of possible obstruction or pathology, she again remembered the pre-operative conversation with the patient. She paused and asked for the circulating nurse to call the attending surgeon back into the room. When he arrived, she was ready to begin closing the abdomen. She gestured to a slight narrowing in the small bowel, "Do you think this is anything to be concerned about?" With a furrowed brow, he leaned over the field and replied, "No…just looks like a peristalsing segment to me." She began closing the abdomen and asked for the attending to stay nearby and verify her closure.

The patient recovered uneventfully in the post-operative period and was discharged home in good condition. Later that week, while reflecting about the case, the chief resident realized she was left with mixed emotions. She felt that through bringing the attending surgeon back into the room and keeping him there, she was able to, in some way, however incomplete, honor the spirit of the patient's desire to have the attending "do" the operation. She also recognized that she had requested his presence at the potential cost of his trust in her clinical acumen. She had known the "narrowed segment" was in fact peristalsing and would not have normally given it any additional consideration. She also felt more than comfortable closing the abdomen with a junior resident and had done so many times. After some deliberation, she decided to discuss the case, her moral distress, and the concerns she had felt at the time with the attending surgeon. She hoped it would be well received.

13.5   Conclusion

In practice, communication surrounding resident involvement in surgery is lacking. Surgeons and trainees commonly adopt a "don't ask, don't tell" practice, despite a demonstrated desire of patients to know. The reasons for this are many, but chief among them is a concern that the information will be met with hesitance, discomfort, and unwillingness to proceed, therein harming the ability of the trainee to learn, and altering the usual flow of care. Data demonstrates not only that patients value the knowledge of the composition of their care team, but that the importance of education is recognized and valued. Blanket statements that simply inform a patient that early learners will be performing operations are, unsurprisingly, often met with reluctance. Therefore, the importance of conversation framing and of a simple discussion including the basics of medical education and experiential learning, cannot be overstated.

Ethically, the responsible surgeon has a duty to ensure the patient understands that trainees will be involved in, and perform under supervision, aspects of their care. Surgeons also should recognize the potential for moral distress that trainees may experience when navigating conversations surrounding involvement in care. The surgeon educator has an obligation to posterity to advocate, within the bounds of reason, for their residents' participation in the operation. When communicated effectively, available evidence suggests that conducting such conversations stands to bolster therapeutic surgeon-patient relationships and benefit trainees, while improving transparency in the field.

13.6   Selected References

- Burke LG, Frakt AB, Khullar D, Orav EJ, Jha AK. Association between teaching status and mortality in US hospitals. JAMA. 2017;317(20):2105–13. https://doi.org/10.1001/jama.2017.5702

    - Medicare claims data was used to examine outcomes following hospitalization at teaching and nonteaching hospitals in the United States. Over 21 million hospitalizations were evaluated, focused on 30 and 90-day mortality in patients treated for several common medical and surgical conditions. There was a statistically significant lower 30-day mortality at teaching hospitals.

- Knifed E, July J, Bernstein M. Neurosurgery patients' feelings about the role of residents in their care: a qualitative case study. J Neurosurg. 2008;108(2):287–91. https://doi.org/10.3171/JNS/2008/108/2/0287

  - Thirty patients, scheduled to undergo elective craniotomy, underwent semi-structured interviews aimed to evaluate their knowledge of and anxiety associated with resident involvement in care. Key findings included: patients who were well educated had low levels of anxiety associated with resident participation and patients desired to meet residents prior to their operations.

- Porta CR, Sebesta JA, Brown TA, Steele SR, Martin MJ. Training surgeons and the informed consent process: routine disclosure of trainee participation and its effect on patient willingness and consent rates. Arch Surg. 2012;147(1):57–62. https://doi.org/10.1001/archsurg.2011.235

  - Questionnaires sent to patients scheduled for surgery evaluated their opinions of teaching programs, and willingness to consent to resident involvement in their operations. While patients at baseline were supportive of teaching programs and resident observation, they were less willing to consent to the operation as their knowledge of resident participation increased.

- Sharda RK, Sher JH, Chan BJ, Kobetz LE, Mann KD. A comparison of techniques: informed consent for resident involvement in cataract surgery. Can J Ophthalmol. 2012;47(2):113–7. https://doi.org/10.1016/j.jcjo.2012.01.017

  - Researchers compared three different methods of discussing trainee involvement in care prior to patients undergoing cataract surgery. Methods that carefully discussed resident participation, including a standardized script, introduction of the resident (if present), and assurance of staff oversight, were met with high rates of patient consent. Methods that simply asked for consent (yes/no) were met with much lower rates of consent.

- Bryan AF, Bryan DS, Matthews JB, Roggin KK. Toward autonomy and conditional independence: a standardized script improves patient acceptance of surgical trainee roles. J Surg Educ. 2020;77(3):534–9. https://doi.org/10.1016/j.jsurg.2020.01.015

  - Patients scheduled to undergo general surgery were consented either in the usual fashion (with minimal and non-standardized discussion of resident participation in care) or with the addition of a standardized script meant to prompt discussion of resident participation in care. Researchers found that patients in the intervention arm were more likely to say that residents should be able to perform portions of their operation, and that care team roles were more adequately explained to them.

References

1. Burke LG, Frakt AB, Khullar D, Orav EJ, Jha AK. Association between teaching status and mortality in US hospitals. JAMA. 2017;317(20):2105–13. https://doi.org/10.1001/jama.2017.5702.
2. Keeler EB, Rubenstein LV, Kahn KL, et al. Hospital characteristics and quality of care. JAMA. 1992;268(13):1709–14.
3. Meguid RA, Brooke BS, Chang DC, et al. Are surgical outcomes for lung cancer resections improved at teaching hospitals? Ann Thorac Surg. 2008;85(3):1015–25. https://doi.org/10.1016/j.athoracsur.2007.09.046.
4. Zafar SN, Shah AA, Hashmi ZG, et al. Outcomes after emergency general surgery at teaching versus non-teaching hospitals. J Trauma. 2015;78(1):69–77. https://doi.org/10.1097/TA.0000000000000493.
5. Kiran RP, Ali UA, Coffey JC, Vogel JD, Pokala N, Fazio VW. Impact of resident participation in surgical operations on postoperative outcomes: National Surgical Quality Improvement Program. Ann Surg. 2012;256(3):469–75. https://doi.org/10.1097/SLA.0b013e318265812a.
6. Edelstein AI, Lovecchio FC, Saha S, et al. Impact of resident involvement on orthopaedic surgery outcomes: an analysis of 30,628 patients from the American College of Surgeons National Surgical Quality Improvement Program database. JBJS. 2014;96(15):e131. https://doi.org/10.2106/JBJS.M.00660.
7. de Santibañes M, Alvarez FA, Sieling E, et al. Postoperative complications at a university hospital: is there a difference between patients operated by supervised residents vs. trained surgeons? Langenbeck's Arch Surg. 2015;400(1):77–82. https://doi.org/10.1007/s00423-014-1261-z.
8. Jonsen AR, Siegler M, Winslade WJ. Clinical ethics. A practical approach to ethical decisions in clinical medicine. 8th ed. McGraw Hill Medical; 2015.
9. Beauchamp TL, Childress JF. Principles of biomedical ethics. 8th ed. Oxford University Press; 2019.
10. Kant I. Groundwork for the metaphysics of morals. 1785.
11. O'Neill O. Some limits of informed consent. J Med Ethics. 2003;29(1):4–7. https://doi.org/10.1136/jme.29.1.4.
12. Kravetz AJ, Anderson CI, Shaw D, et al. Patient misunderstanding of the academic hierarchy is prevalent and predictable. J Surg Res. 2011;171:467–72. https://doi.org/10.1016/j.jss.2010.07.052.
13. Knifed E, July J, Bernstein M. Neurosurgery patients' feelings about the role of residents in their care: a qualitative case study. J Neurosurg. 2008;108(2):287–91. https://doi.org/10.3171/JNS/2008/108/2/0287.
14. Porta CR, Sebesta JA, Brown TA, et al. Training surgeons and the informed consent process: routine disclosure of trainee participation and its effect on patient willingness and consent rates. Arch Surg. 2012;147(1):57–62. https://doi.org/10.1001/archsurg.2011.235.
15. Nguyen T-N, Silver D, Arthurs B. Consent to cataract surgery performed by residents. Can J Opthalmol. 2005;40(1):34–7. https://doi.org/10.1016/S0008-4182(05)80114-0.
16. Wisner DM, Quillen DA, Benderson DM, Green MJ. Patient attitudes toward resident involvement in cataract surgery. Arch Ophthalmol. 2008;126(9):1235–9.
17. Sharda RK, Sher JH, Chan BJ, et al. A comparison of techniques: informed consent for resident involvement in cataract surgery. Can J Ophthalmol. 2012;47(2):113–7. https://doi.org/10.1016/j.jcjo.2012.01.017.
18. Bryan AF, Bryan DS, Matthews JB, Roggin KK. Toward autonomy and conditional independence: a standardized script improves patient acceptance of surgical trainee roles. J Surg Educ. 2020;77(3):534–9. https://doi.org/10.1016/j.jsurg.2020.01.015.

Chapter 14
Can Professionalism Be Taught During Residency?

Kinga B. Skowron Olortegui ⓘ **and Christian Fernandez Olortegui** ⓘ

Abstract Professionalism is the conduct by which we define our role to our community. Lapses in professionalism have real consequences for the surgeon, patient care staff, students, and, most importantly, patients. Teaching of professionalism has traditionally occurred in a hidden curriculum via apprenticeship. Increasingly, attention is drawn to the importance of formal education of professionalism during graduate medical education. In this chapter, we review the various methods for teaching professionalism during residency.

Keywords Professionalism · Surgical culture · Surgical education · Medical ethics

> **Case**
> A senior surgeon walks into an operating room to begin his case. His usual scrub nurse is not present on this day, and a new nurse introduces himself. The operation begins uneventfully. Bleeding is encountered and the surgeon asks for a particular clamp. The scrub nurse is unfamiliar with the item and fumbles to find it. The surgeon is frustrated and throws the incorrect clamp he is handed. The senior resident presses laparotomy pads into the wound to temporize the bleeding. The correct clamp is found, the bleeding is controlled, and the remainder of the case completed in a tense atmosphere. Two

K. B. Skowron Olortegui (✉)
Section of Colon & Rectal Surgery, Department of Surgery, MacLean Center for Clinical
Medical Ethics, University of Chicago Medicine, Chicago, IL, USA
e-mail: kskowron@bsd.uchicago.edu

C. F. Olortegui
Department of Radiation Oncology, Thomas Jefferson University Hospital,
Philadelphia, PA, USA
e-mail: christian.fernandez@jefferson.edu

© The Author(s), under exclusive license to Springer Nature
Switzerland AG 2022
V. A. Lonchyna et al. (eds.), *Difficult Decisions in Surgical Ethics*, Difficult
Decisions in Surgery: An Evidence-Based Approach,
https://doi.org/10.1007/978-3-030-84625-1_14

instrument counts are incorrect, but a third count is correct. The student thinks she saw something blue out of the corner of her eye inside the wound but is nervous to say something in case she is wrong; the surgeon must have seen it if it was there. The wound is closed. One week later, the patient has high fevers, tachycardia and leukocytosis; workup ultimately reveals a retained foreign body. The patient is taken back to the operating room for re-exploration, a laparotomy pad is removed from the surgical wound, and after a long course of antibiotics, the patient is discharged to a rehabilitation facility. The student was considering surgery prior to this rotation, but now does not feel that she belongs in this field.

14.1 Introduction

What is professionalism, and why does it matter? The concept is the basis of the trust placed in surgeons by their patients and the greater community. Patients must feel that their surgeon will at all times act in their best interest in order to trust them. Thus, professionalism is the complex intersection of clinical competence, ethics, respect for others, integrity, duty for altruistic service to individuals and society, and physician self-care and well-being. Maintenance of a high standard for these attributes is how a profession maintains autonomy and self-regulation without intervention from societal or external regulatory bodies. This concept is important enough to warrant a position among the six core competencies by the Accreditation Council of Graduate Medical Education (ACGME) for all U.S. residents (see Table 14.1) [1]. It has been addressed by the American College of Surgeons (ACS) Task Force on Professionalism in a formal Code of Professional Conduct [2, 3].

Nevertheless, it is not hard to imagine the above scenario, and perhaps many of us have witnessed a similar situation or heard of this happening. How did this happen? One can certainly imagine that the surgeon felt that he was doing his best for the patient, and felt that to do his best, he needed to have his instruments. Unfortunately, he did not express this in a professional manner. The involved staff

Table 14.1 Core competencies of the ACGME [1]

ACGME Core Competencies	Assessment Method Examples
Patient Care	Direct Clinical Observation, OSCEs
Medical Knowledge	Standardized Exams
Practice-Based Learning and Improvement	Portfolios, Patient Records Review
Interpersonal and Communication Skills	Direct Clinical Observation, Situational Judgement Tests
Professionalism	Direct Clinical Observation, Multisource Feedback
Systems-Based Practice	Quality Improvement Projects, Multisource Feedback

were distressed, and their usual flow disrupted; ultimately, this patient was harmed. The spirit of the team was damaged, and the medical student was turned away from this specialty as a career choice.

Various contributors can promote unprofessional behaviors, aside from work-related pressures. Mental health, substance abuse, physical health, financial stressors, marital issues, fatigue, and social isolation may contribute to unprofessional behavior [4]. The recent increase in awareness of wellness and self-care among medical centers and surgical departments strives to address these personal factors. However, as members of the common profession, we are also all responsible for identifying a colleague who may be struggling and helping them to identify resources for help.

Unprofessional behavior has real potential to harm patients. In a recent report in JAMA Surgery, authors correlated event reports made by colleagues of unprofessional behavior by surgeons with the outcomes of their patients using the National Surgical Quality Improvement Program database. Research coders reviewed the reports and categorized unprofessional behaviors into four domains (see Table 14.2): poor or unsafe care, disrespect of coworkers, lack of integrity, and lack of responsibility. The patients of surgeons who demonstrated unprofessional behavior had a higher risk of complications (10.7% risk for surgeons with no reports, versus 14.1% for surgeons with >4 reports, $p < 0.001$) [5]. The vast majority of disciplinary actions by state medical boards are due to unprofessionalism, and this has been correlated in several studies with professionalism lapses while those physicians were in medical school [6, 7]. This suggests that an individual's trouble with the behaviors key to professionalism often exist before they begin their practice and could perhaps be remedied while they are in training. Besides action by medical boards, other direct and indirect consequences include poor patient care, litigation, and loss of trust of peers.

As demonstrated in our case and in the JAMA Surgery article above, there is tremendous overlap between professionalism and ethics. Inherent in care of patients are concepts of respect for a patient's autonomy, truthfulness during the informed consent process, prompt disclosure of medical information and responsibility for medical error. Physicians who fail to demonstrate professionalism are inherently disregarding ethical principles. The surgeon who disregards sterile technique, for example, is endangering his patient and violating the patient's trust that their doctor would do their best on their behalf when they are at their most vulnerable. Thus, professionalism is at its core an embodiment of clinical medical ethics.

Table 14.2 Categorization of Unprofessional Behaviors as defined by Cooper et al. [5]

Unprofessional Behavior	Examples
Poor or Unsafe Care	Disregard for Sterile Technique
Disrespect of Coworkers	Name Calling
Lack of Integrity	Falsifying Patient Encounter Information
Lack of Responsibility	Refusal to Comply with Hospital Policy

Many complaints with the topic of "professionalism" are that it is broad and overall, poorly defined. Yet somehow, we seem to know "unprofessional" behavior when we see it. Who better to identify unprofessional behavior than the omnipresent observers among us: medical students. In a survey of third-year medical students at the University of Southern California, 53% of medical students reported having witnessed unprofessional behavior by faculty on their surgery rotation [8]. When asked to describe these events, the majority were a deficiency in "respect for others." Importantly, reflection on student evaluation focusing on professionalism is a valuable feedback mechanism and has the potential to drive improvement within a department [9]. It is understandable that students who witness these events might be turned away from considering surgery as their career.

Knowing the importance of professionalism for our patients, our students, and colleagues, we must place importance not just in identifying the concept, but in teaching it. In this chapter, we will review the current literature regarding the teaching of professionalism in medicine and surgery, in order to understand whether this complex concept can be taught and if so, how best to teach it.

14.2 Search Strategy

This discussion is based upon the results of a literature search utilizing the PubMed, Institute of Education Services (ERIC), MedEdPortal and Google Scholar databases. The search was limited to English language publications available beginning in January 2000. Search terms included combinations of professionalism, surgical education, surgery, medical education, and surgical culture.

14.3 Discussion

As we embark upon the topic, let us review the importance of professionalism in our case and its impact on ethical principles (see Table 14.3). The core ethical principles—Beneficence, Nonmaleficence, Respect for Autonomy, and Justice—are all at risk if not protected by professionalism. If the surgeon's behavior results in patient harm, whether directly or indirectly (as in the example in our case, through a missed opportunity to report an error noticed by a fearful observer), this violates the principle of beneficence, or the goal of improving the condition of the patient. Similarly, nonmaleficence, or preventing harm from befalling the patient, is violated by unprofessional behaviors, as demonstrated by Cooper et al. [5]. Respect for patient autonomy is an undisputed facet of ethics. By consenting to surgery, patients express their acceptance of the risks and benefits of the procedure as outlined by their surgeon. A surgeon whose behavior results in increased risk for the patient is violating this principle, as added risk was not fully disclosed or agreed upon. Lastly, the principle of justice provides the expectation that the surgeon will set aside any personal

Table 14.3 Ethical principles in relation to professionalism

Beneficence
How can this patient benefit by the surgical treatment offered?
Avoidance of unnecessary risk as a result of unprofessional surgical environment
Nonmaleficence
How can harm be avoided?
Creating an environment such that errors are reported or prevented
Respect for Autonomy
Have all risks and benefits been adequately explained to the patient?
Behavior that increases the risk of a procedure violates the patient's autonomy
Justice
Does the patient have fair access to excellent care?
Every patient deserves access to quality care unaffected by extraneous unprofessional behaviors

conflicts of interest in the care of their patient. In our case, the surgeon lost sight of the goal of fair access to excellent care by fixating on the particular instrument, reducing the quality of care for their patient. Thus, teaching professionalism during training in order to prevent cases such as ours is an imperative of sound training in clinical medical ethics.

Unlike anatomy and physiology, professionalism is a challenging construct to define. Expectations of our profession may evolve in response to social challenges and needs of our communities. Most of us have learned a concept of professionalism through personal experiences inside and outside of medicine and have formed a personal framework for this from teachers who served as our role models [10]. What exactly constitutes professionalism may differ regionally, and students arrive to residency with variable expectations as to what it actually means [11]. In the classic assessment of socialization of surgeons, Charles L. Bosk defined types of error a trainee may commit, which might constitute lapses in professionalism [12]. Technical and judgment errors were forgivable, while normative (lapses in character) and quasi-normative (violating cultural norms particular to a given practice) errors were unforgivable and often resulted in a resident's dismissal from the program. Looking at Bosk's thesis through a modern lens, one would agree that normative errors constitute violations of modern professionalism, while quasi-normative errors fall in an unclear "gray area." While the ACS has defined the current basic tenets of professionalism, such influences (e.g., cultural, generational, quasi-normative) make it challenging to teach formally.

To define the methods by which professionalism may be learned, Ong et al. performed a systematic scoping review of medical school training programs [13]. After a qualitative review of 162 studies, the authors defined three broad categories of teaching: informal curricula, hidden curricula and formal curricula. We will review each of these further and discuss specific teaching strategies key to each. Importantly, the authors were able to define barriers and enablers to effective training in professionalism. Barriers exist at system, institution, faculty and individual levels. Examples of this are student observation of unprofessional behavior undermining formal professionalism curricula (system), lack of faculty development or administrative support for professionalism training (institution), lack of understanding of the topic (faculty), disinterest or skepticism among the learners (individual). These may be counteracted by enablers, which include active learner involvement in the process and creation of a feedback mechanism to discuss deficiencies in the training. Ong et al. ultimately described a model incorporating the importance of various available curricula into a stepwise longitudinal program, culminating in reflective practice of the learner.

In a review of the effectiveness of various professionalism curricula in residency, Berger et al. identified significant variability in types of curricula and teaching methods used among the 50 studies included in their systematic review [14]. The majority (56%) employed small-groups discussion teaching strategies; other common strategies were didactics, reflection exercises, and simulation. Half of the curricula employed multiple modalities for teaching. Of the 50 studies included, 35 demonstrated statistical analysis of their outcome data, and 20 (57%) reported a statistically significant positive effect in effectiveness of professionalism training. Programs which addressed knowledge and definition of professionalism were the most likely to succeed, while programs which attempted to alter behavior and patient outcomes were the least effective.

If individual behavior is the most challenging aspect to affect, perhaps we should ask ourselves why. Within surgery, our "surgical culture" may undermine professionalism among trainees. In interviews of surgical trainees, Patel et al. identified that residents felt the need to portray the surgical stereotypes—confident, assertive, and decisive. However, this pressure resulted in major gaps in professionalism. Residents felt the need to fabricate patient details in order to appear confident, remained silent to avoid revealing gaps in knowledge, and avoided calling for help during times of uncertainty [15]. This is alarming, as such failures may have real consequences for patient outcomes and violate our primary tenet of "do no harm." It is imperative that we break these stereotypes and promote a culture that prioritizes professionalism over these outdated and faulty ideals. These stereotype pressures are fundamentally at odds with professionalism, and by promoting and teaching tenets of professionalism, we can weed out such harmful behaviors from surgical training.

Before we begin exploring types of teaching, it is important that we discuss the weight of the *null curriculum* [16]. The concept refers to that which is *not* taught. If a concept does not earn a place in teaching or discussion, learners receive the message that it is not important, and therefore do not spend energy learning it and cultivating it as a skill. Thus, in order to teach the tenets of professionalism, residency programs and hospitals should at the very least name the concept and in some way draw attention to the idea that it is an important component of who we are as surgeons.

14.3.1   The Hidden Curriculum

We have all experienced the "hidden" curriculum in our training. This is the unstated and implicit transmission of beliefs, attitudes and behaviors [17]. This is the passing on of cultural norms and values particular to the "culture" of surgery. It is contrasted by explicit teaching in the form of lectures or seminars on a given topic. When surgical training developed principally under an apprenticeship model, the hidden curriculum was the primary means of passing on learned experiences from the mentor to the mentee. The protégée would carry on the perspectives and behaviors adopted in modeling their teacher, often learned by observation without formal description of the process. This method of teaching is inherently fraught with potential pitfalls. The exact expectations are not made clear to the trainee. There are certainly cultural, race, and gender influences which may influence the trainee's perception of the mentor's behaviors. Without explicit instruction, bad behaviors may be implicitly encouraged and learned.

The hidden curriculum is not simply a thing of the past. Hafferty et al. noticed a recent rise of "On Doctoring" courses through American medical schools [17]. Ostensibly, these courses teach skills including patient interviewing, physical diagnosis, oral presentation, basics of clinical documentation and communication. However, authors noted that much more is taught in these courses. The subtext of the way such courses are conducted inculcate the students into the professionalism expectations of that particular institution. Teachers who take time to impress upon students the importance of a patient-centered interview or the value of addressing their own emotions or stress during a difficult interview bring the concepts of professionalism to the level of a skill equally important to physical diagnosis or efficient history-taking. Meanwhile, other teachers inadvertently minimize these skills with comments such as "this is obvious stuff" or "let's get through this so you can get to the important class."

The hidden curriculum, when utilized appropriately, can be used to teach the concept of professionalism (see Table 14.4). Rogers et al. described their method for harnessing this as a tool, implemented with medical students during their surgery clerkship over a two-year period [18]. The students were asked to write three essays during their rotation: the first, describing an event which they perceived to be a positive example of professionalism during their clerkship, the second, a negative example of professionalism, and lastly, a third essay describing whether their definition of professionalism changed. Following this reflection, students participated in a session where they shared their experiences and discussed the definition of professionalism. Students were able to give examples of the behaviors which they hoped to model in their careers, and negative behaviors which they hoped to avoid. Authors reported high student satisfaction with the program. When physicians are active and mindful of their words and actions this method of teaching has a profound impact on their trainees.

Table 14.4 Summary of curricular styles for teaching professionalism [13]

Hidden curriculum
Implicit demonstration of behaviors in the course of clinical training (positive and negative)
• Reflection exercises
• Small group discussion focused on interpretation of observed behaviors
Informal curriculum
Encouragement of professionalism through explicit demonstration of positive behaviors
• Active role-modeling with expert mentor
• Small group discussions regarding specific topics (highlighting basic tenets of professionalism)
Formal curriculum
Detailed explanation and demonstration of expected positive behaviors, observation, instruction and feedback toward correction and improvement
• Lectures
• Small group discussions
• Observed practice, simulation
• Objective Structured Clinical Examination (OSCE)

14.3.2   Informal Curricula and Active Role-Modeling

Breaking tradition of the apprenticeship model with its widespread use of the hidden curriculum can seem like a daunting task. However, several major academic medical centers have been able to do this with tremendous success. Perhaps the best first step is to harness the power of the hidden curriculum, but incorporate explicit demonstration and encourage active modeling after exemplary mentors. In doing so, an "informal" curriculum arises: formal concepts or rubrics are taught by ad hoc interactions with positive role models, during which professional behaviors are clearly identified and promoted (see Table 14.4).

The University of Washington School of Medicine began by creating the "Colleges program" for teaching professionalism to medical students [19]. Thirty faculty were identified as outstanding clinicians, and assigned students in small groups, with whom they would meet regularly over the course of the students' four-year program. The faculty developed benchmarks which must be covered over the course of the curriculum: altruism, honor, integrity, compassion, communication, respect, accountability, responsibility, scholarship, excellence and leadership. In the first year, the groups learn concepts in various formats, including lectures, small-group discussions, and written reflections. In the second year, they accompany the mentor to the bedside. There, they observe the mentor's interactions with patients, practice skills with the mentor observing, and engage in informal discussions of their observations. After success with the Colleges program for students, the

University developed formal programs, including those for resident and faculty training as well. This has resulted in engagement of all stakeholders on campus, such that the authors describe an "ecology of professionalism" throughout the institution, prioritizing the tenets of professionalism in all interactions.

While formal curricula are certainly ideal and as they lend themselves to standardization, as the University of Washington experience demonstrates, an informal yet active curriculum can serve as an important steppingstone for progress. Programs without sufficient resources for formal curricula may employ a model of active role models who meet with learners to discuss certain key topics on an informal basis. Identifying and encouraging positive behaviors can amplify those over negative behaviors, which may be implicitly encouraged by a hidden curriculum.

Role-modeling as a teaching method fall under the concept of social learning or learning through observation. This requires several components for success [20]. First, the learner must commit attention to the desired behavior. This can be achieved with guidelines of situations that the students should see during the encounters. Next, the learners need to internalize the behavior they have seen and be able to reproduce it. Students and residents have opportunity to practice during the course of their patient encounters on the wards. Lastly, the learners need to be motivated to copy the behavior. This can be in the form of evaluations or recognition for model behavior.

The University of Texas Medical Branch at Galveston (UTMB) is another example of informal curricula and active modeling, which notably utilized motivation as a key component [21]. The experience of UTMB began in a "top down" fashion. In 1997, the newly appointed president of the university announced an initiative to apply professionalism in a comprehensive fashion through every level of the university. This began by informal round table and luncheon meetings with members of the university at all levels, in which formal initiatives were developed. Thus, stakeholders were involved in developing and implementing curricula which would be applicable to the resources and limitations of their particular department. The university developed two key motivators for professionalism: a mechanism by which negative behaviors may be reported, as well as an annual brochure titled *Professionalism and You* in which positive models are highlighted. Over time, this has resulted in a formal curriculum for medical students, as well as formal programs for other groups in the medical center.

With this institutional buy-in, a remarkable change happened. Comparing surveys of students over the years, reports of professionalism rose dramatically. In 2002, 86% of students reported that they were treated with respect by faculty; by 2007, that number rose to 93%. Similarly, 52% of faculty reported that their supervisor was compassionate and 59% that their supervisor treated them with respect in 2002, versus 75% and 78%, respectively, in 2007. As we can see by these examples, raising awareness on the topic of professionalism can have a positive effect throughout a medical center. As these efforts are relatively young, we do not know the objective effects of these types of changes on patient care qualifiers and outcomes. However, the currently available results are encouraging.

14.3.3 Formal Curricula and Simulation

Many reports in the literature describe formal curricula for teaching professionalism in the graduate medical education setting. Formal curricula are based on defined goals, with structured objectives and provision of materials through which to achieve those goals [17]. While observation was a foundation of the methods discussed previously, lectures, active practice, case-based discussion, video demonstration, role-playing, feedback and practice improvement are the core of a formal curriculum [22]. Of course, a thorough curriculum requires significant infrastructure for success. Residents require protected time and financial investment for infrastructure, requiring departmental support. As alluded to in some of the preceding examples, formal curricula often grow and build on prior experience once a need is recognized. This systematic process is important for the success of a formal curriculum. This progresses in a stepwise fashion (see Table 14.5): (1) problem identification and needs assessment; (2) targeted needs assessment for the specific learners; (3) building of goals and objectives; (4) educational strategies; (5) implementation; and (6) evaluation and feedback [23]. Steps 1 and 2 are perhaps the most important, as they engage stakeholders and focus the scope of the proposed curriculum, particularly important given time constraints in a busy residency.

Simulation is a major component of formal instruction in this realm. Current surgical residents have experience with simulation for technical skills; extending this tool to non-technical skill development is reasonable [24]. Simulation allows components of professionalism to be elicited in realistic scenarios, during which residents may practice positive, ideal responses in a safe setting. Key elements of successful simulation include repetitive practice, feedback, and curriculum integration [25]. There is a large body of literature describing the use of simulation as a component of formal professionalism curricula, with a broad range of techniques and success [26]. In a review of the literature, Wali et al. described very creative

Table 14.5 The six step approach to medical education curriculum development by Thomas et al. [23]

Components of Curriculum Development	Details
Problem Identification and General Needs Assessment	Defining the greater deficit in healthcare, current efforts, and ideal approach
Targeted Needs Assessment	Identifying the target learner group, their respective needs, and their environment
Goals and Objectives	Developing overarching, broad learning goals and the discrete, measurable learning objectives to fulfill the goals
Education Strategies	Methods that achieve the goals and objectives
Implementation	Execution of the education strategies
Evaluation and Feedback	Assessing the successfulness of the curriculum and utilizing that information to improve it

methods of incorporating simulation in teaching professionalism, including "secret shopper" standardized patients in the emergency department who would elicit specific issues recently covered in didactic sessions with emergency medicine residents. However, reports of these curricula were variable and often lacked specific details regarding feedback and assessment mechanisms, making implementation based upon these prior experiences challenging.

Perhaps the most thoroughly developed formal curriculum is the Surgical Professionalism in Clinical Education (SPICE) program at The New York University Department of Surgery, a targeted professionalism curriculum for surgical residents [27]. Residents in the first, second and third year undergo a pre-curriculum Objective Structured Clinical Examination (OSCE) in which standardized patients simulated clinical encounters (for example, reporting wrong-sided hernia surgery to a patient) and rate them specifically in the areas of professionalism: accountability or sensitivity to the patient, for example. Over the course of the year, the residents experience six interactive sessions teaching skills specific to these types of encounters. The topics are advanced communication skills (managing difficult situations), admitting mistakes, delivering bad news, interdisciplinary respect, working across language and cultural barriers, and self-care. The residents then repeat the OSCE after this training. In their report of fifteen residents who completed the program in its entirety, the authors noted that the professionalism score rating of "well done" improved from 36% to 45.7% ($p = 0.011$). The authors later reported on their experience after 7 years of the curriculum and noted a significant improvement in professionalism scores of residents prior to the curriculum (38% "well done" in 2007) compared with residents who had completed the curriculum for 3 years (59% "well done" in 2014, $p < 0.001$) [28]. Due to this success, the curriculum has been incorporated into the American Board of Surgery Surgical Council on Resident Education (SCORE) curriculum for residents.

Another excellent example of a thorough professionalism curriculum for surgical residents is the Human Emotion and Response in Surgery (HEARS) curriculum at the University of Massachusetts [29]. In order to develop the curriculum, a panel of surgeons, education specialists and chief residents attended a full-day retreat to review the needs assessment of the department, including options for simulation and assessment. They developed a curriculum for first- through second-year residents, which would cover the topics perceived as lacking in their residency training: patient communication/empathy, teamwork, stress and time management, patient education, and difficult patient interactions. These topics were taught in 5 three-hour faculty-lead sessions per year over 2 years. Residents watched video vignettes and responded in a written format to the scenarios, both before and after the didactic sessions. In each of the areas, residents felt better prepared for similar real-world scenarios. Some limitations of this curriculum include lack of practice and feedback. For example, residents rated the "teamwork" session as less helpful because of lack of practice with nursing or other staff during these sessions. Similarly, practice and feedback from standardized patients would improve the effectiveness of a patient communication seminar. As authors report, they are continually adjusting the curriculum based upon resident feedback and available resources given the constraints at one medical center. This example in particular demonstrates the utility of systemic curriculum inquiry for the development and improvement of a professionalism curriculum [23].

Returning back to our case of the surgeon throwing surgical tools, how can observers respond to the situation of unprofessional behavior? Providing the staff and the students opportunities to report these behaviors in an anonymous fashion allows for both a correction mechanism and a potential deterrence. Debriefing opportunities in a safe space after such events for the staff, most notably the resident and student, would allow for discussion and processing of the events. This may have salvaged the student's interest in surgery and could have provided the student the timely opportunity to reveal their suspicion of a retained sponge. The combination of enforcement mechanisms and discussion opportunities allows for these moments of unprofessional behavior to become moments of improvement and learning [18].

14.4   Conclusion

While the concept of teaching professionalism is young, it is a growing field. Teaching methods range from traditional techniques (harnessing of a hidden curriculum, engaging positive role models) to innovative (formal curricula and abundant use of simulation). The methods discussed here are summarized in Table 14.4. Depending on the specific circumstances of a residency or hospital, any combination of these techniques may be utilized. In reference to the professionalism principles outlined by the ACS, Table 14.6 provides suggestions for how these might be addressed during residency education, either independently or within a curriculum, depending on the need. Definitive outcome data regarding success of the various curricula discussed are forthcoming, as the reported programs continue to grow and reassess their effectiveness. As we reviewed earlier, the impact of professionalism education is likely to be experienced by surgeons beyond residency. Thus, the long-term impact of these curricula should be assessed by evaluating surgeons in practice who have completed these programs during residency. However, the techniques described here certainly are promising, and demonstrate positive results thus far, suggesting that professionalism, like any other important pillar of medical education, can and should be taught.

Table 14.6 ACS principles of professional conduct [30] and suggestions for teaching

Surgeon-based
Component of professionalism:
Scientific knowledge
Surgical competence
Honesty
Self-regulation
Maintain trust by managing conflict of interest
Professional responsibilities
Primacy of patient welfare
Suggestion for Teaching:
Lectures
Technical skill simulation
Case-based discussion
Wellness seminars, distribution of available resources
Mentorship
Inter-disciplinary communication workshop
Patient-based
Component of professionalism:
Social justice
Patient autonomy
Patient confidentiality
Appropriate relations with patients
Suggestion for Teaching:
Lectures
Case- or video-based discussions
Standardized patient-based simulation
Objective Structured Clinical Examination (OSCE)
System-based
Component of professionalism:
Improving quality care
Improving access to care
Just distribution of finite resources
Suggestion for Teaching:
Lectures
Participation in quality improvement project
Participation in quality improvement committee

14.5 Selected References

- Cooper WO, Spain DA, Guillamondegui O, et al. Association of Coworker Reports About Unprofessional Behavior by Surgeons With Surgical Complications in Their Patients. JAMA Surg 2019;154:828.

  Authors correlated increased event reports of unprofessional behavior by surgeons with worse outcomes of their patients using the National Surgical Quality Improvement Program database.

- Hochberg MS, Kalet A, Zabar S, Kachur E, Gillespie C, German RS. Can professionalism be taught? Encouraging evidence. Am J Surg. 2010;199:86–93.

  Authors report on their professionalism curriculum in an American surgical residency program, demonstrating a positive improvement in the core competencies of Professionalism and Communication after completion of the program.

References

1. Accreditation Council for Graduate Medical Education. ACGME common program requirements (residency). February 3, 2020; effective July 1, 2020. https://www.acgme.org/Portals/0/PFAssets/ProgramRequirements/CPRResidency2020.pdf. Accessed 12 Dec 2020.
2. Gruen RL, Arya J, Cosgrove EM, et al. Professionalism in surgery. J Am Coll Surg. 2003;197:605–8. https://doi.org/10.1016/s1072-7515(03)00588-x.
3. ACS Task Force on professionalism. Code of professional conduct. J Am Coll Surg 2004;199:734–735. doi:https://doi.org/10.1016/j.jamcollsurg.2004.08.009.
4. Seehusen DA. Understanding unprofessionalism in residents. J Grad Med Educ 2020;12:243–246. https://doi.org/10.4300.jgme-d-19-00668.1.
5. Cooper WO, Spain DA, Guillamondegui O, et al. Association of Coworker Reports about Unprofessional Behavior by surgeons with surgical complications in their patients. JAMA Surg. 2019;154:828–34. https://doi.org/10.1001/jamasurg.2019.1738.
6. Krupat E, Dienstag JL, Padrino SL, et al. Do professionalism lapses in medical school predict problems in residency and clinical practice? Acad Med. 2020;95:888–95. https://doi.org/10.1097/acm.0000000000003145.
7. Papadakis MA, Hodgson CS, Teherani A, Kohatsu ND. Unprofessional behavior in medical school is associated with subsequent disciplinary action by a state medical board. Acad Med. 2004;79:244–9.
8. Sullivan ME, Trial J, Baker C, et al. A framework for professionalism in surgery: what is important to medical students? Am J Surg. 2014;207:255–9. https://doi.org/10.1016/j.amjsurg.2013.08.027.
9. Biagioli FE, Rdesinski RE, Elliot DL, Chappelle KG, Kwong KL, Toffler WL. Surgery clerkship evaluations drive improved professionalism. J Surg Educ. 2013;70:149–55. https://doi.org/10.1016/j.jsurg.2012.06.020.
10. Park J, Woodrow SI, Reznick RK, Beales J, MacRae HM. Observation, reflection, and reinforcement: surgery faculty Members' and Residents' perceptions of how they learned professionalism. Acad Med. 2010;85:134–9. https://doi.org/10.1097/acm.0b013e3181c47b25.
11. Dilday JC, Miller EA, Schmitt K, Davis B, Davis KG. Professionalism: a Core competency, but what does it mean? A survey of surgery residents. J Surg Educ. 2018;75:601–5. https://doi.org/10.1016/j.jsurg.2017.09.033.
12. Bosk CL. Forgive and remember: managing medical failure. University of Chicago Press; 1979.

13. Ong YT, Kow CS, Teo YH, et al. Nurturing professionalism in medical schools. A systematic scoping review of training curricula between 1990–2019. Med Teach. 2020;42:636–49. https://doi.org/10.1080/0142159x.2020.1724921.

14. Berger AS, Niedra E, Brooks SG, Ahmed WS, Ginsburg S. Teaching professionalism in postgraduate medical education: a systematic review. Acad Med. 2020;95:938–46. https://doi.org/10.1097/acm.0000000000002987.

15. Patel P, Martimianakis MA, Zilbert NR, et al. Fake it 'Til you make it: pressures to measure up in surgical training. Acad Med. 2018;93:769–74. https://doi.org/10.1097/acm.0000000000002113.

16. Flinders DJ, Noddings N, Thornton SJ. The null curriculum: its theoretical basis and practical implications. Curr Inquiry. 1986;16:33–42.

17. Hafferty FW, Gaufberg EH, O'Donnell JF. The role of the hidden curriculum in "on doctoring" courses. AMA J Ethics. 2015;17:129–37. https://doi.org/10.1001/virtualmentor.2015.17.2.medu1-1502.

18. Rogers DA, Boehler ML, Roberts NK, Johnson V. Using the hidden curriculum to teach professionalism during the surgery clerkship. J Surg Educ. 2012;69:423–7. https://doi.org/10.1016/j.jsurg.2011.09.008.

19. Goldstein EA, Maestas RR, Fryer-Edwards K, et al. Professionalism in medical education: an institutional challenge. Acad Med. 2006;81:871–6. https://doi.org/10.1097/01.acm.0000238199.37217.68.

20. Horsburgh J, Ippolito K. A skill to be worked at: using social learning theory to explore the process of learning from role models in clinical settings. BMC Med Educ. 2018;18:156. https://doi.org/10.1186/s12909-018-1251-x.

21. Smith KL, Saavedra R, Raeke JL, O'Donell AA. The journey to creating a campus-wide culture of professionalism. Acad Med. 2007;82:1015–21. https://doi.org/10.1097/acm.0b013e318157633e.

22. Deptula P, Chun MBJ. A literature review of professionalism in surgical education: suggested components for development of a curriculum. J Surg Educ. 2013;70:408–22. https://doi.org/10.1016/j.jsurg.2012.11.007.

23. Thomas PA, Kern DE, Hughes MT, Chen BY, editors. Curriculum development for medical education: a six-step approach. 3rd ed. Johns Hopkins University Press; 2016.

24. de Montbrun S, MacRae H. Simulation in surgical education. Clin Colon Rectal Surg. 2012;25:156–65. https://doi.org/10.1055/s-0032-1322553.

25. Issenberg BS, McGaghie WC, Petrusa ER, Gordon DL, Scalese RJ. Features and uses of high-fidelity medical simulations that lead to effective learning: a BEME systematic review. Med Teacher. 2005;27:10–28. https://doi.org/10.1080/01421590500046924.

26. Wali E, Pinto JM, Cappaert M, et al. Teaching professionalism in graduate medical education: what is the role of simulation? Surgery. 2016;160:552–64. https://doi.org/10.1016/j.surg.2016.03.026.

27. Hochberg MS, Kalet A, Zabar S, Kachur E, Gillespie C, German RS. Can professionalism be taught? Encouraging evidence. Am J Surg. 2010;199:86–93. https://doi.org/10.1016/j.amjsurg.2009.10.002.

28. Hochberg MS, Berman RS, Kalet AL, Zabar S, Gillespie C, Pachter HL. Professionalism training for surgical residents: documenting the advantages of a professionalism curriculum. Ann Surgery. 2016;264:501–7. https://doi.org/10.1097/sla.0000000000001843.

29. Larkin AC, Cahan MA, Whalen G, et al. Human emotion and response in surgery (HEARS): a simulation-based curriculum for communication skills, systems-based practice, and professionalism in surgical residency training. J Am Coll Surg. 2010;211:285–92. https://doi.org/10.1016/j.jamcollsurg.2010.04.004.

30. Barry L, Blair P, Cosgrove E, et al. One year, and counting, after publication of our ACS "code of professional conduct". J Am Coll Surg. 2004;199:736–40. https://doi.org/10.1016/j.jamcollsurg.2004.08.004.

Chapter 15
Surgical Training During a Pandemic

Xavier Pereira ⓘ and Mindy B. Statter ⓘ

Abstract The COVID-19 pandemic caused by the severe acute respiratory syndrome coronavirus-2 (SARS-CoV-2) has caused an unprecedented public health crisis with challenges that can be categorized as operational, technological, knowledge-based, and ethical. The ethical challenge for trainees has been the abrupt transition from patient-centered ethics to public health ethics. This chapter will explore the impact of the COVID-19 pandemic on the surgical residency construct, the residency "life cycle", and the individual resident as a member of the surgical workforce, as a trainee, and their personal well-being.

Keywords COVID-19 · Pandemic · Surgical training · Moral distress
Self-compassion

> **Case**
> Mr. C was one of the four patients assigned to this resident in the all COVID-19 makeshift intensive care unit. This particular unit, staffed by surgical residents and attending surgeons, was housed within a new pediatric hematology infusion floor. The colorful, child-like art freshly painted on the walls was more therapeutic to providers than the unconscious patients they cared for. Earlier in the week, Mr. C was one of the first COVID-19 patients to undergo a bedside tracheostomy at the hospital. The resident participated in the procedure despite the fact that it had not been well studied in patients with coronavirus and concerns surrounding the high risk of transmission to providers continued to surface. The procedure allowed Mr. C's sedation to be decreased and his mental status gradually improved; he was now following simple commands

X. Pereira · M. B. Statter (✉)
Department of Surgery, Montefiore Medical Center, New York City, NY, USA
e-mail: xpereira@montefiore.org; mstatter@montefiore.org

© The Author(s), under exclusive license to Springer Nature
Switzerland AG 2022
V. A. Lonchyna et al. (eds.), *Difficult Decisions in Surgical Ethics*, Difficult
Decisions in Surgery: An Evidence-Based Approach,
https://doi.org/10.1007/978-3-030-84625-1_15

and nodding his head to answer simple questions. Yet, there was no family in sight to celebrate this victory. Due to restricted visitation families were not allowed to visit their loved ones and relied on video calls and frequent dialogue with providers. Each day the resident video-conferenced the patient's family at the same time, 3 p.m. On this particular afternoon Mr. C's eyes were glued to the screen and his family's voices seemed to bring a grin to his face, a first for Mr. C. It was hard to spend more than a few minutes per patient on these calls in the fast-paced setting of an ICU. During this call one of the nearby patients began showing signs of instability and other providers were rushing to the bedside. Annoyed that the family was not satisfied, the resident left the tablet propped up on the side rail facing the patient and left to tend to his unstable patient.

15.1 Introduction

15.1.1 Impact of the Pandemic on the Surgical Residency Construct

The COVID-19 pandemic caused by the severe acute respiratory syndrome coronavirus-2 (SARS-CoV-2) has caused an unprecedented public health crisis. With health care delivery systems prioritizing COVID-19 both patient care processes and surgical education have been disrupted. The challenges faced in this pandemic can be categorized as operational, technological, knowledge-based, and ethical (see Table 15.1). Operationally, there is the challenge of availability of "space, stuff, and staff"—personal protective equipment (PPE), equipment (ventilators, dialysis machines, and hospital beds) and pairing supply with demand [1]. Due to the surge of patients, surgeons and trainees were redeployed to new specialties and departments. The strain on resources has forced hospitals to implement unfamiliar practices such as cancellation of elective operations, non-essential clinic visits, and restricted visitation policies. It became necessary to balance patient needs versus contagion risk from aerosol-generating procedures such as endoscopy, bronchoscopy, intubation, and tracheostomy. Elective surgery was postponed in order to manage the PPE supply, but most importantly, to manage staff and resource supply. Technologically, many elements of clinical care were rapidly transitioned to telemedicine, including communication with patients' families. Academic activity and education have transitioned from being conducted in-person to remotely. Innovation has included modification of best practices for laparoscopy. The knowledge-based challenges include the evolving development of institutional protocols and best practices based on new data that continue to be published and shared [2]. Ethically, surgeons and trainees during this pandemic have been forced to shift from patient-centered ethics to public health ethics [3].

Table 15.1 Ethical principles in conflict during the pandemic

Respect for autonomy	Surgeons and trainees during the peak of the pandemic were in positions where they could not respect all of their patient's wishes and experienced discomfort with this shift from shared decision making to paternalism. Inability to effectively advocate for their patients.
Beneficence (maximizing benefit) vs. Non-maleficence (minimizing harm)	Surgeons and trainees in their fiduciary role, were faced with reconciling their commitment to patient care with personal risk to themselves and their loved ones. Surgeons and trainees were faced with providing care to COVID and non-COVID patients that was not up to standard of care. Due to workforce restructuring, surgeons and trainees were deployed to unfamiliar units, often practicing outside of one's scope of practice. Faced with uncertainty due to lack of experience with this novel coronavirus, applying standard algorithms, e.g., for respiratory failure, were not successful. Maximizing benefit with intubation and ventilatory support was later found to be harmful to patients. Trainees assisted in performing high risk surgical procedures, such as tracheostomies, to expedite the transfer of patients to the floor and "unload" the intensive care units only to find out later that the patient expired. The residents were faced with the conflict of providing care, being beneficent, and concomitantly doing a disservice to the patient, non-maleficence. Surgeons and trainees were faced with the duty to provide care despite institutional heterogeneity in the standardization of PPE use and availability. This caused a sense of inequity and raised concern about potentially increased exposure at certain practice sites. Surgeons and trainees were faced with performing futile CPR in the setting of cardiac arrest from refractory respiratory failure with associated non-reversible multisystem organ failure creating additional COVID exposure to providers without benefit to the patient.
Justice	The standard of care was impacted by the allocation of limited resources, e.g., intensive care unit space, ventilators, and hemodialysis machines, creating conflict around the principle of distributive justice.

15.2 Search Strategy

A PubMed search was performed utilizing the key words COVID-19, pandemic, coronavirus, surgical training. Thirty published articles and articles in press from March 2020 were reviewed.

15.3 Discussion

This chapter is a review of the impact of the COVID-19 pandemic on the surgical residency construct, the residency "life cycle" and the individual resident as a member of the surgical workforce, as a trainee. The shared personal experiences of the Montefiore general surgery residents during the peak of the outbreak in New York

City, specifically the Bronx, where Montefiore is located, will illustrate the impact of the COVID-19 pandemic on the well-being of the individual resident.

Globally, in response to the pandemic, novel approaches were employed to meet the demands of the high COVID-19 patient volumes. General surgery teams were restructured to provide ongoing care, prioritize workforce safety and well-being, with flexibility and sustainability of the workforce, and compliance with physical distancing. At the University of California San Francisco Health System (UCSF) the Department of Surgery combined general surgery services, and as volume decreased, resident staffing was reduced by 67%. The resident rotation schedule was adjusted to ensure that residents remained at a single hospital to prevent cross-contamination across sites. Similarly, attendings were assigned to cover only one hospital. It was emphasized that "in this time of uncertainty, we are all in this together and we need to develop a new level of trust with our colleagues…" accentuating that it was essential that there was a level of trust between providers that everyone was prioritizing what was right for patients and staying within the parameters of the case triage system [4].

Caring for patients balances the ethical principles of beneficence, maximizing benefit, and nonmaleficence, minimizing harm. Surgeons and trainees were faced with providing care to COVID and non-COVID patients that was not up to the usual standards of practice. In managing COVID patients at the initial peak of the outbreak there was significant uncertainty due to the lack of experience with this coronavirus; applying standard algorithms for respiratory failure were not successful. Maximizing benefit with intubation and ventilatory support was later found to be harmful to patients. Non-COVID patients had biopsies of masses postponed, timely tumor resections after completing chemotherapy were deferred. The standard of care was impacted by the allocation of limited resources, e.g., intensive care unit space and ventilators, creating discordance with the ethical principle of distributive justice (see Table 15.1).

Leadership became aware of the unique policies and microenvironments within which their faculty and residents practiced. Lack of standardization of PPE use across practice sites caused a sense of inequity and concern about potentially increased exposure at certain sites. In their fiduciary role, surgeons and trainees were faced with reconciling their commitment to patient care with their moral duties to self and their families. When developing a guideline for the use of laparoscopy during the pandemic, leadership developed one that would work in all practice environments, despite variations in equipment, supplies, and vendors [4].

The use of HIPAA-compliant texting applications and other methods of digital communication was essential to safe transition of patient care while avoiding face-to-face contact and imperative to the maintenance of mandated confidentiality [5].

Workforce restructuring included the development of specific teams and strategic appropriation of resources to facilitate care. As an example, a "Surgical Workforce Access Team" (SWAT) provided a specialized team with the skill set to efficiently perform bedside procedures, e.g., arterial, central venous, and hemodialysis catheters. This effort offloaded procedural work from the emergency medicine, critical care, and medicine departments supporting colleagues, reducing health care personnel exposure, and economizing personal protective equipment [6]. Workforce restructuring also included the deployment of surgeons and trainees to novel, unfamiliar units often practicing outside one's scope of practice creating disharmony in balancing beneficence and nonmaleficence.

As systems prepared and responded to the COVID-19 pandemic, there were different approaches to the surgical hierarchy. The restructuring of the Emory University Department of Orthopedic Surgery residency training more closely resembled a military hierarchy. Their strategy included patient and provider safety, ongoing provision of necessary care, system sustainability, system tolerance of uncertainty and flexibility as circumstances evolve, and preservation of command and control. This latter point is a departure from the typical lead-from-the front surgical mentality, in order to protect the thought leaders and experienced decision-makers [7]. In contrast, in Singapore, senior members of the surgical department rotated alongside junior surgical staff members serving in equal capacity at the frontline, despite the heavier administrative burden on the senior staff. This "flattening of the hierarchy" and leading by example lifted morale and instilled confidence among the junior members [8]. However, this boosting of team morale with institution leadership leading by example and joining the frontline, regardless of hierarchy, was countered in an invited commentary:

> While this gesture is commendable, it should be weighed in the context of risk-to-benefit ratio of potentially exposing a senior member of the institution to the disease, whose role may not be easily replaceable…potentially creating more harm to the situation…The need to seek unity as one healthcare system is the irony amidst the social distancing and isolation that we must now observe. …Trust in the institution and system to prioritize its staff welfare and safety remains core and vital to achieving unity [9].

15.3.1 Impact of the Pandemic on the Residency "Life Cycle"

The surgical residency, like all resident training programs, has a 'life cycle." July heralds the start the academic year, with the influx of new trainees attending orientation and their predecessors advancing to the next PGY-level. Medical students plan away-rotations to experience a program first-hand, and by performing well, hope to be highly considered during resident recruitment. The recruitment process begins in the fall, with departments holding pre-interview social events, in-person interviews, resident tours, and group ranking meetings. Residents are required to take Fundamentals of Laparoscopic Surgery (FLS) and Fundamentals of Endoscopic Surgery (FES) which involves travel to a testing site. Fellowship interviews in the winter and spring involve significant travel by residents.

In June, chief resident preparation for graduation includes completing applications for the American Board of Surgery Qualifying Exam. The milestone of graduation, the culmination of five or more years of clinical training and research, is celebrated at a departmental graduation ceremony attended by the faculty, the graduating residents, their families, spouses, partners, and the junior residents. Due to the concern for viral transmission and restrictions on meeting size, and the risk of travel from cities with high COVID-19 case numbers, all of these activities within the life cycle of the surgical residency have been affected—cancelled or modified to virtual formats.

At Montefiore morale boosting social events celebrating residency milestones such as the "I survived July" party held the last Friday of the month and the post-American Board of Surgery In-Training Examination (ABSITE) party were cancelled.

The interview seasons of surgical fellowships has been significantly affected by the pandemic. Fellowship interviews have universally moved to videoconferencing or teleconferencing. While virtual fellowship interviews still require applicants to ask for protected time from their training programs, days are no longer lost to travel and there is an overall net recuperation of resident clinical productivity. In addition, virtual interviews reduce additive costs to student debt; an applicant would have spent approximately $6000 for live interviews applying for surgical fellowships in 2020 [10].

For each fellowship program new to virtual recruitment, there is a significant upfront investment. In contrast to time saved for the interview applicants, there may not be savings in faculty and staff time due to the time needed for troubleshooting connectivity problems with technical support staff and training faculty in using virtual platforms. Program hard costs, not including personnel effort, is approximately $8400. There are concerns about the equivalency of virtual interviews to live, in-person recruitment [11].

Recommendations for conducting virtual interviews include:

1. Pre-interview preparation of stakeholders including program administrators, interviewers, and information technologists (IT) regarding logistics [11].
2. Preparation of staff and faculty to become more facile with the videoconferencing platform [10].
3. Fellowship applicants and faculty members should prepare for virtual interviews as they would for live interviews. Fellowship programs should accommodate applicants whose home environment may not be appropriate for the interview or may need modifications of their interview days due to clinical responsibilities during the pandemic and recovery [10].
4. Pre-produced videos can be used to highlight traditionally unique "live" aspects of the recruitment, e.g., campus, hospital, city tours. Websites can be supplemented with narrated slide shows and podcasts instead of hardcopy program materials.[13] Detailed written program information should be provided in advance of the virtual event; this allows for meaningful use of interface time during interview [11].
5. Designating a 'Master of Ceremonies' (MC) during the interview, whose responsibilities include appropriate muting of participant microphones, progressing through the designated activities and calling on individual applicants and program representatives to avoid multiple simultaneous speaker [11].

6. Having a 1-hour unscripted question and answer session between the applicants and fellows; applicants submit typed questions through the teleconferencing platform in order to facilitate aggregation of similar questions; and moderating a question queue to minimize downtime; the MC selects the questions, and the fellows respond [11].
7. Post-interview follow-up with the applicants shortly after the conclusion of interviews [11].

During the pandemic communications from regulatory bodies have identified issues related to resident education and wellness. The Accreditation Committee for Graduate Medical Education (ACGME) acknowledged the critical role of the graduate education community in the nation's response to the COVID-19 pandemic, suspending many accreditation-related activities to allow programs to focus on the needs of patients and the careful and appropriate integration of residents into that process:

> The ACGME recognizes that residents have been redeployed to support the critical services of the hospital as a result of the pandemic and may not be able to achieve the minimum number of visits/cases as specified in the time-based and volume-based specialty specific requirements. Visit/case minimums were established for program accreditation and were not designed to be a surrogate for the competence of an individual graduate. Program directors, with consideration of the recommendations of the program's Clinical Competency Committee, were entrusted to assess the competence of an individual resident as one part of the determination of whether that individual is prepared to enter the unsupervised practice of surgery [12].

The COVID-19 pandemic may be an opportunity for educational reform. Progression in time-based surgical training is dependent upon exposure to and performance of specified visit/case minimums in the elective setting which were eliminated during the pandemic. By restructuring training and transitioning from time-based to competency-based, time-variable graduate medical education each physician graduates from residency, or fellowship to unsupervised practice when the necessary competencies are achieved [13].

The mission of the American Board of Surgery (ABS) includes "…protecting the public and enhancing the profession" via "…tools of oversight of resident training and supervision, administration of specialty examinations, and initial confirmation and maintenance of certification [2]." The ABS stated that their role "…is to minimize concerns trainees have about examinations and certification processes, so trainees can appropriately focus on resource-stricken patient-care and self-care throughout the pandemic [2]." The training requirements for chief residents completing training in 2020 were modified allowing for non-voluntary offsite time used for clinical or educational purposed to be counted as clinical time and accepting a 10% decrease in total operative case numbers [2].

15.3.2 Impact of the Pandemic on the Individual Resident

15.3.2.1 Moral Distress, Moral Residue, and Moral Resilience

In shifting from patient-centered ethics to public health ethics tension is experienced among the needs of individual patients versus the community, patient-centered care versus the common good, and patient preference versus fair resource allocation [18]. Our residents confronted death on an unprecedented scale and were not adequately trained for the work delegated to them during this pandemic (see Table 15.2) [1].

Table 15.2 Contributors to moral burden among surgical trainees during the pandemic

Fiduciary role vs. Personal safety	Residents were anxious and fearful of getting sick and spreading the virus at home, and anxious observing the spread of the pandemic nationally and internationally. Their anxiety was attributable to reconciling their duty to care for patients with personal safety and the health of their loved ones. Residents were frustrated with institutional heterogeneity in providing PPE This lack of equity put them at increased risk of exposure to COVID-19. Residents were often deployed to new settings and needed to assume new roles including that of palliative care provider. Residents perceived a lack of fairness when general surgery residents were performing increasing numbers of tracheostomies compared to the otolaryngology residents. They felt they carried a greater burden of responsibility and were subjected to greater personal risk.
Impact upon professional identity as surgeons	Generally, "action-oriented", in control, adhering to a strong work ethic, a true sense of belonging at work was challenged by not operating due to cancellation of elective cases and deployment to unfamiliar units. Residents, who often work collaboratively, were split up during the pandemic contributing to isolation.
Impact upon moral integrity	Residents were witnessing death at unprecedented rates. Death affected their medical community and the other communities to which they belong. Amplification of unresolved grief has contributed to moral distress. Residents admitted to habituation to the "code" announcement. Residents felt powerless witnessing so many critically ill and rapidly deteriorating patients requiring often unsuccessful resuscitation. Residents became frustrated with the disease progression—not seeing patients improve and leave the intensive care unit or the hospital. The patients became homogeneous—same comorbidities, same difficult course. Residents were frustrated with the inability to provide care due to unavailable resources. Residents experienced discordance with their values. They seized the opportunity to operate, performing tracheostomies and percutaneous endoscopic gastrostomies, but questioned whether these procedures were of any benefit to the patient. Residents expressed frustration with their inability to advocate for patients. Residents expressed sadness in seeing patients lose control over decision-making and were uncomfortable with the shift to a greater level of paternalism. Residents expressed sadness in seeing patients die alone.

Moral uncertainty occurs when the agent, the clinician, does not know the ethically correct course, but perceives uncertainty, a sense that something is not right. A moral dilemma occurs when two or more opposing actions can be equally justified and the agent, unable to carry out both actions, faces the dilemma of choosing which ethical course to follow [14]. In 1984 Andrew Jameton introduced the concept of "moral distress" to characterize circumstances in which "one knows the right thing to do, but institutional constraints make it nearly impossible to pursue the right course of action" [15]. Moral distress is the result of a perceived violation of one's core values and duties, concurrent with a feeling of being constrained from taking ethically appropriate action. Emotional (psychological) distress describes emotional reactions to situations but does not necessarily involve violation of core values and duties. Moral distress is a relational experience shaped by multiple contexts, including the socio-political, and cultural context of the workplace environment. Moral agency based on the virtue of integrity is essential to medicine. One of the most important moral products of professional integrity is the sense of self-worth that results from commitments to intellectual and moral excellence in the care of patients. Individual integrity generates one's self-worth as a human being—mattering in the lives of others. A consequence of moral distress, the perceived violations of core values and duties, is that individual moral concerns can remain unaddressed leading to erosion of moral integrity [16]. Moral distress differs from emotional distress; moral distress is destructive to the moral agency and integrity of health care providers. Experiences of moral distress compromise providers' core values which are the fundamental ingredients of their moral, professional, and individual integrity [17]. Frustration, anger, anxiety, guilt, compromised integrity, and psychological disequilibrium characterize moral distress [14]. The awareness that one has become morally undone in response to violations of individual or professional integrity generates worse psychological outcomes such as depression, burnout and dangerous patient care [16].

Sources of moral distress fall into three categories: clinical situations, factors internal to the caregiver, and factors external to the caregiver but inherent in the environment in which the moral distress occurs. Moral distress occurs most commonly in clinical situations when a caregiver perceives care to be unnecessary, unwarranted and futile. Trainees often know the patient and family well, gather much of the information the team needs to formulate a care plan, and then find themselves marginalized at the time of decision-making. Their moral distress may also result from being expected to implement a treatment plan contrary to their ethical beliefs. An internal source of moral distress can be only knowing partial information of a complex case or being unaware of events that took place when the caregiver was absent. The distress may be ameliorated once all facts are known [16]. External factors include limited resources, expressed and unexpressed biases, and institutional constraints [18].

Moral distress can be exacerbated by external forces outside the constraints of the hospital and direct patient care. At home, residents experience moral distress as they weigh the risk of transmission to family members while fulfilling their roles as healthcare providers. Isolating from loved ones at home is not always a feasible option given the financial, time-related, and social constraints of surgical training. As close relatives fall ill, often in geographically distant locations, residents are left without the option to travel and support their loved ones. These external factors cause an unintended isolation from residents' support systems in a time of increased moral distress and moral injury.

Challenges to professional integrity can occur repeatedly; while each episode may seem manageable, their cumulative effect may not be, resulting in moral residue [16]. Moral residue describes the lingering feelings after a morally problematic situation has passed. Moral residue is dependent upon repeated experiences of moral distress. Moral distress is associated with feelings of powerlessness, and inability to fix a wrong, anger, and frustration [19]. The true focus of moral distress and the repetitive nature resulting in moral residue implicates a systemic, multidisciplinary, organizational issue. Ethics consultation services must be aware of the difference between the classic ethical dilemma and moral distress because there may be a failure to identify and treat the problem. The strategies for addressing moral distress are not necessarily the same as reasoning through a moral dilemma [19]. The difference between burnout, a work-related syndrome characterized by emotional exhaustion, depersonalization, and a decreased sense of personal accomplishment, and moral injury is important because using different terminology reframes the problem and the solution. Burnout suggests that the problem resides within the individual, implying deficiency in the individual's resilience to withstand the work environment. In contrast, moral distress and moral injury describe the challenge of simultaneously knowing what care patients need but being unable to provide it due to constraints that are beyond one's control [20].

15.3.2.2 Strategies for Addressing and Mitigating Moral Distress

Antidotes to moral distress include moral agency and moral community. Moral agency implies self-directed capacity or choice to act and is characteristically exercised in the context of deeply interconnected relationships. Solutions to moral challenges are actuated collaboratively through collective effort. Moral resilience is the capacity to restore, sustain, or deepen integrity in response to moral distress and includes self-awareness, and self-regulation skills such as mindfulness, and empathy [21]. There will be post-pandemic growth. As surgeons we are action-oriented, we are defined by our work ethic, and have a true sense of belonging at work. This pandemic has somewhat disrupted that sense of purpose. As stated by Victor Frankl, MD, psychiatrist, and Holocaust survivor, "Those who have a 'why' to live, can bear with almost any 'how'" [22]. Finding meaning in work cultivates resiliency. What distinguishes resilient individuals is the way they view the world—their framing lens—their mindset is a growth mindset that aligns their personal values with work that shapes their actions. A growth mindset leads to optimistic ways of explaining adversity which leads to perseverance [23]. Limited resources expressed and unexpressed biases, institutional constraints, and personal values can result in discordance; dissonance leads to moral distress. Adopting an ethical mindset, being aware of the conflict between two or more ethical principles that can cause moral distress, can mitigate harmful consequences [18].

15.3.2.3 The Role of "Moral Distress Rounds"

Montefiore Medical Center is located in the Bronx, a borough that is racially diverse and predominantly low-income and the hardest-hit borough in New York during the pandemic. At the peak of the COVID-19 outbreak the Bronx had the highest number of coronavirus related cases, hospitalizations, and deaths. During this pandemic we have all become aware of how susceptible we are to multiple losses daily—loss of financial security, loss of social and physical connections, loss of general safety, and loss of autonomy to move around the world. Visitation has been limited or prohibited for hospitalized patients. For bereaved individuals, funerals and burials have been postponed or held remotely.

Clinicians were isolating themselves from their own families indefinitely because of the concern of potentially spreading infection. Working behind the barriers of personal protective equipment (PPE) has increased the sense of distance between provider and patient as well as between colleagues. It has been necessary to attend to both physical and emotional safety [24]. Altruistic goals can become overshadowed by the realization of significant personal health risk [18].

For trainees who are vulnerable to the power differential in surgical hierarchies, experiences of moral distress can be seminal events that can impact their future practice behavior [14]. The resident's sense of responsibility is substantial whether or not that individual participated in the resource allocation decisions or had to uphold the decisions with the patient and family [18]. Being able to express concerns or distress can have utility, allowing individuals to tap into the shared experiences of personal suffering, and one's imperfections can become critical points for self-kindness that can strengthen empathy when helping others [25].

Moral distress rounds (see Table 15.3) were held to provide the Montefiore general surgery residents with a safe space to reflect and share their experiences during the pandemic. The purpose of the surgery moral distress rounds was first to revive a

Table 15.3 Role of moral distress rounds

Moral distress rounds	Held virtually during the peak of the pandemic, provided the residents with a safe space to foster reflection, connectedness, and bolster resilience
Purpose of rounds	1. Revive a sense of community among all of the residents 2. To share experiences to reinforce the common humanity—we are all in this together 3. To re-invigorate a sense of purpose, belonging, and conformation of our identity as surgeons.

sense of community among all the residents, second to share experiences to rein-force the common humanity—we are all in this together, and third to re-invigorate a sense of purpose, belonging, and a confirmation of our identity as surgeons. Their insights, lessons learned, and candid revelations as they faced the challenges to their moral integrity as surgeons, their responsibility to their patients, and their personal safety are shared in this section. Moral distress rounds fostered reflection, connect-edness, and bolstered resilience.

Grief was and is inherently a part of the COVID-19 pandemic affecting patients, families, and providers. Anticipatory grief is the normal mourning that occurs when death is expected. Providers have been experiencing death at unprecedented rates. The experience of death becomes more personal as it affects the provider's medical community and the other communities that providers belong to. Anticipatory grief results from uncertainty as well as trying to make sense of what is coming. For patients, families, and providers there is the uncertainty of disease progression and how they will be impacted by changing hospital policies. Many providers tend to put aside their own feelings and emotions, prioritizing patient care and well-being, using avoidance strategies or compartmentalization to continue treating patients which can lead to unresolved grief. With the unprecedented amount of death during this pandemic unresolved grief has been amplified and can contribute to moral dis-tress [24].

Prior to the first rounds the residents were asked to reflect upon how the pan-demic had affected each of them as an individual, as a surgical trainee, and as a member of the surgical workforce. When prompted with the question, "What are you feeling?" the first feeling expressed was *anxiety*.

Anxiety—and the associated fear of getting sick, having other residents get sick, spreading the virus at home, and watching the pandemic spread across one's home country with concern for family and friends residing there. Anxiety was attributed to their reconciling their duty to care for patients and their personal safety and the health of their family and loved ones. "Hearing code announcements so frequently contributed to anxiety. Now you don't even pay attention". The habituation to the code announcement is an example of how moral residue can develop. Moral distress occurs with feelings of powerlessness as residents witness so many critically ill and rapidly deteriorating patients require often unsuccessful resuscitation. The cumula-tive effect of these repetitive episodes of moral distress contributes to the develop-ment of moral residue impacting professional integrity. One junior resident stated that she has had heightened anxiety since starting training and now everyone else's anxiety is elevated—"they have caught up to my level of anxiety". This exemplifies that there is not the usual emotional containment and that emotions are on the surface.

Loneliness—"What we do day-to-day is collaborative—we are split up. We are not having in-depth discussions with colleagues, consultants, and nurses." This iso-lation altered their identity as surgeons. Several expressed feeling overwhelmed working in a new environment—surgical residents have been deployed to other units to provide much needed care to COVID-19 patients and have assumed new roles within surgical settings.

These new roles include that of the palliative care provider. Four key aspects of palliative care are instructive to surgeons:

1. Using serious illness communication strategies to disclose prognosis and establish goals of care. These strategies include the use of templates, which provide a prepared script and imparts confidence when having potentially emotionally laden conversations.
2. Treating total pain. As surgeons we commonly assess and treat physical pain. Patients with serious illness experience total pain which includes physical, psychological, social, and spiritual components.
3. Caring for the family unit—The rapid progression of the illness, the restricted visitation, and difficulties in keeping families informed produced stress for patients, families, and providers.
4. Supporting clinicians to cope with the challenges of being deployed to areas outside their specialty, working under adverse conditions, fearing becoming sick and possibly spreading COVID to their families and loved ones [26].

Frustration in several aspects was shared—in their role, they are not operating. This is linked to their loss of identity as surgeons. Elective surgery was cancelled. "In the beginning of the ICU rotation I felt demoted to intern-being told what to do—this did eliminate some burden of responsibility however it became rote, boring." Frustrated with the disease progression—not seeing patients improve and leave the ICU. They are frustrated with "taking care of a lot of patients that are the same"—the patient population has become homogeneous—"The same comorbidities, same difficult course—you think they can be extubated, and then they fail—we seem to not be fixing anything." This aspect of frustration illustrates the conflict between beneficence and nonmaleficence. Frustration with the institutional heterogeneity in providing personal protective equipment (PPE). Frustration with resource allocation—many of the patients in the ICU go into renal failure and peritoneal dialysis is not effective—these patients need hemodialysis. There is only one hemodialysis machine, and it comes down to deciding who is the sickest, who will benefit the most. "Disturbing—I felt torn after putting myself in the position of the family member and wanting to offer this therapy [hemodialysis] but felt helpless because it was not available to every patient." When confronted with the inability to provide care due to unavailable resources, the lack of distributive justice, the residents perceived frustration.

They expressed frustration in the constant comparison to other services, hospitals within our health care system, and other health care systems. These repeatedly highlighted inconsistencies added to anxiety, doubt, fear, and uncertainty. Feeling 'taken advantage of'—lack of fairness—doing the work of other services—"Why wasn't ENT doing the trachs [tracheostomies]?" Although not vocalized, their frustration arises from the conflict between beneficence and the duty to care, and the concern for their own safety, and the perception that they carried a greater burden of responsibility and were subjected to greater personal risk. Frustrated in not operating but when the opportunity arose to perform "tracheostomies and PEGs" [tracheostomies and percutaneous endoscopic gastrostomies] they questioned "why?" "It was fun to be operating but did these procedures benefit the patient?" Several patients soon died after the procedures. The senior residents countered with the fact the by performing these procedures the patients could then go to the floor and unload the intensive care unit. The residents were faced with the ethical conflict of being beneficent in performing the operative procedure and concomitantly doing a disservice to the patient. Moral distress is invoked when there is the desire to operate and actively engage in patient care however the care is perceived as unwarranted or futile.

They expressed frustration in their ability to advocate for their patients. "A mother and daughter both had COVID-19—their husband/father died at home. The mother had a pneumoperitoneum from a perforated duodenal ulcer and was in the telemetry unit—the daughter was admitted to the floor. We [second and fourth year residents] wanted to take the daughter to see her mother prior to surgery—it could be the last time they see each other. Because of the restricted visitation policy, the residents were told by the nursing manager that the daughter could not visit her mother. The residents explained that since both were COVID (+) there was no risk that they could make each other sick. They transported the daughter to see her mother because "it was the right thing to do".

As illustrated by the case, the difficulty in making connections with families—having "tough conversations in a new format". "Spending 20 minutes on an iPad so that the family can talk to the patient"—caused initial "annoyance" but later realization that this could be the last conversation the family has with this person. With lack of visitation, it was difficult to update families in a timely fashion, and it was difficult for families to grasp how sick their family member was. For these reasons trying to persuade frightened families to accept DNR status was frequently unsuccessful [1].

Discordance with their values—"doing things that felt wrong". "Contrary to what we had previously learned and did in managing patients—now we needed to adapt". "Not coding patients feels wrong". Cardiac arrest resulting from respiratory failure refractory to ventilatory support with associated multisystem organ failure is not reversible and the provision of chest compressions and defibrillation is medically futile. Most crisis plans explicitly include the right to withhold CPR when it cannot benefit the patient. During this pandemic, a decision not to initiate CPR was not an instance of withholding life-saving care from vulnerable individuals but was both rational and empathic in a futile situation. The New York crisis plans, however, failed to support its doctors in making decisions not to resuscitate [1]. Performing ineffective CPR created additional risk of COVID exposure to providers without benefit to the patient exemplifying the conflict of beneficence and the risk to personal safety.

They expressed *sadness* in seeing patients losing their control over decision-making. Moral distress is experienced with the shift to a greater level of paternalism in contrast to our current shared decision-making paradigm. Now we are in positions where we cannot respect all our patient's wishes [3]. They also expressed sadness in seeing patients dying alone. "It is disheartening seeing so many bad outcomes. Patients leave the hospital after the successful management of a surgical problem only to return with COVID-19—seeing patients going to rehab only to return sick with COVID-19—not seeing our interventions have a positive impact."

Gratitude was shared—"Being grateful for having a job—many people have lost their jobs—and to be able to do a lot of good with our skills." "Going to work gave structure to the day—a sense of purpose. "Grateful for having the opportunity to work with people from other departments, traveling nurses—nice change—opportunity to develop new relationships. "Being around travelers and volunteers— change in the regular staffing provided "newfound passion and energy." They were also grateful "for being given more autonomy and developing confidence."

Pride after receiving external validation and positive feedback from other departments for both surgical and non-surgical skills—"glad to have a surgeon on the team". "I feel very invested in my patients—when the sedation was lightened, I helped him 'talk' with his family via iPad and learned he had a nickname."

The residents vocalized *appreciation* for their attendings and "their willingness to step up and learn new things" to care for patients. Deployment to a new arena can be a positive challenge and give one an appreciation for the "space, stuff, and staff" available to you prior to the pandemic. Being out of one's comfort zone can be a growth experience.

And *uncertainty*—"We are taking a huge risk which has not yet been completely measured." We must acknowledge stress, pressure, and sacrifice and accept that we cope differently.

Compassion is the desire to minimize the suffering of others; self-compassion re-orients that desire to minimize one's own suffering. Self-compassion can bolster resilience. Self-compassion is a construct of three components: self-kindness, common humanity, and mindfulness. Self-kindness refers to the tendency to be caring and understanding with ourselves rather than harshly critical or judgmental. Self-compassion means acceptance of our imperfections. When external life circumstances are difficult, as during a pandemic, a self-compassionate person will respond with concern and comfort rather than a stoical 'just grin and bear it' approach [27]. The sense of common humanity central to self-compassion is the recognition that all people fail, make mistakes, and feel inadequate. When difficult life circumstances are framed in light of the shared human experience, one feels connected and less isolated when experiencing suffering.

Recognizing our shared common humanity reminds us that we are all in this together. *Mindfulness* emphasizes balanced awareness of emotional distress in order to analyze an experience with greater objectivity and perspective. The self-compassionate person approaches their problems with equanimity. Mindfulness prevents 'over-identification' where people go beyond an objective assessment of their responsibility to criticism, and self-blame. When we are kind to ourselves, clearly seeing ourselves as part of a larger, interconnected whole, we feel safe, valuable, accepted, and secure. Self-compassionate people show greater emotional stability, greater optimism, and greater life satisfaction. Self-compassion acknowledges that we are human, imperfect, experience suffering, and are worthy of compassion. Self-compassion provides emotional resilience when the self is seen as part of a greater interconnected whole [28].

15.3.2.4 The Value of "Moral Distress Rounds" on Resident Well-Being—A Resident's Perspective

Surgical residency is rigorous. Over a period of years trainees amass a large volume of clinical knowledge, master a wide variety of technical skills, and accrue surgical judgment. By the nature of this training, surgical residents are vulnerable to moral distress, moral injury, and moral residue. Prior to the pandemic, moral distress rounds have been used in our program as group-based discussions focusing on clinical ethical dilemmas and have provided solace in coping with the loss of a long-standing patient, or a beloved fellow resident. Moral distress rounds also provide the communication tools to frame and conduct palliative care discussions with sensibility and empathy. The discussions, moderated by a surgical attending with an expertise in ethics, are fluid and adaptable to the needs of its participants.

The COVID-19 pandemic has brought unique challenges to the paradigm of surgical training, the roles of trainees, and the delivery of healthcare. The pandemic was an unprecedented source of difficult ethical situations where residents were left with significant moral burden. Moral distress rounds seemed as important as ever. In compliance with conducting academic activity remotely, the discussions went on to take a virtual format. Usually, they began with a reflection on a given topic surrounding the pandemic, but the discussions evolved to address the many needs of the participants. Moral distress rounds during the pandemic were therapeutic to most residents. It was the only time we could, in some way, be together in a time where we had been forced apart.

For some, voicing the many challenges they faced during the pandemic was therapeutic. For others, the validation came from listening to their colleagues. We learned about the disease together and shared a sense of ineptitude because of how little we actually understood it. We grieved the losses of patients and even of colleagues. We shared the few success stories with hope to keep the rest motivated. It was helpful to reframe moral dilemmas with the perspective of different individuals. In doing so we channeled negative feelings into opportunities for learning and growth. It was helpful to unintentionally practice learned optimism—seeing individual defeats as temporary, local and reversible. Moral distress rounds gave us moral resilience and moral grit at an unimaginably difficult time.

15.4 Case Concluded

The resident returned to the room 30 min later and saw multiple family members smiling and rejoicing as Mr. C joined them in singing—softly mouthing the lyrics to his favorite Bob Marley song. They could be seen trying to squeeze onto the frame to interact with him. It was time to move on to the next room. That night, Mr. C was transferred to the floor and died overnight of unknown complications. The family and ICU providers were left with little explanation.

15.5   Conclusion

How do we maintain the integrity of surgical training while protecting trainees and simultaneously ensuring the sustainability of a critical workforce for our healthcare systems? A group of surgical trainees at different stages of training, surgeons, and program directors from the United States and Canada collaborated to provide the following lessons:

1. Trainee wellness and safety must remain a priority.
2. Restructuring of workflow and use of surgical residents to provide needed support in different areas should be anticipated and developed with the aim to protect and preserve the surgical workforce while providing unique opportunities for education. Leading by example and role-modelling leadership in response to the pandemic, attendings can inspire and foster effective skills in future surgical leaders.
3. Restructure surgical learning. The formal educational curriculum should not be abandoned. Programs should provide increased support for trainees' clinical development in non-clinical skill, addressing teamwork development, crisis management, leadership, and residents as educators. Professional development can be supported in terms of research and academic productivity, career planning, or financial literacy. An important consideration is the diminished capacity for learners to take part in educational opportunities due to competing professional and personal priorities, e.g., ongoing 'frontline' service or coping with the impacts of illness, caregiver responsibilities, and financial considerations. All restructured curricula should be sensitive to the vulnerability of trainees during a crisis within a traditional surgical hierarchy.
4. Adapt current educational milestones.
5. Prepare for post-COVID-19. Surgical systems will face backlogs of clinical and operative cases, and this will necessitate a restructuring of clinical and academic curricula [29].

During this pandemic, as members of the surgical workforce and as trainees, our residents were challenged operationally, contended with disrupted education, and ethically, faced the transition from patient-centered ethics to public health ethics. Surgical residents are instilled with accountability. Our residents provided care that was optimally not the standard of care during normal times for an unprecedented number of critically ill patients and witnessed death on an unprecedented scale, challenging their values and moral and professional integrity. We must be cognizant that the consequence is moral distress and moral residue. Post-pandemic surgical training must safeguard the well-being of trainees and provide the tools for moral resilience. This can be fostered with compassion, self-compassion, and an environment that allows for raising ethical concerns.

15.6 Selected References

- Lancaster EM, Sosa JA, Sammann A, et al. Rapid response of an academic surgical department to the COVID-19 pandemic: implications for patients, surgeons, and the community. J Am Coll Surg. 2020;230:1064–73. https://doi.org/10.1016/j.jamcollsurg.2020.04.007

  – The strategy of a single academic health system to address the four critical issues faced by surgery departments during the COVID-19 pandemic: developing a cohesive leadership team and system for frequent intra-departmental communication; ensuring adequate hospital capacity to care for the influx of COVID-19 patients; safeguarding personal protective equipment to protect patients and providers; preparing for an unstable workforce due to illness and competing personal priorities and concerns, such as childcare.

- Coons BE, Tam SF, Okochi S. Rapid development of resident-led procedural response teams to support patient care during the coronavirus disease 2019 epidemic a surgical workforce activation team. JAMA Surg. 2020;155(8):683–4.

  – An example of workforce restructuring during the COVID-19 pandemic with the creation of a "Surgical Workforce Access Team" (SWAT) to help offload procedural work from the emergency medicine, critical care, and medicine departments. Bundling procedures such as placement of central venous catheters, arterial lines, urinary catheters, nasogastric tubes, was an efficient way to minimize personal protection equipment (PPE) usage and personnel exposure to COVID-19.

- Wallace CL, Wladkowski SP, Gibson A, White P. Grief during the COVID-19 pandemic: considerations for palliative care providers. J Pain Symptom Manag. 2020;60:e70–6. https://doi.org/10.1016/j.jpainsymman.2020.04.012

  – Grief is inherently a part of the COVID-19 pandemic affecting patients, families, and providers. With the unprecedented amount of death during this pandemic unresolved grief has been amplified and can contribute to moral distress. Provider well-being is emphasized as is the need to address the vulnerability of surgical residents to moral distress.

- Cooper Z, Bernacki RE. To face coronavirus disease 2019, surgeons must embrace palliative care. JAMA Surg. 2020;155:681–2. https://doi.org/10.1001/jamasurg.2020.1698

  – The COVID-19 pandemic has presented surgeons and trainees with structural, clinical, and ethical challenges as well as an unprecedented opportunity to embrace palliative care. Four instructive aspects of palliative care are: Using communication strategies to disclose prognosis and establish goals of care; treating total pain; caring for the family unit; and supporting clinicians well-being, and resilience in the maintenance of an able workforce.

References

1. Powell T, Chuang E. COVID in NYC: what we could do better. Am J Bioeth. 2020;20:62–6. https://doi.org/10.1080/15265161.2020.1764146.
2. Fong ZV, Qadan M, McKinney R, et al. Practical implications of novel coronavirus COVID-19 on hospital operations, board certification, and medical education in surgery in the USA. J Gastrointest Surg. 2020;24:1232–6. https://doi.org/10.1007/s11605-020-04596-5.
3. Angelos P. Surgeons, ethics, and COVID-19: early lessons learned. J Am Coll Surg. 2020;230(6):1119–20. https://doi.org/10.1016/j.jamcollsurg.2020.03.028.
4. Lancaster EM, Sosa JA, Sammann A, et al. Rapid response of an academic surgical department to the COVID-19 pandemic: implications for patients, surgeons, and the community. J Am Coll Surg. 2020;230:1064–73. https://doi.org/10.1016/j.jamcollsurg.2020.04.007.
5. Nassar AH, Zern NK, McIntyre LK, et al. Emergency restructuring of a general surgery residency program during the coronavirus disease 2019 pandemic: the University of Washington experience. JAMA Surg. 2020;155(7):624–7. https://doi.org/10.1001/jamasurg.2020.1219.
6. Coons BE, Tam SF, Okochi S. Rapid development of resident-led procedural response teams to support patient care during the coronavirus disease 2019 epidemic: a surgical workforce activation team. JAMA Surg. 2020;155(8):683–4.
7. Schwartz AM, Wilson JM, Boden SD, Moore TJ, Bradbury TL, Fletcher ND. Managing resident workforce and education during the COVID-19 pandemic: evolving strategies and lessons learned. JBJS Open Access. 2020;5(2):e0045. https://doi.org/10.2106/JBJS.OA.20.00045.
8. Ahmed S, Tan WLG, Chong Y-L. Surgical response to COVID-19 pandemic: a Singapore perspective. J Am Coll Surg. 2020;230(6):1074–7. https://doi.org/10.1016/j.jamcollsurg.2020.04.003.
9. Chia CLK. Being a surgeon in the pandemic era. J Am Coll Surg. 2020;230(6):1077–9. https://doi.org/10.1016/j.jamcollsurg.2020.04.010.
10. Tseng J. How has COVID-19 affected the costs of the surgical fellowship interview process? J Surg Educ. 2020;77(5):999–1004. https://doi.org/10.1016/j.jsurg.2020.05.018.
11. Day RW, Taylor BM, Bednarski B, et al. Virtual interviews for surgical training program applicants during COVID-19: lessons learned and recommendations. Ann Surg. 2020;272(2):e144–7. https://doi.org/10.1097/SLA.0000000000004064.
12. Nasca TJ. ACGME response to the coronavirus (COVID-19). Published March 18, 2020. https://www.acgme.org/Newsroom/Newsroom-Details/ArticleID/10111/ACGME-Response-to-the-Coronavirus-COVID-19. Accessed 14 Jan 2021.
13. Goldhamer MJE, Pusic MV, Co JPT, Weinstein D. Can COVID catalyze an educational transformation? Competency-based advancement in a crisis. N Engl J Med. 2020;383(11):1003–5. https://doi.org/10.1056/NEJMp20118570.
14. Hamric AB, Davis W, Childress MD. Moral distress in health-care providers: what it is and what can we do about it? The Pharos. 2006;69(2):16–23.
15. Jameton A. Nursing practice: the ethical issues. Prentice Hall; 1984.
16. Thomas T, McCullough LB. A philosophical taxonomy of ethically significant moral distress. J Med Philos. 2015;40:102–20.
17. Hamric A. Empirical research on moral distress: issues, challenges, and opportunities. HEC Forum. 2012;2:39–49.
18. Williams RD, Brundage JA, Williams EB. Moral injury in times of COVID-19. J Health Serv Psychol. 2020;46:65–9. https://doi.org/10.1007/s42843-020-00011-4.
19. Epstein EG, Hamric AB. Moral distress, moral residue, and the crescendo effect. J Clin Ethics. 2009;20(4):330–42.
20. Dean W, Talbot S, Dean A. Reframing clinician distress: moral injury not burnout. Fed Pract. 2019;36(9):400–2.
21. Rushton CH, Carse A. Towards a new narrative of moral distress: realizing the potential of resilience. J Clin Ethics. 2016;27(3):214–8.

22. Frankl V. Man's search for meaning. Beacon Press; 2006.
23. Duckworth A. Grit: the power of passion and perseverance. Scribner; 2016.
24. Nouwen HJM. The wounded healer. 2nd ed. Image Doubleday; 2010.
25. Wallace CL, Wladkowski SP, Gibson A, White P. Grief during the COVID-19 pandemic: considerations for palliative care providers. J Pain Symptom Manag. 2020;60:e70–6. https://doi.org/10.1016/j.jpainsymman.2020.04.012.
26. Cooper Z, Bernacki RE. To face coronavirus disease 2019, surgeons must embrace palliative care. JAMA Surg. 2020;155:681–2. https://doi.org/10.1001/jamasurg.2020.1698.
27. Neff KD. Self-compassion, self-esteem, and well-being: self-compassion, self-esteem, and well-being. Soc Personal Psychol Compass. 2011;5(1):1–12. https://doi.org/10.1111/j.1751-9004.2010.00330.x.
28. Leary M. Don't beat yourself up. Aeon Newsletter. Published June 20, 2016. https://aeon.co/essays/learning-to-be-kind-to-yourself-has-remarkable-benefits. Accessed 14 Jan 2021.
29. Daodu O, Panda N, Lopushinsky S, Varghese TK, Brindle M. COVID-19—considerations and implications for surgical learners. Ann Surg. 2020;272:e22–3. https://doi.org/10.1097/SLA.0000000000003927.

Part IV
Medical Discrepancy/Medical Error

Chapter 16
Surgical Disclosure of Errors

Puneet Singh 🄳

Abstract There is an increasing recognition of the frequency of medical errors and their disclosure to the patient as an ethical duty of the physician. Disclosure conversations should include the details of the error and treatment, a sincere apology and future preventive measures. Surgeons most often discuss the medical facts of the error but may not address the latter two components leading to patient dissatisfaction. Training leads to increased surgeon confidence. In addition, providing emotional support for the surgeon is important since they may experience negative effects as the "second victim." When error disclosure practices are implemented in concert with health care systems that create a safe and transparent environment, the disclosure process is improved and benefits all stakeholders.

Keywords Error · Disclosure · Near miss · Honesty · Truth-telling Communication

Case

Dr. X was called by the ER one night on general surgery call to assess a 60-year-old obese male with abdominal pain and several days of diarrhea. He was recently treated with antibiotics for a joint infection. On physical exam, he was hemodynamically stable but his abdomen was distended with evidence of peritonitis. An upright chest x-ray demonstrated free air under the diaphragm and his white blood cell count was elevated. Dr. X was concerned about fulminant *Clostridium difficile* colitis with colon perforation and recommended an exploratory laparotomy, total abdominal colectomy with end

P. Singh (✉)
Department of Breast Surgical Oncology, Division of Surgery, University of Texas MD Anderson Cancer Center, Houston, TX, USA
e-mail: psingh6@mdanderson.org

© The Author(s), under exclusive license to Springer Nature
Switzerland AG 2022
V. A. Lonchyna et al. (eds.), *Difficult Decisions in Surgical Ethics*, Difficult
Decisions in Surgery: An Evidence-Based Approach,
https://doi.org/10.1007/978-3-030-84625-1_16

ileostomy. After an informed consent discussion, the patient agreed to proceed. The operation lasted a few hours and went as planned. On post-operative day two, the patient was noted to have worsening abdominal pain and the ileostomy appeared dusky in color.

16.1 Introduction

"Error is an inherent feature of human behavior..." [1]

The 1999 report *To Err is Human* by the Institute of Medicine shed light on medical errors in American health care and that these were more prevalent than previously recognized [2]. The report defined medical errors as "the failure of a planned action to be completed as intended or the use of a wrong plan to achieve an aim." Errors are costly and can result in death, disability, loss of productivity, increased health care costs, loss of patient trust in the system and decreased satisfaction among patients and physicians. Medical error can be categorized as serious error, minor error or near miss which has the potential to cause harm but does not by chance or timely intervention [3]. Operating rooms, along with intensive care units and emergency rooms, are settings which have higher rates of errors with the possibility of significant consequences. Surgeons are acutely aware of this and the culture of surgery incorporates evaluation of errors and complications. In the book *Forgive and Remember*, sociologist Charles Bosk describes the role of the surgeon versus the internist and its relationship to the patient's outcome [4]. An internist whose patient dies is asked by colleagues "What happened?" compared to the surgeon who is asked "What did you do?" highlights the direct responsibility a surgeon has to the patient's outcome. Morbidity & Mortality (M&M) conferences are a long-standing, integral part of surgery departments and are an opportunity to review cases and discuss error prevention strategies. Disclosure of errors to patients is an ethical responsibility of the physician as it respects patient autonomy and places honestly and transparency upfront (See Table 16.1). This chapter will detail the evolution of

Table 16.1 Key Components of Error Disclosure [22]

Acknowledgement	Provide details regarding the error and future treatments or necessary care. This upholds the ethical principles of beneficence, non-maleficence and autonomy allowing the patient to actively participate in their care
Apology	Honest and sincere which puts the patient's interests before personal interests. An apology demonstrates respect for autonomy and emphasizes beneficence and non-maleficence
Acquisition	Analyze the error and identify strategies for prevention and improvement which upholds the principle of justice

Note: The surgeon should be candid, transparent and use simple language during the disclosure conversation in addition to informing the patient in a timely manner

disclosure in modern health care, the differences in patient and surgeon perspectives on error disclosure, how to close the disclosure gap and review the case presented at the beginning.

16.2 Search Strategy

A systematic search in the National Library of Medicine (pubmed.gov) from inception to October 7, 2020 was conducted. Searches were not restricted by language or study type. References of the included articles were also searched manually. The search terms included "error," "surgical error," "disclosure," "I'm sorry" and were searched using different combinations of terms. There were 22 relevant articles selected for inclusion.

16.3 Discussion

16.3.1 History of Disclosure

In the past, professional organizations and hospitals advised physicians not to inform patients of adverse events which could bring about malpractice lawsuits. When patients became aware of adverse events, health care organizations would deny and vigorously defend them. In 1987, after medical error occurred in two separate cases at the Lexington Veterans Affairs Medical Center (VAMC), a committee was formed to evaluate these events [5, 6]. Initially, the goal was to assist the defense in lawsuits however, upon discovering that these errors were due to mistakes that the patient or family were not aware of, the committee and VAMC administration decided that there was a fiduciary duty to the patient as caregiver. They disclosed the errors, and the process of humanistic risk management became known as the Lexington model [5]. Honesty and error disclosure was championed by Steve Kraman and Ginny Hamm at the Lexington VAMC and they demonstrated that over a 7-year period, liability payments were moderate despite a system that seemingly encouraged malpractice claims and settlements were similar to other peer institutions. Furthermore, the patient's best interest was supreme and they received just compensation for errors [5].

Different schools of philosophy exist and can be applied in medical ethics however deontological ethics are most applicable when discussing disclosure. Deontological ethics, as described by Immanuel Kant, is a duty-based moral philosophy [1]. The sense of duty or obligation is the moral worth of an action rather than the outcome or consequences of the action. In the modern era of shared decision-making and respect for persons, most physicians and surgeons believe in a duty to disclose error. There is recognition that is it their duty to place the interests of the patient and the profession over their own but how disclosure is performed varies significantly. Surgeons may "choose their words carefully" [7] and/or categorize errors as high or low harm limiting their disclosure to those that are high harm [8]. Although the moral imperative to inform patients of medical errors exists, there remains a gap between acknowledgement of the duty and fulfilling it.

16.3.2 The Patient Perspective

Patient autonomy hinges on physicians being honest regarding the diagnosis, treatments and any errors that may occur. Informing a patient of medical errors allows the patient to be an active participant in the decision-making for management of the error. This also applies to near misses where there is no apparent harm; it is possible that the patient may experience sequelae of the near miss and should be aware of it but more importantly, transparency is essential to patient trust. Furthermore, there may be significant liability if a patient discovers an error of which they are not informed. Patients desire acknowledgement and an explanation of the adverse event which includes information, emotional support and an apology [9]. Wu and colleagues asked adult volunteers to watch scripted videos of physicians disclosing errors and found that a complete apology and acceptance of responsibility were associated with better ratings and greater trust [10]. Interestingly, the volunteers' perception of what was said was more important than what was actually said. The other component of disclosure that patients specifically want to know is how the error will be prevented in the future which is often missing during the disclosure [8]. In a 2012 study by Iedema and colleagues, 100 patients and family members were interviewed about errors in health care [11]. Few conversations met their expectations for basic information and an apology. Despite physician acknowledgement that error disclosure is ethical, patients do not always feel that it is done adequately.

16.3.3 The Surgeon Perspective

Surgeons have embraced a culture of continual learning and improvement most notably in the format of M&M conferences. Though there are favorable attitudes toward error disclosure, surgeons do not always inform patients of all the details. A culture of silence still exists in surgery and there are a number of contributing factors [12]. Barriers to disclosure and transparency can include judgment-related issues such as less severe complications or near misses, difficult to correct errors or feeling less responsible for the error [9]. Adverse events are a known source of distress for health care workers. Psychological and emotional impacts on the surgeon can be significant and include shame, embarrassment and fear of losing reputation or patient trust. Surgeons who experience this phenomena have been referred to as the "second victim" and this is associated with feelings of guilt, burnout and depression [8, 13]. A survey of surgical and non-surgical residents at two academic medical centers demonstrated that surgical residents who witnessed more instances of colleagues being treated harshly for errors, believed they were more likely to be treated harshly if they admitted to committing an error, and were less likely to express their concerns to colleagues [14]. The punitive nature existing within surgical hierarchy may further diminish transparency particularly among trainees. Another major barrier is fear of litigation. While 50% of lawsuits arise due to a medical error, 95% of surgical complications never lead to a lawsuit [12]. In addition, lack of training in appropriate error disclosure and breaking bad news can also be a challenge for surgeons [9]. Whether these are perceived or actual barriers, only 30% of errors are disclosed [15]. The lack of disclosure to patients is termed a disclosure gap. This is a real phenomenon that must be addressed.

When surgeons disclose medical errors, the conversation may be factually accurate but vague and incomplete. Chan et al. conducted a study of 30 academic surgeons who were observed discussing errors with standardized patients [16]. The participating surgeons did the best with explanation of the medical facts surrounding the error but only used the word error or mistake in 57% of conversations. They took responsibility in 65%, provided an apology in 47% and validated the patient's emotions in 55% of cases. Discussion of prevention was rare seen in only 8% of conversations and in only 20%, a second opinion or transfer of care was offered. A more recent survey study of 35 VAMC surgeons demonstrated that the vast majority described why the event happened, expressed regret and concern for the patient's wellbeing and treatment strategies to address the adverse event [8]. Nearly all disclosed the error within 24 h. Fewer surgeons apologized or discussed if the error was preventable and any prevention strategies that could or would be applied. The authors also found factors that led to surgeons being more negatively impacted by the event: not discussing preventability, a very serious event as determined by the surgeon or difficulties with communication. Quality improvement efforts on disclosure increased surgeon wellness. This study highlights surgeons as the second victim when errors occur.

Gallagher et al. conducted a survey study of physicians and surgeons using standardized scenarios [3]. The use of the word error occurred at similarly low rates as previously mentioned studies and specifically, 56% mentioned an adverse event but not an error. They also found that error disclosure was significantly different depending on how apparent the error was to the patient described in the scenarios. Surgeons had greater intention to disclose but provided less information compared to medical physicians. In addition, 58% of medical physicians explicitly stated the error compared to 19% of surgeons ($p < 0.001$). Among the entire survey population, favorable attitudes toward disclosure, prior positive experiences with these conversations or a feeling of responsibility were associated with greater disclosure of information. The results of these studies indicate that training and support for error disclosure can be beneficial for both the surgeon and the patient.

16.3.4   Guidelines for Communication

The previous sections have discussed how and why error disclosures may not be adequate from the viewpoint of the two primary stakeholders. While there may be other stakeholders including health care organizations, family members, community members, the surgeon-patient relationship is supreme. Guidelines and training on having these discussions can improve the experiences of the patient and the surgeon. The National Quality Forum maintains a list of serious reportable errors to increase accountability and their Safe Practices program provides information for physicians and health care organizations on addressing unanticipated outcomes [17]. Various other organizations including the Massachusetts Coalition for the Prevention of Medical Errors and Canadian Patient Safety Institute have established guidelines for error disclosure [18, 19]. Important components include frankness, using simple and straightforward language, providing details of the error and associated treatments, an honest apology and how the physician/team/health care organization will learn and prevent the error from happening again. More simply, this can be summarized as the three A's: acknowledgement, apology and acquisition of data to improve [1]. Furthermore, training in error disclosure, especially during residency, can have a positive impact. Newcomb et al. published a study of residents at a single institution who underwent didactic education and then practiced discussing errors with standardized patients [15]. Self-assessment using a "Disclosure of Complication Checklist" demonstrated that residents stated they completed the tasks and had improved confidence though they rated competence as low. The study results indicate that young surgeons benefit from training and may need multiple opportunities to practice these skills just as with technical skills.

An important aspect of communication in any surgeon-patient relationship is candor. Robert Wheeler defines candor as "full disclosure of truth, motivated by wishing to confer benefit on the person to whom the information is being disclosed" [20]. In the setting of an error, the surgeon knows the full truth and has a duty to be candid with the patient, respecting their autonomy. This is the opposite of spin where selective truths are revealed in an attempt to deceive. While the threshold of which errors to disclose, especially those with low harm or near misses, is analogous to the decision and discussion of specific risks in informed consent, truth telling is critical when an error occurs. Candor can strengthen the surgeon-patient relationship and it has been shown that patients are more likely to continue with a physician who discovers and discloses errors [10].

16.3.5   Facilitating the Disclosure Process

The primary responsibility of disclosure lies with the surgeon, however other stakeholders, particularly health care organizations and government, can facilitate the process. Approximately 30 states have enacted laws that are referred to as "I'm sorry" laws with the basic premise that a physician's disclosure and apology is inadmissible as evidence of liability in a lawsuit [21]. On a more local level, health care systems should take the lead in creating safe environments for disclosure and transparency to occur. This culture benefits the patient and the physician and ultimately, builds trust on multiple levels. Most organizations have legal and risk management systems in place and a number of venues to discuss errors, perform root cause analyses and other quality assurance and improvement efforts. The National Quality Forum's Safe Practices program has additional measures that can strengthen the disclosure process. These include education and training on disclosure, tracking unanticipated outcomes for errors that should be disclosed, providing 24/7 support for physicians to be coached prior to disclosure and emotional support following an error or near miss to alleviate the symptoms of being the "second victim." [17] Having physicians be involved in prevention and improvement efforts can provide a meaningful opportunity for processing the error. Assessing patient satisfaction particularly if the disclosure met their values and expectations can be challenging but involving patients and family members on committees to improve the process can be a constructive step. Though supporting the patient and physician are the top goals of these programs, there are important financial benefits for health care systems. Similar to the financial benefits seen at the Lexington VAMC including lower average settlements and reduced litigation costs, the University of Michigan reported that their program decreased pending lawsuits and led to savings of $2 million annually in litigation costs [17]. Justice for a patient who suffers a medical error may involve a monetary settlement but past concerns about increasing costs to the hospital with disclosure have not borne out upon evaluation. Incorporating best practices for disclosure allow for the ethical imperative to be met with additional downstream, operational and financial advantages for health care systems.

16.4 Case Conclusion

Dr. X assessed the patient and recommended an immediate return to the operating room for exploration. He found that the ileostomy was twisted, resulting in ischemia. He was able to resect the ischemic portion and mature a new ileostomy that, this time, was properly oriented. The patient returned to the general floor clinically stable.

The error in this case was that the end ileostomy was twisted during the initial operation resulting in strangulation and ischemia of the bowel. While it is obvious to the patient that he is undergoing a second surgery, it is critical that Dr. X be honest about the reason. The informed consent discussion for any operation includes the diagnosis or at least what is known at that time. Once Dr. X discovered the etiology of the ischemic ileostomy, he should disclose this as an error to the patient including the critical elements discussed in the chapter: sequelae of the error and/or any additional treatments that may be needed, a sincere apology, and preventive measures to be taken.

In acknowledging the error, Dr. X should use plain language that makes it clear to the patient that this was a technical mistake and not just describe the findings of an ischemic ileostomy which could mislead the patient to believe this was due to factors outside the control of the surgeon. He can then discuss with the patient how he managed the twisted bowel intra-operatively and that the additional resection was small and unlikely to affect overall small bowel function. He should also discuss avenues to review the error such as at an M&M conference and how this event will change his practice. Ultimately, Dr. X has a duty to the patient to be candid about the error and take responsibility.

16.5 Conclusion

Patients are autonomous individuals who should be aware of medical errors and be involved in the decision-making surrounding an error. Surgeons desire to uphold their ethical duty to disclose medical errors and with appropriate education and support, can do this in a manner that puts the patient and profession first and preserves the surgeon-patient relationship.

16.6 Selected References

- Gallagher TH, Garbutt JM, Waterman AD, et al. Choosing your words carefully: how physicians would disclose harmful medical errors to patients. Arch Intern Med. 2006;166(15):1585–1593. doi:https://doi.org/10.1001/archinte.166.15.1585

    - Landmark study that assessed medical and surgical physicians' attitudes and approaches to error disclosure using a survey tool and highlighted the need for disclosure standards and training.

- Kraman SS, Hamm G. Risk management: extreme honesty may be the best policy. Ann Intern Med. 1999;131(12):963–967.

    - This is the earliest published example of a humanistic risk management model; it describes the history and development of the Lexington VAMC model of error disclosure.

- Lipira LE, Gallagher TH. Disclosure of adverse events and errors in surgical care: challenges and strategies for improvement. World J Surg. 2014;38(7):1614–1621. doi:https://doi.org/10.1007/s00268-014-2564-5

    - A review article that summarizes challenges and barriers surgeons face with disclosure, the disclosure   gap, and strategies to improve.

- National Quality Forum (NQF). *Safe practices for better healthcare—2010 update: a consensus report.* National Quality Forum; 2010. Accessed January 19, 2021. https://www.qualityforum.org/Publications/2010/04/Safe_Practices_for_Better_Healthcare_–_2010_Update.aspx

  - This report describes in detail the issues associated with error disclosure including challenges and lists best practices for individual physicians and institutions.

References

1. Bernstein M, Brown B. Doctors' duty to disclose error: a deontological or Kantian ethical analysis. Can J Neurol Sci. 2004;31(2):169–74. https://doi.org/10.1017/S0317167100053816.
2. Kohn LT, Corrigan JM, Donaldson MS, editors. To err is human: building a safer healthcare system. National Academy Press; 2000.
3. Gallagher TH, Garbutt JM, Waterman AD, et al. Choosing your words carefully: how physicians would disclose harmful medical errors to patients. Arch Intern Med. 2006;166(15):1585–93. https://doi.org/10.1001/archinte.166.15.1585.
4. Bosk C. Forgive and remember: managing medical failure. 2nd ed. The University of Chicago Press; 1979.
5. Kraman SS, Hamm G. Risk management: extreme honesty may be the best policy. Ann Intern Med. 1999;131(12):963–7.
6. Eaves-Leanos A, Dunn EJ. Open disclosure of adverse events: transparency and safety in health care. Surg Clin North Am. 2012;92(1):163–77. https://doi.org/10.1016/j.suc.2011.11.001.
7. Mavroudis C, Mavroudis CD, Naunheim KS, Sade RM. Should surgical errors always be disclosed to the patient? Ann Thorac Surg. 2005;80(2):399–408. https://doi.org/10.1016/j.athoracsur.2005.05.023.
8. Elwy AR, Itani KMF, Bokhour BG, et al. Surgeons' disclosures of clinical adverse events. JAMA Surg. 2016;151(11):1015–21. https://doi.org/10.1001/jamasurg.2016.1787.
9. Lipira LE, Gallagher TH. Disclosure of adverse events and errors in surgical care: challenges and strategies for improvement. World J Surg. 2014;38(7):1614–21. https://doi.org/10.1007/s00268-014-2564-5.
10. Wu AW, Huang IC, Stokes S, Pronovost PJ. Disclosing medical errors to patients: it's not what you say, it's what they hear. J Gen Intern Med. 2009;24(9):1012–7. https://doi.org/10.1007/s11606-009-1044-3.
11. Iedema R, Allen S, Britton K, Gallagher TH. What do patients and relatives know about problems and failures in care? BMJ Qual Saf. 2012;21(3):198–205. https://doi.org/10.1136/bmjqs-2011-000100.
12. Stahel PF, Flierl MA, Smith WR, et al. Disclosure and reporting of surgical complications: a double-edged sword? Am J Med Qual. 2010;25(5):398–401. https://doi.org/10.1177/1062860610370989.
13. Scott SD, Hirschinger LE, Cox KR, McCoig M, Brandt J, Hall LW. The natural history of recovery for the healthcare provider "second victim" after adverse patient events. Qual Saf Health Care. 2009;18(5):325–30. https://doi.org/10.1136/qshc.2009.032870.
14. Martinez W, Lehmann LS. The "hidden curriculum" and residents' attitudes about medical error disclosure: comparison of surgical and nonsurgical residents. J Am Coll Surg. 2013;217(6):1145–50. https://doi.org/10.1016/j.jamcollsurg.2013.07.391.
15. Newcomb AB, Liu C, Trickey AW, Dort J. Tell me straight: teaching residents to disclose adverse events in surgery. J Surg Educ. 2018;75(6):e178–91. https://doi.org/10.1016/j.surg.2018.08.006.

16. Chan DK, Gallagher TH, Reznick R, Levinson W. How surgeons disclose medical errors to patients: a study using standardized patients. Surgery. 2005;138(5):851–8. https://doi.org/10.1016/j.surg.2005.04.015.
17. National Quality Forum (NQF). Safe practices for better healthcare—2010 update: a consensus report. National Quality Forum; 2010. https://www.qualityforum.org/Publications/2010/04/Safe_Practices_for_Better_Healthcare_–_2010_Update.aspx. Accessed 19 Jan 2021.
18. Massachusetts Coalition for the Prevention of Medical Errors. When things go wrong: responding to adverse events. A Consensus Statement of the Harvard Hospitals; 2006. http://www.macoalition.org/documents/respondingToAdverseEvents.pdf. Accessed 19 Jan 2021.
19. Canadian Patient Safety Institute. Canadian Disclosure Guidelines: Being Open With Patients and Families. 2011. http://www.patientsafetyinstitute.ca/en/toolsResources/disclosure/pages/default.aspx. Accessed 19 Jan 2021.
20. Wheeler R. Candour for surgeons: the absence of spin. Ann R Coll Surg Engl. 2014;96(6):420–2. https://doi.org/10.1308/003588414X13946184903405.
21. Delbanco T, Bell SK. Guilty, afraid, and alone—struggling with medical error. N Engl J Med. 2007;357(17):1682–3. https://doi.org/10.1056/NEJMp078104.
22. Levinson W, Yeung J, Ginsburg S. Disclosure of medical error. JAMA. 2016;316(7):764–5. https://doi.org/10.1001/jama.2016.9136.

Chapter 17
Disclosing Errors of Others

Lulia A. Kana ⓘ, Emily Marchiano, Andrew G. Shuman,
and Norman D. Hogikyan

Abstract Surgeons have an ethical obligation to disclose their medical errors to patients. Doing so honors the sacred trust at the core of the surgeon-patient relationship. While the ethical and professional considerations surrounding personal errors are clear, disclosing errors of others is inherently more complicated. The calculus surrounding errors of others incorporates multiple practical and ethical dimensions, and the current literature finds less willingness or sense of obligation among physicians to do so. In this chapter, we advocate a proactive approach to error disclosure. We discuss the incidence and significance of medical errors, examine the ethical arguments surrounding the disclosure of errors made by colleagues and/or at other institutions, and narrate systems-level processes to support the disclosure of such errors to patients, providers, and institutional regulatory bodies.

Keywords Clinical ethics · Error disclosure · Professionalism · Surgeon-patient relationship · Peers' medical error

L. A. Kana
University of Michigan Medical School, Ann Arbor, MI, USA
e-mail: lkana@med.umich.edu

E. Marchiano
Department of Otolaryngology-Head and Neck Surgery, Michigan Medicine,
Ann Arbor, MI, USA
e-mail: emarchia@med.umich.edu

A. G. Shuman · N. D. Hogikyan (✉)
Department of Otolaryngology-Head and Neck Surgery, Center for Bioethics and Social Sciences in Medicine, Michigan Medicine, Ann Arbor, MI, USA
e-mail: shumana@med.umich.edu; nhogikya@med.umich.edu

© The Author(s), under exclusive license to Springer Nature
Switzerland AG 2022
V. A. Lonchyna et al. (eds.), *Difficult Decisions in Surgical Ethics*, Difficult
Decisions in Surgery: An Evidence-Based Approach,
https://doi.org/10.1007/978-3-030-84625-1_17

Case

A middle-aged patient presented to voice clinic with persistent dysphonia following a left hemithyroidectomy for benign disease that was performed one year ago at another institution. The patient had been told by her surgeon that the dysphonia was likely due to intubation and was just "one of those things." Evaluation in the voice clinic found a severely hoarse vocal quality and left vocal fold paralysis consistent with left recurrent laryngeal nerve injury.

17.1 Introduction

A surgeon has an ethical obligation to disclose medical errors to patients. Doing so honors the sacred trust at the core of the surgeon-patient relationship. This is rooted fundamentally in truth-telling, a moral action characterized as "right and obligatory" by Beauchamp and Childress in their classic text on Biomedical Ethics [1]. Principles of beneficence and nonmaleficence are embraced, in that open and honest investigation of adverse events allows institutions and practitioners to leverage negative patient experiences to improve patient safety (Table 17.1). Knowledge of errors additionally enables informed, autonomous decisions about future care, and the justice principle is supported by, among other things, fostering appropriate compensation when indicated (see Table 17.1). While this approach to medical errors is not universally followed, the ethics are self-evident, and the financial and legal advantages have also been established [2, 3].

Medical errors are prevalent in healthcare and contribute to thousands of patient deaths in the United States every year [4]. While medical errors are often discussed in relation to inpatient hospital care, such errors can also impact other aspects of healthcare systems, including outpatient clinics, pharmacies, and homecare

Table 17.1 Ethical principles in relation to disclosing errors of others

Principle	Application
Autonomy	Knowledge of errors made by colleagues/institutions empowers patients to make informed, autonomous decisions about future medical care.
Beneficence	Open and honest investigation of medical errors made by colleagues/institutions allows practitioners to leverage negative patient experiences to improve patient safety.
Nonmaleficence	Disclosure of errors safeguards patients against future harm and can mitigate psychological and emotional stress that may be precipitated by a lack of transparency. On the other hand, surgeons also have an obligation not to disparage the skills of another surgeon for malicious reasons.
Justice	Disclosure of medical errors made by colleagues/institutions can ensure rightful compensation, fiscally or otherwise, to patients when indicated and address inherent biases that may adversely engender errors and nondisclosures.

facilities, contributing to growing economic healthcare costs, decrease in patient satisfaction and trust, and distress for providers [4].

Given the prevalence of medical errors in medicine as well as the ethical dilemmas surrounding this topic, it behooves surgeons to develop an understanding of the ethical underpinnings surrounding error disclosure. In this chapter, we will discuss the incidence and significance of medical errors, examine the ethical arguments surrounding the disclosure of errors made by colleagues and/or at other institutions, and discuss systems-level processes to support the disclosure of such errors to patients, providers, and institutional regulatory bodies.

17.2   Search Strategy

We utilized the following search terms in PubMed: truth disclosure[mh] OR candor[ti] OR candour[ti] OR forthright[ti] OR honest[ti] OR honesty[ti] OR truth[ti] OR truthful[ti]) AND (medical errors[mh] OR error[ti] OR errors[ti] OR mistake[ti] OR mistakes[ti]) AND (ethics[sh] OR history[sh] OR ethic[ti] OR ethical[ti] OR ethics[ti] OR historical[ti] OR history[ti])) OR ((error[ti] OR errors[ti] OR mistake[ti] OR mistakes[ti]) AND (disclose[ti] OR disclosing[ti] OR disclosure[ti] OR disclosures. This resulted in 473 texts. Titles were reviewed for relevancy and abstracts identified were further explored. The references of articles deemed to be relevant were included for evaluation and then additional texts were identified thereafter.

17.3   Discussion

17.3.1   Medical Errors

In the Institute of Medicine's *To Err is Human*, the definition of an error is "the failure of a planned action to be completed as intended or the use of a wrong plan to achieve an aim." [4]. Injuries that occur as a result of medical management rather than from an underlying disease process are termed adverse events, and events due to errors are considered preventable adverse events [4]. Quantifying incidence of adverse events has been examined globally through large retrospective reviews of patient outcomes, including incidence data from Australia (16.6%), [5] Canada (7.5%), [6] and the United Kingdom (10.8%) [7]. Examining data from New York, Utah, and Colorado revealed that more than 40% of adverse events were classified as operative [8, 9]. Given the current legal tort system in healthcare, surgeons are vulnerable and fearful of litigation, collectively contributing to systemic challenges that discourage error disclosure [10].

17.3.2 Error Disclosure: Personal Errors

It is widely recognized that physicians have an ethical obligation to disclose medical errors made by themselves to patients. Doing so honors the trust that is at the heart of the doctor-patient relationship. According to the American Medical Association, in order for patients to be fully informed and engaged in their care, patients are entitled to information, including knowledge of medical errors [11]. Furthermore, the American College of Surgeons Code of Professional Conduct states that surgeons have a responsibility to "fully disclose adverse events and medical errors" [12].

Current literature documents patients' desire for disclosure of errors with a focus upon nature and causality of the error and how consequences and incidence will be mitigated and prevented in the future [13]. It is therefore not surprising that the most common reason for patients to pursue litigation against physicians is due to a lack of communication surrounding the circumstances of an error [14]. Honesty and integrity, hallmarks of any honorable profession, are at the heart of personal error disclosure and may even discourage patients from seeking legal recourse in such situations.

In 2001, the University of Michigan adopted a transparent, principle-based, and proactive approach to patient injuries and malpractice claims [2]. This approach acknowledged that medicine is inherently dangerous and that avoidable medical mistakes can lead to unintended outcomes even with the best of intentions. Adverse events were openly and honestly discussed with patients and families, with a focus on learning and improving safety, as well as apologizing and offering fair compensation when appropriate. Implementation of this methodology has, among other things, led to a reduction in institutional malpractice claims. Then-Senators Obama and Clinton highlighted this as a model for (still-awaited) tort reform [3]. This approach is now embodied in a best-practice toolkit [15].

While specific details of self-error disclosure may vary, there is no ethical debate about the obligation to do so. But what is a subsequent or co-treating physician to do about recognized errors by other providers and/or at other institutions? What if, as in the index case, the clinical facts indicate that the patient has been harmed and that other providers or institutions have not been forthright or have intentionally misled the patient? What are the professional and moral obligations of the subsequent treating physician? In the remainder of this chapter, we examine the ethical discourse surrounding disclosing errors of others to patients, providers, and institutions.

17.3.3 Error Disclosure: Errors of Others

While the American Medical Association's stance on disclosure of personal errors to patients is clear, the disclosure of errors made by other providers is less instructive [11]. When a medical error is identified by a professional, the association recommends the provider to report incompetent/impaired colleagues and also encourages having the referring provider disclose their error to the patient [11].

Physicians hold conflicting views regarding their obligation to disclose errors made by other physicians and to whom this obligation is directed. One study found that physicians varied in their methods of disclosure but tended to lean towards partial/non-disclosure to the patient, with some citing that the physician who made the error should instead be responsible for disclosure [16]. Another survey of physicians revealed that disclosure of errors made by other clinicians was found to be event, physician, and/or organization-dependent, with over half of participants stating they would not disclose such to the patient [17]. This position does not directly conflict with the American Medical Association's stance on this topic, which urges the provider to encourage the referring provider to disclose to the patient [11]. But it is simultaneously a position that is difficult to support with a valid ethical argument.

The American College of Surgeons proclamations regarding Surgeons and Society state that every surgeon has a responsibility to safeguard patients from harm due to impaired or incompetent colleagues and to both participate in institutional peer review processes and assist impaired surgeons in receiving appropriate care and support for their condition [12]. Reflecting the potential for misuse of this principle, it is also stated that surgeons are not to disparage the actions or skills of another surgeon for malicious reasons [12]. The complex and at-times conflicting ethical and personal professional considerations at play in these situations will be readily apparent to both medical physicians and surgeons. Prominent among these is recognition that lack of presence in the moment significantly limits contextual and possibly also factual understanding of a medical error. This in part engenders the strong tradition of loyalty to other physicians and recognition that as physicians we are human, and we all make mistakes.

The characterization of an error and the role or not of a provider's negligence leading to negative outcomes may be somewhat ambiguous in a given situation. Morreim breaks this down by grading adverse outcomes into five levels (see Table 17.2) [18]. An adverse outcome is not synonymous with an error, nor is a difference in professional practice equivalent to incompetence [18]. She argues that the care by a physician is not judged based on outcomes but by the reasoning behind such a decision and skill involved in performing specific tasks [18]. In order to accurately grade an event into one of the aforementioned levels, it can be argued that the role of the physician must be clearly known first, and as a result, it would be

Table 17.2 Levels of adverse outcomes

Level 1	Negative outcomes occurring not due to a faulting physician
Level 2	Correct decision-making leading to an unforeseen/unexpected negative outcome
Level 3	Differing practice patterns within the standard of care that cause negative outcomes
Level 4	Poor, though not egregious, judgement/skill from a physician with no concerning practice pattern
Level 5	Significant and egregious deviations from the expected standard/quality of care

Adapted from Morreim [18]

difficult to do so unless the provider directly involved with the case was present at the time of the event. As a result, the situational factors of such circumstances merit discussion.

Healthcare is often delivered through a network of consulting physicians at different institutions, further adding to complexity in assigning responsibility and blame [19]. It can be difficult to discern the details of an encounter from viewing medical records alone as conversations between providers and patients as well as steps for disclosure may not have been thoroughly documented [19]. During procedures, a supervising physician may be unaware that an error had occurred if he or she was not directly responsible for or proximately involved in it. This explains the tendency of physicians who may prefer recusing themselves from disclosing errors of other physicians. Further, because patients may want information surrounding the error, how such a situation will be prevented in the future, and the implications of the error moving forward [13], this information can be difficult to provide from a physician who was not present in the case.

Additionally, it may be challenging for a physician to surmise which team member was responsible for an error or injury and how exactly it might have occurred. Several studies have explored provider-provider expectations with regards to error disclosure. One report found that providers have an expectation from their colleagues to report errors to them first rather than to patients directly and likewise prefer to report errors made by other physicians to their peers first and advise them to discuss the error with their patient [20]. In another study, when providers were asked about previous treatments that involved a medical error by another physician, participants stated concerns that pursuing such disclosure directly to patients would unnecessarily cause damage by inducing worry as well as harming collegial relationships [16]. These data contextualize the reticence that exists in the medical community with regard to addressing and exposing errors of others.

While the impact of healthcare fragmentation complicates disclosing documented or suspected errors of others, the fiduciary nature of the medical profession as a whole necessitates that physicians safeguard patients against incompetence [18]. In a qualitative study examining patients' preferences surrounding error disclosure of inter-system medical error discovery, it was found that patients express a desire to have a subsequent treating physician disclose errors made by referring providers [21]. Furthermore, patients considered inter-system medical errors to be the same as those that were self-discovered [21]. Similar to the ethical principles supporting disclosure of one's own errors as outlined above, participants cited their belief that the medical profession depends on honesty and transparency to promote fully informed actions by patients [21].

As such, patients are entitled to information that may specifically pose a risk to their well-being, and ethical and professional duty mandates that physicians are not ambiguous in exposing errors of others even when it is practically difficult or uncomfortable to do so. Importantly though, because of the inherent uncertainties in fully understanding such errors, the process of error disclosure should promote an environment of transparency that is rooted in patient safety and quality of care through both communication with the patient as well as respectful communication with the involved colleague. Providing emotional support to both the patient and the provider/care team involved in the error should be embedded in this care model. The discovering provider should, where appropriate, invoke a tone of uncertainty inherent in not having been present, suggesting that the patient further discuss with their previous physician the specific aspects of the care in question. The subsequent treating physician may also have concerns about quality of care without line of sight to define a specific error, and/or be asked for a second opinion in which the patient is still considering additional care under the previous physician or institution.

In such cases, it is incumbent upon the subsequent physician to provide honest guidance without malice. This can be accomplished in most cases in a diplomatic manner that emphasizes advantages of alternative care settings or approaches, rather than focusing upon impugning the reputation of others. While there is certainly an element of information manipulation with this approach, it can accomplish the goals of quality of care while acknowledging uncertainties inherent in assessing potential errors of others. Notably though, if there is concern for truly and consistently substandard care, it only addresses the particular patient in question while doing nothing for future patients at a previous treating institution.

To protect future patients, the professional duty of the discovering provider to report circumstances of the case "up the chain" merits discussion. Promoting the integrity of the medical profession as an institution can be seen as an additional duty of a physician in this context. In *The Road to Character*, David Brooks writes of an individual's responsibility to institutions in which we work as "accepting the gifts of the dead, taking on the responsibility of preserving and improving an institution and then transmitting that institution, better, on to the next generation...commitments to something that transcends a single lifetime...an inheritance to be passed on and a debt to be repaid" [22].

Morreim [18] wrote about responding to unethical or incompetent colleagues. While doing so is both difficult and important, it also requires "courage, integrity, and wisdom" [18]. She opines that fear of "being either the agent or the recipient of unfair accusations and reprisals" can be a strong incentive to ignore this type of problem but also feels that there is no choice but to act [18]. She continues: "One's own professional integrity is compromised when one permits the integrity of one's profession to be compromised. And the care of all patients is jeopardized if physicians do not care about their own profession" [18].

According to the American Medical Association's code of ethics, physicians who believe a colleague is incompetent or has engaged in unethical behavior have an obligation to report this circumstance, and they advocate a graduated approach beginning with notifying the related clinical authorities, institutional peer review body, or state society, with reporting to state licensing boards or other higher authorities being an option for the most serious or recalcitrant circumstances [11]. Institutional programs, professional societies, and state oversight bodies are a means to monitor the skill and conduct of providers. However, there still exists the potential for errors of lesser gravity to occur. Given medicine's long-standing history of self-governance, it has been argued that only physicians can reasonably gauge a colleague's competence [18]. Thus, physicians have a duty to maintain public trust of physicians and overall safety of patients by disclosing the errors of colleagues.

17.3.4   Systems-Level Process Improvement

Strategies to overcome the disclosure gap in medical error reporting have recently been proposed to streamline the process. For example, a "disclosure time out" can provide a space for the surgical team to establish clarity and consensus regarding an adverse event and institutions may also look to invest in disclosure coaches, or professionals who are well-versed in the optimal delivery of disclosure and dialogue with patients and families, to assist in preparing for these conversations [23].

To address medical error reporting on an institutional level, an ethical framework was proposed for how and why institutions should address interfacility medical error discovery. Physicians are identified as key players in addressing the gap that exists about medical error discovery between healthcare institutions [24]. The authors argue that disclosing errors ultimately ensures optimal patient care through the promotion of feedback loops, identifies gaps in the current method, ensures collaboration amongst institutions through open communication, and instills accountability amongst providers to promote increased transparency [24].

Multidisciplinary professionals proposed an outline for how to practically manage the disclosure of medical errors made by other physicians [25]. In their proposal, they suggest utilizing provider-provider discussions to initiate the conversation and assembling institutional-level support to install a disclosure coaching program to promote a "just culture" [25]. This "just culture" is an attempt to balance the accountability of individuals and the system when approaching problems in healthcare in order to move away from an environment that places individual blame towards one that embraces collective responsibility [26]. However, while such strategies have been proposed, eventual broad implementation is a moving target.

Finally, while the ethical obligations in support of error disclosure should not be conflated with a physician's legal obligations, there may be state or other regulations governing legal obligations for disclosure. Therefore, in addition to understanding the ethical obligation towards disclosure of medical errors of others to patients and institutions, it behooves surgeons to also understand their obligations towards error disclosure from a legal standpoint. For example, under the Michigan Public Health Code, physicians are mandated to report another licensed health professional to the Michigan Department of Licensing and Regulatory Affairs for various reasons, including incompetence, substance abuse, fraud, and unprofessional conduct [27]. Thus, a provider has a duty in this regard and those who fail to do so may suffer legal repercussions.

Case Resolution

In our index case, the high likelihood of surgical error was disclosed to the patient, and relevant surgical anatomy was discussed in order to contextualize the disclosure and logical nature of this conclusion. Uncertainty as to the mechanism of nerve injury (e.g., transection versus retraction injury) was acknowledged. Any questions were answered in a forthright and transparent manner. Written correspondence detailing the findings and the discussion with the patient was sent to the referring and primary care physicians with whom the patient was encouraged to have further discussions regarding the circumstance.

17.4   Conclusion

Surgeons have a clear ethical and moral obligation to disclose errors. The professional considerations surrounding one's own errors are clear although specifics of disclosure will vary by individual and institution. Disclosing errors of others is inherently more complicated. The moral calculus surrounding errors of others incorporates multiple practical and ethical dimensions, and current literature finds less willingness or sense of obligation among physicians to do so. Nevertheless, a surgeon's ethical obligation to disclose the errors of others must supersede any arguments to the contrary. Such disclosures should acknowledge, as appropriate to the situation, any uncertainties inherent in not being present at previous care, be respectful and professional, and include communication with involved physicians. The formidable potential significance of reporting such errors to oversight bodies mandates diligent and thoughtful case by case consideration with cases of clear surgeon incompetence, impairment, or willful deception to likely be the primary situations when this avenue should be pursued. Ongoing systems-level recommendations and innovations are rightfully guided by the principle of creating a culture that embraces collective rather than individual responsibility and in doing so, encourages reporting errors of others.

17.5   Selected References

- Dossett LA, Kauffmann RM, Lee JS, et al. Specialist physicians' attitudes and practice patterns regarding disclosure of pre-referral medical errors. Ann Surg. 2018;267(6):1077–83. https://doi.org/10.1097/sla.0000000000002427.

  - A qualitative study exploring cancer specialists' attitudes and practices with regards to pre-referral medical error disclosure.

- Antunez AG, Saari A, Miller J, Dossett LA. Patient preferences in cases of Intersystem Medical Error Discovery (IMED). Ann Surg. 2021;273(3):516–22. PMID:31348037.

  – A qualitative study exploring patients' perspectives surrounding the disclosure of inter-system medical error discovery cases.

- Antunez AG, Shuman AG, Jagsi R, Dossett LA. Ethical duty of health care systems to address interfacility medical error discovery. J Am Coll Surg. 2018;227(5):543–7. https://doi.org/10.1016/j.amcollsurg.2018.08.184.

  – An ethical framework for how and why institutions should address interfacility medical error discovery.

References

1. Beauchamp TL, Childress JF. Principles of biomedical ethics. 9th ed. Oxford University Press; 2019.
2. Boothman RC, Imhoff SJ, Campbell DA Jr. Nurturing a culture of patient safety and achieving lower malpractice risk through disclosure: lessons learned and future directions. Front Health Serv Manage. 2012;28(3):13–28.
3. Clinton HR, Obama B. Making patient safety the centerpiece of medical liability reform. N Engl J Med. 2006;354(21):2205–8. https://doi.org/10.1056/NEJMp068100.
4. Kohn LT, Corrigan JM, Donaldson MS. To err is human: building a safer health system. National Academies Press; 2000.
5. Wilson RM, Runciman WB, Gibberd RW, Harrison BT, Newby L, Hamilton JD. The quality in Australian health care study. Med J Aust. 1995;163(9):458–71. https://doi.org/10.5694/j.1326-5377.1995.tb124691.x.
6. Baker GR, Norton PG, Flintoft V, et al. The Canadian adverse events study: the incidence of adverse events among hospital patients in Canada. CMAJ. 2004;170(11):1678–86. https://doi.org/10.1503/cmaj.1040498.
7. Vincent C, Neale G, Woloshynowych M. Adverse events in British hospitals: preliminary retrospective record review. BMJ. 2001;322(7285):517–9. https://doi.org/10.1136/bmj.322.7285.51.
8. Leape LL, Brennan TA, Laird N, et al. The nature of adverse events in hospitalized patients. Results of the Harvard Medical Practice Study II. N Engl J Med. 1991;324(6):377–84. https://doi.org/10.1056/nejm199102073240406.
9. Thomas EJ, Studdert DM, Burstin HR, et al. Incidence and types of adverse events and negligent care in Utah and Colorado. Med Care. 2000;38(3):261–71.
10. Lipira LE, Gallagher TH. Disclosure of adverse events and errors in surgical care: challenges and strategies for improvement. World J Surg. 2014;38(7):1614–21. https://doi.org/10.1007/s00268-014-2564-5.
11. American Medical Association. Code of Medical Ethics overview. https://www.ama-assn.org/delivering-care/ethics/code-medical-ethics-overview. Accessed 25 Oct 2020.
12. American College of Surgeons. Statements on principles. https://www.facs.org/about-acs/statements/stonprin#code. Accessed 25 Oct 2020.
13. Gallagher TH, Waterman AD, Ebers AG, Fraser VJ, Levinson W. Patients' and physicians' attitudes regarding the disclosure of medical errors. JAMA. 2003;289(8):1001–7. https://doi.org/10.1001/jama.289.8.1001.

14. Liebman CB, Hyman CS. A mediation skills model to manage disclosure of errors and adverse events to patients. Health Aff. 2004;23(4):22–32. https://doi.org/10.1377/hlthaff23.4.22.
15. Agency for Healthcare Research Quality. Communication and Optimal Resolution (CANDOR) toolkit. https://www.ahrq.gov/patient-safety/capacity/candor/index.html. Accessed 21 Feb 2021.
16. Dossett LA, Kauffmann RM, Lee JS, et al. Specialist physicians' attitudes and practice patterns regarding disclosure of pre-referral medical errors. Ann Surg. 2018;267(6):1077–83. https://doi.org/10.1097/sla.0000000000002427.
17. Mazor K, Roblin DW, Greene SM, Fouayzi H, Gallagher TH. Primary care physicians' willingness to disclose oncology errors involving multiple providers to patients. BMJ Qual Saf. 2016;25(10):787–95. https://doi.org/10.1136/bmjqs-2015-004353.
18. Morreim EH, Am I. My brother's warden? Responding to the unethical or incompetent colleague. Hastings Cent Rep. 1993;23(3):19–27.
19. Rubin MA, Friedman DI. The ethics of disclosing another physician's medical error. Continuum: Lifelong Learn Neurol. 2015;21(4):1146–9. https://doi.org/10.1212/con.0000000000000198.
20. Asghari F, Fotouhi A, Jafarian A. Doctors' views of attitudes towards peer medical error. Postgrad Med J. 2010;86(1012):123–6. https://doi.org/10.1136/qshc.2007.025015.
21. Antunez AG, Saari A, Miller J, Dossett LA. Patient preferences in cases of Inter-system Medical Error Discovery (IMED). Ann Surg. 2021;273(3):516–22. PMID:31348037
22. Brooks D. The road to character. Random House; 2015.
23. Souter KJ, Gallagher TH. The disclosure of unanticipated outcomes of care and medical errors: what does this mean for anesthesiologists? Anesth Analg. 2012;114(3):615–21. https://doi.org/10.1213/ane.0b013e3182228604.
24. Antunez AG, Shuman AG, Jagsi R, Dossett LA. Ethical duty of health care systems to address interfacility medical error discovery. J Am Coll Surg. 2018;227(5):543–7. https://doi.org/10.1016/j.amcollsurg.2018.08.184.
25. Gallagher TH, Mello MM, Levinson W, et al. Talking with patients about other clinicians' errors. N Engl J Med. 2013;369(18):1752–7. https://doi.org/10.1056/nejmsb1303119.
26. Marx DA. Patient safety and the "just culture": a primer for health care executives. Trustees of Columbia University; 2001.
27. Schulte DJ. Ask our lawyer: physicians and self-regulation. In: Michigan Medicine Magazine. Michigan State Medical Society. 2019. https://www.msms.org/About-MSMS/News-Media/Michigan-Medicine-Magazine/May-June-2019/Ask-Our-Lawyer-Physicians-and-Self-Regulation. Accessed 21 Nov 2020.

Chapter 18
Expert Witness Testifying Against Colleagues

Alberto R. Ferreres (iD)

> *"Testifying in court is among the most demanding work that I do, both technically and ethically. It requires thinking through not just the details of the case, but also how I stand philosophically about statistics, and how I stand ethically and morally. And that is why I find it a welcome challenge."* [1]
>
> —*Joseph B. Kadane, Professor of Statistics, Carnegie Mellon University*

Abstract Performing the task of an expert witness in the field of medical and surgical malpractice litigation takes on great ethical and moral responsibilities. Providing medical expert witness (MEW) is part of the scope of medical practice both in the field of Medicine and Surgery. In order to be a MEW and able to judge the doings of a colleague, the expert witness needs to confirm his credentials of training, license, board certification and reliability. The importance of the MEW testimony lies upon the fact that it will set the standard of care criteria applicable in the particular case under scrutiny. The MEW needs to act in accordance with the four ethical principles of beneficence, non-maleficence, respect of patient autonomy and justice. Following these moral imperatives, he/ she is able to interpret to the judge and jury the facts of the case.

Keywords Medical expert witness · Testimony · Ethics · Malpractice
Professional liability · Standard of care

A. R. Ferreres (✉)
University of Buenos Aires, Buenos Aires, Argentina

University of Washington, Seattle, WA, USA
e-mail: aferre17@uw.edu

© The Author(s), under exclusive license to Springer Nature
Switzerland AG 2022
V. A. Lonchyna et al. (eds.), *Difficult Decisions in Surgical Ethics*, Difficult
Decisions in Surgery: An Evidence-Based Approach,
https://doi.org/10.1007/978-3-030-84625-1_18

Case

Dr. Helen Jones is a well-respected, board certified academic gastrointestinal surgeon who primarily focuses on the treatment of biliary and pancreatic cancer diseases, having completed a fellowship at a top institution. She has endured a stormy divorce and her children's educational debt and home mortgage are worrying her. She has been approached by a local law firm to hire her services in a case against Dr. Philip Austin, a well-known hepatopancreatobiliary (HPB) surgeon in private practice in the same city. Upon reviewing the medical records and pertinent documents, including the depositions from both sides and additional documentation, and having been offered an exorbitant fee schedule, she decides to accept the role of a medical expert witness. She is conflicted as she does consider Dr. Austin to be a top surgeon in his field of practice. The case revolves around the death of a 69-year-old lady with a cardiac history who had undergone a Whipple procedure. She died on her 30th postoperative day due to an acute myocardial infarction. She is uncomfortable confronting Dr. Austin's actions in front of the jury, but the offered fee substantially exceeds her expectations. In her mind, she believes Dr Austin has not been negligent in his management of the case, but she chooses to be on the plaintiff's side for, if not her, another physician will be employed in this role.

18.1   Introduction

Most, if not all, decisions regarding medical liability are performed by judges or lay jurors. Since neither of them are educated in the medical field, they depend upon the testimony and opinion of the medical expert witnesses (MEW) in order to get knowledge and a complete understanding of the matters under discussion. The great military surgeon Ambroise Paré (1510–1590) astutely observed that "… judges rule according to how they are informed by the experts" [2]. The role of the MEW is of paramount importance to defend the rights of patients harmed with disability or even death and also of physicians, who although performing under the umbrella of their expertise, may have had failures or unexpected outcomes. The purpose of the MEW is to illustrate to the judges and juries what the defending practitioner did, what should have been done or not under the particular circumstances of the case and if that behavior is consistent with negligence due to breach of the standard of care [3].

A MEW, also known as a skilled witness, is a physician qualified, by reason of his or her education, training, skills, knowledge and expertise to testify on a particular medical situation involving the patient and his or her physician under certain and determined circumstances of time, place and surrounding features. Their role is to decipher, evaluate, assess, criticize or agree with the medical conduct and decisions in cases of alleged malpractice, including negligence, imprudence or unskillfulness, based on the facts provided by the medical records and witnesses. The role played by the medical records is of the utmost importance and will allow the MEW to perform the task. Ideally that person should have knowledge of that particular field of medical topic in discussion. For their time and expertise, the MEW is entitled to a fee or honorarium surrendered by the party who hires him or her. However, there are legal systems where side expert witnesses, guided by an impartial approach, coexist with the official expert witnesses. It is important to distinguish the role of a standard witness (also known as a fact witness), who provides only facts from that of the expert witness, who is skilled in some appropriate field or discipline and thus is able to provide opinion about the facts that have been collected and knowledge and the critical assessment of those collected facts. The MEW provides assessment if the physician at trial performed within the appropriate standard of care, despite not having been present during the delivery of the health care that is now the subject of malpractice [4].

Challenges to the ethical principles as described by Tom Beauchamp and James Childress may be encountered during the activity of the medical expert witness in court [5]. The four ethical principles (justice, autonomy, beneficence and nonmaleficence) offer a systematic approach to Medical Ethics and serve as a frame for solving conflicts. A typical challenge, confronted by all the four ethical principles, is linked to the truthfulness and impartiality the MEW must keep in mind when performing the testimony. The principlist approach serves as a list of moral and ethical criteria which assist in solving conflicts in the work of a medical expert witness. Each principle may be linked to different aspects in the field of expert witness testimony and thus helps in developing a typology, as can be seen in Table 18.1, which will serve as a guideline for discussion.

18.2   Search Strategy

A search using the following MeSH terms (ethics, surgical ethics, expert witness, expert witness testimony, malpractice litigation, ethical conflicts, standard of care) was performed in these databases: Pubmed, Medline and LiLacs. The years of search spanned from 1995–2020. References included within the retrieved publications were further assessed and those considered the most appropriate have been included in the chapter's list of references.

18.3   Discussion

The well-known 1767 English legal case of "*Slater vs Baker & Stapleton*" contributed not only to the development of the informed consent process but more significantly it laid the foundations of the standard of care concept as well as the role of

Table 18.1 Typology of ethical topics in the expert witness activity

Principle	Topics
Justice	– Medical/ surgical diligence and expertise – Admissibility of the MEW testimony – Honesty – Truthfulness and impartiality – Reliability – Definition and assessment of the standard of care – Assessment of potential harms
Respect for autonomy	– Avoidance of "hired guns" – Disclosure of the expert own experience – Recognition of pressure from either party
Beneficence	– Medical/ surgical diligence and expertise – Definition and assessment of the standard of care – Appropriateness of the testimony – Truthfulness and impartiality – Reliability – Accountability
Non-Maleficence	– Medical/ surgical diligence and expertise – Definition and assessment of the standard of care – Appropriateness of the testimony – Truthfulness and impartiality – Reliability – Not contingent on final results of claim – Avoidance of hindsight bias

Source: Author's own work

the expert witness. Baker, a surgeon, and Stapleton, an apothecary, were summoned by Slater, who had suffered a fracture of his leg. Due to poor healing, Baker and Stapleton decided to refracture the bone and apply a device to stretch and straighten the fracture. When expert witnesses were called to offer their testimony, they considered that the therapeutic management had been contrary to standard practice and that both professionals have acted contrary to the rule of the profession and performed what no surgeon ought to have done. The ruling stated, "Physicians and surgeons were to be judged by the usage and law of surgeons … the rule of the profession as testified to by surgeons themselves" [6].

Years ago, because of a so-called "conspiracy of silence", hiring an expert physician to testify and provide standard of care guidelines for the plaintiff was difficult. The situation has reversed, since the economic compensation may be pretty beneficial, as in the case of the theoretical Dr. Jones.

The role of the MEW should be considered within the scope of medical practice and accordingly, subject to scrutiny in two ways: in the legal scenario by a potential accusation of false testimony; and in the professional arena by peer review. The resolution of medical malpractice claims relies on the expert witness testimony which helps the judge and jury to understand medical topics, which may be complex. The MEW is invaluable to educate the court on the science and practice of Medicine and Surgery. Thus, there is an ethical duty imposed on the MEW for the provided testimony to be truthful, fair and unbiased so it may achieve validity, objectivity and soundness in front of the court.

The ethical aspects and moral obligations of the MEW must be highlighted since testimony which is unethical and untruthful may lead to flawed sentences. Some examples include testimony which just represents the opinion of the expert witness and is not grounded on medical records or facts; the lack of a precise causal relationship; testimony definitively mistaken or biased or against accepted variations within the standard of care or influenced by a hindsight bias. These are all examples where truth has not been the beacon of the MEW's assessment and opinion. The MEW may be confronted by ethical or moral dilemmas, represented by the decision-making quandary between two or more plausible moral imperatives.

Although medical malpractice litigation seems to be a present epidemic with worldwide expansion and compromises many fields of medical practice (mainly, surgery, anesthesia, gynecology, obstetrics and neonatology), its incidence was also high in the early twentieth century [7].

The declaration of medical professional liability is based on the following points, which need to be proven through substantial evidence during the process:

1. Duty: represented by the standard of care which should have been provided in a similar case under similar circumstances by similar physicians
2. Breach of duty: the assessment of the magnitude, level or degree of that violation of duty
3. Damage: represented by harm, disability or death of the patient
4. Causal relationship: comprises three aspects: between the breach of duty and the damages, chronological and topographical.

Since the judge and jury are lay personnel, the legal system, based either on common law (British tradition) or codified law (Roman and French tradition) rely upon experts to illustrate and educate about the above-mentioned points. There may be civil cases against a physician, where the discussion is about the monetary compensation for an inflicted harm, or criminal, where the physician's freedom and punishment is at stake. In many countries, mainly in those with codified laws, professional liability claims may advance in both jurisdictions.

The whole system of expert witness testimonies is grounded upon the fact that the MEW should be independent, neutral, unbiased and adjusted to right when offering expert counsel in a sincere and reliable way with the sole objective of providing truth and better judgment. However, in real life things may not be so straightforward; the role of the MEW is not that of an advocate but of an educator on topics in which the judge and the jury are not familiar. In adversarial systems, such as the

American one, the plaintiff's attorney is devoted to winning the case more so than being worried for finding the real truth of the facts [8].

From an ethical standpoint, the duties of a MEW arise from the following two conditions:

- The implicit moral contract amongst the members of the medical profession and between them and the society, which overlays the foundations of the physician's responsibility to the entire society, to Medicine as a whole and to the self-regulation of the medical profession.
- The professional duty to use scientific knowledge entrusted to physicians to serve others, including those involved in a litigation process, the administration of justice and society in its totality.

The ideal circumstance should be that in which the MEW plays his/ her role role with full trust from the public, but society should also be concerned if the judiciary is targeting the moral and ethical responsibilities involved in their activity. Gross holds a very strong view regarding the role of the expert witness: "to put it bluntly, in many professions, service as an expert witness is not considered honest work, the contempt of lawyers and judges for experts is famous" [9].

18.4 Justice

The foremost objective of a trial is to find the truth, grasp and shed light about the medical facts of the care of a patient under particular circumstances of time, place and person and thus provide justice to both parties. There are several topics which compromise the ethical principle of justice in the performance of Dr Jones and which emerge clearly from the typology offered in Table 18.1. The Courts consider the MEW as an expert in the medical field with a specific background and knowledge grounded in his or her training, skill or abilities. The role of the MEW is completely different from that of the percipient witness, in the sense that the latter one provides information about what has been seen, heard or experienced, meanwhile the MEW provides an expert opinion based on the assessment of the medical records and other proofs.

The goals of the MEW are [10]:

- Provide a reliable and trustworthy opinion about the presumed existence of malpractice
- Define the standard of care in the precise circumstances which surround the case
- Describe precisely if the physician's demeanor adjusted itself to the established standard of care
- Specify the harm suffered by the patient and the severity of disability
- Detail the causal, topographical and chronological relationships between the delivery of care and the definitive clinical outcome

The qualifications of a MEW include professional competence, intellectual accuracy, precise data analysis and recollection and unbiased methodology to perform judgments. In many countries, each side hires its own expert, while in other systems these party or side experts work alongside official experts, appointed by the courts, providing impartial and unbiased opinions. This last situation may provide unbiased, objective and prevalent opinion about a given subject. The accuracy, reliability and truthfulness of the expert testimony may be affected by the collected facts, the medical record documentation and personal factors of the expert witness (qualifications, reasons and motives, biases and personal interests). The MEW final report should be based on the collected evidence of the medical case, which pertains the review and thorough assessment of all the medical records, taking into account that these have been completed by the physicians involved in the claim.

The US Federal Rule of Evidence 702 establishes the requirements of the expert witness testimony: "If scientific, technical, or other specialized knowledge will assist the trier of fact to understand the evidence or to determine a fact in issue, a witness qualified as an expert by knowledge, skill, experience, training or education may testify in the form of an opinion or otherwise" [11].

It further adds the requirements that:

- The testimony is based on sufficient facts or data,
- The testimony is the product of reliable principles and methods, and
- The expert has reliably applied the principles and methods to the facts of the case. [11]

The admissibility of the expert witness testimony was expounded by the American court system through different precedents including the following:

- The Frye standard (1923): refers to a case where the admissibility of a blood pressure deception test in evaluating truthfulness of a response of a witness was in discussion. The Court considered that expert opinion based on a scientific technique is admissible only when the technique is generally accepted as reliable in the relevant scientific community, which was not the case in this court proceeding [12].
- The Daubert standard (1993) defined the benchmark for the acceptance of expert testimony in federal courts. It was linked to birth defects which were considered the result of the prenatal use of bendectin (combination of doxylamine, dicyclomine and pyridoxine) widely used for the treatment of nausea and vomiting during pregnancy until 1983 [13]. But the assumptions about the side effects of bendectin were dismissed since this position did not meet the "general acceptance in the scientific community' standard. The Supreme Court of Justice set the guidelines to assess the appropriateness of the expert witness methodology. The guidelines encompass the following five elements:

  (a) Whether the theory or technique in discussion has undergone test
  (b) If it has been exposed to peer review and/or publication
  (c) The potential rate of error associated with its use
  (d) Existing standards and/or regulations regarding use or operation
  (e) Predominant acceptance within the academic circle

The Daubert standard was further confirmed and expanded by two additional cases: *General Electric Co v Joiner* in 1997 [14] and *Kumbo Tyre Company v Carmichael* two years later [15].

In accordance with these guidelines the testimony of Dr Jones cannot rely solely on her opinion, but needs to be based on scientific evidence in order to be accepted in court, since the other party may request a Daubert challenge to contest her testimony.

The definition of the standard of care and its application to a particular situation represents the core issue in every professional liability claim and is also encompassed by an ethical approach with proper observance of the ethical principles. Establishing if the standard of care in a particular case defines the case at hand or not, and therefore represents a breach of the duty of care, is of paramount importance for the final determination of the case.

The development of the concept of standard of care derives from two legal cases. The first one is not related to the medical field, but with the sinking of two barges guided by tugboats. The *T.J. Hooper* case (1932) dealt with the plaintiff's 2 barges were towed by the defendant's tugboats (TJHooper and Montrose). The case started with the cargo owners sueing the owner of the barges which sank during a storm, and then repeated the action against the owner of the tugs towing the barges. All the vessels were found to be unseaworthy. Also, the tugs were negligent for failure to be rigged with reliable radios, which may have aided them during the storm. Judge Hand considered that there are precautions so imperative that if the utility of a safety safeguard outranks the cost of it, then it is negligent not to carry the safety safeguard. This case is regarded as the initial cornerstone in the legal appreciation of custom and standard of care, considering that if there is a practice that is reasonable but not universally "customary" it may still be used as a measure of the standard of care [16].

In the second case, the plaintiff Barbara Helling sued her team of ophthalmologists, Thomas Carey and Robert Laughlin. The patient, who was 32 years old when diagnosed with glaucoma, sued the ophthalmologists for medical malpractice, alleging that she suffered severe and permanent eye damage as result of the ophthalmologists' negligence in failing to timely perform a pressure test for glaucoma [17]. Although the expert witness considered that as the patient was under 40 years and the incidence of glaucoma among this age group was very low (1 in 25000), it was not standard to test patients under 40 years with a tonometry test. Both the trial and appellate courts ruled in favor of the ophthalmologists, but the Supreme Court of the State of Washington overruled in favor of the plaintiff, deciding that being that the test was readily available, inexpensive and harmless, it should have been performed. Justice Hand's decision in the T.J.Hooper case was quoted in this sentence, which also mentions a court decision by Justice O W Holmes from 1903: "What usually is done may be evidence of what ought to be done, but what ought to be done is fixed by a standard of reasonable prudence, whether it usually is complied with or not" [18].

This approach set a worrisome precedent for medical malpractice cases [19], but in more recent cases there is a constant effort to ensure that jurors understand that the concept of standard of care is not equal to perfection in practice. It should be acknowledged that the standard of care should not be associated with a perfect and ideal care, or of care with a perfect result or even with the personal approach of the expert witness. It is more reasonable to refer to an appropriate standard of care, thus allowing a range of therapeutic options, and not the personal preference or inclination of the expert witness, as in the case in discussion. The difference between malpractice and maloccurrence should also be emphasized, representing the latter in any bad or undesirable outcome unrelated to the quality of care provided.

In the 1985 case of *Hall v Hilbun*, the Mississippi Court sentence provided a new approach in the definition of the standard of care in the present era. Patient Terry Hall's husband filed a malpractice claim against Dr. Hilbun, the surgeon who had operated on her due to a small bowel obstruction, dying because of respiratory failure after the operation. In addition, the autopsy revealed a retained sponge, but which had not contributed to her death. Dr. Hoerr, a retired surgeon from Cleveland was summoned as expert witness but was initially disqualified because he was not familiar with the local standard of care. In the appeal, the state Supreme Court provided the adoption of a national standard of care: "Given the circumstances of each patient, each physician has a duty to use his or her knowledge and therewith treat through maximum reasonable medical recovery, each patient, with such reasonable diligence, skill, competence and prudence as are practiced by minimally competent physicians in the same specialty or general field of practice throughout the United States, who have available to them the same general facilities, services, equipment and options" [20].

What happens when the MEW does not abide by the principles? Traditionally judicial immunity had been granted to expert witness testimony, by application of the US Supreme Court ruling in *Mitchell v Forsyth*, which established differences between qualified and absolute immunity. This distinction endorsed the activity of many "hired guns" providing opinion without grounds and justification [21]. The need of accountability regarding the consequences and substance of the expert witness testimony started to be challenged in the *Brousseau v Jarrett* case [22]: the plaintiff suffered personal injuries in a hit-and-run collision. The defendant was a surgeon hired to manage the injuries and was requested to prepare reports about the disability of the plaintiff for medico-legal purposes. His last report stated there was no residual disability from the accident, which did not correspond to the sequelae and the severe nature of the injuries. The defendant, hired by insurance companies to provide medical reports detailing harm and disability, did so in a fashion negating the real sufferings of the victims, a situation that was duly recognized by the court.

Meanwhile in *Hart v Brown* the obligation of the MEW to provide "an unbiased and fair evaluation of another physician's care of a patient" was highlighted [23]. The expert testified as to the chance that seven year old Kathleen Hart's twin was a potential kidney donor for her sister, the urgent need for renal transplantation and the safety of the procedure to the donor.

Some years later the Fifth Circuit Court of Appeals raised the concern about an unlawful and unethical behavior stating: "Experts whose opinions are available to the higher bidder have no place testifying in a court of law before a jury and with the imprimatur of the trial judge's decision that he is an expert", when reviewing the claimed loss of inheritance of three children whose parents were among the 138 killed passengers of Pan American World Airways flight 759, after takeoff from New Orleans airport in 1982. The estimations were performed by an economist appointed as expert witness for the plaintiff side and were judged to be so excessive as to require a new trial [24].

The moderate to poor agreement among expert witnesses when confronted to professional liability claims is not only a major concern for the administration of justice but also for scientific and academic institutions since truthfulness, reliability, fairness and trustworthiness represent a priority not only for those involved but also for the society as a whole [25, 26].

18.5 Autonomy

Due to the absence of physician-patient relationship, the MEW should follow the ethical principle of autonomy being free from any type of coercion; this right of self-determination explains that the beacon should be to avoid any type of pressure from either party. In the case under discussion, Dr Jones has undoubtedly recognized the pecuniary benefit she would receive if she testified against Dr. Austin.

The MEW should be free to accept or decline a case if they consider that their testimony will not be useful for the side they represent. Quite different is the situation when official expert witnesses are appointed by the Courts. There is another implicit trait in this principle of autonomy applied to the expert witness activity and that is the disclosure of the expert's own experience. This duty is a right for both sides, and should be considered a mandatory imposition from the judiciary. Of course, the MEW needs to prove the qualifications and background, his or her expertise in a particular topic should be reliably accredited, the current keeping of competence should be appropriately certified and he or she should be able to inform the conclusions of their assessment in a clear and accurate fashion. In the case, Dr Jones is unquestionably an expert in the matter of discussion, but with a particular self-interest in the final result.

The appearance of "hired guns" is represented by those experts whose medical opinions depend on which side is hiring them. The characteristic features include frequent expert witness activity and high fees. Oddly, defense "hired guns" are better considered than plaintiff ones, since professional "esprit de corps" may be considered more acceptable than pecuniary compensation. Nonetheless, both versions should be utterly dismissed, and the MEW should not be an advocate of any side and their fee should not be contingent on the final outcome [27]. However, the critical and sometimes negative opinion of the expert witness should be appreciated by the plaintiff, particularly in the initial stages, since it may help to formulate a different strategy, or even an out- of- court settlement.

18.6 Beneficence and Nonmaleficence

The activity of the MEW confronts ethical challenges which must be taken into account in order to achieve an ethically sound and justifiable course of action in the activity [28]. These entangle implications and potential consequences for all those involved in the litigation: plaintiff and defendant, the administration of justice and the MEW himself/ herself. An inappropriate testimony is that which is biased, false, not grounded on the facts of the medical record does not benefit any of the above mentioned parties. In this sense, Dr Jones should be aware of all the consequences of providing a testimony which may not be verifiable or agreed upon. The moral imperative is the recognition of the rights of all parties summoned in the trial, and the MEW has a preeminent role as a justice collaborator to make things clear to judges and jurors. If Dr. Jones is solely pursuing an economic benefit, she needs to recognize that her behavior may be prone for later audit and review and charges may be even pressed on her person. The behavior of the MEW should be virtuous, and among those virtues of a good physician the following should be mentioned: fidelity to trust and promise, benevolence, effacement of self-interest, compassion and caring, intellectual honesty, justice and prudence [29]. With the same understanding, Jonsen contemplates that the first conflict a physician encounters is between altruism and self- interest, applicable to the dilemma of Dr Jones [30]. These virtues should guide Dr. Jones as an expert witness, in the same fashion she needs to observe and follow them in everyday surgical care with patients. It is her clinical expertise and her position as a physician that allow her to offer an expert opinion in aforementioned case.

The colleagues, the professional associations, the courts and the society should play an active role to correct unethical expert testimonies, lacking all the mentioned characteristics. If the MEW review is inaccurate, biased, not adequately grounded in its conclusions or lacking scientific methodology, it should undergo review and if inappropriate, even subjected to sanctions and/or fines. A final aspect of the ethics surrounding the activity of the MEW refers to the relationship between physicians, their associations and the society to which they belong. The MEW is not just a physician acting on his or her own, but should be considered as one entitled with the corresponding moral authority to illustrate the knowledge of the medical profession about different topics in the field where they apparently achieve expertise and wisdom.

The role of the MEW is to be a judge of peers, providing the required and necessary advice to those who will judge other physician's behavior, assisting with the correct understanding of the medical facts surrounding a particular medical case. The MEW needs to approach every case with autonomy and an impartial view, dissect and appraise the facts and the data in a systematic fashion, meticulously, objectively and dispassionately, without consideration to the consequences on either side. Two circumstances should be prevented from occurring: the failure to forward satisfactory evidence to support their conclusions and the failure to demonstrate their whole understanding of a particular medical case.

A very important and useful element which aids in the ethical assessment and evaluation is represented by the guidelines and recommendations enacted by professional associations for those members serving as expert witness. In that sense the American Medical Association [31], the American College of Surgeons [32], and many others have issued their rulings [33, 34]. In the case of the American College of Surgeons, the statement underlines the obligation of the task to serve as an expert witness as well as the qualifications to act as one, and the standards of fairness and honesty.

18.7 Case Conclusion

After discussing all these concepts, the best course of action for Dr. Jones may be to decline the proposal to be an expert witness for the plaintiff side. Her knowledge and expertise agree that the late complication was not due to the performance and the standard of care delivered by Dr. Austin but due to the cardiac background of the patient and unrelated to the Whipple procedure. The indication was clear and well grounded, the expertise of Dr. Austin is well recognized, the postoperative management was according to appropriate standards of care and the institution where he works is also widely recognized as outstanding.

18.8 Concluding Remarks

Our recommendations for the ethical activity of the medical expert witness (MEW) include the following:

- Every physician has an ethical obligation to assist in the administration of justice, by providing truthful and non-biased opinion about the delivered standard of care and the relationship between that care and the final outcome.
- The MEW testimony should not be contingent upon the financial compensation or the case outcome or the side which hires the expert.
- The MEW should not be an advocate for either party, but needs to collaborate in the finding of the truth surrounding the case and thus with the administration of justice system.
- The MEW role imposes recent and substantive expertise in the medical field of discussion, accountability and thus, their testimony may be subjected to professional peer review if requested
- The opinions should be unbiased, based upon the experience on the matter of the MEW and supported by solid references of the medical literature.
- The MEW should strive to provide objective, thorough, truthful, impartial testimony and thus collaborate with the integrity of the whole judicial process.

18.9   Selected References

- Andrew LB. Expert witness testimony: the ethics of being a medical expert witness. Emerg Clin N Am. 2006; 24: 715–731. https://doi.org/10.1016/j.emc.2006.05.001.

  - The author highlights the educational role of the expert witness and the ethical implications embodied in the provided counsel to judges and jurors. She insists on the need to overthrow the conspiracy of silence, common in many professions. The qualifications of an expert are clearly enumerated. The author focuses on the topics of dishonest statements, financial influences, and the consequences of unethical experts and what recourse is available to those affected by unethical expert witness testimony.

- Ferreres AR. Ethical issues of expert witness testimony. World J Surg. 2014; 38: 1644–1649. https://doi.org/10.1007/s00268-014-2641-9.

  - This is an overview of the ethical conflicts encountered by the surgical expert witness in daily practice and provides a background regarding the admission of the expert testimony in court.

- Kass JS, Rose RV. Ethics case: ethical challenges for the medical expert witness. AMA J Ethics. 2016;18: 201–208. https://doi.org/10.1001/journalofethics.2016.18.3.ecas1-1603.

  - Using a case example, the authors describe ethical appeals in five different categories when physicians are confronted with the task of assuming the role of a medical expert witness.

References

1. Kadane JB. Ethical issues in being an expert witness. Law, Probability and Risk. 2005;4:21–3. https://doi.org/10.1093/lpr/mgi004.
2. Hamby WB. Ambroise Pare, surgeon of the renaissance. WH Green; 1967.
3. Andrew LB. Expert witness testimony: the ethics of being a medical expert witness. Emerg Clin N Am. 2006;24:715–31. https://doi.org/10.1016/j.emc.2006.05.001.
4. Ferreres AR. Ethical issues of expert witness testimony. World J Surg. 2014;38:1644–9. https://doi.org/10.1007/s00268-014-2641-9.
5. Beauchamp TL, Childress JF. Principles of biomedical ethics. 8th ed. Oxford University Press; 2019.
6. Slater v Baker & Stapleton, 95 Engl Rptr 860, 2 Wils, KB 359, 1767.
7. Stetson HG, Moran JE. Malpractice suits, their cause and prevention. N Engl J Med. 1934;210:1381–5.
8. Amon E. Expert witness testimony. Clin Perinatol. 2007;34:473–88. https://doi.org/10.1016/j.clp.2007.03.016.
9. Gross SR. Expert evidence. Wis L Rev. 1991;1991:1113–232.

10. Bal BS. The expert witness in medical malpractice litigation. Clin Orthop Relat Res. 2009;467:383–91. https://doi.org/10.1007/s11999-008-0634-4.
11. Testimony by Experts. 28 USC 702 (2010).
12. Frye v United States, 293 F. 1013 (DC Cir. 1923).
13. Daubert v Merrell Dow Pharmaceuticals, Inc., 509 U.S. 579 (1993).
14. General Electric Co. v Joiner, 522 U.S. 136 (1997).
15. Kumho Tire Co. v Carmichael, 526 U.S. 137 (1999).
16. The T.J. Hooper, 60 F:2d 737 (2d Cir.), cert. denied, 287 U.S. 662 (1932).
17. *Helling v Carey*, 83 Wash. 2d 514, 519 P.2d 981 (1974).
18. *Texas & Pac. Ry. v Behymer*, 189 US 468, 470 (1903).
19. Torts – Medical Malpractice – Sources of a Physician's Standard of Care: The Medical Profession or the Courts—*Helling v. Carey*, 1975 BYU L Rev. (1975);572.
20. Hall v Hilburn, 466 So. 2d 856 (Miss. 1985).
21. Mitchell v Forsyth, 472 US 511 (1985).
22. Brousseau v Jarrett, 73 Cal App 3d 864, 141 Cal Rptr 200 (1977, 3rd Dist).
23. Hart v Brown, 103 Cal App3d 947, 163 Cal Rptr 356 (1980, 1st Dist).
24. Eymard v Pan Am World Airways re Air Crash Disaster, 795 F2d 1230, 1234 (5th Cir 1986).
25. Posner KL, Caplan RA, Cheney FW. Variation in expert opinion in medical malpractice review. Anesthesiology. 1996;85:1049–54. https://doi.org/10.1097/00000542-199611000-00013.
26. De Reuver PR, Dijkgraaf MGW, Gevers SKM, Gouma DJ; for the BILE Study Group. Poor agreement among expert witnesses in surgical malpractice. Ann Surg. 2008;248:815–820. https://doi.org/10.1097/SLA.0b013e318186de35.
27. Gomez JCB. Silencing the hired guns: ensuring honesty in medical expert testimony through state legislation. J Leg Med. 2005;26:385–9. https://doi.org/10.1080/01947640500218356.
28. Kass JS, Rose RV. Ethics case: ethical challenges for the medical expert witness. AMA J Ethics. 2016;18:201–8. https://doi.org/10.1001/journalofethics.2016.18.3.ecas1-1603.
29. Pellegrino ED. *Humanism and the physician*. University of Tennessee Press; 1979.
30. Jonsen AR. Watching the doctor. New Engl J Med. 1983;308:1531–5.
31. American Medical Association. Code of medical ethics. https://www.ama-assn.org/topics/ama-code-medical-ethics. Accessed 30 May 2020.
32. American College of Surgeons. Statement on the physician acting as an expert witness. https://www.facs.org/about-acs/statements/8-expert-witness. Accessed 30 May 2020.
33. American Academy of Pediatrics Committee on Medical Liability. Guidelines for expert witness testimony in medical malpractice litigation. Pediatrics. 2002;109:974–9.
34. American College of Emergency Physicians. Expert witness guidelines for the specialty of emergency medicine revised 2015. https://www.acep.org/patient-care/policy-statements/expert-witness-guidelines-for-the-specialty-of-emergency-medicine/. Accessed 9 June 2020.

Part V
Cultural/Religious Diversity

Chapter 19
Acceptance or Refusal of Surgery Due to Religious or Cultural Reasons

M. Jeanne Wirpsa ⓘ

Abstract The United States is witnessing an unprecedented increase in religious and cultural diversity. The highly rational, positivistic, and evidence-based practice of medicine inevitably clashes with practices of and normative claims made by members of these communities. While no comprehensive data exists on the prevalence of ethical conflicts featuring religious or cultural reasons for refusal or acceptance of surgery, studies suggest that these cases rarely end well. Health outcomes for patients suffer; surgeons fail to honor the core values of their profession leading to high levels of moral distress. This chapter uses two cases involving patients from different religious and cultural backgrounds—a Pentecostal African American woman and a young man from a faithful Islamic family—to uncover the normative assumptions of Western medicine, specifically the limitations of the conventional principle-based approach used in surgical ethics. In order to successfully cross the divide between the culture of medicine and religious conceptions of the body, health, illness, and healing, surgeons are invited to cultivate cultural and epistemic humility rather than attempt to understand every aspect of their patient's religious beliefs or cultural norms. Clinical ethicists, community leaders, clergy, healthcare chaplains, and religious scholars are among those who may serve as cultural brokers in these challenging cases.

Keywords Culture · Religion · Refusal of treatment · Cultural humility Cross-cultural medicine

M. J. Wirpsa (✉)
Northwestern Memorial Hospital, Chicago, IL, USA

MacLean Center for Clinical Ethics, University of Chicago, Chicago, IL, USA
e-mail: jwirpsa@nm.org

© The Author(s), under exclusive license to Springer Nature
Switzerland AG 2022
V. A. Lonchyna et al. (eds.), *Difficult Decisions in Surgical Ethics*, Difficult
Decisions in Surgery: An Evidence-Based Approach,
https://doi.org/10.1007/978-3-030-84625-1_19

19.1   Cases

Case #1

Mrs. Williams is a 64-year-old African American woman who resides on the South side of Chicago but is employed part-time in housekeeping for one of the large downtown office buildings. When her co-workers notice she is increasingly fatigued and protecting her left arm, they suggest she go see a doctor. Instead, Mrs. Williams talks to her godmother, an elder in the Holiness Church, who instructs her to study scripture, pray, and attend a special worship service where members lay on hands and anoint with healing oils.

A few months later, Mrs. Williams goes to the emergency department when the pain is too much to bear. Imaging reveals a 5 cm tumor in her left breast. The oncologist recommends surgical removal of the tumor—a mastectomy—followed by chemotherapy and/or radiation. He fears it might be a triple negative breast cancer, a most aggressive and life-threatening form of the disease. Mrs. Williams will not, however, consent to a biopsy nor further therapy.

Mrs. Williams closes her eyes and spiritedly proclaims, "I am healed by the stripes of Jesus. In Jesus' name." Flustered, the oncologic surgeon shows her the scans, reiterates the aggressive nature of her cancer, and provides statistics to support his dire prognosis if her cancer is left untreated. Mrs. Williams responds, "I understand what you are saying. I've been around the block a few times, young man. But hear me when I say, no one is going to cut on me." He sends her home with pain medication and a follow-up appointment—which she never keeps.

Case #2

Zahid is a 26-year-old unmarried Iranian man and a devout Muslim who lives with his extended family in a suburb of Los Angeles. He has advanced interstitial lung disease, goes into respiratory failure and is emergently placed on VV ECMO. For two months the team and family agree to aggressive, life-prolonging care hoping Zahid will either recover or be a candidate for lung transplant. As a complication of prolonged ECMO support, Zahid suffers severe limb ischemia. Zahid's condition deteriorates; he requires CVVH and vasopressors. Lung transplant is no longer an option.

In a series of goals of care conversations with Zahid's father, older brother, and uncles, the vascular surgeon and critical care team explain that Zahid will need amputation of his left foot and sections of both arms. If he can be weaned from ECMO and survives to discharge, he probably will be vent dependent. They invite the family to tell them about Zahid, his life prior to this illness, healthcare preferences, and religious beliefs related to end-of-life medical care. They ask what Zahid would want if he could speak for himself.

Zahid's father does not tell them about Zahid's wishes. Instead, he calmly proclaims, "Allah, the Merciful, will decide his fate, not the doctors." The team pushes Zahid's father to consider if this formerly athletic, independent young man would want to live with this level of dependence and impairment. The family responds that "We will carry him around if need be and care for him night and day. We will attend to his every need. It is our duty. We cannot decide otherwise." The vascular surgeon considers the amputations inappropriate in the context of Zahid's impending demise; she is reluctant to perform the requested surgery.

19.2 Introduction

A vast body of literature in anthropology, religious studies, and bioethics is devoted to exploring the complex interplay between religion, culture and medicine. Probably best known to both the general public and healthcare providers is Anne Fadiman's seminal work, *When the Spirit Catches you and You Fall Down*, which documents the tragic consequences of the clash between a Western scientific understanding of illness and healing and that of a Hmong family [1]. Equally ubiquitous in healthcare is knowledge of the Jehovah's Witnesses' refusal of blood transfusions. The highly organized advocacy of this religious community not only encouraged the development of techniques to support bloodless surgeries but, more significantly, has led to religiously informed requests for/or refusals of medical care being granted a privileged, non-negotiable status.

Organ transplantation, reproductive health, orthopedics, cardiology, and end of life medical decision making, to mention just a few specialty areas in surgery, bear the imprint of a heightened attention to the influence of culture and religion. Many pre-surgical screening protocols either ask the patient directly about specific cultural practices that may impact care or disclose product information (e.g., bovine or porcine components) considered potentially relevant for informed consent by patients from certain religious sects [2]. Surgeons temporarily delay high risk procedures to accommodate religious rituals aimed at providing families spiritual peace. Pediatric ENT surgeons are no longer surprised (even if dismayed), when parents refuse implantation of a cochlear device to restore hearing for their deaf child on the grounds they reject the dominant assumptions about body, health and wholeness of the "ableist" culture [3].

The proliferation of international medicine, medical missionary programs, and global efforts to eradicate disease occasion unprecedented ethical concerns about the imposition of Western bioethics frameworks, moral relativism, and provider conscience as illustrated in literature on Xenotransplantation [4], Gender

Transformation Surgery [5], and Female Genital Mutilation [6], to mention a few highly controversial areas of care.

The cases of Mrs. Williams and Zahid—oft encountered by this ethicist chaplain—provide an entry point to discuss difficult ethical dilemmas faced by surgeons when adult patients from diverse cultural and religious backgrounds present for care (pediatric care falls outside the scope of this discussion). Mrs. Williams forgoes recommended life-saving surgery in favor of divine healing, and possibly, because of community beliefs about how cancer spreads, reinforced by distrust in the healthcare system. Zahid's father, on the other hand, requests life-altering amputation and continued use of advanced medical technology to prolong his son's life citing the authority of Islamic teachings and familial duty. In both cases, cultural norms and expectations are inextricably interwoven with religiously grounded ethical principles.

I will discuss limitations of the conventional principle-based approach to medical ethics when clinicians are confronted with acceptance or refusal of surgery due to culture or religion and suggest strategies for negotiating ethical conflicts. How does a surgeon respect patient autonomy, for example, when a culture employs a relational rather than individualistic understanding of personhood? Surgical informed consent (or refusal) requires the ability to rationally weigh benefits and burdens of a medical intervention as well as an appreciation that the medical information provided pertains to their own body. What happens if a patient's reason is perceived as "irrational" or they claim divine healing when the clinician has evidence of advanced disease? How can shared decision making (which requires a respectful consideration of the values of the patient in the context of the clinical assessment and recommendation of the medical team) proceed when the two parties inhabit foreign conceptual and discursive worlds? These are core ethical concepts that are challenged in the care of persons from diverse cultural and religious backgrounds.

I am not aiming to provide definitive views of any one religious tradition, denomination, or sect nor capture the richness, variations, and dynamic nature of a specific cultural framework or culture in general (see Table 19.1). Moreover, a presupposition throughout this chapter is that Western medicine and bioethics—and surgery and surgical ethics as subspecialties therein—are cultures with their own norms, values, systems of relationships, role expectations, epistemology, and conceptual frameworks for understanding the body, disease, and healing [7].

19.3 Search Strategy

To supplement my knowledge of foundational literature on culture, religion and medicine in general and to identify recent publications specific to the intersection of surgical consent/refusal and religion/culture I conducted a search using PubMed and SCOPUS. The search was limited to 2010–2020. The following combinations of search terms were selected: (1) Patient, refusal of surgical treatment AND

Table 19.1 Religious demographics, United States 2015

Religion	Percentage of US population
Evangelical protestant	25.4
Unaffiliated	22.8
Catholic	20.8
Nothing in particular	15.8
Mainline protestant	14.7
Historically black protestant	6.5
Agnostic	4
Atheist	3.1
Jewish	1.9
Mormon	1.6
Other faiths	1.5
Muslim	0.9
Jehovah witness	0.8
Buddhist	0.7
Hindu	0.7
Don't know	0.6
Orthodox Christian	0.5
Other Christian	0.4
Other world religions	0.3

Modified from "Religious Landscape Study." Pew Research Center, Washington, D.C. (May 12, 2015). https://www.pewforum.org/religious-landscape-study/

religion; (2) Patient, refusal of surgical treatment AND culture; (3) Racial Disparities AND Surgery; (4) Racial Disparities AND Cancer AND Refusal of treatment; (5) Islam and Surgery; (6) Surgical Ethics AND Religion; (7) Surgery AND Cultural Competence. The following terms were excluded: Jehovah's Witness; Pediatrics; Children; Provider, Refusal of Treatment.

19.4 Discussion

19.4.1 Culture, Religion, and Medicine: Intersection and Embeddedness

There is a notable lack of consensus on definitions of religion and culture. Anthropologist Clifford Geertz' foundational descriptions suffice to orient our readers to their complex and dynamic interrelatedness:

> Culture denotes a historically transmitted pattern of meanings embodied in symbols, a system of inherited conceptions expressed in symbolic forms by means of which men [sic] communicate, perpetuate, and develop their knowledge about and attitudes toward life.

> [R]eligion is a system of symbols which acts to establish powerful, pervasive and long-lasting moods and motivations in men [sic] by formulating conceptions of a general order of existence and clothing the conceptions with such an aura of factuality that the moods and motivation seem uniquely realistic. [8]

Religious leaders explicate religious "conceptions of a general order of existence", core theological principles, scripturally-sourced ethical directives, and ethical-legal frameworks in order to provide guidance to adherents about what is of value, virtuous, permissible, obligatory or forbidden in healthcare. How persons integrate these teachings into their everyday health behavior and medical decisions depends on a number of factors including level of adherence to the tradition, the cultural weight of folk beliefs, socio-economic location, level of education, personal experience with illness and healing, gender norms, and the historic narrative of the relation between a population and the healthcare system (see Fig. 19.1).

Mrs. Williams brings to her interaction with the surgical oncologist a culturally transmitted belief about how cancer is spread; as a result, she concludes that surgical intervention will make matters worse rather than better. She does not have the opportunity in the encounter described above to discuss her core belief in the power of Jesus to heal, her trust in the cultural institution of the Black Church, respect for

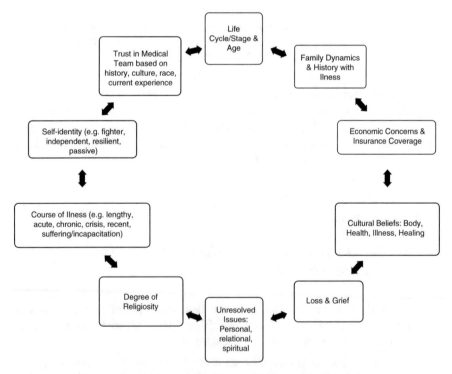

Fig. 19.1 Complex intersection between culture, religion, individual demographics & life-experience

the wisdom of elders, and informal but binding "familial" relationship to her godmother.

Mrs. Williams is far from unique: Studies confirm that African Americans are significantly more likely than whites to hold folk beliefs such as "air causes cancer to grow" as well as the specific religious belief that "God is in control of cancer", with strong associations found between these beliefs, race, and late stage cancer presentation and opposition to surgical treatment [9]. While other beliefs such as the sanctity of the body in turn may motivate healthcare seeking behavior, the higher prevalence of delays in seeking treatment and outright refusals of surgical treatment for breast, pancreatic, lung, and colon cancer among African Americans (when compared to whites, Asians or Latino) should provoke attention to the impact deeply embedded cultural beliefs and a pervasive distrust of US healthcare system have on health outcomes [10, 11].

Hayward et al. convincingly demonstrate that even African Americans who do not affiliate with "theologically conservative" Black churches, which grant the locus of control over health and healing to an "external" divine source, bear its imprint in their high prevalence of acceptance of health fatalism. Lower levels of education and health literacy further mediate a loss of control over health, potentiating attraction to religious world views that confer alternative forms of control [12]. Religiously grounded refusals or, contrarily, requests to continue life-prolonging interventions in the post-surgical period even when the medical team assesses they offer little to no meaningful benefit, certainly may be based on core, potentially inviolable tenets of a faith tradition; they may also be, as the study by Courtwright et al suggests, the only "legitimate" and ethically authorized way of claiming agency within the healthcare system for members of marginalized groups [13].

Religious grounding for health behaviors and decisions often eludes providers, as the case of Zahid illustrates. Surgeons operating in the Western world are likely to be familiar with the high priority in Islam given to protecting, promoting and saving life (most often seen in requests for so-called "futile" treatment or challenges to the definition of death by neurological criteria). As a result, they will honor, albeit reluctantly and with no small amount of moral distress, requests to provide life-prolonging surgical interventions. However, they are unlikely to recognize the claim to "familial duty" for the sacred obligation it is. A detailed exploration of the rights and responsibilities of parents and children in the Quran and Hadith can be found in the rich Islamic bioethical literature; suffice it to say, an Islamic theological anthropology posits a relational understanding of the human person arising from the primary relationship with God. The duty to care for one's children by providing food, clothing, health, education, inheritance, and spiritual instruction as well as the specific duty to attend to their health and well-being both through prayer and/or medical attention cannot be extricated from duties owed by the faithful to God [14].

The vascular surgeon and critical care team approach the family looking for them to exercise "substituted judgement", that is, to tell the team what Zahid would want if he could speak for himself. This commonly employed first step in shared decision making with a proxy decision maker relies upon a conception of human beings as individuals with authority over their own bodies and lives, articulated as the principles of autonomy and self-determination. The father sidesteps the very question suggesting that Zahid's preferences are not relevant to this faithful Islamic family. Whether Zahid shares the father's framework for decision making is unknown; the question no longer can be posed directly to him. An impasse occurs because the medical team does not recognize the very different approach to medical decision making based on familial duty and sacred obligations brought to the table by Zahid's family.

19.4.2 The Culture of Medicine and the Limits of a Principle-Based Approach to Surgical Ethics

The culture of biomedicine proffers

> a naturalist cosmology that divides the material and biological from the spiritual and supernatural; a positivist and atomistic universalism that reduces the human to biological animals with secondary qualitative differences like rationality, culture and belief; and a concept of the autonomous individual as rational agent, responsibility to work on the health of the body as a project. [7]

In order to successfully interface with patients from diverse cultural and religious backgrounds, surgeons need to first acknowledge their claims to "truth" and conceptualization of the human body, disease, and medicine for what they are—one epistemological framework among other possible ways of knowing.

Farr Curlin, a leader in the field of religion, bioethics and medicine, contends:

> Religious concepts expose the limits of "medical ethics" particularly when they critique as false what the culture of medicine takes for granted as true. Whether advanced by Jewish, Christian or Muslim scholars, religious accounts of medical ethics all seem to criticize conventional medical ethics for being captive to an imagination in which nothing beyond the immanent is morally significant. [15]

Religious texts contain truth not verifiable through reason, evidence, or the logic of cause and effect. In some traditions, moral obligations are revealed directly to an inspired holy person while in others they are mediated through the application of ethical-legal codified texts to specific cases by clergy or religious legal experts. In some traditions, religion and scientifically based medical truths conflict; in others, they seamlessly co-exist with the divine as author and arbiter of all aspects of existence.

In our first case (see Table 19.2), Mrs. Williams claims, "I am healed." The surgeon, however, sees a tumor on his scan; biopsy results no doubt would yield confirmation of his "truth" in the form of cancerous cells clearly distinguishable from normal ones. Mrs. Williams attributes the *fait accompli* of healing to a historical and supernatural event—the suffering and death of Jesus, the central act of healing in Christianity (the stripes refer to Jesus' flogging at the hands of Pontius Pilate)—rather than to medicine. The surgical oncologist clings to the facts before him as he

Table 19.2 Application of conventional medical ethics principles to illustrative cases

Autonomy	Although Mrs. Williams' belief that she has been healed may lead the surgeon to question her decisional capacity, autonomy asks that "non-rational" religious beliefs be respected if they are a core part of a patient's identity and worldview. The concept of autonomy is called into question by the relational and theological approach to decision making used by Zahid's family—what Zahid would want is of little concern to the family. The principle of autonomy could also be cited to ethically support honoring specific medical requests by Zahid's family arising from their Islamic tradition (eg. duty, quality of life, and bodily integrity)
Beneficence/ Non-maleficence	The oncologic surgeon has an obligation to provide Mrs. Williams with his expert clinical assessment of her condition and to offer treatment options that will promote her well-being. The vascular surgeon faced with amputation of multiple limbs fears her intervention will cause more harm than good in the context of Zahid's quickly deteriorating condition
Justice	Distrust of the medical system in the context of a history of unequal access to healthcare and disparities in health outcomes for African Americans in the US raises the principle of justice to the fore in the case of Mrs. Williams. For Zahid, justice might easily be misconstrued as requiring clinicians approach care and decision the same for all patients, when it is best understood to require accommodation of cultural differences

reiterates evidence to convince her to seek treatment. In so doing, he not only fails to validate her faith but forecloses possible negotiation between the two competing frameworks.

A surgeon's obligation to ensure that patients who deviate from recommended therapies fully understand the potential consequences of their decisions logically follows from the epistemological assumptions embedded in the culture of medicine. As Huijer et al highlight in their study comparing the perspectives of patients who refuse surgery to that of their providers:

> [Surgical informed consent] implies having information on a certain problem, being well-informed about the advantages and disadvantages, and balancing the pros and cons against each other. If the pros are heavier than the cons, you should make that decision. [16]

In other words, a patient cannot have "good reasons" to refuse treatment if there is a reasonable chance of recovery. Lack of training in attending to religiously based claims, among other non-medical forces at play in refusals of surgical treatment for cancer or other maladies, impedes the development of trust, undermines shared decision making, and potentiates non-adherence with the medical plan: Mrs. Williams does not return for her follow-up appointment.

The vascular surgeon and critical care team in our second illustrative case also fail to appreciate the broader ontology of healing embraced by Zahid's family. Expert consideration of Zahid's case—lab values, data indicating multiple organ failure, lack of lung recovery while on ECMO, and deterioration of tissues caused by inadequate blood circulation—provides sound clinical basis for them to consider amputation to prevent additional harm to the entire biological system, even as they predict the imminent cessation of his bodily functioning; in other words, death appears inevitable. While they do not hammer the family with these facts in the segment of the case cited, they base their concerns about disability, dependence, and benefits vs. harms of treatment on Western medical values that narrate the goal of medicine itself and what makes life worth living. A life with severely limited functional and cognitive abilities, not to mention the degree of suffering Zahid would have to endure for a long shot at survival itself, violates the core values or aims of medicine to cure disease, restore bodily systems, preserve rationality, and promote individual agency.

Refusal to amputate Zahid's limbs based on clinical judgement that it is medically inappropriate may be claimed by the vascular surgeon as her ethical prerogative. Withholding a surgical intervention that is "strictly futile"—meaning it will not achieve the purpose for which it is intended or may precipitate physiological deterioration—is clearly ethically justifiable. Refusal to amputate based on a personal value judgment about quality of life or that it offers no "meaningful benefit" would be harder to justify especially if the critical care team conceded to the family's request to continue life-prolonging interventions such as CVVH or ECMO [17, 18].

The Islamic tradition, among other religions and non-Western cultures, provides an alternative framework to inform goals of medicine and for understanding disability, quality of life, and bodily integrity—with considerable, nuanced variability among its distinct branches or schools. Padela and Quraeshi emphasize the importance of bringing together clinicians and religious scholars to support decision makers given the complexity of these concepts within Islam and the need for clinical expertise on the intended goal of a proposed medical intervention and the evidence supporting its therapeutic value [19]. For example, clear distinctions exist within the tradition between violating bodily integrity to increase personal attractiveness, improve quality of life, fix a defect or abnormality, and when necessary to preserve life. Similarly, if parts of the body are lost in order to honor higher sacred goods of preserving life or religious faithfulness (such as in circumcision following the example of the Prophet Mohammed), any resulting alteration in physical appearance or so-called "disability" should not occasion a sense of feeling deficient as it might within Western dominant culture [20].

Finally, within Islam there is wiggle room rarely known by surgeons and critical care physicians in the West that might support forgoing life-prolonging medical interventions. This rich tradition contains theological tenets that have the potential to support setting limits on aggressive medical care including: How Islam defines a life worth medically maintaining; scriptural references for direct healing by Allah; and, the promise of reward in the afterlife for abstaining from seeking medical treatment entirely [19]. Not surprisingly, devout Muslims are not always aware of this complex array of beliefs, thereby leading them to insist clinicians "do everything" even when the available interventions have little chance of saving the patient's life.

19.4.3   Strategies for Negotiating Surgical Acceptance or Refusal Based on Culture or Religion

When faced with the religious testimony of a Mrs. Williams or the sacred duty to care of Zahid's family, surgeons commonly respond in one of two ways: by ignoring the request/refusal; or, respecting it at face value. In my 26 years of experience as a healthcare chaplain and clinical ethicist, I have met only a handful of surgeons prepared to engage in a deeper exploration of beliefs and ethical frameworks that directly contradict their own, an observation regrettably supported by research literature [21].

Cultural competency training and programs to advance literacy in religion and medicine are a needed corrective to the current gap in knowledge and skill among surgeons. Cultivating epistemic and cultural humility is needed to successfully negotiate these ethical conflicts. The knowledge, virtue, and skill for successful cross-cultural care may best be gained by paying attention first to the dominant narratives of the West and of Western medicine about what it means to be human, what constitutes illness, health and healing, and the aim of medicine itself; only then is the surgeon sufficiently self-aware and humble to respectfully solicit and listen to the life stories of patients, their illness narratives, the historical narratives of a community, and orally transmitted cosmologies or sacred written texts. Cultural humility asks that medicine no longer regard persons with diverse cultures and religious frameworks as the "Other" but rather see that each actor is located in a complex set of narratives with normative force [22]. In responding to claims of faith healing or hope for a miracle, clinicians are reminded that demonstrating respect for a belief does not equal agreement or abandonment of one's own framework. Validation serves as a starting point for exploring how the person of faith conceptualizes disease, health and healing and opens the door to see what, if any, role Western medicine might play within that religious framework [23].

Consider for a moment if the oncologic surgeon had responded to Mrs. Williams by first bracketing his own need to convince her of the medical facts. By validating her faith with simple statements like, "It sounds like your faith centrally informs how you view healing and medicine. Can you tell me more?" a climate of respect would be created, a foundational step toward cultural exchange and deliberation. He might have followed up with questions about the prevalence of miracles in her faith tradition or solicited her views on the relationship between God's healing activity and the use of medications. He also might have acknowledged the pervasive distrust of the healthcare system among African Americans based upon this community's historical treatment of neglect and exploitation. Finally, having established a modicum of rapport he might actually have the opportunity to inquire about her specific resistance to surgical treatment—"cutting"—thereby potentiating discussion of alternative cancer treatment modalities such as radiation or chemotherapy. Additional visits might have included the presence of Mrs. William's pastor, godmother or elders from the church, or a professionally trained healthcare chaplain who may present an alternative view of Pentecostal Holiness teachings that allows for a complimentary relationship between faith and medicine.

Unfortunately, the initial response from the surgical oncologist did not employ any of these strategies. Mrs. Williams did not return for medical treatment for her cancer until a few days before her death when her family brought her in unresponsive. An ethics consult was requested to negotiate a conflict between elders in the family ready to accept her decision to rely upon faith for healing and the younger generation requesting the medical team intervene to do everything to save her life. The ethicist supported the religious request to honor Mrs. William's consistently expressed wish to "let God's will be done." She died with her pastor, family, and church elders praying for healing.

If aware of her own biases about dependence, disability, and quality of life, the vascular surgeon might have shared why she was reluctant to subject Zahid to multiple amputations. Subsequently, she could have solicited insight into beliefs the family (rather than Zahid) held about caring for one another, the limits of that duty, and what gives meaning to an individual life within Islam. If then the surgeon had refused to operate on the grounds it was "medically inappropriate" [17]—a right surgeons frequently exercise [18]—the values informing her own position would be on the table, replacing the presumptive stance of value-neutrality. To honor her own estimation of proportional benefit, the surgeon would be ethically permitted but not obligated to transfer care to another surgeon. For pragmatic reasons, transfer may prove difficult as another surgeon in the same setting would hesitate to override the clinical evaluation of a colleague.

Would Zahid's family then have continued to insist on continuing ECMO, ventilation, CVVH and other life-prolonging medical interventions? Would they have demanded amputation of limbs on the grounds that surgery aligns with the overarching goals of care they established for Zahid? Consulting with Islamic religious scholars, clergy, or a bioethicist familiar with the nuances of Islamic teachings on end of life care might have yielded possible avenues for an informed discussion of the efficacy of the proposed intervention in the context of what is obligatory, permissible or forbidden within the family's Islamic ethical-legal framework [19]. Institutional policies and state laws may also have supported the surgeon and critical care team in unilaterally setting limits on life-prolonging medical interventions, thereby lifting the burden of decision making entirely from the family.

Zahid's condition deteriorated shortly after the family met with ethics and the health care teams, leaving no time for the above interventions. No limbs were amputated; the request to provide all other life-prolonging interventions was honored. ECMO failed and Zahid suffered a series of cardio-pulmonary arrests. After 4 rounds of CPR lasting 30 minutes the attending physician called the time of death. The family who was present throughout expressed their deepest gratitude; they later reported being at peace. Zahid's body was removed directly from the intensive care unit as male elders chanted verses from the Quran. Leadership requested an ethics debrief to mitigate high levels of moral distress of the bedside clinicians and the code team.

19.5   Concluding Remarks

A failure of moral imagination is at the center of most ethical conflicts featuring religious or cultural differences. Only if surgeons acknowledge that their scientific approach to understanding the human body, disease, and healing is part of a circumscribed, particular culture—the culture of medicine—will they be able to approach the diverse world views of their patients with genuine curiosity and respect. To consider that one's *"view of reality is only a view, not reality itself"* requires a degree of epistemic humility not customarily cultivated in medicine [1]. Curiosity and respect do not free surgeons from accountability to the core values of their profession; but they create a bridge where a chasm of distrust once stood and, therein, pave the way for dialogue, negotiation, and possible resolution.

19.6   Selected References

- Barnes LL, Laird LD. Anthropologies of medicine, religion, and spirituality. In: Balboni MJ, Peteet JR, editors. Spirituality and religion within the culture of medicine: from evidence to practice. Oxford; 2017. p. 275–91.

  - A conceptual framework for understanding biomedicine as "culture" as a prerequisite for successful provision of care to persons from diverse religious and cultural backgrounds.

- Curlin F. Religion and spirituality in medical ethics. In: Balboni MJ, Peteet JR, editors. Spirituality and religion within the culture of medicine: from evidence to practice. Oxford; 2017. p. 179–94.

  - Documents common ethical dilemmas involving religion and argues that conventional medical ethics fails to account for normative claims of religious traditions.

- Fadiman A. The spirit catches you and you fall down: a Hmong child, her American doctors, and the collision of two cultures. Macmillan; 2012. p. 276.

  - A tragic story of cultural misunderstanding between the family of a young Hmong child with epilepsy and the medical profession in a small county hospital in California.

- Hayward RD, Krause N, Pargament K. The prevalence and antecedents of religious beliefs about health control in the US population: variations by race and religious background. J Relig Health. 2017;56:2194–211. https://doi.org/10.1007/s10943-017-0391-3.

  - Descriptive analysis of core cultural and religious beliefs of racially diverse patients with a focus on frameworks positing the locus of control for health outcomes in external or divine sources.

- Padela AI. Islamic medical ethics: a primer. Bioethics. 2007;21(3):169–78. https://doi.org/10.1111/j.1467-8519.2007.00540.x.

  - An overview of the emerging field of Islamic Medical Ethics with attention to historic sources in Islamic law, literature on moral formation, and application to contemporary issues such as abortion and end of life care.

References

1. Fadiman A. The spirit catches you and you fall down: a Hmong child, her American doctors, and the collision of two cultures. Macmillan; 2012. p. 276.
2. Jenkins ED, Yip M, Melman L, Frisella MM, Matthews BD. Informed consent: cultural and religious issues associated with the use of allogeneic and xenogeneic mesh products. J Am Coll Surg. 2010;210:402–10. https://doi.org/10.1016/j.jamcollsurg.2009.12.001.
3. Pass L, Graber AD. Informed consent, deaf culture, and cochlear implants. J Clin Ethics. 2015;26(3):219–30.
4. Paris W, Seidler RJH, FitzGerald K, Padela AI, Cozzi E, Cooper DKC. Jewish, Christian and Muslim theological perspectives about xenotransplantation. Xenotransplantation. 2018;25(3):e12400. https://doi.org/10.1111/xen.12400.
5. Bizic MR, Jeftovic M, Pusica S, et al. Gender dysphoria: bioethical aspects of medical treatment. BioMed Res Int. 2018;13:9652305. https://doi.org/10.1155/2018/9652305.
6. Nabaneh S, Muula AS. Female genital mutilation/cutting in Africa: a complex legal and ethical landscape. Int J Gynecol Obstet. 2019;145(2):253–7. https://doi.org/10.1002/ijgo.12792.
7. Barnes LL, Laird LD. Anthropologies of medicine, religion, and spirituality. In: Balboni MJ, Peteet JR, editors. Spirituality and religion within the culture of medicine: from evidence to practice. Oxford; 2017. p. 275–91.
8. Geertz C. The interpretation of cultures. Basic Books; 1973.
9. Polite BN, Cipriano-Steffens T, Hlubocky F, et al. An evaluation of psychosocial and religious belief differences in a diverse racial and socioeconomic urban cancer population. J Racial Ethnic Health Disparities. 2017;4(2):140–8. https://doi.org/10.1007/s40615-016-0211-6.
10. Lu PW, Fields AC, Yoo J, et al. Sociodemographic predictors of surgery refusal in patients with stage I-III colon cancer. J Surg Oncol. 2020;121(8):1306–13. https://doi.org/10.1002/jso.25917.
11. Restrepo DJ, Sisti A, Boczar D, et al. Characteristics of breast cancer patients who refuse surgery. Anticancer Res. 2019;39(9):4941–5. https://doi.org/10.21873/anticares.13682.
12. Hayward RD, Krause N, Pargament K. The prevalence and antecedents of religious beliefs about health control in the US population: variations by race and religious background. J Relig Health. 2017;56:2194–211. https://doi.org/10.1007/s10943-017-0391-3.
13. Courtwright AM, Romain F, Robinson EM, Krakauer EL. Ethics committee consultation due to conflict over life-sustaining treatment: a sociodemographic investigation. AJOB Empirical Bioethics. 2016;7(4):220–6. https://doi.org/10.1080/23294515.2015.1111956.
14. Padela AI. Islamic medical ethics: a primer. Bioethics. 2007;21(3):169–78. https://doi.org/10.1111/j.1467-8519.2007.00540.x.
15. Curlin F. Religion and spirituality in medical ethics. In: Balboni MJ, Peteet JR, editors. Spirituality and religion within the culture of medicine: from evidence to practice. Oxford; 2017. p. 179–94.
16. Huijer M, van Leeuwen E. Personal values and cancer treatment refusal. J Med Ethics. 2000;26(5):358–62. https://doi.org/10.1136/jme.26.5.358.
17. Bosslet GT, Pope TM, Rubenfeld GD, et al. An official ATS/AACN/ACCP/ESICM/SCCM policy statement: responding to requests for potentially inappropriate treatments in inten-

sive care units. Am J Respir Crit Care Med. 2015;191(11):1318–30. https://doi.org/10.1164/rccm.201505-0924st.
18. Wicclair MR, White DB. Surgeons, intensivists, and discretion to refuse requested treatments. Hastings Cent Rep. 2014;44(5):33–42. https://doi.org/10.1002/hast.356.
19. Padela AI, Qureshi O. Islamic perspectives on clinical intervention near the end-of-life: we can, but must we? Med Health Care and Philos. 2017;20(4):545–59. https://doi.org/10.1007/s11019-016-9729-y.
20. Alahmad G, Dekkers W. Bodily integrity and male circumcision: an Islamic perspective. JIMA. 2012;44. https://doi.org/10.5915/44-1-7903.
21. Changoor NR, Udyavar NR, Morris MA, et al. Surgeons' perceptions toward providing care for diverse patients: the need for cultural dexterity training. Ann Surg. 2019;269(2):275–82. https://doi.org/10.1097/sla.0000000000002560.
22. Derrington SF, Paquette E, Johnson KA. Cross-cultural interactions and shared decision-making. Pediatrics. 2018;142(suppl 3):S187–92. https://doi.org/10.1542/peds.2018-0516j.
23. Bibler TM, Shinall MC Jr, Stahl D. Responding to those who hope for a miracle: practices for clinical bioethicists. Am J Bioethics. 2018;18(5):40–51. https://doi.org/10.1080/15265161.2018.1431702.

Chapter 20
Subtle Approach to the Mores of the Navajo Nation

Erica C. Bennett ⓘ and Ethan Paddock

Abstract Physicians frequently care for patients whose cultural, religious, or social backgrounds differ from our own. If these differences are not attended to, the substantial variety in patient values, beliefs, and behaviors related to health and healthcare may result in conflict, misdiagnosis, poor adherence to recommendations, suboptimal outcomes, or decreased patient satisfaction. Cultural, ethnic, or racial discordance between patients and physicians has an impact on communication related to healthcare, and barriers can be due to differences in language, religion or spirituality, family involvement in decision-making, responses to inequities in care, and lack of trust.

This chapter explores the mores of the people of the Navajo Nation, the *Diné*, and how culture may influence healthcare discussions and decision-making as we highlight a brief history of the Navajo Nation, present-day social determinants of health, and health inequities. We discuss how the concepts of positive and negative thinking may influence medical management and examine culturally competent strategies to improve communication with and advocacy for patients and lessen the effect of cultural and racial discordance between patients and healthcare workers.

Keeping in mind variation of individual patient views, understanding more about the beliefs and customs of the *Diné* and the Navajo Nation's beginning as well as its current place in the United States, may assist in a thoughtful approach to caring for patients from a culture or background different from one's own as we strive to eliminate health disparities.

Keywords Navajo · *Diné* · Bioethics · Cross-cultural · Racial concordance · Health inequities · Positive thinking · Cultural competence · Cultural humility

E. C. Bennett (✉) · E. Paddock
Department of Surgery, Division of Otolaryngology – Head and Neck Surgery,
University of New Mexico, Albuquerque, NM, USA
e-mail: ebennett@salud.unm.edu

© The Author(s), under exclusive license to Springer Nature
Switzerland AG 2022
V. A. Lonchyna et al. (eds.), *Difficult Decisions in Surgical Ethics*, Difficult
Decisions in Surgery: An Evidence-Based Approach,
https://doi.org/10.1007/978-3-030-84625-1_20

273

Case

Faith was a one-month-old girl with a diagnosis of trisomy 13 (Patau syndrome) admitted to the Newborn Intensive Care Unit (NBICU) at an academic medical center in Albuquerque, New Mexico. She had severe hypotonia, an atrial septal defect, microphthalmia, and cleft lip and palate. She was ventilator dependent and unable to be weaned. The overall prognosis was poor with only a 5–10 percent chance of living past her first year. The family lived in Tohatchi, NM, an extremely rural town in the Navajo Nation with no running water in their home and electricity provided by a diesel generator. In this town, there were very few medical services, and no home nursing care. The NBICU team offered several options to the parents. An alternative feeding route, tracheotomy, ventilator dependence, and a possible cardiac procedure would be necessary to consider discharge to home. The option of withdrawing care was also explained.

The health care providers were concerned about the 165-mile distance between the hospital and the home, a three-hour drive. The interventional teams were consulted, including Cardiology, Otolaryngology-Head and Neck Surgery, and Pediatric Surgery. When the providers attempted to discuss the benefits and risks of tracheotomy, gastrostomy, and cardiac catheterization, the family did not wish to hear the risks. The surgical teams were concerned about their ability to obtain a *truly* informed consent for the procedures and the difficulties in caring for a tracheostomy in a rural area with reduced access to emergency and specialty care. The parents became upset during these interactions and did not want to discuss any further. Since conversations with providers did not go well, the family was considering transfer to another facility for a second opinion.

The Neonatology team offered a family meeting. The parents requested the participation of extended family members. Contact was made with Native American Health Services through the hospital who offered a patient advocate and interpreter for the meeting. The parents invited the paternal grandparents, maternal grandmother, both great grandmothers, and 2 great aunts. Medical teams included Neonatology, Dysmorphology, Neurology, Cardiology, Pediatric Surgery, and Otolaryngology. The neurologist was also a member of the Ethics Consult service. A social-worker and discharge planner were included. The Navajo medical student on the Pediatric Otolaryngology service was also invited.

20.1 Introduction

Discussing complex medical and surgical information is difficult, but when required between people of different cultures, beliefs, and daily practice patterns, it is even more challenging. Understanding where differences are, on what they are based,

Table 20.1 Navajo
words [1–8]

Diné	The Navajo people
Diné Bizaad	Navajo language
Diyin Dine'é	Holy people, holy spirits
Naabeehó Bináhásdzo	Navajo Nation
Hózhó or Hózhoni	Balance, peace, beauty, harmony
Hózhooji	The Beauty Way
Hózhooji nitsihakees	"think in the beauty way"
Hózhooji saad	"talk in the beauty way"
Doo'ájíniidah	"don't talk that way!"
Hataałii	Chanter, singer, medicine person
Bilagáana	European, Caucasian, White man
Dikos Ntsaaígíí-19	COVID-19
K'é	Family, kinship, compassion, caring, kindness, respect
Kiva	Round room used for ceremonies
Hogan	Traditional/sacred Diné home

and being able to employ and engage people competent in both cultures may allow true communication to occur.

This chapter explores the mores, traditions and customs, of the people of the Navajo Nation, the *Diné*. We outline a brief history of the Navajo Nation, present-day social determinants of health, structural and health inequities for Navajo residents, and some of the traditional and contemporary beliefs of some Navajo people (see Table 20.1. Navajo Vocabulary). Maintaining a positive outlook and hope through words and actions is central to Navajo culture. The traditional Navajo belief system holds the idea that thoughts and language have power to shape and influence reality and may affect the outcome of future events. The belief that thinking negative thoughts or speaking negative ideas or sentiments can be causative is held by many cultures and may influence discussions of surgical care, informed consent, and advance directives. The definition of "family" and who is involved with major healthcare decisions also varies across cultures. Some patients may wish to complement allopathic treatments with traditional healing methods or spiritual care based on cultural beliefs.

There is very little written literature about Native American peoples' beliefs and views on healthcare. However, there is more literature about the *Diné,* compared to other tribes, perhaps due to the unique geographic location and large size of the Navajo Nation, allowing greater language and cultural retention [9]. Based on the 2010 United States (US) census, the Navajo Nation is home to almost 50% of those who identify as *Diné* (Navajo) and the largest number of persons who associate with one tribe [10]. At least 50% of the population speaks fluent Navajo, and a high percentage of tribal members participate in traditional Navajo customs [9]. The relative concentration of healthcare services on and bordering the Navajo Nation also allows a focused population of patients to interview, care for, and foster relationships with. This can lead to a better understanding of cultural practices, which is helpful in developing culturally sensitive communication skills and surgical care.

In caring for people from some cultures, it may be necessary to further contemplate the four principles of biomedical ethics and how their application may differ with regard to communication and treatment to assure beneficence, non-maleficence, autonomy, and justice for *all* patients. With the use of an illustrative case, this chapter examines some culturally competent strategies to improve communication with and advocacy for patients. We also consider focused efforts to lessen the effect of cultural and racial discordance between patients and healthcare workers.

We hope that this chapter will provide a glimpse into the wonderful, rich Navajo culture, which is based on tradition and a belief system that may contrast with US healthcare education and policies and can be used to help guide surgeons and other healthcare providers to a better understanding of how culture and medical decision-making intersect. As we each strive to become culturally competent *and* practice cultural humility in providing surgical care, we can endeavor to improve healthcare for patients of *all* cultures and backgrounds and move us closer toward the goal of eliminating health disparities.

20.2 Search Strategy

Given the relative paucity of scientific evidence about the subject of this chapter, alternative sources of information were utilized, and timeframe was expanded beyond a typical evidence-based search, 1995–2021. Sources and methods used were PubMed, WorldCat, Google Scholar, official Navajo Nation websites, news interviews, and personal communication in the form of a grand rounds lecture. What is notable, yet not surprising, is that the themes and conclusions of the most recent articles have not changed in 25 years. The importance of integrating a culturally competent approach to treatment and communication with culturally diverse populations runs throughout the literature. We are still talking about the identical structural inequities leading to health disparities today.

20.3 Discussion

20.3.1 Background

20.3.1.1 Population Demographics

There are 574 federally recognized ethnically, culturally, and linguistically diverse Indian Nations in the US (variously called tribes, nations, bands, pueblos, communities, and native villages). Each has their own land base, culture, government, and language. Each is very distinct in *every* way. Additionally, there are state recognized tribes throughout the US acknowledged by their respective state governments [11].

The Navajo people are called *Diné*, which means "the People" in *Diné Bizaad*, the Navajo language. Anthropologists and historians believe that the Navajo first arrived in the southwestern US from what is now known as western Canada between 900 and 1300 AD. They came in contact with Pueblo Indians who lived in the area around 13–1400 AD, from whom they learned farming. The Spaniards made contact around 1581 AD and brought sheep, goats, and horses to the region. There is an extensive history of warfare with the Spanish and the Pueblo Indians. By 1700, the Navajo were living in the area of the present-day Navajo Nation (see Fig. 20.1) defined by Four Sacred Mountains created by the "Holy People", *Diyin Dine'é,* for the Navajo people.

- Video 20.1: Navajo traditional teachings. Landmarks of Navajo Nation, August 17, 2020. Accessed 1 March 2021. https://www.youtube.com/watch?v=vBradAQqt6I
- Video 20.2: Navajo traditional teachings. Native American (Diné) Story of the Beginning, January 11, 2021. Accessed 1 March 2021. https://www.youtube.com/watch?v=Gu9d3QGPLfU
- Video 20.3: Navajo traditional teachings. Two types of Europeans… First encounter with Native Americans (Diné), November 16, 2020. Accessed 1 March 2021. https://www.youtube.com/watch?v=atW-R6QZms0

In 1864, they were forced from this land on the "Long Walk", 300 miles to the Bosque Redondo Reservation in Fort Sumner, New Mexico (NM) and imprisoned by American soldiers. They were allowed to return in 1868, after a peace treaty was signed. Those who survived the imprisonment and travel returned to their sacred

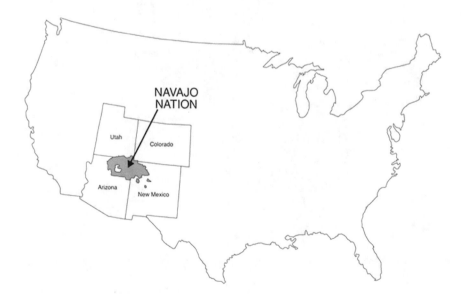

Fig. 20.1 Map of the Navajo Nation within the United States

land [12]. The results of the "Long Walk" are still discussed today through stories and teachings to Navajo youth. "The physical genocide of the 1800's, followed by the cultural genocide of the 1900's left behind a tribe whose roots and foundation were shattered". What has resulted is a deep historical grief, anger, mistrust, and misunderstanding [1]. Native Americans were not granted US citizenship until 1924.

- Video 20.4: Navajo traditional teachings. The Long Walk, May 11, 2018. Accessed 1 March 2021. https://www.youtube.com/watch?v=wDb5Wc8HgOo

Today, Navajo Nation (*Naabeehó Bináhásdzo*) is the largest Indian reservation. The sovereign nation, created in 1923, covers portions of northeastern Arizona (AZ), southeastern Utah, and northwestern NM, borders Colorado, and is over 27,000 square miles in size (over 17 million acres, approximately the size of West Virginia). The Navajo Nation is larger than 10 of the 50 United States (see Fig. 20.2). The Navajo people farmed and raised goats and sheep and eventually developed a barter economy, exchanging rugs and silverwork with white traders. In the Four Corners region, oil and mineral exploration began in the 1920s and uranium mining in the 1940s, which improved the wealth of the Nation but caused contamination of water and other environmental damage (see Fig. 20.3). The Navajo Nation now has a population of greater than 250,000 and serves over 300,000 registered tribal members and is the second largest Native American population after the Cherokee Nation [2].

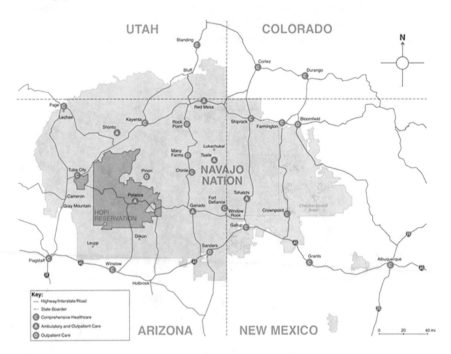

Fig. 20.2 Map showing the Navajo Nation and Hopi reservation and highlighting healthcare services

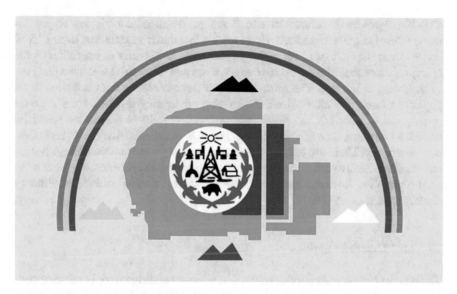

Fig. 20.3 Navajo Nation Flag. The Navajo Nation flag has a pale buff color background, bearing a map of the Navajo Nation in the center. The original area of the 1868 reservation is dark brown, while the much larger current borders are copper. Surrounding the map are the four sacred mountains in each cardinal direction: black (representing the north), turquoise (representing the south), white (representing the east), and yellow (representing the west). These 4 colors form a recurring theme in the legends of the Navajo, beginning with the Navajo creation story. In it, the world began as a black island floating in the mist. Above it are 4 clouds: black, white, blue (turquoise), and yellow. The story describes the colored clouds as successive worlds and narrates the themes of birth, propagation, flood, escape, and continuing life. Arching over the mountains and map is the rainbow of red, yellow, and blue, with red outermost in reverse sequence from the Navajo Nation seal. The rainbow symbolizes Navajo sovereignty. Centered on the map is a white disk bearing corn stalks and three domestic animals from the Navajo Nation seal representing the Navajo livestock economy. Symbols of other aspects of the Navajo economy: a traditional Hogan, modern home, oil derrick, forestry, mining (symbolizing the resource potential of the Navajo Nation), and fishing and hunting (recreational economy). At the top near the sun, the modern sawmill symbolizes the progress and industry characteristic of the Navajo Nation's economic development [12]

20.3.1.2 Social Determinants of Health

Social determinants of health are the nonmedical factors that impact health [13]. The Navajo Nation has poverty rates more than twice as high as the other portions of AZ. Forty-four percent of tribal members live in poverty and half were unemployed before the COVID-19 pandemic. The median income is $27,389 per year and 57% of individuals have an income less than $10,000 per year [10]. Thirty percent of households on the Navajo Nation lack running water, electricity, and/or indoor plumbing. Many members drive an average of 2 hours to obtain water. Sixty percent of residents have no internet, causing digital social isolation with no access to emergency alerts, public health announcements, news, virtual schooling, and limited emergency health care command operation responses [14]. To combat the

COVID-19 pandemic, schools have tried to expand online learning through providing wireless hotspots to students. However, the fact that many students live in "dead zones" from the cellular tower highlights the serious disparity of education on the Navajo Nation. Families would have to travel several miles to a local town that provides access to internet. The infrastructure of Navajo Nation does not allow for a physical address for many, therefore limiting emergency services, routine postal routes, and contact tracing. Food insecurity on Navajo Nation is worsened by decreased farming, lack of water access, and lack of refrigeration due to no household electricity. There are only 13 full-service grocery stores on the Navajo Nation and residents need to drive an average of 3 hours to obtain groceries. The remaining food sources are fast food restaurants and gas station convenience stores, limiting *healthy* food choices [10, 14, 15].

20.3.1.3 Health Inequities

The Navajo Nation suffers from health disparities in addition to or because of poverty and its location in a water, food, and technological desert [14]. The Indian Health Service (IHS), established in 1951, is an agency within the Department of Health and Human Services that is responsible for providing federal health services to American Indians and Alaska Natives. The Navajo Area IHS (NAIHS) provides inpatient, emergency, outpatient, public health, and other services through 12 health care centers including 4 full-service inpatient hospitals with *only* 400 hospital beds and 40 intensive care beds. There is chronic underfunding of the IHS with yearly average per capita expenditure of $4,078, which is less than half of the funds spent for non-Native Americans. An average of $9,726 is spent for non-Native Americans, $9404 for Veterans Affairs patients, and $13,185 for Medicare patients [5, 14]. The people of the Navajo Nation also have poor health status with an average life expectancy of only 73 years (5.5 years fewer than other races) and unintentional injury, heart disease, and cancer are the leading causes of death [5, 13, 14]. There are also high rates of comorbid diseases with Navajo adults being more than 2 times more likely as white adults to have type 2 diabetes. In 2018, 48% of American Indians had BMI of 30 or greater [5]. In the Navajo Nation, there are 523 abandoned uranium mine and mill sites which have contaminated soil and water supplies and are implicated in high rates of cardiovascular disease, hypertension, diabetes, kidney disease, anemia, gastrointestinal cancers, and various pregnancy disorders, such as preeclampsia and preterm labor [16].

20.3.1.4 *Dikos Ntsaaigii-Na haʹstʹeʹiʹtsʹaʹadah* (COVID-19)

The Navajo Nation led the country in per capita infections of COVID-19 early in the global pandemic, and the disease has devastated the elder population. Cases were at the highest per capita rate in the US in mid-May 2020 [2]. At that time, the Navajo Nation's infection rate was 2,304 cases per 100,000 people, or one in every 43 persons had been infected with SARS-CoV-2. As of February 10, 2021, there had been 28,994 cases of COVID-19 and 1,075 deaths, or one death per 27 cases. As of February 2021, the NM cumulative age-adjusted case rate for American Indian or Alaska Native persons was 15,379/100,000 or one case per 6 to 7 persons, which is about 2–3 times higher than any other racial/ethnic group in NM [17]. In Arizona, only 5.3% of the population are American Indian or Alaska Native but 8% of COVID-19 deaths were in these populations [18]. In the state of New Mexico, only about 10% of the population are Native American but this demographic accounted for 33% of all coronavirus cases in May 2020 and 29% through February 2021 [10, 17]. All US indigenous tribes are disproportionally affected by COVID-19. For most Native American communities, including the Navajo, structural and health inequities are major factors, but cultural practices may also contribute to high rates of infection. For example, the importance and frequency of large gatherings for ceremonies and celebrations in addition to the handshake being the traditional method of greeting. These factors have aided in the rapid spread of coronavirus [13, 14]. Devastation from infectious diseases is not new to the Navajo Nation. Diseases that were introduced to Native American populations during European colonization were devastating due to immunological naivety. Smallpox caused mortality rates greater than the warfare and enslavement that followed [13]. The 1918 Spanish influenza pandemic infected 24% of Native Americans resulting in a loss of 2% of the Native American population, the highest death rate of any racial/ethnic group and thousands of Navajo persons were lost [13]. In 1993, the Sin Nombre hantavirus spread through Navajo Nation with a 75% mortality rate [1, 13]. During the H1N1 Influenza A pandemic, the Native American population had a 4 times higher mortality rate than all other US racial and ethnic groups combined [13]. For many communities including the Navajo people, structural and social factors cumulatively increase the transmission rates of infections. Frequent travel is essential to border towns, such as Gallup and Farmington, NM, Page and Flagstaff, AZ which provide employment and supplies for those who live on the Navajo Nation. Lack of delivery options for groceries or other goods and the need to travel outside the Nation increases contact and makes self-isolation difficult. Personnel are less able to work from home due to job types, such as blue-collar professions, and poor access to the internet [14]. Close-knit families living in multigenerational homes, lack of plumbing and running water for hand washing in 30% of homes, and a paucity of emergency services on Navajo Nation contribute. Many households lack physical addresses, and the telecommunication infrastructure is poor resulting in emergency medical services decreased ability to find homes. Poor access to health care, high rates of comorbid conditions, paucity of professional caregivers, deficient funding for health care centers, and a shortage of intensive care beds contribute to a high rate of mortality. Since the elderly are at higher risk of poor outcomes with COVID-19, there is intense worry among the *Diné* about losing elders with specialized knowledge. For example, each medicine person (*Hataałii*) specializes in different and unique ceremonies and this knowledge may die with the person and be forever lost, since wisdom is handed down *only* verbally to learners. Over the last several decades, the tribe has gone from 1000 *Diné* medicine people to just 300, and the coronavirus threatens the few who remain. The elders and medicine persons who depart take an encyclopedia of information with them, so the tribe is rushing to educate the younger population and reconnect youth with elders. Traditional medicine apprenticeships are offered through the 6 campuses of *Diné College* on the Navajo Nation and groups are creating digital files on cultural practices, so the expertise is not lost forever. Due to pandemic-related stay-at-home orders and curfews with difficulty accessing stores, there has also been a resurgence of farming to improve upon the scarcity of healthy food [19].

Although Native American communities have struggled with reducing the spread of COVID-19, they have exceeded other US states in vaccination rates, likely due to cultural cohesiveness and a centralized healthcare system, the IHS [20–22]. Almost every US tribal member has been affected by or lost family members in the pandemic and considers protecting family and tribal elders a cultural responsibility [20]. United, with a common goal, tribes are striving to inform members with consistent information regarding COVID-19 vaccine facts through coordinated public relations campaigns in partnership between government officials, IHS, tribal health care employees, and tribes [20]. There has been a unified communication process across the Navajo Nation with the Navajo President's Office using social media, radio, and a bilingual approach [20]. Navajo Nation President, Jonathan Nez, publicly received the vaccinations to increase confidence in their safety for the *Diné*. Support for the vaccines has been discussed in public town hall meetings with tribal leaders and respected health experts to allow for questions [22]. Well-respected and trusted tribal elders and medicine men and women were enlisted to record radio broadcast messages to encourage vaccination [22]. A more streamlined Navajo vaccination program was made possible with the decision to use the centralized IHS system of hospitals and clinics for extensive vaccine clinics and drive-through sites [22]. Public health nurses and community health representatives are identifying tribal elders without transportation to clinic sites and are vaccinating them in their households [20]. By mid-April 2021, 86.5% of the Navajo population had at least one dose and 37% were fully vaccinated, and 12 of the 15 counties with the highest vaccination rates in the US contain Indian reservations or Alaskan Native communities where IHS or tribal clinics are the primary source of healthcare [20, 22, 23].

Due to the physical distancing requirements and decrease in health care providers in the Navajo Nation due the pandemic, the tribe has expressed interest in tele-education, tele-traditional medicine, and tele-monitoring to decrease health inequities on the Navajo Nation. Some traditional Navajo healers are using virtual platforms for tele-traditional medicine, however, concerns about barriers with internet access and technologic literacy remain [14]. While over 1.2 million persons on US tribal lands lack basic access to mobile technology and quality Internet capability, advancing tele-health services is improbable. The Navajo Nation has been allocated funds from the Coronavirus Aid, Relief, and Economic Security (CARES) Act to increase Internet services, broadband expansion and mobile towers, but much more funding for infrastructure is needed to improve health equity [14].

20.3.1.5 Cultural Difference

Culture is shaped by mores (values, beliefs, norms, and practices) that are shared by members of a cultural group and guide thinking, doing, and being. Culture becomes a patterned expression of who we are and is passed down from one generation to the next. Cultural values are unique principles of a particular culture that become acceptable as they are practiced over time. Persons in the general US society and many who work in the US healthcare system may have differing views based on cultural values related to health care decisions, life, and death.

Individuality

Health care providers should not assume that all patients from a particular group or culture are of the same mind [3]. Native Americans are not one people or culture, and we cannot generalize about individuals. Beliefs, traditions, rituals, and ceremonies among tribes vary widely. The culture of each nation or tribe also reflects the influences of assimilation and acculturation, which may be the result of relocation, forced education in boarding schools, and competing religious missionary efforts in American history. These events resulted in a heterogeneous belief system among the Native American community [9]. Based on the 2010 US Census population count, 47% of Navajo tribal members lived on the Navajo Nation, 10% in larger towns bordering Navajo, 26% in metropolitan areas throughout the US, with large populations in Phoenix, AZ and Albuquerque, NM, and 17% in other areas of the US [10]. Knowing whether a patient resides or was raised on the Nation of Navajo versus a large metropolitan area, may help to inform the approach a health care provider takes during interactions and difficult medical discussions. However, even if a person was raised in a large urban area, influences of culture may still have an effect on beliefs and identity [24].

Some Navajo patients have multiethnic and multicultural families with members of other Native and non-Native peoples who practice different religions. It is common to have a family in which some segments are Christian while others maintain traditional Navajo religious beliefs in the multiple generations of a matrilineal family [4]. An individual may also be influenced by the push and pull of traditional and modern beliefs. Allopathic therapies may be acceptable with the addition of traditional and/or Christian ceremonies to ward off evil, harm, and negativity to protect the individual and family [4].

These factors may influence how a patient and family process medical decision-making and combine to define the individual's preferences with regard to health, values, and behavior. A family may have traditional cultural beliefs combined with varying religious beliefs and a contemporary context, resulting in a spectrum that needs to be explored to provide good communication with each patient [5, 6]. Getting to know each patient and family will guide the methods for discussing medical information.

Positive Thinking

In the traditional Navajo belief system, thoughts and language shape and influence reality and may affect future events. For Navajo people, it is believed that your words carry power, hence the act of discussing something can make it happen and may influence the outcomes of medical interventions [3]. *Hózhó* or *hózhóni* is the central concept in Navajo culture and its meaning is approximated by combining the concepts of beauty, blessedness, goodness, balance, order, harmony, peace, and everything that is positive or ideal. *Hózhó,* the "beauty way of life", defines the traditional Navajo way of thinking, speaking, behaving, and relating to other people and the surrounding world and living a balanced and harmonious life [1, 7]. In general, Navajo people believe health is maintained, or restored, through positive language, termed *hózhoojí* [7]. The Navajo phrases *hózhoojí nitsihakees* and *hózhoojí saad* literally translate to "think in the beauty way" and "talk in the beauty way". Positive thoughts are important in all things and negative thoughts and ideas are avoided [5]. Many Navajo persons refrain from thinking or speaking in a negative way and maintain a positive outlook and hope. The Navajo phrase, "*Doo'ájíniidah*" has literal translation "don't talk that way!" Speaking about potential future harm will either call upon the negative result that is discussed or will make it more likely to occur [8]. This positive thinking has sometimes been misinterpreted by others that the Navajo people are intensely afraid of death. On the contrary, they have tremendous respect for life and the preservation until old age would be ideal [9]. The belief that talking about bad things can be causative is held by many other cultures, such as people in Greece, China, Italy, Korea, Mexico, and the Horn of Africa [7].

- Video 20.5: Navajo traditional teachings. Walk In Beauty, October 8, 2018. Accessed 1 March 2021. https://www.youtube.com/watch?v=ruYNl-emEic
- Video 20.6: Navajo traditional teachings. Traditional Native American Beauty Way Prayer, September 7, 2020. Accessed 1 March 2021.https://www.youtube.com/watch?v=nwegDq6quQY

Family Structure

According to laws in the US, there are strict definitions of "family", *k'é*. Immediate blood-relations, family members by marriage or adoption, and legally appointed powers-of-attorney are allowed to make decisions about individual patients. Many cultures have differing family structures that do not adhere to these rules. Native American tribes may be matriarchal, bilinear, or patriarchal, but in most tribes, the wisdom and experience of elders are honored and respected. The *Diné* are a matriarchal and clan society, emphasizing the importance of the maternal lineage. The lineage of the clans is passed down through women and women have authority over property and are custodians of the children. A clan is a small tribe within a tribe [1]. The Navajo tribe has more than 100 clans from differing areas of the Navajo Nation with unique meanings and histories. Each person belongs to four different clans, derived from family linage. The individual's primary (or first) clan is from the mother's female linage (grandmother, great grandmother, etc.). The second is from the father's primary clan, third from the maternal grandfather's primary clan, and forth from the paternal grandfather's primary clan. These clans are used to identify family members or establish kinship with one another. Therefore, a person/patient may have many "mothers", "aunts", and "siblings" who are influential in upbringing and decision-making throughout one's life. Separate clans are interwoven by cross-membership in other groups, forming a complex network and may inform the decision-makers for health care choices. In each family or clan, one elder may be designated as the final decision-maker [6, 25]. The *Diné* also have a close-knit extended family with many multigenerational households due to culture but also structural inequities on the Navajo Nation. Extreme poverty necessitates shared homes or close proximity of small households on one plot of land owned by the family. The definition of "family" and who is involved with major decisions regarding health care varies across cultures. Allowing participation of non-conventional family members in decision-making is crucial to cultural competence in treating many patients [1, 6].

- Video 20.7: Navajo traditional teachings. *K'é* Navajo kinship, September 19, 2017. Accessed 1 March 2021. https://www.youtube.com/watch?v=IO2y36hnzLc

Traditional Medicine

The *Diné* value living in harmony with everyone and everything, people, the land, and animals [1]. This is called "Walking in Beauty", a world view in which everything in life is connected and influences everything else and is a path to health, healing, and life [1]. Traditional Navajo religion involves worship of the winds and watercourses and a number of divine beings who are believed to intervene occasionally in human affairs. These entities are frequently invoked, offerings are made to them, and ceremonies are performed to continue to live a life of balance and harmony (*hózhó*). Songs, chants, dances, prayers, sweat baths, and sand paintings also form portions of the intricate religious rituals [6]. Traditional Navajo customs may partially or completely inform an individual patient's culture or may have no influence at all based on individual and/or family belief.

- Video 20.8: Explore documentary films. Becoming a Diné Navajo Medicine Man, June 18, 2015. Accessed 1 March 2021. https://www.youtube.com/watch?v=gwTt6wIQnVk
- Video 20.9: Navajo traditional teachings. Medicine Man Training, May 11, 2018. Accessed 1 March 2021. https://www.youtube.com/watch?v=-f6rhOpNxsk

Traditional Navajo healers are called *Hataałii* or "singers", also known as medicine men (or women), and use chanting, singing, praying, and herbs to create medicinal elixirs or ointments, and "cleansers" to perform healing ceremonies and blessing rites intended to protect and cure the body, mind, and spirit. The *Hataałii* sees a person not simply as a body, but as a whole being, connected to other people, families, communities, the planet, and universe. All of these relationships need to be in harmony to be healthy [1]. In traditional Navajo medicine there are no disease names. Sickness is a result of things falling out of balance, of losing one's way on the path of beauty. Religion and medicine are combined [1]. Illness is thought to be caused by transgressions against the supernatural, witchcraft, or violation of taboo [26] and by imbalance with an animal or bird or caused by the wind, dirt, or the season. The word "taboo" can be defined as not being acceptable to talk about or do and is a strong cultural warning or prohibition against an action [26]. Violating a taboo may have a negative effect on the family and community, not only the individual's mores. *Bilagáana* (European-American or white man) illness are the names and causes of allopathic diseases. Diseases may be attributed to contamination and oppressive social conditions resulting in loss of traditions by having to live according to the "white man's" philosophy, eating processed foods, or exposure to environmental pollutants. Traditional healers and ceremonial interventions may be needed to correct for contamination caused by contact with non-Navajo blood, breath, organs, and medical personnel. This type of background information for a particular culture may be beneficial in working with indigenous populations across the globe [4]. For Navajo patients, traditional healers may be requested to reverse taboo or for protection ceremonies. Patients or families may wish to consult with a traditional healer combined with contemporary allopathic medical treatments [27]. Often the songs of the medicine man can inspire hope and compliment treatment with biomedical medicine [1]. Having a ceremony before surgery or other treatment may result in a calm patient who is a better candidate for surgery. Navajo healers practice a viable and real medicine that works with the patient's mind as well as the body [1]. It is therefore important to realize that using "science" to try to talk patients out of their beliefs will be ineffectual when used alone. Allowing traditional medicine to come alongside science may be an effective holistic approach.

- Video 20.10: Alvord LA. The healing properties of Navajo ceremonies, January 4, 2016. Arizona State University Libraries. Accessed 1 March 2021. https://www.youtube.com/watch?v=93LiJFvjZsg&t=2056s

Allopathic Treatments

Traditional Navajo believe that each person has a predetermined life span or limit. There is also belief in an afterlife in which a person returns to the spirit world to be with the "holy people or *diyin dine'é*" and will need the tools to reside there, including an intact, uncontaminated body, "the sacred gift". Taboo procedures, such as autopsy or organ transplantation, either as a recipient or donor, may hinder the journey process after death. Organ transplantation, blood transfusion, cardiopulmonary resuscitation (CPR), and even some surgical treatments may be difficult to accept, because they may interfere with one's predetermined life limit by extending it [4].

- Video 20.11: Navajo traditional teachings. Life Does Not End: Navajo Beliefs on After Life, September 2, 2019. Accessed 1 March 2021. https://www.youtube.com/watch?v=FIqjccc35JE

Organ transplantation is a particular conundrum. Belief that the body should remain intact to enter the spirit world, mistrust of the ethical process of organ procurement, and uncertainty about the safety and quality of deceased organs are concerns. On the other hand, patients have expressed that their family and loved ones were the primary motivation to pursue transplant, in addition to improved quality of life by avoiding dialysis and dietary restrictions. Although a more modern cohort of patients may *accept* transplants, there remains a resistance to organ *donation*. An organ, blood, or breaths received in CPR may be contaminated by the donor's spirituality, personality, or physical ailments and may be acquired by the recipient. Donated organs or breaths given in CPR are also thought to give away a part of the Navajo donor, therein, a piece goes to and stays with the recipient. Navajo patients with traditional beliefs would rather accept blood or organs from someone living, as opposed to deceased, and in their own kinship, however, some may not wish to burden family members by taking an organ they may need in this life or the afterlife. Patients also express that some taboos of accepting allopathic treatments can be remedied with ceremony and asking for permission and protection and are, therefore, rendered less objectionable [4, 28].

20.3.2 Principles of Medical Ethics in Surgical Care and Cultural Difference

In caring for people from some cultures, it may be necessary to further contemplate the four principles of clinical medical ethics and how their application may differ with regard to communication and treatment to assure autonomy, non-maleficence, beneficence, and justice for *all* patients. Belief systems, family structure, communication styles, characteristics and temperament of individuals, and distrust of the healthcare system can position cultures such as the *Diné* in conflict with the classic intention of the four principles of clinical medical ethics as outlined by Beauchamp and Childress (see Table 20.2) [29].

20.3.2.1 General Concepts

Many aspects of surgical care, such as obtaining informed consent and advance directives, involve outlining negative consequences, risks, and possible dire scenarios. Having belief in the causal efficacy of stating future harms, some patients may ask that their healthcare providers avoid these negative discussions and doing so may uphold non-maleficence. Some traditional Navajo persons would like to avoid "*Doo'ajiniidah*", negative thoughts, and wish for *hózhoojí*, positive language and thinking to maintain *hózhó* [8]. The belief of creating negative outcomes by voicing them also exists in other cultures and is known as the *Nocebo Effect* and refers to adverse outcomes produced by negative expectations for an event, procedure, or treatment [30]. This may lead to some patients experiencing anxiety or

Table 20.2 Ethical principles [29]

1. **Respect for autonomy**—A norm of respecting and supporting autonomous decisions, may have different a meaning for some cultures and people, depending on decision-making participants and styles.
2. **Non-maleficence**—A norm of avoiding the causation of harm, must be of particular focus in conversations, evaluations, treatment options, and post-operative care in Navajo and other patients.
3. **Beneficence**—A group of norms pertaining to relieving, lessening, or preventing harm and providing benefits and balancing benefits against risk and costs, needs careful consideration to avoid biases and inequity in care.
4. **Justice**—A group of norms for fairly distributing benefits, risk, and costs, should be maximized to provide a purposeful reduction of inequity in healthcare for disparate communities.

other adverse outcomes, if aware of serious side effects or risks of surgery [31]. Some patients expect to hear a complete list of possibilities and to be *fully* informed. Others wish only to gather basic information and avoid conversations about advance directives or specific scenarios and negative outcomes. This dichotomy may be particularly evident between Navajo patients with traditional beliefs and those from a more progressive background, emphasizing the need to individualize dialogue with each patient.

20.3.2.2 Trust

Historically, the education system was used to forcibly acculturate Native Americans by removing them from their families, tribes, and land, assigning them European-American names, prohibiting them from speaking their languages, sending children to boarding schools, and generally stripping away every aspect of indigenous culture [28]. Healthcare institutions, both historically and in the present, have not always shown themselves to be worthy of trust, which is a critical element in cross-cultural cooperation. Experimental treatments and inequity in medical and surgical care for ethnic minorities are well documented. Until disparities in access and quality of care are eliminated or at least greatly reduced, simply encouraging Native Americans and other ethnic minorities to be more *trusting* of recommendations provided by non-Native physicians is likely to fail [32]. Attention to culturally competent communication is a first step in inspiring trust.

20.3.2.3 Patient Autonomy

In the United States healthcare system, the value of autonomous decision-making is strongly held. Autonomy is defined as a norm of respecting and supporting independent decisions [29], permitting control over one's body according to an individual's personal values and beliefs. How does autonomy differ in a maternal, family-based culture? For many American Indians, autonomy is not an *individual* concept as decision-making lies in the community. Since the Navajo family composition can be quite complex and elders held in high regard, many health decisions may be made together with multiple family members, *and* families may make decisions *for* individual members (see Chap. 19).

20.3.2.4   Advance Directives

In 1991, the United States legislature implemented the Patient Self-Determination Act (PSDA) that requires health care organizations and encourages patients to create advance directives (ADs) [8]. Initially, ADs were viewed as a solution for decreasing the use of costly, life-sustaining technology, which did not maintain life at a quality level. Individuals, regardless of race, ethnicity, culture, and cultural heritage, fear that life-extending technology might increase suffering without ultimately resulting in sustained and prolonged life. The PDSA was adopted by the Indian Health Service in 1992 with the proviso that "Tribal customs and traditional beliefs that relate to death and dying will be respected to the extent possible when providing information to patients on these issues." [8] However, if a healthcare provider honors her Navajo patients' *Doo'ajiniidah* request, these patients may not receive sufficient information needed to make informed decisions. Navajo patients with traditional beliefs may not wish to participate in the discussions concerning dire circumstances necessary for advance directives that are mandated by the PSDA, for they may believe that talking about the possibility of becoming terminally ill and/or in a persistent unconscious state will either cause them to suffer this fate or make it more likely [8]. For some, an advance directive is considered a death warrant and a violation of fundamental tribal views and is perceived to be detrimental not only to the individual but to the family and community [7, 33].

20.3.2.5   Informed Consent

As surgeons trained in the US, we are taught to explain every risk and possible bad outcome of each treatment option. Not doing so can put us at risk for litigation, if complications occur. Fully "informing" our patients of not only the benefits and alternatives to surgery but also the risks involved in having or declining surgical treatment is the key portion of obtaining informed consent. In the same way discussing advance directive choices regarding end-of-life care may cause distress for those who wish to only discuss positive ideas, the informed consent process can be problematic and may result in a patient losing trust in their care. On one hand, most persons value autonomy, and so value giving informed consent to treatment to protect it. On the other hand, a view of causation may preclude a patient from talking or thinking about "negative things," and so may prevent giving *truly* informed consent for treatment [8].

20.3.2.6 Treatment

Pain Assessment

There are several studies that show ethnic disparities in assessment and treatment of postoperative pain [34]. Expression of pain is a complex interaction between biologic, psychosocial, and cultural factors and may be more subtle in Navajo and other Native patients. Commonly used assessment instruments may not accurately reflect the degree of experienced pain. While various pain scales exist, their reliability and validity across different racial/ethnic backgrounds remains to be determined [34]. When given numeric pain scale options, some Native American patients may tend to choose favorite or sacred numbers instead of the number that accurately indicates their level of pain. There can also be a difference in *communication* of pain. Many indigenous tribal beliefs about causes of illness and pain are related to imbalance between the spiritual, mental, physical, and social interactions of the individual and are to be endured. Courage and humble, soft-spoken stoicism should not be misconstrued as absence of pain. There is also evidence that subtle symptoms and the use of descriptive words by Native American patients to describe pain can be used as an indicator for the presence of pain. Due to the combination of the above factors, there is a need to assess acute postsurgical pain differently for some patients to avoid maleficence by undertreating pain. Attention should be given to nonverbal cues, as well as universal objective indicators of pain, such as tachypnea, tachycardia, diaphoresis, pallor, or increasing blood pressure [34].

Withdrawal of Treatment

As in our case of Baby Faith, families are often opposed to withdrawal of treatment for diagnoses with poor prognosis and limited life expectancy. People of many backgrounds prefer to choose life-sustaining treatments, including surgery, which may allow for improvement of disease or discharge home. It was difficult to find evidential information in the literature concerning this subject with regard to Navajo tradition. There are some reports about other cultures that approximate the Navajo concept of avoiding interference with one's predetermined life limit and preserving hope in deciding to continue treatment [4]. Many Christian religions also discourage withdrawal of care or hastening death. Since it is difficult to provide a definitive prognostic estimate for a diagnosis due to phenotypic variability and severity of disease processes, life expectancy projection cannot be exact, complicating decision-making for patients and families. Families have stated that letting a patient die is not their decision to make, which has been expressed by other groups who have beliefs that "only God has knowledge about and power over life and death" [32]. Despite the reasons, we should attempt to understand and accommodate desires for continued or more aggressive care, and use respectful negotiation when treatment is contraindicated or seems medically futile [32].

20.3.3   Cultural Competence and Cultural Humility Improvement Strategies

Physicians frequently care for patients whose cultural, religious, or social backgrounds differ from our own. If these differences are not attended to, the substantial variety in patient values, beliefs, and behaviors related to health and healthcare may result in conflict, misdiagnosis, poor adherence to recommendations, suboptimal outcomes, or decreased patient satisfaction. Cultural, ethnic, or racial discordance between patients and physicians has an impact on communication related to healthcare, and barriers can be due to differences in language, religion or spirituality, family involvement in decision-making, responses to inequities in care, and lack of trust. Biases in treatment recommendations, pain assessment, and outcomes can be mitigated if we use an individualized, culturally competent method of providing care, which has been shown to improve outcomes in many disciplines and should be a part of modern-day medical care [3, 35]. Focused improvement strategies for individuals, medical education, hospitals and health systems, and the broader society can be used to improve culturally competent communication and care for patient populations. "To effectively reach populations affected by disparities, providers need to have a personal understanding of the communities and people within those populations—who they are, what matters to them, and how they can be supported in building a stronger foundation for health." [24]

20.3.3.1   Individual Provider Strategies

Unconscious Bias Awareness and Training

Individual surgeons and other healthcare practitioners should familiarize themselves with cultural competence *and* cultural humility and strive to understand and practice both. We should *embrace* implicit bias training, awareness of biases, and make a conscious effort to lessen them and endeavor to be knowledgeable about and accepting of other cultures. Lead by example with professional behavior and compassion for cultural difference with emphasis on beneficence, non-maleficence, autonomy, and justice [3]. Implicit bias is likely the most common form of bias among healthcare providers, but *explicit* bias is also persistent, and efforts are needed to minimize its occurrence as well. We also need to enhance *structural* competence among healthcare providers, which refers to increasing awareness of how racism is embedded in our culture and institutions and shapes not only behavior of individuals but also the ways in which policies and procedures in medical and other social institutions have initiated and sustain racial inequality. Therefore, effectively addressing implicit bias also requires identifying and dismantling institutional legacies and social consequences. This will require changes not only in the individual behavior of providers but also policy changes across many domains of healthcare and other social institutions [36].

Communication Strategies and Ethical Principles

Good communication is critical for caring for all patients but can be more difficult with those from different cultural backgrounds. Cultural differences can lead to the need to alter the typical manner of pre- and post-operative discussions, which are often blunt and directly goal oriented. Awareness of the differences between cultures can enhance communication and using interpreters and lay medical advocates improves quality of care. "Increased awareness of social cues that communicate respect to Indigenous people, attending to these during medical history-taking, physical exams and delivery of treatment, ensuring that patients will be treated with respect and dignity, and that there will be time to answer questions" are helpful practices [24].

Four-Step Approach

Carrese's 2000 article describes a four-step guide for communicating with Navajo patients based on conversations with Navajo informants and can be adapted for use with many patients of differing backgrounds (see Table 20.3) [3]. The overarching premise of the approach is to interact while applying the Navajo concept of *k'é*, compassion, caring, kindness, and respect, especially when discussing negative information. Getting to know the patient and family and communicating awareness of potential differences in culture will allow them to have more confidence in the care. These methods can be beneficial in connecting with *all* patients.

The first step in the guideline is to *ask permission* to discuss negative information, which goes hand in hand with the second step of *rapport building*. Rapport is cultivated by (1) establishing a trusting relationship, (2) facilitating involvement of family members, (3) warning the patient about the nature of the discussion and communicating that no harm is intended *while* asking permission to discuss negative things, and (4) facilitating the involvement of a patient advocate and interpreter and

Table 20.3 Carrese's four step approach [3]

First Step—Ask permission to discuss negative information
Second Step—Build Rapport
 1. Establish a trusting relationship
 2. Involve family members
 3. Warn about the nature of the discussion
 4. Use a patient advocate, interpreter, traditional healers
Third Step—Communication
 1. Use the k'é concept to communicate
 2. Do not rush
 3. Maintain a positive focus
 4. Refer to a third party when discussing risks or prognosis
 5. Review the patient's story in a circuitous fashion using positive language
Fourth Step—Follow-through and continued care

traditional healers, if the patient desires. The third step involves specific techniques for *communication*. (1) Communicate information in a caring, kind, respectful manner, *k'é*. (2) Do not rush the interaction and allow enough time for the conversation and questions. (3) Maintain a positive focus, keeping in mind *hózhoojí*, using positive concepts and words. (4) Refer to third parties rather than to the patient directly when discussing prognosis, risks, or other potentially negative information; "Some people with this diagnosis had these treatments." "The types of problems we have seen may include bleeding, transfusion, or need for more surgery." (5) Review the patient's story in a circuitous route from symptoms, physical findings, and study results, then meander to the most likely conclusion, rather than stating the facts and diagnosis bluntly. Use positive language for wishing these things were not happening. Using positive action words and third person language are techniques that uphold non-maleficence. The fourth step involves *follow-through* and the physician's responsibility to the patient and family after negative information has been shared. Continue to care for the patient, communicate hope, and invite traditional healing and other methods of care, especially for those with a poor prognosis. Outline the options and continue to convey a positive message in positive language to maintain *hózhó*. "In the Navajo way there is always something to be done" [3]. As an example:

> If you say, *"This medicine is for your high blood pressure, and you've got to take it like this, and if you don't, one of these days you're going to get worse, and maybe a year later or two you're going to be dead,"* then right there, that guy's going to back off from you. That's the negative aspect. If instead you say, *"If you follow this example, you will get better, you will feel better, you will feel good."* Then the Navajo patient may actually follow the recommendation to take the medication. *"Mention the positive thing. That's what people want to hear. (Traditional healer)* [3]

Hypothetical Case Approach

Another strategy to preserve non-maleficence is using a hypothetical case to inform the patient and family about the procedure, treatment plan, or prognosis. This technique acknowledges the patient's and family's realistic fears, respects the need for indirect discussion, and invites further questions. Direct confrontation may frighten or offend the patient, and sensitivity and skill are essential to gauge the degree of information sought. Responses to inquiry may be indirect or phrased as hypothetical, according to the wishes of the patient and family [3].

Ask, Tell, Ask Approach

The physician should regularly seek feedback from the patient and family to assess their understanding of the proposed treatment plan or progression of the disease and to determine need for additional information [32]. Ask patients what they want to hear, tell them what they are comfortable hearing, and then ask what they understand and repeat as the conversation progresses [37].

Modified Informed Consent

There is some literature proposing modifying informed consent (IC) by withholding negative information, such as risks, out of respect for the wishes for some people to avoid negative thinking, including in Navajo culture [8, 30, 38]. Some authors recommend either providing only basic information about a treatment unless asked for more [30] or tailoring a discussion to each specific patient, termed "contextualized informed consent" [39]. Asking about the preferred mode of decision-making will allow the patient to know you are aware of potential cultural differences. The patient may wish to have family, tribal elders, and/or a spiritual healer or *Hataałii* participate in the discussion. Determine and document who may not want to hear about the negative risks. Prioritize positive thinking during discussion of risks and document any modification the IC process. Customizing the information given to provide maximal transparency with the least potential harm may uphold non-maleficence and avoid the nocebo effect [31]. Since the primary motivation behind informed consent is the protection of patients, then through the principle of beneficence, withholding nocebogenic information may be appropriate. Clinicians should be aware of the impact of their conversations on patients' experiences and endeavor to shape their discussions to optimize outcomes while maintaining patient autonomy [39].

20.3.3.2 Medical Education Improvements

Improving diversity in the healthcare workforce will likely need to start with societal changes and improved institutional inequities in the US education system. Medical schools should strive for admissions that reflect the diversity of the population served. Mentoring and recruitment needs to begin in early education, high school or earlier, to attract students to medical disciplines, especially surgical specialties, by developing mentorship and pipeline programs to foster diversity. The diversity among surgical residents and practicing surgeons should be a focus in residency recruitment and admissions, since there continues to be a paucity of black, indigenous, and people of color (BIPOC) in surgical residencies and, subsequently, surgical practice [40]. A diverse workforce improves patient-provider racial and cultural concordance. Research indicates that racial concordance between a patient and a clinician is associated with better communication, overall health outcomes, higher levels of patient satisfaction with care, and superior adherence to provider recommendations. Therefore, as the US population becomes increasingly diverse, with the current BIPOC populations becoming the majority of the US population in less than 25 years, ensuring the increasing diversity of health care providers is in the best interest of national health care delivery [36].

20.3.3.3   Health Systems Strategies for Cultural Competence (see Table 20.4)

Diversify the Workforce

Hospitals and health systems should increase educational opportunities in medical disciplines for diverse populations and recruit *actively* for medical providers, physicians, and nurses with differing backgrounds that reflect the local population and/or population at large. Hospitals should recruit and cultivate a diverse workforce with intention and provide educational competencies not only in compliance, HIPAA, patient safety, but also in cultural competence and communication. They should require courses on common cultural traditions in the region and emphasize using customized techniques with patients. *Diné* College offers cultural orientation courses for non-Navajo medical workers, as an example. Outline potential differences in various patient populations and emphasize the need to inquire with the patient and family their preferred communication style, type of care, other healing methods or holistic care they prefer. Require that staff are educated on implicit and explicit biases and cultural and structural competence. Maintain ongoing evaluation and training on potential for bias and strategies to eliminate or diminish the influence of biases on behavior and patient care. Deliberately recruit and hire health care workers who strive for inclusion and cultural openness. Be sure this is part of the interview and hiring requirements with ongoing training and evaluation.

Table 20.4 Healthcare systems strategies for cultural competence and humility [1, 4, 5, 7, 8, 21, 24, 30, 31]

Diversity the workforce
1. Increase educational opportunities for diverse populations
2. Actively recruit diverse employees
Cultivate cultural competence and cultural humility
1. Required courses for employees
2. Implicit bias training
3. Ongoing evaluation of competence
Hire bilingual, bicultural staff
1. Training in interpretation
2. Employ and use patient advocates
3. Always use an interpreter
Allow for traditional or alternative healing
1. Consult local populations on wishes/needs
2. Hire or contract with traditional healers to provide care on site
3. Provide spaces for traditional healing practices/ceremonies
Hospital policy changes
1. Advance directive requirement
2. Family member definitions
3. Allow for a designee to make decisions

Interpreters and Patient Advocates

Hospitals should hire bilingual, bicultural staff and train them in medical translation/interpretation for the common racial and ethnic groups in the region of practice. Create paid job positions for patient advocates with background and understanding of the patient populations cared for. Assure that these positions are *paid* and not on a volunteer positions to promote longevity and provide income [24]. Providers should always avoid the use of family members as interpreters and insist on using medical interpretation during interactions with Navajo and other non-English speaking patients. Many patients may speak English, but pride may impede the request for an interpreter [5]. Patient advocates and interpreters understand the Navajo positive speaking and culture and can enhance interactions [32].

Traditional Healing

Healthcare facilities that care for populations of American Indian patients should employ and/or development consultation contracts with traditional healers and provide spaces for traditional healing. Hospitals should facilitate the use of traditional Native healers as a complement to allopathic medicine and recognize the importance of spiritual traditions when setting up prevention programs, screenings and health care services [24]. In 1996, the Navajo Nation was granted funds from the US Department of Veterans Affairs to finance traditional healing services. The Indian Health Service (IHS) has made efforts to incorporate Navajo opinions into its operations to make facilities more accessible to Navajo practitioners. One of the first examples of this cooperation is the Chinle Health Care Facility in AZ which created an Office of Navajo Healing to build a bridge between biomedicine and traditional Navajo medicine. They offer traditional counseling and care and arrange herbalists and ceremonial practitioners and have a hogan (traditional dwelling and ceremonial structure) at the facility. Other centers have integrated traditional practices in treatment with medicine persons as permanent staff members, hogans and healing rooms on site, facility doors facing east, Navajo artwork, and *Diné Bizaad* signage [1, 4]. At the University of New Mexico Hospital, there is a non-denominational meditation space with respect for differing religions and beliefs. There are Native American patient advocates and interpreters on staff through the office of Native American Health Services.

Hospital Policy Considerations

Health systems should consider policy revisions to incorporate a culturally competent organizational strategy [7]. Revising policies on *requiring* advance directives, family member definitions, and requirements for decision-makers may be appropriate. Some patients may want an advance directive and others prefer a more stepwise decision-making algorithm, making choices as only necessary. Policy should allow patients to designate decision-makers and how involved they are in healthcare choices. Some elders of many cultures will prefer to have a designee hear the "bad news" and make decisions about informing the patient.

20.3.3.4   Societal Advocacy

Healthcare leadership, especially physician leaders, in medical schools and hospitals should (1) work to increase diversity in the health system, intentionally and actively, (2) take a proactive role in learning, researching, publishing, and educating others about structural and institutional racism, cultural competence, and cultural humility, (3) use knowledge learned to inform health policies and for advocacy and mentorship to ensure and improve justice and equity in medical care, and (4) continue to support elevation, appointment, and election of persons underrepresented in medicine to medical leadership positions and elected offices.

20.3.4   Return to the Case

The Navajo patient advocate, *Diné* interpreter, and the medical teams met for pre-conference planning and various aspects of communication with Navajo families were examined. The advocate stressed the importance of shaking hands with a light touch, as opposed to a vigorous tight firm grip, as a necessary and respectful greeting in Navajo culture. The concept of positive thinking and avoidance of negative thinking and ideas were discussed. Use of the third person when naming risks was emphasized to avoid seeming to wish harm on the patient [3]. The Navajo medical student was elected to take the lead on discussing the proposed procedures. She was given the risk and benefit information and was assured the specialists would be present to answer more detailed questions.

The family meeting began with a prolonged introduction of all the participants to the family by the *Diné* interpreter. The interpreter, advocate, and medical student were noted to shake the hands of all of the family members before beginning. The dysmorphologist began with a detailed description of Patau syndrome. The interpreter repeated the details in Navajo for the elder family members, as the parents spoke both English and Navajo. She also occasionally paused to explain some Navajo traditions and common wishes to the medical team. In discussing the symptoms and prognosis of the syndrome, the team was very careful to frame the information and statistics to a third party. "Some patients have a short life and develop very serious medical problems."

The baby's current problems were outlined and described. The potential future associated problems were explained very delicately in the third person, prefacing each problem with "some patients have developed…". The discharge planner and social worker clarified requirements for care at home with regard to plumbing, electricity, home care services. They offered to help obtain housing in Albuquerque, close to the medical center. The family stated that this was not an option due to their wishes to stay close to their extended family and community.

The benefits of tracheostomy and gastrostomy surgery were listed. The medical student then *asked permission* to discuss the risks of the surgical procedures. The family granted this discussion. Each statement was prefaced by *positive action words* and was stated in the *third person*. "*We do not wish* for any of these problems to happen, but *some patients have had* bleeding, collapse of the lung, infection, and the trach tube can get plugged or fall out." With the "stomach feeding tube, in other patients *we have seen* infection in the belly, leakage of stomach fluids, infection of the skin. We *hope* that none of these difficulties will happen."

The subject of an advance directive was brought up, and the family did not wish to make specific plans for negative outcomes and preferred to make decisions in a stepwise fashion at the time choices are needed. Withdrawal of care was also mentioned. "In similar situations, some parents have chosen to remove the breathing tube and let nature take its course." The parents asked, "Let her die? We cannot let her die. This is not up to us. We need to do everything we can to take her home." The family did not wish to discuss this any further. The family members had many questions, which were slowly, thoughtfully, and comprehensively answered.

The family stated they would like some time to think things over and asked the patient advocate about the availability of a traditional healer who could go to their daughter's bedside. This was not available, therefore they wished to consult with a medicine woman at their home in Tohatchi.

The medical team members continued to round on the patient and visit with the parents daily, answering questions about the medical status and potential surgeries. The team members kept in mind the methods of discussing the negative information in the *third person* and emphasizing that they did not wish any poor outcomes and hoped for only benefits. The care teams and family all perceived improved communication and trust.

After discussion with extended family members and consultation with a traditional healer, the parents decided to stay at the facility, again expressing wishes to do anything necessary to take Faith home. They gave consent for the surgical procedures. They had discussions with the social worker about the availability of extended family members to help with 24-hour care and their comfort with their local health facility and transfer to Albuquerque, if necessary.

The medical team members felt satisfied that the family understood the benefits *and* risks of the recommended treatments, giving *true* informed consent. The individuals learned valuable skills in communication with Navajo families, but more importantly, culturally competent skills that may be applied to *all* patients.

20.4 Conclusion

Medical decision-making can be incredibly complex for patients and families as many belief systems, traditions, fears, and hopes combine. As surgeons and other healthcare providers, we should listen, learn and gather liaisons, interpreters, family members, and any other tools at our disposal to assist in understanding and communicating with patients. Further, we should treat every patient as an individual and keep an inclusive attitude to maximize beneficence, minimize maleficence, support and encourage autonomy, and protect and enhance justice and equity for those we care for. Deliberate attention to inclusion and embracing cultural difference will allow for improved care for marginalized populations.

We hope that the ideas and evidence presented in this chapter can inform surgeons and other health practitioners how to tailor discussions regarding surgical care to the individual, taking into account the background, culture, and belief-systems of the patient. The people of the Navajo Nation are the most written about US indigenous group, therefore, discussing some aspects of this unique culture can serve as an example in the examination of communication approaches that can be used with patients. This informed methodology can be applied to *every* encounter with patients and families in medical practice. Cultural competence and humility can and should be learned, taught, and customized for a surgeon's patient population and practice setting (see Table 20.5). Ask respectful questions, *listen* to answers, keep a receptive mind, communicate in a kind and thoughtful manner, and walk gently during difficult conversations. The use of interpreters, patient advocates, consultation with traditional healers, and being open to perspectives divergent from our own beliefs will assist us in providing culturally competent care. As we each strive to become culturally competent *and* practice cultural humility in providing surgical care, we can endeavor to improve healthcare for patients of *all* cultures and backgrounds and move us closer toward the goal of eliminating health disparities.

Table 20.5 Cultural competence versus cultural humility [41–43]

Cultural competence	**Cultural humility**
A necessary foundation for cultural humility	Requires the components of cultural competence
Both cultural competence and humility require:	**Cultural humility also requires:**
1. **Developing cultural self-awareness** What is my culture and how does it influence the ways I view and interact with others? a. Becoming aware of your own often ill-defined and multidimensional cultural identities, attitudes, beliefs, and behaviors b. Identifying and examining your own personal biases, stereotypes, and prejudices c. Considering the impact cultural differences might have on your interactions with BIPOC (Black, Indigenous, and People of Color), their families, and their communities	1. **Humility in *continually* engaging in individual honest, courageous, self-reflection and self-critique as *lifelong* learners and thoughtful practitioners** a. Committing to lifelong, infinite learning with patients, communities, colleagues, and ourselves b. Actively engaging in ongoing processes that change in response to new situations, experiences, and relationships c. Continuously identifying and examining our own patterns of unintentional and intentional racism, classism, and homophobia

(continued)

Table 20.5 (continued)

2. **Gaining cultural knowledge**	2. **Understanding and equalizing power imbalances that exist in the dynamics of physician-patient communication**
What are other cultures like and what strengths do they have? a. Being comfortable with "not knowing"—Balancing your expert knowledge with being open to learning from patients and community and their lived experiences b. Developing skills for communication and interaction across cultures c. Being curious about other cultures, asking questions, reading about other cultures, viewing films and documentaries, studying another language, attending classes and workshops about other cultures, etc. d. Attending cultural events and festivals e. Establishing trusting relationships with community or patient advocates who are able to provide insights into cultural norms, family practices, communication styles, traditions, etc. f. Understanding the principles of trust, respect for diversity, equity, fairness, and social justice	How can I use my understanding of my own *and* other cultures to identify and work to disrupt inequitable systems? a. Studying the history of race and racism in the US and understanding how it disproportionately impacts BIPOC b. Awakening ourselves to the position of power physicians potentially have over all patients, especially in the context of wealth, race, ethnicity, class, linguistic capability, and sexual orientation c. Completing racial equity or implicit bias training d. Using patient-directed/focused interviewing and care, understanding that every patient's story is unique and only they know it. Ask questions and keep an open mind to learn about her needs and wishes and how little or how much culture has to do with that particular clinical encounter. e. Learning to develop and evaluate culturally relevant and appropriate health programs, materials, and interventions
	3. **Holding the health and/or educational systems accountable for providing inclusive and equitable programs and services** How can I work on an institutional level to ensure that the systems I am part of move toward greater inclusion and equity? a. Serving on an equity team b. Collecting and analyzing data about practices, programs, services, and community partnerships through an equity lens c. Analyzing policies for bias and rewriting them to make them reflective of the cultures, customs, behaviors and information needs of various patients and community members d. Holding institutions and systems accountable for providing inclusive care e. Developing and maintaining mutually respectful, beneficial, non-paternalistic partnerships with communities on behalf of individuals and defined populations.

Adapted from [42]. Video 20.12: "Cultural Humility: People, Principles and Practices," a 30-minute documentary by San Francisco State professor Vivian Chávez, August 9, 2012. Last accessed 28 February 2021. https://www.youtube.com/watch?v=SaSHLbS1V4w&t=689s

20.5 Selected References

- Alvord LA, Van Pelt EC. The scalpel and the silver bear. The first Navajo woman surgeon combines western medicine and traditional healing. Bantam Books;1999.

  - The first Navajo woman surgeon takes us on her journey to combine modern medicine and traditional healing while working in the Navajo Nation in Gallup, NM.

- Bird ME, Bowekaty M, Burhansstipanov L, Cochran PL, Everingham PJ, Suina M, eds. Eliminating health disparities. Conversations with American Indians and Alaska natives. ETR Associates; 2002.

  - Interviews with public health experts provide background information on existing disparities and recommendations to improve future practice and outcomes.

- Navajo Traditional Teachings, youtube.com. https://www.youtube.com/c/NavajoTraditionalTeachings/videos. Accessed 1 Mar 2021

Acknowledgements We would like to thank Nizhoni Denipah, MD for her kind mentorship and contributions to this work and Lori Arviso Alvord, MD for her inspiring narrative and mentorship of underrepresented students to pursue higher education.

References

1. Alvord LA, Van Pelt EC. The scalpel and the silver bear. The first Navajo woman surgeon combines western medicine and traditional healing. Bantam Books; 1999.
2. The Navajo Nation Government. History. https://www.navajo-nsn.gov/history.htm. Accessed 1 Mar 2021
3. Carrese JA, Rhodes LA. Bridging cultural differences in medical practice. The case of discussing negative information with Navajo patients. J Gen Intern Med. 2000;15(2):92–6. https://doi.org/10.1046/j.1525-1497.2000.03399.x.
4. Schwarz MT. "I Choose Life": contemporary medical and religious practices in the Navajo World. University of Oklahoma Press; 2008.
5. Begay M. COVID-19 in the remote Navajo Southwest. Lecture presented at: University of New Mexico Internal Medicine Grand Round; May 18, 2020; Albuquerque, NM.
6. Clements PT, Vigil GJ, Manno MS, et al. Cultural perspectives of death, grief, and bereavement. J Psychosoc Nurs Ment Health Serv. 2003 Jul;41(7):18–26.
7. Carrese JA, Rhodes LA. Western bioethics on the Navajo reservation, benefit or harm? JAMA. 1995;274(10):826–9. https://doi.org/10.1001/jama.1995.03530100066036.
8. Taylor JS. Autonomy and informed consent on the Navajo Reservation. J Soc Philos. 2004;35(4):506–16. https://doi.org/10.1111/j.1467-9833.2004.00250.x.
9. Pesantubbee M. Negotiating advance directives in a Navajo context. In: Knepper TD, Bregman L, Gottschalk M, editors. Death and dying. An exercise in comparative philosophy of religion, vol. 2. Switzerland: Springer Nature; 2019. p. 51–61. https://doi.org/10.1007/978-3-030-19300-3_4.

10. Navajo Division of Health, Navajo Epidemiology Center. Navajo Nation population profile 2010 US census. Navajo Nation; 2013. https://www.nec.navajo-nsn.gov/Portals/0/Reports/NN2010PopulationProfile.pdf. Accessed 10 Feb 2021.
11. National Congress of American Indians. Tribal Governance. https://www.ncai.org/policy-issues/tribal-governance. Accessed 13 Feb 2021
12. Discover Navajo. Yá'át'ééh Welcome to the Navajo Nation! Navajo History. https://www.discovernavajo.com/navajo-culture-and-history.aspx. Accessed 10 Feb 2021
13. Kakol M, Upson D, Sood A. Susceptibility of southwestern American Indian tribes to coronavirus disease 2019 (COVID-19). J Rural Health. 2021;37(1):197–9. https://doi.org/10.1111/jrh.12451.
14. Begay M, Kakol M, Sood A, Upson D. Strengthening digital health technology capacity in Navajo communities to help counter the COVID-19 pandemic [published online ahead of print February 12, 2021]. Ann Am Thorac Soc. https://doi.org/10.1513/AnnalsATS.202009-1136PS.
15. MacKenzie OW, George CV, Pérez-Escamilla R, et al. Healthy stores initiative associated with produce purchasing on Navajo Nation. Curr Dev Nutr. 2019;3(12):nzz125. https://doi.org/10.1093/cdn/nzz125.
16. Bird ME, Bowekaty M, Burhansstipanov L, Cochran PL, Everingham PJ, Suina M, editors. Eliminating health disparities. Conversations with American Indians and Alaska natives. ETR Associates; 2002.
17. Shaefer J. When an infant dies: cross cultural expressions of grief and loss. In: National Fetal Infant Mortality Review Program Bulletin, from the Third National Conference of the National Fetal Infant Mortality Review Program. 1999 July.
18. Colclough YY. Native American death taboo: implications for health care providers. Am J Hosp Palliat Care. 2017 Jul;34(6):584–91. https://doi.org/10.1177/1049909116638839.
19. Williams DH, Shipley GP. Cultural taboos as a factor in the participation rate of native Americans in STEM. Int J STEM Educ. 2018;5(1):17. https://doi.org/10.1186/s40594-018-0114-7.
20. Keddis M, Finnie D, Kim W. Native American patients' perception and attitude about kidney transplant: a qualitative assessment of patients presenting for kidney transplant evaluation. BMJ Open. 2019;9(1):e024671. https://doi.org/10.1136/bmjopen-2018-024671.
21. Dashner-Titus EJ, Hoover J, Li L, et al. Metal exposure and oxidative stress markers in pregnant Navajo Birth Cohort Study participants. Free Radic Biol Med. 2018;124:484–92. https://doi.org/10.1016/j.freeradbiomed.2018.04.579.
22. New Mexico Department of Health. COVID-19 epidemiology reports. New Mexico COVID-19 cases update: demographics. https://cv.nmhealth.org/epidemiology-reports/. Accessed 22 Mar 2021.
23. Arizona Department of Health Services. Data dashboard, demographics/COVID-19 deaths. https://www.azdhs.gov/preparedness/epidemiology-disease-control/infectious-disease-epidemiology/covid-19/dashboards/index.php. Accessed 30 Mar 2021
24. Morales L. Navajo Nation loses elders and tradition to COVID-19 [transcript]. Weekend Edition Sunday. National Public Radio. May 31, 2020.
25. Krisst R. Navajo outpacing states in rate of vaccinations. NavajoTimes. March 9, 2021. https://navajotimes.com/reznews/navajo-outpacing-states-in-rate-of-vaccinations/. Accessed 14 Apr 2021
26. Delkic M, Ngo M. The once-battered Navajo Nation has gained control of the virus, for now. Covid-19: with Big Vaccine Push, Navajo Nation Has Tamed Virus. New York Times. April 12, 2021. Accessed 14 April 2021. https://www.nytimes.com/live/2021/04/04/world/covid-vaccine-coronavirus-cases
27. Whelan R. Native-American tribes pull ahead in Covid-19 vaccinations. Wall Street Journal. April 10, 2021. Accessed 14 April 2021. https://www.wsj.com/articles/native-american-tribes-pull-ahead-in-covid-19-vaccinations-11618047001
28. In numbers: tracking COVID-19 Across the Navajo Nation. NavajoTimes. April 14, 2021. https://navajotimes.com/coronavirus-updates/covid-19-across-the-navajo-nation/. Accessed 14 Apr 2021.

29. Beauchamp TL, Childress JF. Principles of biomedical ethics. 8th ed. Oxford University Press; 2019.
30. Kagawa-Singer M, Blackhall LJ. Negotiating cross-cultural issues at the end of life: "You got to go where he lives". JAMA. 2001;286(23):2993–3001. https://doi.org/10.1001/jama.286.23.2993.
31. Lasser J, Gottlieb MC. Facilitating informed consent: a multicultural perspective. Ethics Behav. 2017;27(2):106–17. https://doi.org/10.1080/10508422.2016.1174121.
32. Agozzino E, Borrelli S, Cancellieri M, Carfora FM, Di Lorenzo T, Attena F. Does written informed consent adequately inform surgical patients? A cross sectional study. BMC Med Ethics. 2019;20(1):1–8. https://doi.org/10.1186/s12910-018-0340-z.
33. Giger JN, Davidhizar RE, Fordham P. Multi-cultural and multi-ethnic considerations and advanced directives: developing cultural competency. J Cult Divers 2006;13(1):3–9. PMID: 16696539.
34. Lee E, Teeple M, Bagrodia N, Hannallah J, Yazzie NP, Adamas-Rappaport WJ. Postoperative pain assessment and analgesic administration in native American patients undergoing laparoscopic cholecystectomy. JAMA Surg. 2013;148(1):91–3. https://doi.org/10.1001/jamasurg.2013.6828.
35. Giger JN, Davidhizar RN. Transcultural nursing: assessment and intervention. Mosby Year Book; 2004.
36. Williams DR, Cooper LA. Reducing Racial inequities in health: using what we already know to take action. Int J Environ Res Public Health. 2019;16(4):606. https://doi.org/10.3390/ijerph16040606.
37. Gawande A. Being mortal. Profile Books; 2014.
38. Hall A. What the Navajo culture teaches about informed consent. HEC Forum. 2002;14(3):241–6. https://doi.org/10.1023/a:1020577030697.
39. Wells RE, Kaptchuk TJ. To tell the truth, the whole truth, may do patients harm: the problem of the nocebo effect for informed consent. Am J Bioeth. 2012;12:22–9. https://doi.org/10.1080/15265161.2011.652798.
40. Schwartz JS, Young M, Velly AM, Nguyen LHP. The evolution of racial, ethnic, and gender diversity in US otolaryngology residency programs. Otolaryngol Head Neck Surg. 2013;149(1):71–6. https://doi.org/10.1177/0194599813485063.
41. Tervalon M, Murray-García J. Cultural humility versus cultural competence: a critical distinction in defining physician training outcomes in multicultural education. J Health Care Poor Underserved. 1998;9(2):117–25. https://doi.org/10.1353/hpu.2010.0233.
42. Chávez V. Cultural humility: people, principles and practices. San Francisco State University. August 9, 2012. https://www.youtube.com/watch?v=SaSHLbS1V4w&t=689s. Accessed 28 Feb 2021
43. Cooke NA. Project READY: reimagining equity & access for diverse youth. Module 8: cultural competence & cultural humility. https://ready.web.unc.edu/section-1-foundations/module-8/. Accessed 28 Feb 2021

Electronic Links

Tribal Governance. National Congress of American Indians. https://www.ncai.org/policy-issues/tribal-governance. Accessed 13 Feb 2021.
YÁ'ÁT'ÉÉH. Welcome to the Navajo Nation! Discover Navajo. Navajo History. https://www.discovernavajo.com/navajo-culture-and-history.aspx. Accessed 10 Feb 2021.
Welcome to the Navajo Nation Government. History. https://www.navajo-nsn.gov/history.htm. Accessed 1 Mar 2021.

Navajo Nation population profile, 2010 US census. https://www.nec.navajo-nsn.gov/Portals/0/Reports/NN2010PopulationProfile.pdf. Accessed 10 Feb 2021.

Project READY: reimagining equity & access for diverse youth, module 8: cultural competence & cultural humility. https://ready.web.unc.edu/section-1-foundations/module-8/. Accessed 28 Feb 2021.

"*Cultural humility: people, principles and practices*," is a 30-minute documentary by San Francisco State professor Vivian Chávez, August 9, 2012. https://www.youtube.com/watch?v=SaSHLbS1V4w&t=689s. Accessed 28 Feb 2021.

NMDOH, Covid-19 epidemiology reports, New Mexico Covid-19 Cases Update, Demographics. https://cv.nmhealth.org/epidemiology-reports/. Accessed 10 Feb 2021.

Arizona Department of Health Services, data dashboard, demographics/COVID-19 deaths. https://www.azdhs.gov/preparedness/epidemiology-disease-control/infectious-disease-epidemiology/covid-19/dashboards/index.php. Accessed 10 Feb 2021.

youtube.com, Navajo traditional teachings. https://www.youtube.com/c/NavajoTraditionalTeachings/videos. Accessed 1 Mar 2021.

Erica Bennett is a pediatric otolaryngologist who has practiced at the University of New Mexico for the past 15 years and has had the privilege of getting to know and caring for many families, including those from the Navajo Nation and surrounding tribes.

Ethan Paddock is a member of the Navajo Nation who graduated from the University of South Dakota Sanford School of Medicine and is an Otolaryngology-Head and Neck Surgery resident at the University of New Mexico. He has ambitions to serve a Native American community in the future.

Chapter 21
Surgery on the Incarcerated Patient

Todd D. Beyer and Megan K. Applewhite ⓘ

Abstract There are 2.3 million people incarcerated in the United States prison system, and there is very little information known about their healthcare as it relates to surgery. The incarcerated patient experiences and physicians witness delays in care, barriers to delivery of the standard of care. There are significant challenges to studying outcomes in this vulnerable population, which is disproportionately made up of racial and ethnic minorities. Here, we take a detailed look into each of these topics and expand on literature-based descriptions and the authors experiences to provide a comprehensive overview of care of the incarcerated surgical patient. As physicians and surgeons, it is our ethical obligation to better understand opportunities for improvement in access to care, provide equivalent operations and postoperative attention, as well as strive for robust data collection to prove equivalent excellent outcomes in the incarcerated population.

Keywords Incarcerated patients · Surgery on inmates · Surgery in vulnerable populations · Barriers to care of inmates · Implicit bias

T. D. Beyer
Department of Surgery, Albany Medical College, Albany, NY, USA
e-mail: beyert@amc.edu

M. K. Applewhite (✉)
Department of Surgery, Alden March Bioethics Institute, Albany Medical College, Albany, NY, USA
e-mail: applewm@amc.edu

© The Author(s), under exclusive license to Springer Nature Switzerland AG 2022

V. A. Lonchyna et al. (eds.), *Difficult Decisions in Surgical Ethics*, Difficult Decisions in Surgery: An Evidence-Based Approach, https://doi.org/10.1007/978-3-030-84625-1_21

305

Case
A 45-year-old male inmate presented to the surgery clinic with a five-year history of symptomatic cholelithiasis manifested with intermittent biliary colic. His pain typically lasted about 20 min following ingestion of fatty food, but he had several occasions of prolonged pain associated with low grade temperatures, which resolved within 36 h. Including his current several hour-long unrelenting episodes of pain, he had been managed by the infirmary physician and had never been to the hospital. He had mild essential hypertension well-controlled on single agent therapy. His past medical, surgical, and family history were unremarkable. Following an outpatient surgical consultation, he underwent elective laparoscopic cholecystectomy and was admitted for pain management, given the complexity of the case with significant inflammation and involvement of surrounding structures from previous episodes of acute cholecystitis.

21.1   Introduction

There are 2.3 million people incarcerated in the United States prison system, with racial and ethnic minorities being disproportionately represented. Black Americans make up 13% of the United States population, but make up 40% of adults in U.S. jails, state, and federal prisons as opposed to white Americans, who make up 64% of the U.S. population and just 39% of the incarcerated population [1]. Because of mandatory minimum times of many prison sentences, the number of individuals who will require medical and surgical care during their time in prison is significant. One out of every eight people will undergo surgery during the time they are incarcerated in the U.S. prison system [2, 3].

Aside from this datum out of the Bureau of Justice Statistics, very little is known about the surgical care of these individuals, including their indications for surgery, their operations, any variation in care during their surgeries, and, most importantly, their outcomes [4]. In the 2003 landmark Institute of Medicine Report, *Unequal Treatment*, it was found that racial and ethnic minorities receive lower quality healthcare even when controlling for access-related factors such as insurance status and income [5]. Therefore, in addition to being vulnerable due to their incarceration, the known discrepancies in care experienced by ethnic minorities compounds the potential for substandard care in this patient population.

Critical to rectifying this discrepancy in healthcare is admitting that the chasm exists, identifying systematic ways to remove barriers to care, and empowering surgeons to collect and publish outcomes data. These steps will ensure outcomes equivalent to those in the general population.

21.2   Search Strategy

A literature search was performed in PubMed; a review of the Bureau of Justice Statistics was completed to gather data on individuals who had surgery while incarcerated. The focus of data collection was: indications for and outcomes of surgery, ethical challenges in studying the inmate population, and barriers encountered in the perioperative period. Keywords included but were not limited to: "incarcerated patients", "surgery on inmates", "surgery incarcerated patients", "surgical outcomes in incarcerated patients" "surgical outcomes inmates", "surgery in vulnerable populations", and "barriers to care of inmates." Due to the paucity of data, there was no limitation to years of the search.

21.3   Discussion

21.3.1   Paucity of Data in a Large Population

In 2016, the United States held 21% of the world's prisoners while only 4.4% of the world's population [6, 7]. With greater than two million people incarcerated in the United States prison system, and the long duration of sentences, not only do chronic medical health problems precipitate during incarceration, but surgical problems do also. Exactly what surgical problems inmates incur is not known. Inmates are not included in any national surgical databases [4] and securing data at the individual hospital level is dependent on an institutional review board that would see value in the research for this population, as well as a high enough census of incarcerated patients having surgery to be able to power a study.

Obtaining primary data at the level of the infirmary, the initial presentation, and an understanding of the disease progression is challenging. In contrast, there is a body of literature addressing the topics of palliative, hospice, and end of life care in the incarcerated patient population. Here, the risk of isolation has a significant impact. McParland and Johnston examined 23 studies and identified the importance of relationships between providers and inmates near end of life, the value of hospice volunteers, and the counter-productiveness of the prison environment toward end-of-life goals [8].

Inmates are a vulnerable population for research due to historic abusive research practices that exploited these individuals in reprehensible ways. The Terre Haute Prison Experiments were conducted at the U.S. Penitentiary in Terre Haute, Indiana in 1943 and 1944 under the direction of the Venereal Disease Research Laboratory of the US Public Health Service. The objective was to determine the effectiveness of treatments for sexually transmitted diseases in order to be able to minimize the impact on infected U.S. military personnel during World War II. After volunteering, inmates were intentionally infected with *Neisseria gonorrhoeae*. Consent was obtained to participate in the study, however, intentionally inflicting disease in a vulnerable population in exchange for $100, a certificate of merit, and a letter of commendation for the parole board following their participation is a breach of ethics in medical research [9].

Another study done at the Rankin Farm prison in Mississippi promised to pardon inmates in exchange for experimenting on them by inducing the disease pellagra. Following "successful" contraction of the disease, the subjects were pardoned by the Governor. One inmate said he had been through "a thousand hells" and another said he would choose a "lifetime of hard labor" rather than go through such a "hellish experiment" again [10, 11]. These exploitations and others dictate the need for stringent protections for inmates when it comes to research.

Due to the added regulatory standards that need to be satisfied in order to proceed with even retrospective data analysis in the inmate population, surgical outcomes studies are very sparse. Not having any knowledge of the surgical problems inevitable to arise in this vulnerable population makes them even more vulnerable, as surgeons lack the data to know if any systems barriers, implicit bias, or structural limitations are affecting the healthcare and surgical care of inmate patients.

21.3.2 Altered Preoperative Care

In the preoperative period, from the initial symptom manifestation to the day of surgery, there are increased security measures imposed by local, regional, and state policies that are intended to protect the safety of both the hospital workers and the incarcerated patients that make caring for these individuals challenging. In our institution, inmates are transported to specialty surgeon clinics accompanied by at least two corrections officers, who are present in the room throughout the visit. While this is meant to protect all involved, it also limits the privacy of the patient encounter and impairs the surgeon-patient relationship. When an operative problem is confirmed, surgery is scheduled through a process that is subject to more regulatory protocols than standard operating room scheduling. Therefore, the patient is frequently not operated on as expeditiously as compared to the general population, and as a general rule, is not allowed to know the date or time of the next hospital appointment or even the operative date. A qualitative study from London described:

> (F)ive experiences that challenged the 'equivalence of care' for prisoners: security overriding healthcare need or experience, security creating public humiliation and fear, difficulties relating to prison officer's role in medical consultation, delayed access due to prison regime and transport requirements, and restricted (nay, nonexistent) patient autonomy in the management of their own healthcare [12].

In this study, incarcerated patients just accepted a lower standard of care, recognizing they had compromised independence with regard to their healthcare and inability to book their own appointments. The participants in the study also found that physicians would address the correctional officers about the health of patients rather than the patient directly. An individual was going to have surgery and the physician asked the corrections officers about preference for anesthesia type, rather than the patient himself. This idea of loss of autonomy, or compromise of autonomy is one that is especially concerning.

21.3.3 Disease Severity

The challenge of understanding the unique differences that occur in the surgical care of hospitalized inmates is directly related to the lack of quality studies and objective data. It has been well demonstrated in the medical literature that incarcerated patients when compared to non-incarcerated patients suffer from higher rates of hypertension, asthma, arthritis, hepatitis after adjusting for age, sex, race, education, employment, marital status, birth country, and alcohol consumption [13]. Such knowledge about surgical disease severity is unknown.

There are unique environmental factors imposed by living in a prison that may predispose inmates to specific problems. Living in an environment of fear and violence can lead to development of a hypervigilant state. It is known that inmates have a higher prevalence of Post-Traumatic Stress Disorder (PTSD) [14], which, in animal models were found to exhibit a state of immune modulation. These animal models with PTSD were found to have elevated pro-inflammatory cytokines (IFN-γ, IL-6, TNF-α, IL-17), immune stimulatory Th1 and inflammatory Th17 cells [15]. Further studies in Marines found that those with elevated CRP before deployment were predictive of PTSD following deployment, suggesting inflammation may predispose to PTSD [16]. Increased autoimmune disease severity have been anecdotally reported in the inmate patient population. Interspecialty discussions with gastroenterology and endocrine surgery at our tertiary care center, where we care for a large volume of inmate patients, have suggested severe biochemical and symptomatic Graves' disease and inflammatory bowel disease relative to patients in the general population. Prospective research is necessary to prove this anecdotal difference is real, but the importance of identifying elevated risk and more advanced disease is of ethical and clinical importance to this vulnerable group of patients.

21.3.4 Implicit Bias

Incarcerated inpatients are faced with unique barriers to their care that are multifactorial and not encountered by their general population counterparts. One such barrier is implicit bias or having a negative preconceived notion or prejudice of individuals without knowing them. In this case, individuals participating in the care of inmates may have implicit bias against these patients solely because of their incarcerated status.

Hospital employees face combinations of fear and implicit bias when caring for inmates despite the precautions taken for safety and security. In some states, the incarceration history for inmates is public information easily obtained from the internet. Such information includes the reason for conviction, sentence duration, and incidence of repeat offenses. With this available information, the patient's character, morality, and behavior now become a part of their known history and introduces the risk of false assumptions and biases by their healthcare providers. There is data to show that those patients with a criminal record who have recently been released from prison experience discrimination by healthcare workers that may impact healthcare utilization [17], but similar studies in those who are currently incarcerated have yet to be done, based on our literature review. One can imagine, however, that knowledge of criminal history can foster provider fear or mistrust of their patient. However, even without that information, providers may fear for their personal safety when caring for inmates, which can consciously or unconsciously influence their care. It can affect the amount of time the provider spends with the patient, their level of communication with the patient, and/or thoroughness of their history and examination.

Inappropriate and unfounded assumptions made projecting the incarcerated patient's desire not to return to prison post-discharge, educational level, knowledge base of disease and treatment, drug-seeking behavior, tendency for malingering, ulterior motives, or desire to seek care can all affect care, and have no role in the ethical and moral treatment of these individuals. Similar concerns have arisen in studies that examine the delivery of inpatient healthcare to other isolated and vulnerable patient groups, most commonly the mentally ill [18]. If implicit bias is present in medical professionals and trainees who care for patients with mental illness, it may even affect whether psychiatric patients receive certain surgical procedures in addition to their outcomes [19]. In addition to implicit bias, overt prejudice and systemic racism compounds these barriers to care and addressing these deficiencies with implicit bias training is a reasonable place to start on the individual institutional level to achieve equity of healthcare delivery.

21.3.5 Mistrust of the Hospital System

Just as providers may harbor distrust of their incarcerated patient, the patients themselves may possess distrust of their caretakers or the healthcare system in general, a problem that compromises the very essence of the doctor-patient relationship. Why is there mistrust? The life of an incarcerated individual is one without control and with few rights. Inmates can view their right to healthcare as an opportunity to take back some control. They are less often presented with alternatives in healthcare and can view their relationship with their surgeon as a power struggle or confrontation. They fear that their personal health and life will not be held to the same standard and value by medical staff as the lives of non-inmate patients and that as a result their care will be sub-optimal or compromised. Mistrust is further fueled by less contact with their providers and sub-optimal communication [20].

The incarcerated patient population is found less likely to be adherent to recommended medications and medical interventions, partly thought to be due to mistrust of the healthcare system. Cuthbertson, in a study of inmates in Canada, utilized the Trust in Physician Scale as well as a survey of support (Medical Outcomes Study Social Support Survey) to evaluate factors that may contribute to ineffective medical care delivery to the incarcerated patient population [21]. They found that mistrust of physicians among inmates is a common finding, which negatively influences adherence to medication, and that inmate patients experience high rates of lack of social and emotional support throughout treatment for health problems. Inmates seek providers who treat them with respect, are good listeners, and display understanding, just as patients in the general population do.

21.3.6 Modified Policies and Procedures

Policies and procedures implemented by departments of corrections and hospital institutions are meant to maximize the safety of all personnel and the security of the inmates themselves. Such policies exercise control over their hospital stays in a way that can be like prison itself. By design, they also remove personal autonomy. They affect everything from time out of bed, time out of their room, access to other departments within the hospital, access to providers, access to visitors, and knowledge of their care: surgery date, medications, discharge instructions, disposition, and discharge date. These policies and procedures do uniquely impact patient care and its delivery while in the hospital in numerous ways.

While these safety measures certainly have a role to play, one particular point arises in the care of the incarcerated surgical patient, that of being shackled to the operating room table. Concerns for attempted escape or unpredictable behavior that may exist outside of the operating room are extraordinarily unlikely to happen after a general anesthetic is induced, however these restraints are frequently left in place unless the surgeon explicitly asks for them to be removed. Removing the shackles during operations is a humane and compassionate thing to do and honors the trust that the patient puts into the surgeon [22].

It is well established that early ambulation improves postoperative outcomes and is an integral part of recovery pathways. Ambulation reduces the risk of deep venous thrombotic events [23], contributes to reduced time to return of bowel function [24], minimizes atelectasis [25], shortens hospital stay [26], and provides a means of assessment of post-discharge physical therapy needs. Incarcerated patients are faced with barriers to ambulation. In most hospitals, they are shackled to their beds, reside in a locked unit, and/or require corrections officers to ambulate outside of their rooms. This loss of autonomy and ad lib ambulation undoubtedly results in less early ambulation and a risk of unnecessarily poor postoperative outcomes.

The isolation of inmates while in the hospital is a very real phenomenon. Whether they are housed in a secured unit away from the general population or simply integrated in a regular room, yet guarded continuously, the inmate patient is at risk of being physically or functionally isolated from the rest of the hospital and its services. Even if the care of an inmate is not altered in a conscious or deliberate way, inequalities in hospital care do exist, and the onus is on us as a medical society to study and identify potential inequalities based on objective data.

An example of inequality in care is the delivery of inpatient physical and occupational therapy. A patient's physical independence and postoperative needs can not only dictate their timeliness to discharge but also their required resources outside of the hospital. The involvement of physical therapy in a patient's postoperative care not only hastens physical recovery, but also provides a means of critical assessment. Incarcerated inpatients have less access to physical therapy services and expertise. The reasons include the physical barrier that occurs from being in a locked unit, the availability of officers to accompany them to the therapy sessions, and the under-recognized fear of personal safety from the therapists themselves.

Bedside nurses face a set of unique challenges that affect their ability to establish the same type of relationship with the patient if they were not under guard [27]. Nurses have a very close relationship with their patients and are their biggest advocates and motivators to maintain optimism and to progress perioperatively. At the time of surgery, when many patients benefit from frequent attention, the presence of correctional officers, limited mobility of the patient, and potential safety concerns may limit this relationship. The care nurses deliver must overcome the limitations intended for security and barriers encountered, but this requires a cognitive shift in the way that this patient population is viewed and accessed.

The companionship, support, encouragement, improved communication, and advocacy that comes from family members or loved ones at the bedside cannot be under-valued. In most institutions, visits for inmate patients from family or friends are forbidden to maintain security. The isolation that results further impacts inmate patients during a time when they are most vulnerable. If inmates are allowed visits while at the jail or prison, why cannot similar precautions be made to allow visits while in the hospital? The significance of a lack of family presence becomes most evident during times when surrogate decision making is required, such as hospice or end of life care.

21.4 Case Conclusion

This was a technically challenging case given multiple previous episodes of acute cholecystitis, so it took about twice the time of a normal laparoscopic cholecystectomy. Postoperatively, standard mechanical venous thromboembolic prophylaxis was used. The secured unit was at capacity, so he was admitted to the general population floor, which resulted in the need to be restrained to the bed in his room and required a corrections officer and ankle as well as wrist shackles when ambulating. He stayed an extra day for pain control.

On postoperative day two, he was found to be intermittently febrile with temperatures in excess of 102° F. Laboratory studies showed no leukocytosis and normal liver function. His chest x-ray showed no infiltrates or consolidation. Urine analysis, urine culture, and blood culture were all negative, and his wounds were unremarkable. On postoperative day four, with continuing fevers, a lower extremity duplex was performed, which revealed an acute occlusive right sided deep thrombosis of the popliteal vein for which he was started on IV heparin. He was ultimately discharged back to prison on Coumadin and was seen in the postoperative clinic doing well with no concerns. The pathology revealed chronic inflammation of the gallbladder.

21.5 Concluding Remarks

Care of the surgical patient varies dramatically when that individual is incarcerated. Due to a lack of data on surgical indications, disease severity and operative outcomes, the surgical community has a very limited understanding of what problems these individuals face, and how to optimize outcomes. Incarcerated patients have limited autonomy with respect to their operative dates, medications, and postoperative care, which has been found to foster a mistrust with the healthcare system. Policies in place to protect the hospital workers, other inpatients, the greater community, and the patients themselves, impose barriers to optimal care, and should be addressed and discussed to maintain safety but minimize variation in care. Given the overrepresentation of Black Americans in the incarcerated patient population, implicit biases, prejudice, and racism that predisposes them to lower quality healthcare for reasons related to race are compounded by the discrepancies they experience due to being incarcerated. We have a moral and ethical obligation to study, identify, address, and improve the inequities in surgical and medical care of inmates, and failure to do so propagates ongoing vulnerability in this patient population.

21.6 Selected References

- Scarlet S, Meyer AA, Dreesen EB. Lack of information on surgical care for incarcerated persons. JAMA Surg. 2018;153(6):503–4. https://doi.org/10.1001/jamasurg.2018.0314

  – Despite the prevalence of surgical care within the incarcerated patient population, this paper highlights the clear void and need that exists within medical literature regarding surgical outcomes of incarcerated patients.

- Binswanger IA, Krueger PM, Steiner JF. Prevalence of chronic medical conditions among jail and prison inmates in the USA compared with the general population. J Epidemiol Community Health. 2009;63(11):912–9. https://doi.org/10.1136/jech.2009.090662

- – This paper highlights that the prison environment is unique and suggests a causative relationship with disease pathophysiology, severity, and prevalence despite adjustment for demographic differences.

- Scarlet S, Dreesen E. Surgery in shackles: what are surgeons' obligations to incarcerated patients in the operating room? AMA J Ethics. 2017;19(9):939–46. https://doi.org/10.1001/journalofethics.2017.19.9.pfor1-1709

  - – This article emphasizes the idea that procedural measures for safety and security must not compromise the privacy, autonomy, and trust of the incarcerated patient.

References

1. Sakala L. Breaking down mass incarceration in the 2010 census: state-by-state incarceration rates by race/ethnicity. Prison Policy Initiative. May 28, 2014. https://www.prisonpolicy.org/reports/rates.html. Accessed 11 Jan 2021.
2. Kaeble D, Lauren G. Correctional populations in the United States, 2015. Washington, DC: US Dept of Justice, Bureau of Justice Statistics; December 2016. NCJ 250374. https://www.bjs.gov/content/pub/pdf/cpus15.pdf. Accessed 5 Nov 2020.
3. Maruschak L. Medical problems of prisoners. In: Bureau of Justice Statistics. US Department of Justice; 2008. https://www.prisonpolicy.org/scans/bjs/mpp.pdf. Accessed 5 Nov 2020.
4. Scarlet S, Meyer AA, Dreesen EB. Lack of information on surgical care for incarcerated persons. JAMA Surg. 2018;153(6):503–4. https://doi.org/10.1001/jamasurg.2018.0314.
5. Institute of Medicine (US) Committee on Understanding and Eliminating Racial and Ethnic Disparities in Health Care, Smedley BD, Stith AY, Nelson AR, editors. Unequal treatment: confronting racial and ethnic disparities in health care. National Academies Press; 2003.
6. United Nations Department of Economic and Social Affairs. The world population prospects: 2015 revision. United Nations; 2015.
7. Kaeble D, Glaze LE. Bureau of justice statistics. Correctional populations in the United States, 2015. Published December 29, 2016. https://www.bjs.gov/index.cfm?ty=pbdetail&iid=5870. Accessed 5 Nov 2020.
8. McParland C, Johnston BM. Palliative and end of life care in prisons: a mixed-methods rapid review of the literature from 2014–2018. BMJ Open. 2019;9:e033905. https://doi.org/10.1136/bmjopen-2019-033905.
9. Presidential Commission for the Study of Bioethical Issues. "Ethically impossible" STD research in Guatemala from 1946 to 1948. September 2011. https://bioethicsarchive.georgetown.edu/pcsbi/sites/default/files/Ethically%20Impossible%20(with%20linked%20historical%20documents)%202.7.13.pdf. Accessed 11 Jan 2021.
10. Hornblum AM. They were cheap and available: prisoners as research subjects in twentieth century America. BMJ. 1997;315(7120):1437–41. https://doi.org/10.1136/bmj.315.7120.1437.
11. Etheridge EW. The butterfly caste. Greenwood Press; 1972. p. 7.
12. Edge C, Stockley R, Swabey L, et al. Secondary care clinicians and staff have a key role in delivering equivalence of care for prisoners: a qualitative study of prisoners' experiences. EClinicalMedicine. 2020;24:100416. https://doi.org/10.1016/j.eclinm.2020.100416.
13. Binswanger IA, Krueger PM, Steiner JF. Prevalence of chronic medical conditions among jail and prison inmates in the USA compared with the general population. J Epidemiol Community Health. 2009;63(11):912–9. https://doi.org/10.1136/jech.2009.090662.

14. Facer-Irwin E, Blackwood NJ, Bird A, et al. PTSD in prison settings: a systematic review and meta-analysis of comorbid mental disorders and problematic behaviours. PLoS One. 2019;14(9):e0222407. https://doi.org/10.1371/journal.pone.0222407.
15. Wang Z, Caughron B, Young MRI. Posttraumatic stress disorder: an immunological disorder? Front Psych. 2017;8:222. https://doi.org/10.3389/fpsyt.2017.00222.
16. Eraly SA, Nievergelt CM, Maihofer AX, et al. Assessment of plasma C-reactive protein as a biomarker of posttraumatic stress disorder risk. JAMA Psychiat. 2014;71(4):423–31. https://doi.org/10.1001/jamapsychiatry.2013.4374.
17. Frank JW, Wang EA, Nunez-Smith M, Lee H, Comfort M. Discrimination based on criminal record and healthcare utilization among men recently released from prison: a descriptive study. Health Justice. 2014;2:6. https://doi.org/10.1186/2194-7899-2-6.
18. Kopera M, Suszek H, Bonar E, et al. Evaluating explicit and implicit stigma of mental illness in mental health professionals and medical students. Community Ment Health J. 2015;51(5):628–34. https://doi.org/10.1007/s10597-014-9796-6.
19. Li Y, Cai X, Du H, et al. Mentally ill medicare patients less likely than others to receive certain types of surgery. Health Aff. 2011;30(7):1307–15. https://doi.org/10.1377/hlthaff.2010.1084.
20. Feron JM, Tan LH, Pestiaux D, Lorant V. High and variable use of primary care in prison. A qualitative study to understand help-seeking behaviour. Int J Prison Health. 2008;4(3):146–55. https://doi.org/10.1080/17449200802264696.
21. Cuthbertson L, Kowalewski K, Edge J, Courtney K. Factors that promote and hinder medication adherence from the perspective of inmates in a provincial remand center: a mixed methods study. J Correct Health Care. 2018;24(1):21–34. https://doi.org/10.1177/1078345817745613.
22. Scarlet S, Dreesen E. Surgery in shackles: what are surgeons' obligations to incarcerated patients in the operating room? AMA J Ethics. 2017;19(9):939–46. https://doi.org/10.1001/journalofethics.2017.19.9.pfor1-1709.
23. Geerts WH, Pineo GF, Heit JA, et al. Prevention of venous thromboembolism: the Seventh ACCP Conference on Antithrombotic and Thrombolytic Therapy. Chest. 2004;126(3 Suppl):S338–400. https://doi.org/10.1378/chest.126.3_suppl.3385.
24. Lubawski J, Saclarides T. Postoperative ileus: strategies for reduction. Ther Clin Risk Manag. 2008;4(5):913–7. https://doi.org/10.2147/tcrm.s2390.
25. Moradian ST, Najafloo M, Mahmoudi H, Ghiasi MS. Early mobilization reduces the atelectasis and pleural effusion in patients undergoing coronary artery bypass graft surgery: a randomized clinical trial. J Vasc Nurs. 2017;35(3):141–5. https://doi.org/10.1016/j.jvn.2017.02.001.
26. Fisher SR, Kuo YF, Graham JE, Ottenbacher KJ, Ostir GV. Early ambulation and length of stay in older adults hospitalized for acute illness [letter]. Arch Intern Med. 2010;170(21):1942–3. https://doi.org/10.1001/archinternmed.2010.422.
27. Weiskopf CS. Nurses' experience of caring for inmate patients. J Adv Nurs. 2005;49(4):336–43. https://doi.org/10.1111/j.1365-2648.2004.03297.x.

Part VI
Surgical Dilemmas in the Adult Patient

Chapter 22
Surgical Buy-In for Major Operations

Sean C. Wightman ⓘ

Abstract Deep review on the ethics of surgical buy-in and how this conversation, and unwritten contract, frames the informed consent conversation and reveals patients' goals and desires during their post-operative recovery. This chapter looks at the beginning of buy-in, why surgeons seek buy-in, the surgeon's covenant, how patients perceive buy-in, the ethics of buy-in, a postoperative caveat, the conflict around buy-in, a surgeon's time, cashing out, and the solution.

Keywords Ethics · Surgery · Informed consent · Surgical buy-in · Patient autonomy · Surgical consent

Case

A 68-year-old male with a new diagnosis of an advanced, but potentially surgically resectable, esophageal cancer also has known chronic kidney disease. While the patient had some response to neoadjuvant chemoradiotherapy, the patient is reluctant to undergo surgery due to the possible complications. The patient previously decided that he is not interested in pursuing dialysis if ever needed for his own impending kidney failure as the patient had a family member with end-stage kidney disease and dependence on dialysis with a bad experience.

S. C. Wightman (✉)
Division of Thoracic Surgery, Keck School of Medicine, University of Southern California, Los Angeles, CA, USA
e-mail: sean.wightman@med.usc.edu

© The Author(s), under exclusive license to Springer Nature
Switzerland AG 2022

V. A. Lonchyna et al. (eds.), *Difficult Decisions in Surgical Ethics*, Difficult
Decisions in Surgery: An Evidence-Based Approach,
https://doi.org/10.1007/978-3-030-84625-1_22

22.1   Introduction

Embarking on a major operation is a huge endeavor and demands commitment from both the patient and surgeon. Together they make critical decisions in the time before and after an operation. When agreeing to move forward with a major operation, both patients and surgeons contribute a level of dedication to the surgical process and postoperative recovery. While the surgical consent is written out on paper, this commitment to the postoperative recovery—between patient and surgeon—is an unwritten contract. Patients hold a broad range of preferences for post-operative care. Surgical buy-in is an informal commitment between the surgeon and patient where the patient agrees to not only the major operation, but also to the postoperative recovery and any life supported measures necessary.

This chapter will discuss the key areas pertaining to buy-in including the beginning of buy-in, why surgeons seek buy-in, the surgeon's covenant, how patients perceive buy-in, the ethics of buy-in, a postoperative caveat, the conflict around buy-in, a surgeon's time, cashing out, and the solution (see Table 22.1).

22.2   Search Strategy

Using PubMed, papers pertaining to informed consent and surgical buy-in were searched dating back to 2000. Twelve pertinent papers were selected and utilized to review the topic of surgical buy-in for major operations.

22.3   Discussion

22.3.1   The Beginning of Buy-In

The concept of surgical buy-in came about as surgeons were noticed to hesitate to withdraw any needed support for their patients postoperatively. This reluctance even withstood a patient's specific request for support cessation [1]. It was theorized that

Table 22.1 Terminology

Cashing out	The refusal of treatment after a change in values when an initial agreement (buy-in) to continue post-operative care previously existed
Informed consent	Permission for an intervention or treatment after a patient is aware of the risks and potential benefits
Surgeon's covenant	Surgeon commits more than a technical service and agrees to sharing of both the hope and risk of an operation
Surgical buy-in	An informal commitment between the surgeon and patient where the patient agrees to not only the major operation, but also to the postoperative recovery and any life supported measures necessary

the innate characteristic of surgeons to press ahead mandated a forward fight without concession. Due to these notions, in 2010, Schwarze et al. were able to define and further develop the concept of surgical buy-in using in-person interviews [1]. The interviews were conducted after reading two scenarios. One in which surrogates requested withdrawal of life support with a patient unable to participate and a second scenario of a patient with a preoperative advanced directive stating to withdraw prolonged life support [1]. When reviewing the responses, surgeons agreed that discussing the postoperative care was an important part of the informed consent process. Surgeons felt, in general, that these led to a patient-doctor contract—a package deal—that went along with the agreed upon operation [1]. When interviewed, many surgeons felt that getting the patient through the postoperative period was just as important as getting the patient through the operation [1].

Surgical buy-in, an informal contract between patient and surgeon, is completely undocumented. Even if it was written however, like a surgical consent, it could be revoked or changed by the patient or the patient's surrogate at any time. Surgeons were open to negotiate on postoperative care based on patients' preferences, but some areas were non-negotiable depending on the clinical scenario. Surgeons also seemed to have a defined period of time, dependent upon the clinical situation, that a patient must continue postoperative life sustaining interventions [1].

When the interviews were analyzed, it appeared that there were some clear *contributors* to surgeon buy-in (see Table 22.2) [1]. The contributors included the surgeon's responsibility for bad outcomes, the emotional toll of unanticipated outcomes, and the expectation of operative success [1]. Surgeons feel personally responsible for adverse outcomes. Charles Bosk's book, *Forgive and Remember*, articulates how death and complications are handled different across specialties [2]. He states that "when a patient of an internist dies, the natural question his colleagues ask is 'What happened?' When a patient of a surgeon dies his colleagues ask, 'What did you do?'" This statement simply demonstrates that surgeons, by nature, are more personally accountable for the operative and postoperative outcomes. The idea described by Bosk still carries true weekly in medical centers across the world. This theme is actively coached at morbidity and mortality conference by questioning, "what would you have done differently?" [3]. It is taught that a surgeon should feel personal responsibility for surgical outcomes. Surgeons have a sense of responsibility when the expected postoperative outcomes are not achieved; especially if the surgery performed is elective. When an operation is an emergency, complications are more often contributed to the initial insult and the inherent need for the

Table 22.2 Contributors to the surgeon's need for buy-in and consequences of surgeon adherence to buy-in (based on Schwarze [1])

Contributors	Consequences
Responsibility	Decline to operate
Emotional toll	Refuse to withdraw
Expected Success	Negotiate care
	Shift responsibility to patient

operation rather than the performance of the operation itself. The emotional cost causes surgeons to continue to strive for an improved outcome after surgery even if it means enforcing prolonged life support. So, the goal of doing everything may be a defense to avoid an inevitable poor outcome [2].

Similarly, there were also *consequences* of surgeon buy-in discovered in the responses (see Table 22.2) [1]. These consequences were that surgeons declined to operate, refused to withdraw life-sustaining treatment, negotiated postoperative care, and shifted responsibility of poor outcomes to the patient. If patients did not agree preoperatively to certain requirements of postoperative care, for example dialysis, then some surgeons decided not to offer surgery [4]. Surgeons would also refuse to permit withdrawal of care after surgery as they thought some "bumps in the road" should be endured [1]. Furthermore, if surrogates wanted to enact an advance directive limiting postoperative support, surgeons would push back if they thought there was a chance of success [1]. Finally, if a patient wanted to limit postoperative therapy, surgeons often would support the request but then shift ownership and responsibility of subsequent poor outcomes back onto the patient or surrogate.

22.3.2 Why Surgeons Seek Buy-In

Surgeons seek buy-in for various reasons including a pressure to have operative success. Operative success is not judged based on the operating room alone but translates into the patient succeeding postoperatively. To surgeons, a concession on life-sustaining measures could be interpreted as admitting defeat [1].

Surgeons are naturally optimistic. Surgeons believe, at the onset of an operation, that they can see the patient through to recovery. If even remote success was not possible, surgeons would not burden themselves with carrying the patient to the operation and through to the other side. Surgeons are aware that patients are counting and depending on them for surgical success. A rapid road to death after surgery cheats a patient of life they would have otherwise had [5]. So, if a surgeon is going to invest literal blood, sweat, and tears into a patient's major operation and postoperative recovery, a surgeon desires mutual commitment and investment from the patient. In an extreme sense, no surgeon wants to knowingly participate in a patient's demise. And life support cessation, when recovering from a major operation, would normally hasten the patient's death.

When people think about an impending surgery, most people appropriately first consider the patient [3]. But the investment of a surgeon into a complex major operation should not go unnoticed [3]. No surgeon wants to invest and then have the patient quit in defeat in the early post-operative period. Because buy-in is not a literal contract, this scenario may never be able to be completely avoided, but with appropriate preoperative buy-in and outlining the expectations, it can be mitigated. Just as a patient can revoke informed consent at any time, so too can a patient's desire to continue aggressive postoperative care be revoked.

Schwarze et al. used surveys to tease out surgeons' goals when acquiring buy-in. Surgeons rely on buy-in to the point where they are willing to negotiate for it before the surgery. 60% of surgeons noted they would sometimes or always refuse to operate on a patient if the patient requested to limit supportive measures after surgery [4]. If agreed upon postoperative limitations were noted, 20% of surgeons would go as far as to document this contractually in the medical record [4].

It is known that some specialties have publicly reported outcome metrics. Half of the surgeons surveyed felt that outcome metrics weighed in on the need to obtain buy-in. Those surgeons who valued these same outcome metrics were more likely to refuse to operate on a patient who wanted to limit postoperative life sustaining measures as it may adversely affect the reportable metrics [4]. Surgeons who performed higher risk operations were more than twice as likely to intentionally discuss and obtain surgical buy-in [4]. Surgeons who thought patients could rightfully choose to decline life sustaining interventions after a major operation were more likely to clearly obtain an informal contract preoperatively to avoid this conflict scenario [4]. These findings emphasize the surgeon's recognition of a need for a greater commitment by the patients undergoing major operations.

Surgeons seek buy-in to protect the indicated interventions of the postoperative period required to see the patient through a successful recovery. Surgeons want to obtain buy-in to successfully ensure patients are not going to be contradictory; commit to a major operation, but not tolerate less burdensome interventions [4].

22.3.3   The Surgeon's Covenant

While surgeons may ask patients to agree to surgical buy-in, they are also providing an agreement on the surgeon-side, the covenant. This covenant, briefly described by Buchman et al., identifies that the surgeon is committing more than a technical service [6]. In this way, the surgeon shares with the patient both the hope and risk of the operation and hospital course [6]. Although initially stated by Buchman et al., this covenant is more than what was described. The surgeon's commitment to their patients, like the patient's buy-in, is similarly unwritten. A surgeon would not offer an operation unless the surgeon is truly convinced the patient can reasonably recover. Surgeons plan their personal lives, holidays, and vacations around major operations to ensure they are able to see their patients through to recovery on the other side. This covenant makes it hard for surgeons to divert from the final goal of the expected successful intended outcome. Buchman et al. state that "the surgeon is ideally trained to organize and sustain the rescue attempt… [but] poorly positioned to abort the rescue attempt when it has failed [6]." It takes time, reflection, and living the postoperative course alongside a patient to understand a specific patient may not achieve the initially anticipated postoperative success. The willingness for a surgeon to agree to the withdrawal of life sustaining measures may be inversely correlated to both the time the surgeon has known the patient and the responsibility the surgeon feels for the patient's current postoperative decline (see Fig. 22.1) [6]. As it already takes time and reflection to realize the operative and postoperative goals may need to change due to adverse events, it likely takes even longer for a surgeon to consider initiating an end-of-life conversation. Surgeons seek buy-in because

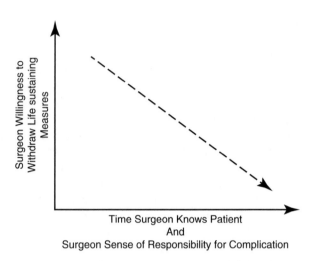

Fig. 22.1 The willingness for a surgeon to agree to withdrawal of life sustaining measures [6]

they are already similarly agreeing to the unwritten surgical covenant for each major operation they perform, and they similarly want to know the patient is committed.

22.3.4 How Patients Perceive Buy-In

Many patients do not understand the large complication profile which accompanies major operations. Patients lean on their medical teams, largely their surgeons, to navigate these grave but potentially reversible complications [7]. Due to trust in their surgeon, many patients rely on the surgeon to work through the postoperative period paternalistically with the patient's best interest in mind. Without the written formalization of buy-in, much of buy-in from the patient's perspective is simply reliance on the surgeon. Ruske et al. looked at patients undergoing vascular surgery procedures and only 14% of those patients were truly informed after being consented for a major operation [8]. The surgeon routine of listing postoperative complications and stating the percent risk often does not translate to how complications would change a patient's life after surgery. This gap in understanding, limited by surgeons' time and patients' medical comprehension, directly impacts patients' perception of buy-in.

22.3.5 The Ethics of Buy-In

Surgeons do not want to agree to perform an operation that can weaken a patient to the point of needing prolonged recovery simply to have the patient withdraw life sustaining support; this scenario leaves the surgeon playing an active role in the

Table 22.3   The Four Boxes model integrating ethical principles [10]

Medical Indications	Patient Preferences
• Medical problem (Acute/Chronic/Emergent) • Goals of treament • Treatment options and alternatives • Likely success of treatment	• Informed of risks • Understands benefits • Patient have decisional capacity? • Preferences • Surrogates
Quality of Life	**Contextual Features**
• Baseline functionality • Current lifestyle and independence • Expected time to recovery • Possible deficits resulting from treatment	• Conflicts of interest • Personal interests • Financial incentives • Professional biases • Research conflicts • Hospital pressures

demise of the patient. That said, it is understood that a patient's values can change over time. What a patient is willing to endure before surgery may not be the same as what she or he is willing to endure immediately postoperatively. It is appropriate to apply the popular Four Boxes model which integrates the ethical principles more comprehensibly (see Table 22.3) [9, 10]. Utilizing this approach would specifically highlight Contextual Features and Patient Preferences. If a patient is not going to fully commit to the needed postoperative recovery, an argument for conservation of resources can be made. The argument is that health care resources should not be invested in a patient needing a major operation if the patient plans to abruptly stop care postoperatively. However, the argument for resources and contextual features cannot *ever* supersede a patient's personal preference and respect for a patient's autonomy. The paternalistic stance of permitting the surgeon to dictate the postoperative plan unilaterally cannot stand alone against a patient's wishes.

22.3.6   A Postoperative Caveat

A large component of obtaining surgical buy-in is to have the patient properly informed of the postoperative expectations and experience. After major surgery, some patients are not decisional. Whether it be due to hemodynamic changes, prolonged intubation, or medication side effects, patients cannot often decide what they want done in the moment after a major operation. Having surgical buy-in up front lets the patient, and surrogates, know what everyone agreed to *prior* to the operation. As said above, this does not mean that values and wishes cannot be changed, but it at least puts everyone present in agreement. Without this preoperative conversation, with both patients and surrogates, surgeons can find themselves having a very different conversation with only the surrogates *after* an operation than the one they were having with the patient *before* the operation. An unforeseen scenario after surgery with a patient who cannot make her or his own decision causes difficult and tragic decisions to fall to surrogates [2]. A surrogate has significant power over the patient during the post-operative period while the patient is not decisional. This period when patients are not able to make sound decisions for themselves underscores the importance of having surrogates present during the preoperative conversations.

Without preoperative surgeon, patient, and surrogate conversations together obtaining surgical buy-in, surrogates alone have the power to make major decisions after surgery. Often, with patients unable to speak, surrogates will permit or refuse treatments for the patient based on previous conversations they personally had with the patient. A surgical buy-in conversation, with all members present, can help pre-empt an unexpected postoperative decision by a surrogate, on a patient's behalf. This avoids surrogate reliance on substituted judgment to make these decisions and approaches a level closer to an explicitly written advance directive.

22.3.7   The Conflict around Buy-In

After surgery, if patients or their surrogates are not willing to press forward with full commitment to recovery, this can create conflict. The conflict arises because, as mentioned above, the surgeon expects a reciprocal commitment from the patient during recovery. Surgeons only agree to perform an operation if there is some level of expected success afterwards. If it was possible to know, with one-hundred percent certainty, that a surgery would be completely unsuccessful, no surgeon would perform it. It is the possibility of life altering successes that drives surgeons to hone their craft and offer this service to patients. So similarly, if a surgeon knew before an operation, that a patient would withdraw all care after an operation, it would be unlikely for a surgeon to agree to perform the operation.

Surgeons resist this abrupt life support withdrawal. To look at surgeons' willingness to withdraw life support, surgeons were provided a scenario where after a non-emergent high-risk operation, the patient's surrogate requested removal of life supporting treatment [4]. The surgeon's willingness to agree to the withdrawal of life support correlated with time. Only 6% of respondents agreed on postoperative day one, 50% by postoperative day 7, 85% by postoperative day 14, and nearly all by postoperative day 35. An abrupt change in postoperative commitment by the patient or surrogate can cause conflict between the surgeon and the patient. This conflict arises when their agreement is violated. As patients' views, desires, and perspectives can change, so can their willingness to endure complications. If and when this changes, it can put a surgeon into a place where she or he would not have ever done the initial operation. But since the surgeon *has* completed the operation, he or she believes, at some level, the patient too should complete the recovery.

At times, there is even conflict with the different hospital teams participating in the care of a patient. When a patient enters the hospital to have an operation, it is rare for any other team to have met the patient preoperatively. The only typical pre-existing physician-patient relationship for the hospital course is between the surgeon and patient. This divide can strain the relationship between the surgeon and other hospital teams when other teams are likely less invested than the surgeon and less known to the patient and surrogates. So, when non-surgical hospital teams are in support of withdrawal of life sustaining measures, this is in absence of the surgeon's context. Buchman et al. discuss this as the SICU (surgical intensive care unit) dilemma [6]. They internally debate who should manage the dying patient and agree it is difficult for the surgeon to envision and fight for anything but the intended postoperative outcome [6]. Alternatively, the intensivist, who largely plays an inpatient role and does not meet the patient preoperatively, needs to exercise caution in the role played to dismantle the agreed upon surgical buy-in as she or he was not there to obtain it initially.

22.3.8 A Surgeon's Time

Preoperative conversations take time. Informed consent for major operations takes more time. While it is understood that full and appropriate preoperative conversations require time to complete, a surgeon's time, like any healthcare provider, is limited. This is not to say that this conversation should not occur; of course, it should. But understanding that a surgeon has limited time to complete true informed consent conversations with patients plays a real part. As patients typically cannot understand when they have heard enough content to be appropriately informed, it is the responsibility of the provider to ensure that this point of adequate informed consent is reached. In the survey mentioned above by Ruske et al., patients were better informed when that conversation came from the attending surgeon [8]. This underscores that while a surgeon's time is limited, it is imperative that this conversation is not delegated to another. Furthermore, in some locations, it is illegal for a surgeon to delegate this task to another provider as they must directly provide the information to the patient [11].

A solution to a surgeon's time is repeat appointments or longer appointments to discuss surgery, but this is again not typically feasible due to a surgeon's time limitations or the acuity of the impending major surgery. It is possible to envision a scenario, with unlimited time, where patients are appropriately informed of the surgery and its postoperative expectations and complications; this is the informed consent surgeons strive to achieve. Surgeons obviously need to prioritize the time necessary to obtain appropriate informed consent; but this is confounded by the vast amount of content required to cover and convey within a surgical conversation as well as a surgeon's availability for a long preoperative conversation.

22.3.9 Cashing Out

Just as quickly as patients can buy-in before an operation, they can also cash-out afterwards [7]. Cashing-out is defined as the refusal of treatment after a change in values when an initial agreement (buy-in) to continue care existed [7]. Patients, in adherence with their respect for autonomy, can change their minds on the care they are receiving. A patient has the ability to revoke a signed consent; so too may they change the informal buy-in contract.

When addressing this issue of cashing-out after surgery, Scheiner and Liaschenko investigated why patients and families change their views. Patients may cash out after living in the postoperative period. The experience of recovering from a major operation may not be what they expected. It is often impossible to completely prepare a patient for postoperative expectations as it would take an understanding of medicine and working in that environment to truly understand. Unless the patient is a surgeon, it would be nearly impossible to obtain a truly informed consent as no dialogue would be sufficiently adequate to ensure the patient comprehends the vast risk profile and life-altering complications from this operation. The lack of true informed consent and understanding of what is expected and required after surgery may lead a patient to change what she or he is willing to undergo to recover. As stated by Scheiner and Liaschenko, "Patients may be able to imagine the experience of a complication, but this does not translate to embodied knowing of the experience [7]." Even if a patient was able to be truly informed, for example if they personally experienced a given complication previously, and even if that exact same complication returned, a patient may still cash out due to a patient's values changing over time.

Cashing out is not uniquely attached to major surgery. Patients can cash out of many planned medical interventions as well [7]. Where, after appropriate information and initially agreeing to a medical therapy, the patient changes their mind for any number of reasons [7]. This could be due to adverse side effects of anything from chemotherapy and antibiotics. The difference is that with medical interventions, there is no surgeon actively performing a task to better the patient. So just as a patient can consent to an operation preoperatively, a patient can withhold life sustaining measures postoperatively. As readily as a patient can buy-in, they can similarly cash out.

22.3.10 The Solution

The solution lies in strong communication and shared decision making. While this requires more preoperative time investment, this is likely worthwhile since the time spent with patients preoperatively can provide insight into the patient's goals. This discussion of goals and concerns can assist in finding what the patient deems acceptable and unacceptable. This will also give the surgeon insight into the patient's values. Although this conversation will further widen the knowledge gap of patients by their surgeon and inpatient providers, and similarly the potential conflict mentioned above, it will give the surgeon the knowledge to appropriately lead the postoperative care in line with the patient's values and wishes.

Taylor et al. identified a framework to enhance surgeon communication preoperatively for major operations [12]. Using a training session, surgeons were educated to communicate best- and worst-case scenarios to their patients preoperatively when framing postoperative expectations [12]. They created a graphic with parallel paths showing surgery versus no intervention. This diagram then depicted the best case, most likely case, and worst case of a surgical path and contrasted it to the best case, most likely case, and worst case of a non-surgical/supportive care path [12]. This tool allowed surgeons to delve into what may be inconsistent with patients' goals postoperatively. Taylor et al. found that utilizing this approach shifted the focus from a complication after surgery to alternatives and outcomes. Using a shared decision-making scoring scale, patients were found to have an improved score leading to improved patient understanding and involvement perioperatively thereby mitigating cashing out.

22.4 Case Conclusion

After meeting the surgeon, the patient appreciated the opportunity to talk about his goals and objectives. The patient understood that the need for perioperative dialysis was a higher probability with his current kidney disease. Through shared decision making and intentional conversation, the surgeon and patient agreed that utilization of dialysis, were it to be needed post-operatively, still was consistent with the patient's desire to attempt to be cancer free.

22.5 Conclusion

The focus on clear tangible disease processes and tangible expectations for surgery and postoperative recovery are imperative in an informed consent conversation. Patient awareness and patient communication are the keys to obtaining maximal buy-in. The surgeon and patient come together and agree on what is permissible and not permissible in the perioperative period. It is innate for surgeons to hope for the best and yet plan for the worst; surgeons never enter an operation without knowing alternate surgical plans. Similarly, surgeons must help the patient plan for possible alternate outcomes. Through an intentional and clear preoperative conversation, a mutually agreed upon surgical buy-in can be attained for major operations.

22.6   Selected References

- Schwarze ML, Bradley CT, Brasel KJ. Surgical "buy-in": the contractual relationship between surgeons and patients that influences decisions regarding life-supporting therapy. Crit Care Med. 2010;38(3):843–8. https://doi.org/10.1097/ccm.0b013e3181cc466b

    – The origins of the concept of obtaining surgical buy-in for the postoperative period.

- Scheiner N, Liaschenko J. "Buying-in" and "cashing-out": patients' experience and the refusal of life-prolonging treatment. J Clin Ethics. 2018;29(1):15–9. PMID: 29565793

    – The descriptive paper on patients changing their goals after an operation—cashing out.

- McKneally MF, Martin DK, Ignagni E, D'Cruz J. Responding to trust: surgeons' perspective on informed consent. World J Surg. 2009;33(7):1341–7. https://doi.org/10.1007/s00268-009-0021-7

    – Based on interviews with surgeons, the following were emphasized: making informed decisions; communicating information and confidence; managing expectations and fears; consent as a decision to trust; and commitment inspired by trust.

Conflict of Interest   The author reports no potential conflicts of interest.

Funding   This manuscript had no outside funding sources.

References

1. Schwarze ML, Bradley CT, Brasel KJ. Surgical "buy-in": the contractual relationship between surgeons and patients that influences decisions regarding life-supporting therapy. Crit Care Med. 2010;38(3):843–8. https://doi.org/10.1097/ccm.0b013e3181cc466b.
2. Bosk C. Forgive and remember: managing medical failure. University of Chicago Press; 1979. p. 30.

3. Angelos P. Complications, errors, and surgical ethics. World J Surg. 2009;33(4):609–11. https://doi.org/10.1007/s00268-008-9914-0.
4. Schwarze ML, Redmann AJ, Alexander GC, Brasel KJ. Surgeons expect patients to buy-in to postoperative life support preoperatively: results of a national survey. Crit Care Med. 2013;41(1):1–8. https://doi.org/10.1097/ccm.0b013e31826a4650.
5. McKneally MF, Martin DK, Ignagni E, D'Cruz J. Responding to trust: surgeons' perspective on informed consent. World J Surg. 2009;33(7):1341–7. https://doi.org/10.1007/s00268-009-0021-7.
6. Buchman TG, Cassell J, Ray SE, Wax ML. Who should manage the dying patient?: rescue, shame, and the surgical ICU dilemma. J Am Coll Surg. 2002;194(5):665–73. https://doi.org/10.1016/s1072-7515(02)01157-2.
7. Scheiner N, Liaschenko J. "Buying-in" and "cashing-out": patients' experience and the refusal of life-prolonging treatment. J Clin Ethics 2018;29(1):15–9. PMID: 29565793.
8. Ruske J, Sharma G, Makie K, et al. Patient comprehension necessary for informed consent for vascular procedures is poor and related to frailty [SAVS abstract 15]. J Vasc Surg. 2020;71:e23–4.
9. Jonsen AR, Siegler M, Winslade WJ. Clinical ethics: a practical approach to ethical decisions in clinical medicine. 8th ed. McGraw Hill Education; 2015.
10. Wightman SC, Angelos P. An organized approach to complex ethical cases on a surgical service. World J Surg. 2014;38:1664–7. https://doi.org/10.1007/s00268-014-2567-2.
11. *Shinal v. Toms*, 162 A.3d 429 (2017).
12. Taylor LJ, Nabozny MJ, Steffens NM, et al. A framework to improve surgeon communication in high-stakes surgical decisions: best case/worst case. JAMA Surg. 2017;152(6):531–8. https://doi.org/10.1001/jamasurg.2016.5674.

Chapter 23
The Changing Ethical Landscape of Cesarean Delivery on Maternal Request

Paul Burcher

Abstract Until recently, cesarean birth was deemed more dangerous than vaginal birth for both woman and fetus, but with surgical advances it is no longer clear than cesarean sections before labor offer greater surgical risks than planned vaginal birth. Cesarean delivery on maternal request (CDMR) began eliciting ethical concerns and controversy beginning approximately twenty years ago. Specialty societies reached differing conclusions at first, but then an ethical consensus seemed to emerge supporting reproductive autonomy and permitting CDMR. More recent evidence has rekindled these discussions as the relationship between multiple cesarean births and maternal morbidity and mortality has been examined, and the impact of elective cesarean birth on the newborn's microbiome has also been raised.

Keywords Cesarean section · Cesarean delivery on maternal request (CDMR) Reproductive autonomy · Shared decision making

> **Case**
> I was asked to see a patient in our office who had requested CDMR (cesarean delivery on maternal request, i.e. an elective cesarean birth) and had already undergone multiple visits for the purpose of establishing informed consent for this procedure. This was a few months after I had authored an article in *Obstetrics and Gynecology* arguing that a patient's request for CDMR during labor could be ethically refused because of concerns regarding the adequacy of informed consent in this setting [1]. But the patient I saw that day had been extensively counseled by multiple physicians, and still was adamant in her

P. Burcher (✉)
Wellspan, York Hospital, York, PA, USA

Pennsylvania State University College of Medicine, Drexel University College of Medicine, York, PA, USA
e-mail: pburcher@wellspan.org

© The Author(s), under exclusive license to Springer Nature Switzerland AG 2022
V. A. Lonchyna et al. (eds.), *Difficult Decisions in Surgical Ethics*, Difficult Decisions in Surgery: An Evidence-Based Approach,
https://doi.org/10.1007/978-3-030-84625-1_23

CDMR request. She had witnessed an older sister give birth vaginally, and she described watching her sister in excruciating pain—a fate she wished to avoid for herself. As I reviewed her chart notes, I noticed one important aspect of the informed consent had not been raised. I asked her one question and based upon her answer then counseled her against going forward with her planned cesarean. She accepted my recommendation and went on to deliver vaginally without any difficulty (and with a good epidural).

23.1 Introduction

The specific circumstances surrounding a patient's request for an elective cesarean are crucial in determining the ethics of a physician's response. This is why I remain leery of last-minute decisions for an elective cesarean delivery: there is simply too much information that needs to be conveyed in both directions for appropriate informed consent. Shared decision making, particularly for an elective procedure with life changing implications, takes time. As in all cases of true shared decision making, the patient needs to convey enough of her lifeworld to the physician so that the doctor can tailor their counseling to the specific needs, concerns, and future that the patient envisions.

Because the reasons and circumstances of each patient request need to be discussed and evaluated individually, the blanket responses of specialty societies seem particularly *not helpful*. FIGO, the International Federation of Gynaecology and Obstetrics, has a position statement against performing CDMR stating that it is a procedure without benefit [2]. A National Institutes of Health (NIH) consensus panel concluded that physicians could accede to requests for CDMR in the setting of adequate informed consent arguing from a position of patient autonomy. The American College of Obstetrics and Gynecology (ACOG) first supported the conclusions of the NIH panel, and then partially reversed themselves several years later [3, 4]. Although they stopped short in the revised committee opinion of forbidding CDMR, they do discourage it and promote vaginal birth as superior to non-indicated cesarean birth [4]. While this newer committee opinion offered no new evidence or citations to explain their reversal, it appears that they read the same evidence differently in their revised statement. The most recent iteration of this committee opinion did not change this stance and continues to advise physicians to counsel patients that vaginal birth is the preferred option if no medical indication for cesarean birth is present [5].

23.2   Search Strategy

The literature review for this chapter was performed using the Medline database in PubMed, Google Scholar, and the ACOG website. Searches for both "elective cesarean" and "cesarean delivery on maternal request" were performed from 1985 to the present.

23.3   Discussion

I will review the history of the controversy surrounding CDMR, and then discuss the relevant ethical issues physicians need to consider when faced with a CDMR request. I believe that the question I asked the patient at the beginning of this chapter is related to the change in stance that ACOG made in relation to this question. It relates to the difference between examining the risks and benefits of the procedure more narrowly or more broadly, including the future consequences for both the woman and the child after an elective cesarean birth.

23.4   The History of CDMR

Cesarean birth did not become a routinely survivable procedure until the twentieth century, but until relatively recently it was still considered the higher risk, more morbid method of childbirth, reserved only for women who could not deliver vaginally, or for fetuses unable to tolerate the rigors of labor [6]. The first journal article that made an argument for non-medically indicated cesarean was in *The New England Journal of Medicine* [7]. Two obstetricians argued that performing elective cesarean births at term would save 5–10 babies for each excess maternal death. They compared the risk of term stillbirths and neurologically injured babies from labor with the maternal risks of cesarean. They did not make the claim that scheduled cesareans were as safe as a vaginal birth, but they did correctly acknowledge that a scheduled cesarean is safer than a cesarean after labor. Looking to the future, they postulated that if the cesarean rate increased to above 27%, a number we currently exceed nationally [8], then scheduled cesareans would actually be safer than planned vaginal birth because the women having cesareans after a trial of labor would have the highest complication rates, thus making planned vaginal birth more dangerous than performing cesareans on every woman at term. Their "evidence" was extrapolations from other studies, none of which directly addressed the risks or benefits of elective cesarean at term. Furthermore, they did not consider the impact of a cesarean birth on the risks to future pregnancies.

Elective cesareans are not necessarily all initiated by patient request, but since respect for patient autonomy is generally accepted as the strongest ethical argument for its permissibility, it is important to distinguish between two types of non-medically indicated cesareans: physician initiated, and patient requested. Kalish surveyed physicians at one large New York hospital and found that 18% of cesarean births during labor were elective, but that physicians initiated almost twice as many as patients did [9]. While it is outside the scope of this chapter it is worth noting that making an ethical argument supporting physician initiated elective cesareans is difficult to imagine. Recommending a surgical approach over physiological vaginal birth without indication, even if one believes that risks and benefits are essentially balanced is inconsistent with respecting patient autonomy, since the patient is likely to not fully appreciate that the recommendation is not arising from medical necessity and is not necessarily in the patient's best interest. If Kalish's results are widely applicable, and I know of no other study that has examined the prevalence of physician initiated elective cesarean, it would represent a relatively frequent example of unethical physician behavior.

The 1990s saw a gradual increase in cesarean birth overall, and in CDMR as well. Estimates of the incidence of CDMR are imprecise because of inconsistencies in coding (and lack of a code specific for CDMR), but by 2004 published estimates varied from 4–18% of all cesarean sections arising from maternal choice [10]. With both the rate of cesarean section and CDMR rising, the NIH convened a scientific panel to explore both the science and the ethics of CDMR. Their conclusions were twofold: firstly, that the science at that time could not provide a convincing answer regarding whether CDMR offered any risks or benefits substantially different than planned vaginal birth, and secondly, that in the absence of obvious differences in outcomes, "After thorough discussion and review, cesarean delivery on maternal request may be a reasonable alternative to planned vaginal delivery." Drs. Minkoff and Chervenak, both prominent obstetrician ethicists reached similar conclusions with the additional proviso that physicians had no obligation to offer CDMR to their patients [11]. Subsequent to these opinions, ACOG then issued a Committee Opinion on Obstetric Practice affirming this same conclusion [4]. The most recent update of this committee opinion did not change their stance [5].

23.5   Reconsiderations of CDMR

23.5.1   Focus on the Mother

After this consensus, the ethical literature on CDMR goes quiet for several years. Then in 2013 two important publications shift the terrain quite substantially. Jeffrey Ecker, Professor of Obstetrics at Harvard Medical School, writing a Clinician's Corner article in JAMA, notes that the balance of risks discussed in the NIH consensus statement and the ACOG Committee Opinion are referring only to the index pregnancy, and that for subsequent pregnancies, "prior cesarean delivery may lead to increased complication rates [12]." Specifically, more than two cesarean births lead to substantial increases in abnormal placentation (placenta previa and accreta) and that an increase in these conditions appears to be increasing maternal mortality in this country. In 2013, ACOG changed the language of the abstract in their Committee Opinion on CDMR as well. They added a new sentence, that can be understood as significantly changing their position, "Given the balance of risks and benefits, the Committee on Obstetric Practice believes that in the absence of maternal or fetal indications for cesarean delivery, a plan for vaginal delivery is safe and appropriate and should be recommended to patients [4]."

Although there are no new references in the Committee Opinion, it is reasonable to assume that like Ecker the shift in thought is related to the increasing incidence of significant maternal morbidity and mortality secondary to abnormal placentations arising from multiple cesarean sections. Increasing cesarean rates since 1998 have correlated with increasing maternal mortality, and some have argued that this relationship is also causal [13, 14]. Solheim et al. argue that elective cesareans should be expected to increase maternal mortality by increasing abnormal placentation in women having multiple cesarean births, and that the full impact of this effect will take several years to be fully seen, since it is third and fourth cesarean births that carry the largest risk [14]. This is why counseling a patient who requests CDMR is both so crucial and also so fraught. One important aspect of assessing the risk/ reward balance of a CDMR decision involves expecting a patient to accurately predict her own future desire for children beyond the current pregnancy. This was the question I asked the pregnant patient at the beginning of this chapter, and she gave a clear, unambiguous answer, "at least four, maybe five." This led to a discussion of increasing surgical risk beyond two cesareans and changed her decision to pursuing a vaginal birth. However, in my experience, many of us are much less clear about our future plans than she was, so a critical aspect of informed consent counseling for CDMR relies upon asking people to predict their own family planning choices in the future.

Admittedly, CDMR only plays a small role in the increase in cesarean births, but some have worried that it also has a multiplier effect by increasing the acceptability of cesareans even in the absence of medical indications for the procedure. In other words, once we accepted that cesareans could be done without a compelling medical reason, we make vaginal birth and surgical birth appear simply as two co-equal choices, weakening the necessity for both patients and physicians to justify their choice. As a practicing obstetrician for the last 25 years, I can affirm that patients and physicians are much more poised to "throw in the towel" during labor as soon as anything appears amiss or even if it just seems to be taking too long. This normalization of cesarean birth goes beyond the quantitative increase that CDMR provides. As Sylvia Burrow writes in the American Journal of Bioethics, it creates a technological imperative that can make vaginal birth actually appear to be an inferior choice because it does not involve a surgical approach to childbirth [15]. Burrow is concerned that what appears to be a turn toward respecting women's autonomy is actually something quite different. One obvious problem besides the allure of technology is that autonomous decision making requires good information regarding risks and benefits, but both the NIH and the ACOG statement acknowledge that in the absence of a randomized controlled trial comparing elective term cesarean to planned vaginal birth we really don't even know which is safer for mother and child even in the index pregnancy. Add to this the distorting media influence that makes vaginal birth appear horrifying or at least really unappealing, and subtle (or not so subtle pressure) from physician or employer that a scheduled surgical birth is really more convenient for everyone, and it becomes quite reasonable to question both the autonomy of the decisionmaker and the informed consent it rests upon [16].

This places physicians in a quandary regarding how to best respect patient autonomy when assessing a patient request for an elective cesarean. If the requisite discussions and information sharing has occurred, should a physician then accede to the request even if they have misgivings regarding either the patient's true understanding of the information, or the external pressures that may be distorting her decision making? Is it possible to question whether a patient's choice is truly autonomous without slipping into paternalism?

For that matter, both ACOG and NIH statements affirm that CDMR is inappropriate for women who desire several children (although no absolute cut-off is given), but they do not then address whether physician refusal in these cases is ethically justified.

23.5.2   *Focus on the Newborn*

While the risk assessment on the maternal side has shifted as attention has moved to subsequent pregnancies, the risk assessment for the newborn born from an elective cesarean has also changed. In the original ACOG and NIH statements, the calculus for the newborn focused on the short-term risks of respiratory problems that are higher in children born by cesarean versus the rare but catastrophic risks associated with birth injuries, particularly neurological injuries that occur more frequently in vaginal birth. Again, without a randomized trial it was deemed impossible to conclude that one method of birth offered greater benefit or less risk to the newborn, so the presumption fell to patient choice. But newer research has identified a number of serious, chronic conditions that are increased in children born by cesarean section, and that are perhaps even more common when the cesarean was not performed after labor [17]. Blustein and Liu in their review of the evidence argued that studies and meta-analyses provided strong evidence that cesarean birth increased risks for asthma, diabetes and obesity [18]. Yuan et al. reported the findings from a large prospective cohort of 22,000 children [19]. They found that children born by cesarean were 64% more likely to experience childhood obesity, and that this risk was even greater when the cesarean section was without indication.

This association is surprisingly biologically plausible. Studies have shown that children born by cesarean have a different, and less diverse, gut microbiome than children born vaginally [20]. Children born vaginally are exposed to maternal intestinal and vaginal flora, whereas cesarean born children have gut flora more consistent with skin flora. Persistence of this difference has been demonstrated even into adulthood [21]. Differences in gut flora have in turn been implicated in increased energy harvest and subsequent obesity [22]. The putative mechanism for increases in asthma and diabetes relate to immunological responses to the exposure to the vaginal microbiome. If this line of research is correct, then unlabored cesarean birth holds greater risk for the newborn than cesareans after a trial of labor because during labor even babies born eventually by cesarean are likely to receive some exposure to vaginal flora once the amniotic sac separating fetus from laboring woman has broken.

23.6 Case Resolution

The one question I asked her during the informed consent discussion was to predict her own future desire for children beyond the current pregnancy. She gave a clear, unambiguous answer, "at least four, maybe five." This led to a discussion of increasing surgical risk beyond two cesareans, specifically the increased risk of placenta accreta after multiple cesarean deliveries, and she opted to attempt vaginal birth, which was successful.

23.7 Conclusions

The evolution in ACOG's position between 2007 and 2013 seems to reflect a growing concern regarding the impact of multiple cesarean births on maternal morbidity and mortality secondary to increases in abnormal placentation. This does not change their original position that for the index pregnancy they did not see any evidence of compelling differences between the risks and benefits of vaginal birth and elective cesarean. The newly identified risks of elective cesarean for newborns, however, changes this calculus. The evidence appears to be building that lack of exposure to maternal vaginal flora has risks that include chronic health conditions for the child. How should we incorporate this into our ethical analysis of CDMR? There are at least two possible answers.

The first answer is to still value the reproductive autonomy of the woman as the ascendant principle in these encounters, and the physician responsibility is unchanged. Our job is to effectively communicate the evidence and help the patient incorporate this information into their own specific circumstances to make a decision that is best for her and her family. While we should be attentive of outside pressures or distorting influences in her responses, our response should be to discuss this with the patient, but not overrule her choices. There is a strong tradition in bioethics to place patient autonomy as the most important of the four bioethics principles, although this was not the original intent of Beauchamp and Childress in their *Principles of Biomedical Ethics* [23, 24]. The paternalistic history of obstetrics and gynecology provides added support for not overstepping the physician role beyond counseling and shared decision making. A recent ACOG Ethics Committee opinion on sterilization counseling affirms this same stance stating that, "Eliminating the risk of regret by limiting patient autonomy generally is considered by bioethicists to be worse than allowing a patient to make a possibly erroneous choice. It is impossible to eliminate regret, as the very fact of being a fully autonomous human being with decisional capacity carries with it the risk of decisional regret [25]."

The counterargument to this line of thinking is that positive assertions of patient autonomy are to be respected by physicians when the request is within medical standards of care and risks and benefits are roughly equal between the possible patient choices. While the first aspect of this is indisputable—CDMR has been widely accepted by the obstetric community for at least the last fifteen years, the emerging evidence on risks to the newborn and to subsequent pregnancies might be evaluated as no longer making it an acceptable choice even in the setting of excellent counseling and informed consent (see Table 23.1).

I do not think that refusing CDMR in a setting of adequate informed consent is an acceptable final position, even in light of recent evidence of increased risks for both the patient and her child. Women are socialized to sacrifice and accept risk for the sake of their children. Most women, upon hearing that their choice of delivery potentially places increased health risks to their child, will change their decision. Those who do not are likely to have compelling personal reasons for their choice which they may not be comfortable sharing. Research has shown that fear of labor

Table 23.1 Ethical principles to consider in performing Cesarean Delivery on Maternal Request

Beneficence	Importance of complete informed consent prior to delivery
	Vaginal birth is superior to non-indicated Cesarean section
	The ethics of physician initiated Cesarean delivery
Non-maleficence	Risks of Cesarean section vs. vaginal delivery must favor the safety of both the patient and the fetus.
	What are future risks of subsequent Cesarean deliveries?
	More than two cesarean births lead to substantial increases in abnormal placentation.
Autonomy	Shared decision making allows for patient input.
	Should CDMR be performed to respect patient autonomy?
	Autonomous decision making requires good information regarding risks and benefits,
	Avoiding paternalism, the physician's role is a delicate balance between counseling and shared decision making.
Justice	Does a physician have the obligation to offer CDMR to the patient?
	Counseling a patient who requests CDMR is crucial.
	Why not perform a scheduled surgical birth as it is more convenient for everyone?
	Should children be exposed to an increased risk of childhood obesity in those born by Cesarean delivery?
	A physician should refuse any requested treatment outside the bounds of his/her professional judgment.

pains and a history of trauma are two of the primary drivers behind a request for CDMR [26]. In any case, the patient must be free to place her reproductive autonomy over the interests of the child so long as it is still a fetus within her. Placing limits on pregnant women's choices because they carry a potential risk to the fetus is a slippery slope headed toward *The Handmaid's Tale* [27].

The history of obstetrics and gynecology is littered with examples of physicians disrespecting patient choices and women's bodily autonomy. From Dr. Marion Sims perfecting his surgical techniques on enslaved women [28], to forced sterilizations [29], to even recent cases of women required to have cesarean births to which they did not consent [30], the history of my profession is that doctors have often claimed to know more about what is best for the patient than the woman herself. We are certainly allowed our misgivings regarding whether the patient is really making the best choice, but ultimately, we should counsel, even recommend when appropriate, but allow the patient to make the choice in her method of delivery—with one exception. Like all medical decision making, if the patient choice, in her specific circumstances, creates unacceptable risks, then physician refusal to participate is appropriate. An elective cesarean in a woman desiring 5 children may very well represent such an example. This is consistent with the positive/negative distinction in respecting patient choices. A well-informed adult patient with decisional capacity has a near sacrosanct right to reject medical or surgical treatments (negative right), but the positive right of requesting treatment is limited by standards of care and medical judgment. A physician can, and should, refuse any requested treatment outside the bounds of their professional judgment, but this should be decided in a careful weighing of risk/benefit (beneficence/nonmaleficence) rather than judgments regarding the prudence of the patient's choice given their life circumstances. While pregnant women often do take additional risks upon themselves for fetal or neonatal benefit, it is hard to conceive that this could play a role in a truly elective cesarean section.

All this leads back to the sentence ACOG added to their committee opinion on CDMR in 2013, "…the Committee on Obstetric Practice believes that in the absence of maternal or fetal indications for cesarean delivery, a plan for vaginal delivery is safe and appropriate and should be recommended to patients [4]." If after thorough counseling including the latest evidence, shared decision making, and a recommendation supporting vaginal birth, a patient still desires CDMR, I believe it is both ethically appropriate to perform it, and furthermore, refusal would constitute an ethically inappropriate lack of respect for her informed choice.

I would like to end on a personal note. I have never refused a request for CDMR, and I have never performed one. I hope that this is not because my counseling was coercive, but rather that the evidence I presented was persuasive. Of course, I will never know the truth, but I certainly have had patients reject other recommendations, and the philosophy that I teach to residents is that it is important to counsel without ego, and respect patient choices that are different than your own thinking. While I do not think that the principle of autonomy should be the deciding principle in many ethical dilemmas, I think at this moment telling women that you cannot respect their informed choice is something our profession must relegate to a historical dustbin.

23.8 Selected References

- FIGO Committee for the Ethical Aspects of Human Reproduction and Women's Health. Ethical aspects regarding cesarean delivery for non-medical reasons. Int J Obstet Gynecol. 1999;64:317–322.

  - FIGO's statement against offering CDMR using beneficence-based reasoning.

- American College of Obstetricians and Gynecologists. ACOG Committee Opinion No. 394, December 2007. Cesarean delivery on maternal request. Obstet Gynecol. 2007;110(6):1501. doi:https://doi.org/10.1097/01.aog.0000291577. 01569.4c (This document has been withdrawn by ACOG; of historic value only).

  - First ACOG committee opinion supporting CDMR with proper consent.

- American College of Obstetricians and Gynecologists. ACOG committee opinion no. 559: Cesarean delivery on maternal request. Obstet Gynecol. 2013;121(4):904–907. doi:https://doi.org/10.1097/01.aog.00004286447.67925. d3 (This document has been withdrawn by ACOG; of historic value only).

  - Revised committee opinion with more neutral wording including recommendation for support of vaginal birth over CDMR.

- Feldman GB, Freiman JA. Prophylactic cesarean section at term? N Engl J Med. 1985;312:1264–1267. doi:https://doi.org/10.1056/nejm1985050931211926

  - Early reference arguing for fetal benefits to elective cesarean.

- Kalish RB, McCullough L, Gupta M, Thaler HT, Chervenak FA. Intrapartum elective cesarean delivery: a previously unrecognized clinical entity. Obstet Gynecol. 2004;103(6):1137–1141. doi:https://doi.org/10.1097/01. aog.0000128118.37737.df

  - Single institution survey that showed high rates of elective cesarean during labor including CDMR.

- Rothenberg KH. National Institutes of Health State-of-the-Science Conference Statement: Cesarean Delivery on Maternal Request. Obstet Gynecol. 2006;107(6):1386–1397. PMID: 16738168.

  - NIH consensus statement concluding that CDMR is permissible with proper informed consent. Justification is primarily autonomy-based.

- Yuan C, Gaskins AJ, Blaine AI, et al. Association between cesarean birth and risk of obesity in offspring in childhood, adolescence, and early adulthood. JAMA Pediatr. 2016;170(11):e162385. doi:https://doi.org/10.1001/jamapediatrics. 2016.2385

  - Large study documenting association between cesarean birth and childhood obesity.

References

1. Burcher P, Gabriel JL, Campo-Engelstein L, Kiley KC. The case against cesarean delivery on maternal request in labor. Obstet Gynecol. 2013;122(3):684–7. https://doi.org/10.1097/aog.0b013e31829d83c2.
2. Committee FIGO. For the ethical aspects of human reproduction and Women's health. Ethical aspects regarding cesarean delivery for non-medical reasons. Int J. Obstet Gynecol. 1999;64:317–22.
3. American College of Obstetricians and Gynecologists. ACOG Committee opinion no. 394, December 2007. Cesarean delivery on maternal request. Obstet Gynecol. 2007;110(6):1501. https://doi.org/10.1097/01.aog.0000291577.01569.4c. First ACOG committee opinion supporting CDMR with proper consent
4. American College of Obstetricians and Gynecologists. ACOG committee opinion no. 559: Cesarean delivery on maternal request. Obstet Gynecol. 2013;121(4):904–7. https://doi.org/10.1097/01.aog.00004286447.67925.d3. (This document has been withdrawn by ACOG)
5. American College of Obstetricians and Gynecologists. Committee on obstetric Prqctice. Cesarean delivery on maternal request. ACOG Committee opinion no. 761. Obstet Gynecol. 2019;133(1):e73–7. https://doi.org/10.1097/aog.0000000000003006.
6. Gabert HA, Bey M. History and development of cesarean operation. Obstet Gynecol Clin N Am. 1988;15(4):591–605. 3067172.
7. Feldman GB, Freiman JA. Prophylactic cesarean section at term? N Engl J Med. 1985;312:1264–7. https://doi.org/10.1056/nejm1985050931211926.
8. Centers for Disease Control and Prevention. National Center for Health Statistics. Births – Method of Delivery. Last modified March 2, 2021. Accessed May 8, 2021. https://www.cdc.gov/nchs/fastats/delivery.htm.
9. Kalish RB, McCullough L, Gupta M, Thaler HT, Chervenak FA. Intrapartum elective cesarean delivery: a previously unrecognized clinical entity. Obstet Gynecol. 2004;103(6):1137–41. https://doi.org/10.1097/01.aog.0000128118.37737.df.
10. Rothenberg KH. National Institutes of Health state-of-the-science conference statement: Cesarean delivery on maternal request. Obstet Gynecol. 2006;107(6):1386–97.
11. Minkoff H, Powderly KR, Chervenak F, McCullough LB. Ethical dimensions of elective primary cesarean delivery. Obstet Gynecol. 2004;103(2):387–92. https://doi.org/10.1097/01.aog.0000107288.44622.2a.
12. Ecker J. Elective cesarean delivery on maternal request. JAMA. 2013;309(18):1930–6. https://doi.org/10.1001/jama.2013.3982.
13. Blanchette H. The rising cesarean delivery rate in America: what are the consequences? Obstet Gynecol. 2011;118(3):687–90. https://doi.org/10.1097/aog.0b013e318227b.
14. Solheim KN, Esakoff TF, Little SE, Cheng YW, Sparks TN, Caughey AB. The effect of cesarean delivery rates on the future incidence of placenta previa, placenta accreta, and maternal mortality. J Matern Fetal Neonatal Med. 2011;24(11):1341–6. https://doi.org/10.3109/14767058.2011.553695.
15. Burrow S. On the cutting edge: ethical responsiveness to cesarean rates. Am J Bioeth. 2012;12(7):44–52. https://doi.org/10.1080/15265161.2012.673689.
16. Campo-Engelstein L, Howland LE, Parker WM, Burcher P. Scheduling the stork: media portrayals of Women's and physicians' reasons for elective Cesarean delivery. Birth. 2015;42(2):181–8. https://doi.org/10.1111/birt.12161.
17. Chu S, Chen Q, Chen Y, Bao Y, Wu M, Zhang J. Cesarean section without medical indication and risk of childhood asthma, and attenuation by breastfeeding. PLoS One. 2017;12(9):e0184920. https://doi.org/10.1371/journal.pone.0184920.
18. Blustein J, Liu J. Time to consider the risks of caesarean delivery for long term child health. Brit Med J. 2015;350:h2410. https://doi.org/10.1136/bmj.h.2410.

19. Yuan C, Gaskins AJ, Blaine AI, et al. Association between cesarean birth and risk of obesity in offspring in childhood, adolescence, and early adulthood. JAMA Pediatr. 2016;170(11):e162385. https://doi.org/10.1001/jamapediatrics.2016.2385.

20. Dominguez-Bello MG, Costello EK, Contreras M, et al. Delivery mode shapes the acquisition and structure of the initial microbiota across multiple body habitats in newborns. Proc Natl Acad Sci. 2010;107(26):11971–5. https://doi.org/10.1073/pnas.1002601107/-/dcsuplemental.

21. Goedert JJ, Hua X, Yu G, Shi J. Diversity and composition of the adult fecal microbiome associated with history of cesarean birth or appendectomy: analysis of the American gut project. EBioMedicine. 2014;1(2–3):167–72. https://doi.org/10.1016/j.ebiom.2014.11.004.

22. Turnbaugh PJ, Ley RE, Mahowald MA, Magrini V, Mardis ER, Gordon JI. An obesity-associated gut microbiome with increased capacity for energy harvest. Nature. 2006;444(7122):1027–31. https://doi.org/10.1038/nature05414.

23. Gillon R. Ethics needs principles – four can encompass the rest – and respect for autonomy should be "first among equals". J Med Ethics. 2003;29(5):307–12. https://doi.org/10.1136/jme.29.5.307.

24. Childress JF, Beauchamp TL. Principles of biomedical ethics. Oxford University Press; 2019.

25. American College of Obstetricians and Gynecologists. Committee on ethics. Sterilization of women: ethical issues and considerations. Committee opinion no. 695. Obstet Gynecol. 2017;129(4):e109–16. https://doi.org/10.1097/aog.0000000000002023.

26. O'Donovan C, O'Donovan J. Why do women request an elective cesarean delivery for non-medical reasons? A systematic review of the qualitative literature. Birth. 2017;45(2):109–19. https://doi.org/10.1111/birt.12319.

27. Atwood M. The Handmaid's tale. Everyman's Library; 2006.

28. Ojanuga D. The medical ethics of the 'father of gynaecology', Dr J Marion Sims. J Med Ethics. 1993;19(1):28–31. https://doi.org/10.1136/jme.19.1.28.

29. Silver MG. Eugenics and compulsory sterilization laws: providing redress for the victims of a shameful era in United States history. Geo Wash L Rev. 2003;72(4):862–92. 16211742.

30. Morris T, Robinson JH. Forced and coerced cesarean sections in the United States. Contexts. 2017;16(2):24–9. https://doi.org/10.1177/1536504217714259.

Chapter 24
Ethics of Fertility Sparing Oncologic Surgery in Women

Tracilyn Hall ⓘ and Claire Hoppenot ⓘ

Abstract Fertility-sparing surgery (FSS) for women with early stage, low-risk gynecologic cancers can allow patients to have spontaneous or assisted pregnancies without compromising oncologic outcomes. However, candidate patients for these procedures must be carefully selected. The clinical medical ethics framework of nonmaleficence, beneficence, autonomy and justice is used to discuss FSS in women with cancers of the ovary, uterus, and cervix. The concept of nonmaleficence can be applied primarily to oncologic and surgical outcomes: FSS should not be recommended if it confers a substantial worsening of survival. The potential for high-risk pregnancy should also be discussed. In terms of beneficence, candidates must have a reasonable expectation that they could conceive based on clinical and social factors. The consent process, a reflection of patient autonomy, must reflect the intricacies of the clinical assessment for both the cancer and fertility. Lastly, it must be addressed that many patients cannot afford the reproductive technology that they would need for reproduction even after FSS. Physicians should be open to discussing FSS options that could provide cancer survivors the option of having children, with a realistic expectation of success and oncologic outcomes.

Keywords Fertility sparing cancer ethics · Fertility cancer ethics
Fertility-sparing surgery · Fertility after ovarian cancer · Fertility after endometrial cancer · Fertility after cervical cancer

T. Hall · C. Hoppenot (✉)
Dan L Duncan Comprehensive Cancer Center, Baylor College of Medicine,
Houston, TX, USA
e-mail: tracilyn.hall@bcm.edu; Claire.hoppenot@bcm.edu

© The Author(s), under exclusive license to Springer Nature
Switzerland AG 2022

V. A. Lonchyna et al. (eds.), *Difficult Decisions in Surgical Ethics*, Difficult
Decisions in Surgery: An Evidence-Based Approach,
https://doi.org/10.1007/978-3-030-84625-1_24

345

Case

TB is a 26-year-old woman with pelvic pain. Imaging showed bilateral complex adnexal masses and labs reveal an elevated cancer antigen (CA125). She and her husband met with Dr. H, a gynecologic oncologist, to review the images. They discussed possible diagnoses, ranging from benign to borderline to invasive ovarian cancer. In the case of borderline or ovarian cancer, full staging surgery would involve removing the uterus and both ovaries, making her unable to have more children. Dr. H asked TB about her family. TB lives with her husband and two small children. She and her husband were thinking of having more children, but more than anything she wanted to be healthy and well for her current children. Dr. H recommended against ovarian stimulation for oocyte retrieval because the ovaries were involved with the tumor. He reviewed that ovarian tissue biobanking was experimental. However, she explained that select borderline and invasive cancers could be treated with a unilateral salpingo-oophorectomy to allow for future fertility. TB told Dr. H that she trusted her completely, and to proceed as she thought was most appropriate based on the intraoperative findings and pathology.

24.1 Introduction

It is estimated that in the year 2020 there will be 89,050 young adult cancers (ages 15–39) diagnosed in the United States [1]. These young patients face many challenges in their cancer treatments, including keeping the ability to create a family. In particular, women with gynecologic cancers are prone to losing fertility since traditional staging and treatment involves removing all the female reproductive organs. However, there are select patients with early, low risk gynecologic cancers who may be candidates for fertility-sparing surgery (FSS). To forgo complete surgical debulking and staging of gynecologic cancer in order to preserve fertility can be a difficult decision. In this chapter, we will explore the ethical considerations inherent in the balance of fertility preservation and cancer treatments, with a focus on women with gynecologic cancers and FSS.

24.2 Search Strategy

PubMed search was performed under an institutional login for publications from 2000 to 2020. Search terms included: "fertility sparing cancer ethics," "fertility cancer ethics," "fertility-sparing surgery," "cancer treatment and fertility," "cancer, pregnancy, and fertility," "fertility preservation," "oncofertility."

24.3 Discussion

24.3.1 Fertility Sparing Surgery

Fertility sparing surgery (FSS) for cancers involving the gynecologic organs involves removing the minimum affected portion of the reproductive tract in hopes of treating the cancer while still preserving enough of the reproductive organs for the patient to have the potential to procreate. Not all patients are candidates for FSS, and selecting the right patient is critical. FSS can be considered for women of reproductive age with early stage, lower risk gynecologic cancers. FSS can include ovarian preservation, uterine preservation, and/or ovarian transposition.

Some women with ovarian or uterine cancer can be offered FSS even if the standard treatment would involve removal of all gynecologic organs [2, 3]. In the case of suspected early-stage ovarian cancer, for example, it is possible to perform a unilateral salpingo-oophorectomy (USO) alone, USO with hysterectomy, or bilateral salpingo-oophorectomy with uterine preservation [2, 3]. During any of these FSS approaches, surgical staging can still be done by performing the omentectomy, lymphadenectomy, and/or peritoneal washings with targeted biopsies.

FSS can also be an option for women with uterine cancer. Women with early low-grade uterine cancer who desire future fertility can consider hysteroscopy and curettage for full uterine evaluation, followed by progestin therapy [3, 4]. Women who are not candidates for progestin therapy can consider ovarian preservation at the time of hysterectomy and staging.

Additionally, uterine preservation can be done for select women with cervical cancer by performing a cervical conization, removing only a portion of the cervix, for low-risk cervical cancer patients with FIGO stage IA1 disease, or with radical trachelectomy for select patients with FIGO stage IA2-IB disease [2, 3, 5]. A radical trachelectomy involves surgically removing the entire uterine cervix as well as the parametrial tissue [2, 6]. A cerclage can then be placed to close the remaining lower uterine segment and allow for pregnancy in the future [2].

Women receiving pelvic radiation likely to induce premature ovarian failure, such as for cervical or colorectal cancer, can also have the ovaries moved out of the radiation field to preserve ovarian function and possibly for oocyte retrieval. Ovarian transposition, also known as oophoropexy, involves surgically moving the ovaries and their blood supply to an area above an intended radiation field [3]. This can be done at the time of other cancer surgery if radiation is anticipated, or as a separate procedure prior to definitive chemoradiation. It is often performed laparoscopically [2, 3].

24.4   Options for Reproduction After Cancer Treatment

Even when FSS cannot preserve spontaneous reproduction, it can allow for reproduction with assisted reproductive technology (ART). The options for women vary
based on anatomy and prior cryopreservation of eggs or embryos (see Table 24.1).
Spontaneous reproduction requires an intact hypo-thalamo-pituitary axis, one ovary
and fallopian tube, and the uterus. In the United States, surrogacy with a gestational
carrier is an option for a woman with intact ovarian function or cryopreserved
oocytes/embryos whose uterus has been removed or radiated [7]. A woman with a

Table 24.1 Fertility preservation options for cancer patients

POTENTIAL Etiology of Infertility Related to Cancer or Treatment	Fertility Preservation Options	Alternative Options for Reproduction	Assistive Reproductive Technology Possibly Needed for Fertility Preservation or Alternative Reproduction
Testicular Failure	1. Sperm Cryopreservation	1. Sperm Donor	1. IUI
	2. Testicular Tissue Cryopreservation[a]		2. IVF
	3. Testicular Tissue Transplantation[a]		3. Embryo Transfer
	4. Testis Xenografting[a]		
Ovarian Failure	1. Oocyte Cryopreservation	1. Oocyte Donor	1. Egg Retrieval
	2. Embryo Cryopreservation	2. Embryo Donor	2. IVF
	3. Ovarian Suppression with GnRH Agonist[a]		3. Embryo Transfer
	4. Ovarian Tissue Cryopreservation		
	5. FSS with Ovarian Transposition		
	6. FSS with Ovarian Preservation		
	7. FSS with Uterine Preservation		
Uterine Dysfunction	1. FSS with Ovarian Preservation	1. Gestational Carrier	1. Egg Retrieval
	2. FSS with uterine corpus preservation		2. IUI
			3. IVF
Any	None	1. No children	Not applicable
	Patient Declines	2. Adoption	

[a]Experimental, IUI = intrauterine insemination, IVF = In vitro fertilization, GnRH = Gonadotropin
releasing hormone, FSS = fertility-sparing surgery

functional uterus and absent ovarian function (premature ovarian failure or no remaining intact ovaries) can use donor eggs with sperm from a partner or donor [7]. Should a woman no longer have functional ovaries or a functional uterus, she could have an embryo from a donor egg and a partner's sperm transferred into a gestational carrier, to provide linkage with paternal genetic material [7].

Several ethical considerations should be reviewed when considering FSS and assisted reproduction. In considering treatment options for cancer patients, nonmaleficence comes first; the effects of both FSS and potential future pregnancy on recurrence and cancer outcomes, as well as the risks of pregnancy itself must be considered. Beneficence, the second pillar of clinical medical ethics, requires consideration of the success of FSS at allowing cancer survivors to have children, ensuring FSS will provide the good that was intended. Third, patient autonomy and consent require adequate patient education of traditional and fertility sparing options, time for patients to consider these options, as well consideration for family influence. Lastly, since FSS often requires the use of ART which have limited availability or can be cost-prohibitive, there is the issue of justice and patient access.

24.5 Ethical Issues

24.5.1 Nonmaleficence

For many patients with gynecologic cancer, FSS can potentially preserve the option of carrying a child and/or having a genetically related child. However, it is critical to select patients for whom an incomplete resection at the time of cancer surgery would not adversely impact cancer outcomes. Oncologic factors such as histology, stage, adjuvant treatments, and prognosis will contribute to whether to offer FSS to a patient and should be reviewed by a multi-disciplinary team that can confirm that the pathology is associated with a "good" prognosis [8]. For example, FSS can be offered to women of reproductive age with early stage (IA1-IB) squamous cell or adenocarcinoma confined to the cervix [2]. For these women, treatment with radical trachelectomy had a low recurrence rate of 3.9% [2]. Patients with other cervical cancer histologic subtypes like clear cell, neuroendocrine, or undifferentiated carcinoma, however, are not traditionally candidates for FSS.

The same principle holds true in uterine cancer, where both stage and histologic subtype must be considered prior to FSS. It is recommended that FSS be limited to grade 1 endometrioid endometrial adenocarcinoma with no evidence of myometrial invasion or metastatic disease [2, 3]. Estrogen and progesterone receptor positivity is also associated with response to progestins [2]. Close follow-up is required to monitor for progression or recurrence, but most recurrences remain curable [2, 3]. Women undergoing FSS for uterine cancer are still recommended to have a hysterectomy after completing their family to prevent later recurrence [2].

When it comes to ovarian neoplasms, FSS is relevant only for early-stage ovarian cancers, and prognosis is closely related to histology. Borderline epithelial ovarian tumors have a 90% ten-year survival. Although up to 18% recur on the contralateral ovary, they can be salvaged with repeat surgery, making FSS the preferred treatment for women wanting fertility preservation in the absence of metastatic disease [2, 3]. Germ cell ovarian tumors of the ovary typically occur in younger women, are often limited to one ovary, and tend to be exquisitely sensitive to chemotherapy (90–95% are curable with chemotherapy even after FSS), making most patients with early germ cell tumor of the ovary good candidates for FSS. Some gynecologic oncologists argue that FSS is the standard of care for women of reproductive age [9]. Ovarian sex cord stromal tumors tend to be diagnosed in an early stage and have an indolent course, which can make pre-menopausal patients' candidates for FSS [3]. However, women with the most common type of ovarian cancer, epithelial ovarian cancers, are rarely candidates for FSS, as most are diagnosed at a late stage. For women with epithelial ovarian cancer, about 25% will present with stage I disease and have a 90% 5-year survival, making them candidates for FSS [3]. In these selected cases, FSS can be considered for reproductive age women with an encapsulated, unilateral ovarian lesion with a normal contralateral ovary, but it is recommended they still receive full staging including pelvic washings, omentectomy, and lymphadenectomy to confirm early-stage disease [2, 10]. Local recurrence can be curable, but peritoneal spread is not, potentially increasing the risk of mortality.

Cancer outcomes for patients undergoing FSS may be tied to surveillance [2]. FSS may confer equivalent outcomes despite increased recurrence only if the recurrence is caught early and a cure is salvaged. For example, early, localized cervical cancer recurrence can be diagnosed on a pap test and treated with surgery or chemoradiation. Contralateral recurrent ovarian tumors can be resected with definitive surgery. Endometrial cancer treated with progestin therapy has a high rate of recurrence that can be diagnosed at an early stage on a routine endometrial biopsy. Therefore, difficulty with follow up can be a relative contraindication to FSS.

FSS in and of itself does not confer a higher surgical risk, since it generally requires removing fewer organs or undergoing a smaller surgery. But surgeons doing certain fertility-sparing surgeries such as trachelectomies, and in particularly vaginal trachelectomies, will tend to be low-volume due to the paucity of good candidates [11]. LeBlanc et al. estimate that based on epidemiologic data, there are about 80 surgical candidates for vaginal trachelectomy each year in France, a country of 64 million people. They suggest developing centralized referral centers that would each do about a quarter of the cases to allow surgeons to have an adequate volume [11]. In the United States, there is no centralized health care to establish such centers, but self-assessment regarding surgical volume and referral options is important to ensure that the surgeries do no harm.

In addition to cancer outcomes, it must also be ensured that pregnancy is safe, both for mother and potential offspring. The risk of pregnancy itself has not been shown to increase cancer recurrence for most cancers, including hormone-sensitive breast cancer, or to incur cancer-related harm to the offspring [12]. Additionally, ovarian stimulation for egg retrieval that had previously been considered a risk factor for epithelial ovarian cancer have not had a similar correlation in more recent studies [3].

In the case of cervical cancer and trachelectomy, there is also the potential for a high-risk pregnancy. A meta-analysis found a 24% rate of miscarriage and 26% rate of preterm delivery after a radical trachelectomy [6]. In another analysis, 38–44% of pregnancies after a radical trachelectomy ended in a pregnancy loss or deliver before 32 weeks [13], which is associated with a higher risk of neurological sequelae for the offspring. With these possible complications of pregnancy, it is recommended that patients consult with a maternal fetal medicine specialist for counseling on the fetal risks associated with preterm birth prior to radical trachelectomy [2].

Another possible harm to future offspring is the potential for losing a parent to a cancer recurrence. However, the burden of the offspring of cancer survivors is not appreciably higher than other children [14]. Robertson et al. argue that the potential to lose a parent falls far short of a "wrongful birth," and that as long as avoidable harms are mitigated, it is better to be born and risk having grief from the loss of a parent than not being born at all [14].

One last aspect to consider avoiding harm when offering FSS is the risk of a hereditary cancer syndrome that could affect the patient by increasing her personal risk for a second cancer, or the risk of passing on a hereditary cancer syndrome. There is debate if conservative FSS should be offered to patients with high-risk cancer genetic syndromes, such as hereditary breast and ovarian cancer or Lynch Syndrome [3, 4]. Having genetic testing will allow couples to consider preimplantation genetic diagnostic testing if patients want to avoid passing on cancer predisposition to offspring.

In summary, nonmaleficence addresses cancer outcomes after surgery and after pregnancy, as well as surgical complications and risk to potential offspring from high-risk pregnancy, shortened lifespan from cancer recurrence, and passing on genetic syndromes.

24.5.2 Beneficence

Beneficence addresses the next ethical concept, which is to do good. The goal of FSS is to assist patients to have one or more live births, and candidates must have a reasonable chance of success based on baseline clinical factors, the effect of prior cancer treatments on fertility, and the type of FSS considered.

Factors related to the potential success of FSS include younger age, prior obstetrical history, no prior infertility, family history, and patient's motivation to preserve fertility [3]. First, the patient's pretreatment fertility potential is directly related to post-treatment fertility potential. But there is an age-related decline in fertility potential in women as they grow older [15]. Younger female patients are also more likely to regain menstrual function and are less like to have ovarian failure after chemotherapy or radiation [15]. It is also well established that obesity, polycystic ovarian syndrome, endometriosis, and other conditions that can be present in cancer patients lower their fertility potential [4]. Additionally, patient factors such as motivation to maintain fertility and compliance should be considered as close follow up is often needed after FSS [2, 4].

Lastly, one must take into consideration pregnancy rates and pregnancy outcomes for cancer survivors. When looking specifically at gynecologic cancers treated with FSS, variable rates of both pregnancy and live birth are again seen. After FSS for cervical cancer, the literature describes a range in pregnancy outcomes that vary based on type of FSS [6]. A meta-analysis by Zhang et al. describes a pooled pregnancy rate of 36% for women who underwent a cervical conization, compared to a pooled pregnancy rate of 21% after radical trachelectomy [6]. Eskander et al. report a 44% pooled pregnancy rate after radical trachelectomy with a live birth rate of 64%, a first trimester loss rate of 19%, and a second trimester loss rate of 10% [2].

For women with uterine cancer treated with a fertility-sparing approach using progestin therapy, Eskander et al. report pooled live birth rates of 47% [2]. When looking at the effect of FSS with hysteroscopic resection of tumors in patients treated for uterine cancer, Laurelli et al. report that the technique does not worsen reproductive outcomes, with a pregnancy rate of 58% and a live birth rate of 53% [4]. The authors also note that 75% of the women treated for endometrial cancer with a fertility sparing approach in this study used ART, which is associated with higher conception and live birth rates than those who rely on spontaneous conception, highlighting the role of ART after FSS [4].

Women with ovarian cancer treated with FSS have been found to have an infertility rate of 11%, which is similar to the general population prevalence of 9% [16]. Eskander et al. report pooled pregnancy rates of 30% for borderline tumors, 41% for malignant germ cell tumors, and 36% for invasive epithelial ovarian cancers [2]. They also report pooled live birth rates of 58% for borderline tumors, 80% for malignant germ cell tumors, and 87% for invasive epithelial cancers. No data was generated in our search of the literature on FSS for the treatment of Krukenberg tumors and subsequent fertility, possibly because of the poor survival outcomes after a Krukenberg tumor.

FSS prior to pelvic radiation has a high success rate, with 50–80% of patients retaining some ovarian function after oophoropexy, including hormone production [2, 3]. In regard to pregnancy, there are reports of up to 68% of patients having at least one pregnancy after oophoropexy and pelvic radiation [17]. Prior to FSS with ovarian transposition, it is important to counsel patients that radiation scatter, alteration to ovarian vascular supply, or ovarian migration can lead to this technique not being successful [3, 5]. It is also important to counsel patients that ovarian function in the form of hormone production does not always equate to fertility retention, but can have benefits on bone health, cardiovascular health, cognitive function, and all-cause mortality.

24.5.3 Consent/Autonomy

The informed consent process, which should allow for patient autonomy and shared decision-making, is difficult in the best of times. Consent for FSS is made more complicated by the amount of information and emotional toll of cancer- and fertility-related decision, the need for intraoperative decision-making, a history of sterilization without consent, navigating family involvement, and defining standard versus experimental treatments.

Young women with a new possible diagnosis of cancer have to weigh cancer treatments with risks and benefits of future fertility. This is a difficult time to be weighing so much information about the future [18]. Not everyone desires fertility [18], and how to separate those who do not from those who are too overwhelmed to consider FSS is difficult. No studies have looked at regret of FSS or loss of fertility despite the option of FSS in cancer patients. A small study of patients who had a trachelectomy for fertility preservation after cervical cancer did show that only about 1/3 of women changed their mind about having children [19]. Studies investigating regret of permanent sterilization with tubal ligation have shown that the risk of regret is increased in younger women, particularly women under the age of 30 [20]. This potential for regret suggests that it should be offered and discussed to all good candidates, especially for patients under the age of 30.

Additionally, there are situations in which the final operative decision occurs while the patient is under anesthesia. For example, a woman with an ovarian mass will discuss the possibilities of an oophorectomy for benign disease versus a hysterectomy with bilateral salpingo-oophorectomy for high-grade serous ovarian cancer. The ultimate decision, however, will occur after the frozen analysis of the pathology, while the patient is asleep. Most of the consent process must thus happen theoretically, prior to the final pathology result. Retrospective interview studies show that patients do not always remember much of the surgical consent discussion, even for a straightforward plan for resection [21]. Consent for young patients in these situations may require multiple discussions and a good knowledge of the patient's priorities so the surgeon can make the appropriate decisions at the time of surgery.

We must also remember the history of sterilization without consent in the United States, particularly for women of color, women with developmental delays, and women who are incarcerated [22]. These are not in the setting of cancer surgery, but the history of sterilization without consent can affect conversations about decisions regarding fertility-preservation. To ensure education of patients about loss of fertility in the setting of hysterectomy, Medicaid has taken steps to require the signature of a separate consent form for a hysterectomy, where the patient acknowledges that the procedure is an irreversible loss of fertility. It is important to tell young patients undergoing gynecologic cancer surgery whether their fertility will be affected, whether options exist to preserve fertility, and what the implications are, both in terms of fertility and cancer outcomes.

Questions of fertility can also be complicated by the direct involvement of a spouse or partner, who may have expectations and hopes of having offspring, as well as the cultural implications of fertility loss. In Saudi Arabia, the involvement is made explicit: the consent of a woman's husband is needed prior to surgery that will affect her fertility [23]. While most countries do not have such an existing law, culturally throughout the world, spouses and parents are involved in a woman's reproductive decisions. Navigating these conversations can again require multiple visits, both with and without the partner or family, as well as a dose of cultural competence.

Lastly, some women are willing to go to great lengths to preserve fertility, and may be willing to pursue experimental treatments, or those outside the standard of care. It is reasonable for women to search for available trials and experimental procedures, as long as they are presented as such, and the standard of care is discussed as well.

24.5.4   Justice

Justice relates to the equitable distribution of medical care. In the setting of a young patient with cancer, justice includes equitable access to FSS, which has been shown to vary. Additionally, many women need assisted reproductive technology to become pregnant after FSS, which can be prohibitively expensive for many families. Lastly, even the option of adoption may be limited for cancer survivors.

Patients cannot benefit from FSS if the option is not presented to them. Data from 50 cancer centers in Italy showed a wide range of rates of fertility-sparing surgery [24]. Almost half of the centers did not have access to assisted reproduction or obstetrics departments that could assist in the counseling of patients [24]. In the United States, a National Cancer Database study revealed a 70% rate of fertility-sparing surgery for ovarian dysgerminomas; age and ethnicity were not associated with fertility-sparing surgery, but women less likely to have fertility-sparing surgery tended to come from lower income neighborhoods and be uninsured [25].

Many fertility-sparing treatments, such as leaving the uterus to allow for an embryo transfer or leaving only an ovary for egg retrieval, require the patient to be able to afford fertility treatments, which are not always covered by insurance and are often expensive. Women with lower income may not be able to benefit from FSS, despite incurring the risk (if there are potential differences in outcome or need for closer surveillance). Advocacy for increased access to fertility treatments for women who have gone through surgery for an oncologic diagnosis could assist those women in having families.

Lastly, child adoption can be a viable option for many women who lost their fertility due to cancer or cancer treatments. However, some adoption agencies may require a certain cancer free interval prior to considering a parent who is a cancer survivor, and it is also important to note that not all agencies can offer cancer survivors protection against discrimination by the parents placing their child up for adoption [7, 26].

24.6   Case Concluded

Patient TB in the example case is typical of a young patient with a suspicious adnexal mass. The final diagnosis occurs after completion of surgery, and the counseling must be conducted in advance. The gynecologic oncologist told TB that she recommended removal of the larger ovary for pathologic evaluation. If the pathology was benign or borderline, it would be safe to proceed with a contralateral cystectomy, leaving the uninvolved portion of the ovary, followed by close surveillance. If the pathology showed cancer, she would undergo a laparotomy and full debulking. TB underwent a laparoscopic oophorectomy and contralateral cystectomy for a borderline serous adenocarcinoma of the ovary. She subsequently was lost to follow-up for 3 years, then came back with a new recurrence on her remaining ovary at the age of 29. In the meantime, she had delivered a baby boy. At this time, she opted for full debulking to decrease the chance of another recurrence.

24.7   Conclusion

Young women with cancer may have options for fertility preservation. However, many women may not prioritize fertility preservation after receiving a new diagnosis of cancer, and many oncologists focus on the oncologic outcomes. However, it is important both to discuss the fertility implications of treatments and surgeries and to offer fertility preservation and FSS with women who are appropriate candidates.

Appropriate candidates for FSS are described in Table 24.2. The concept of non-maleficence can be applied primarily to oncologic and surgical outcomes: FSS should not be recommended if it confers a substantial worsening of survival. Patients who undergo FSS should be screened for compliance for close surveillance and should understand the potential for a high-risk pregnancy due to FSS. Attention should also be paid to indications for testing for genetic syndromes that should be treated with definitive surgery or for which preimplantation testing of embryos could be offered.

The potential benefit of FSS is to provide the patient with a child or children, and candidates must have a reasonable expectation that they would be successful. This includes a clinical evaluation of fertility, including prior pregnancies, co-morbidities associated with decreased fertility, and age. Patients must want to become pregnant, although in certain situations, such as stage I germ cell tumors, the standard of care is shifting for all young women toward FSS regardless of desires for fertility.

Patient autonomy, as reflected in the consent process, must reflect the intricacies of the clinical assessment for both the cancer and fertility. It is complicated by the fact that many patients with adnexal masses, for example, go into surgery without a known diagnosis of cancer, and many of the decisions occur while she is under anesthesia. The preoperative discussion must provide the surgeon with a plan and an understanding of patient priorities for each likely pathology result.

Table 24.2 Criteria for candidates for fertility-sparing surgery

Oncologic factors (non-maleficence)
– Equivalent oncologic outcomes, even if it means closer follow-up and risk for second surgery
– Good prognosis
– Ability to comply with close surveillance
– Willingness to undergo definitive surgery in case of recurrence
Reproductive factors (beneficence)
– Desires future fertility
– Young age
– Reasonable probability of pregnancy based on clinical fertility evaluation
Patient consent (autonomy)
– Understanding of risks and potential benefits
– Understanding of minor deviations from standard of care versus experimental treatments
– Plan for intraoperative decision-making
– Incorporates cultural family influence regarding fertility, if appropriate
Access to care (justice)
– Discuss FSS with all premenopausal patients, and explain whether and why they are a candidate
– Ensure that the patient understands the need for assisted reproductive technology and its financial implications, if appropriate

Justice is always a difficult issue. We currently work at a safety-net hospital system with a large indigent population. Candidates for FSS are limited due to the advanced disease presentation we frequently see. Additionally, there is no option within our system for assisted reproductive technology with reproductive endocrinologists. Most patients are unable to afford out of pocket costs if they go outside the system. Many have unreliable access to care and are at high risk of being lost to follow-up. Cultural and socioeconomic factors play a role in oncologic outcomes, but also in desires and expectations regarding fertility and their family. As gynecologic oncologists practicing in both academic and safety-net systems, it is jarring to see the different opportunities based on socioeconomic status.

Oncologists and surgeons caring for cancer patients should consider fertility preservation and FSS for all patients who would be candidates. Not all patients will desire fertility, and adoption can be an option for women who are not candidates. But surgeons, oncologists, and gynecologic oncologists should be open to discussing options within the resources of their system that could provide cancer survivors the option of having children, with a realistic expectation of success and oncologic outcomes.

24.8   Selected References

- Eskander RN, Randall LM, Berman ML, Tewari KS, Disaia PJ, Bristow RE. Fertility preserving options in patients with gynecologic malignancies. Am J Obstet Gynecol. 2011;205(2):103–110. https://doi.org/10.1016/j.ajog.2011.01.025

  - A review of fertility-preserving options for patients with gynecologic malignancies and associated outcomes.

- Gershenson DM. Fertility-sparing surgery for malignancies in women. J Natl Cancer Inst Monogr. 2005(34):43–47. https://doi.org/10.1093/jncimonographs/lgi011

  - A review of fertility-preserving surgery options for women with gynecologic cancers.

- Zhang Q, Li W, Kanis MJ, et al. Oncologic and obstetrical outcomes with fertility-sparing treatment of cervical cancer: a systematic review and meta-analysis. Oncotarget. 2017;8(28):46580–46,592. https://doi.org/10.18632/oncotarget.16233

  - A comparison of cancer and obstetric outcomes of women with cervical cancer treatments with cervical conization versus radical trachelectomy.

References

1. American Cancer Society. Cancer Facts & Figures 2020. American Cancer Society; 2020.
2. Eskander RN, Randall LM, Berman ML, Tewari KS, Disaia PJ, Bristow RE. Fertility preserving options in patients with gynecologic malignancies. Am J Obstet Gynecol. 2011;205(2):103–10. https://doi.org/10.1016/j.ajog.2011.01.025.
3. Gershenson DM. Fertility-sparing surgery for malignancies in women. J Natl Cancer Inst Monogr. 2005;34:43–7. https://doi.org/10.1093/jncimonographs/lgi011.
4. Laurelli G, Falcone F, Gallo MS, et al. Long-term oncologic and reproductive outcomes in young women with early endometrial Cancer conservatively treated: a prospective study and literature update. Int J Gyn Ca. 2016;26(9):1650–7. https://doi.org/10.1097/igc.0000000000000825.
5. Oktay K, Harvey BE, Partridge AH, et al. Fertility preservation in patients with Cancer: ASCO clinical practice guideline update. J Clin Oncol. 2018;36(19):1994–2001. https://doi.org/10.1200/jco.2018.78.1914.
6. Zhang Q, Li W, Kanis MJ, et al. Oncologic and obstetrical outcomes with fertility-sparing treatment of cervical cancer: a systematic review and meta-analysis. Oncotarget. 2017;8(28):46580–92. https://doi.org/10.18632/oncotarget.16233.
7. Benedict C, Thom B, Kelvin J. Fertility preservation and cancer: challenges for adolescent and young adult patients. Curr Opin Support Palliat Care. 2016;10:87–94. https://doi.org/10.1097/spc.0000000000000185.

8. Bentivegna E, Maulard A, Miailhe G, Gouy S, Morice P. Gynaecologic cancer surgery and preservation of fertility. J Visc Surg. 2018;155(suppl 1):S23–9. https://doi.org/10.1016/j.jviscsurg.2018.03.001.

9. Aviki EM, Abu-Rustum NR. A call to standardize our approach to fertility-sparing surgery in patients with gynecologic cancers. Gynecol Oncol. 2017;147(3):491–2. https://doi.org/10.1016/j.ygyno.2017.11.001.

10. Jiang X, Yang J, Yu M, et al. Oncofertility in patients with stage I epithelial ovarian cancer: fertility-sparing surgery in young women of reproductive age. World J Surg Oncol. 2017;15(1):154. https://doi.org/10.1186/s12957-017-1222-4.

11. Leblanc E, Narducci F, Ferron G, Querleu D. Indications and teaching of fertility preservation in the surgical management of gynecologic malignancies: European perspective. Gynecol Oncol. 2009;114(suppl 2):S32–6. https://doi.org/10.1016/j.ygyno.2009.04.010.

12. Ethics Committee of the American Society for Reproductive Medicine. Fertility preservation and reproduction in patients facing gonadotoxic therapies: an ethics committee opinion. Fertil Steril. 2018;110(3):380–6. https://doi.org/10.1016/j.frtnstert.2018.05.034.

13. Wethington SL, Cibula D, Duska LR, et al. An international series on abdominal radical trachelectomy: 101 patients and 28 pregnancies. Int J Gynecol Cancer. 2012;22(7):1251–7. https://doi.org/10.1097/igc.0b013e318263eee2.

14. Robertson JA. Cancer and fertility: ethical and legal challenges. J Natl Cancer Inst Monogr. 2005;34:104–6. https://doi.org/10.1093/jncimonographs/lgi008.

15. Oktem O, Urman B. Options of fertility preservation in female Cancer patients. Obstet Gynecol Surv. 2010;65(8):531–42. https://doi.org/10.1097/OGX.0b013e3181f8c0aa.

16. Ceppi L, Galli F, Lamanna M, et al. Ovarian function, fertility, and menopause occurrence after fertility-sparing surgery and chemotherapy for ovarian neoplasms. Gynecol Oncol. 2019;152(2):346–52. https://doi.org/10.1016/j.ygyno.2018.11.032.

17. Fernandez-Pineda I, Davidoff AM, Lu L, et al. Impact of ovarian transposition before pelvic irradiation on ovarian function among long-term survivors of childhood Hodgkin lymphoma: a report from the St. Jude lifetime cohort study. Pediatr Blood Cancer. 2018;65:e27232. https://doi.org/10.1002/pbc.27232.

18. Carr SV. Surrogacy and ethics in women with cancer. Best Pract Res Clin Obstet Gynaecol. 2019;55:117–27. https://doi.org/10.1016/j.bpobgyn.2018.11.001.

19. Yahata H, Sonoda K, Okugawa K, et al. Survey of the desire to have children and engage in sexual activity after trachelectomy among young Japanese women with early-stage cervical cancer. J Obstet Gynaecol Res. 2019;45(11):2255–9. https://doi.org/10.1111/jog.14099.

20. Curtis KM, Mohllajee AP, Peterson HB. Regret following female sterilization at a young age: a systematic review. Contraception. 2006;73(2):205–10. https://doi.org/10.1016/j.contraception.2005.08.006.

21. Scheer AS, O'Connor AM, Chan BPK, et al. The myth of informed consent in rectal cancer surgery: what do patients retain? Dis Colon Rectum. 2012;55(9):970–5. https://doi.org/10.1097/dcr.0b013e31825f2479.

22. Reilly PR. Eugenics and involuntary sterilization: 1907-2015. Annu Rev Genomics Hum Genet. 2015;16:351–68. https://doi.org/10.1146/annurev-genom-090314-024930.

23. Muaygil R. Her uterus, her medical decision? Dismantling spousal consent for medically indicated hysterectomies in Saudi Arabia. Camb Q Healthc Ethics. 2018;27(3):397–407. https://doi.org/10.1017/s0963180117000780.

24. Bergamini A, Petrone M, Rabaiotti E, et al. Fertility sparing surgery in epithelial ovarian cancer in Italy: perceptions, practice, and main issues. Gynecol Endocrinol. 2018;34(4):305–8. https://doi.org/10.1080/09513590.2017.1393508.

25. Stafman LL, Maizlin II, Dellinger M, et al. Disparities in fertility-sparing surgery in adolescent and young women with stage I ovarian dysgerminoma. J Surg Res. 2018;224:38–43. https://doi.org/10.1016/j.jss.2017.11.046.

26. Gardino SL, Russell AE, Woodruff TK. Adoption after cancer: adoption agency attitudes and perspectives on the potential to parent post-cancer. Cancer Treat Res. 2010;156:153–70. https://doi.org/10.1007/978-1-4419-6518-9_11.

Chapter 25
Anal Sparing Surgery: Pushing the Limits of Patient Autonomy

Chen Lin ⓘ, Peipei Wang ⓘ, and Bin Wu ⓘ

Abstract With fast-moving scientific and technologic advancement, surgeons in this era may face ever more complicated problems and dilemmas exacerbated by the demands of increasing patient autonomy. This chapter is designed to provide surgeons with some insights to common ethical problems in adult colorectal surgery that they are likely to encounter. We present a case of watch and wait (W&W) strategy versus radical surgery and local excision for rectal cancer with complete clinical response (cCR) after neoadjuvant therapy. It illustrates some of these ethical issues and demonstrates a method for approaching the issue and finding rational solutions in a more evidence-based pattern.

Keywords Anal sparing · Colorectal cancer · Neoadjuvant therapy · Watch and wait · Patient autonomy · Four-Box model of decision-making

Case

An 81-year-old male patient presented with a chief complaint of hematochezia for 2 months. Colonoscopy (Fig. 25.1a) showed a protruding rectal mass 6–8 cm from the anus occupying about one third of the cavity. Pathological results of the biopsy reported moderately differentiated adenocarcinoma. Rectal magnetic resonance (MR) (Fig. 25.2a) demonstrated local thickening of the rectal wall with luminal stenosis, and limited diffusion on diffusion weighted imaging (DWI). The lesion had an obvious enhancement in length of 3.7 cm and the

C. Lin (✉)
Department of General Surgery, Chinese Academy of Medical Sciences, Peking Union Medical College Hospital, Beijing, China

P. Wang · B. Wu
Peking Union Medical College Hospital, Beijing, China

© The Author(s), under exclusive license to Springer Nature Switzerland AG 2022

V. A. Lonchyna et al. (eds.), *Difficult Decisions in Surgical Ethics*, Difficult Decisions in Surgery: An Evidence-Based Approach,
https://doi.org/10.1007/978-3-030-84625-1_25

lower margin was 5.5 cm from the anus. Continuous signal of the wall was interrupted, and a rough serosal surface was found with a clear surrounding fat gap. Small lymph nodes were visible demonstrating a staging of mrT3N1.

The guidelines [1] for patients with locally advanced rectal cancer recommend neoadjuvant chemoradiation before surgery. Preoperative neoadjuvant therapy can reduce the local recurrence rate of patients with locally advanced rectal cancer, may reduce tumor volume, may downstage the tumor and increase the chance of sphincter preservation. Thus, the patient's treatment plan was as follows: Radiotherapy: 50Gy (2Gy/time/day, 5 days a week, 5 weeks in total); Chemotherapy: Xeloda (capecitabine) 850 mg/m^2 bid, day 1–14 with an interval of 1 week, a total of 3 cycles. Re-examination of the patient was performed 8 weeks after radiotherapy. Rectal MR (plain scan + enhanced) showed the aforementioned mid-rectal wall was irregularly thickened, and significantly smaller than before. The tumor volume was reduced by more than 75%.

The College of American Pathologists (CAP) has established a grading system to evaluate the tumor response following neoadjuvant therapy [2, 3]. Our patient had a CAP level 0, complete clinical response (cCR) not excluded, as shown in Fig. 25.2b. Colonoscopy (Fig. 25.1b): at 7 cm from the anus, there was a scar-like formation 1.0 cm in diameter on the posterior wall of the rectum. The surface of the mucosa was smooth. Biopsy showed chronic inflammation of the colon mucosa. Combining rectal MRI and colonoscopy, we concluded a diagnosis of cCR of the lesion.

The current ESMO (European Society for Medical Oncology) and NCCN (National Comprehensive Cancer Network) colorectal cancer diagnosis and treatment guidelines [1, 4] both recommend total mesorectal excision (TME) after neo-adjuvant chemoradiation therapy (nCRT) as standard treatment strategy for locally advanced rectal cancer. Therefore, the patient was informed of the necessity of TME surgery for rectal cancer and the risks of the surgery. TME surgery has the risk of various complications (e.g., anastomotic leakage), and it may also have an impact on rectal and anal control as well as sexual function. In addition, the patient's rectal cancer lesion was located in the middle and lower segment of the rectum. Thus, there's a risk that the anus cannot be preserved during the operation. Abdominoperineal resection (APR) may be required and there might be a need for a temporary/permanent stoma as the patient was told so.

However, the patient, after being informed of a diagnosis of cCR of his rectal cancer, strongly refused to undergo a surgery which may require even a temporary stoma. When questioned, he said that he knew some people who had a similar low rectal cancer and achieved cCR after nCRT; they were in a watch and wait (W&W) strategy and survived well! He stated that he would rather die than have a stoma and he thought he was too old to bear even a laparoscopic surgery. The surgeon who made his preoperative plan was troubled by the patient's refusal of surgery because he truly believed that this would be in the patient's best interests, despite the patient's refusal to undergo this treatment plan.

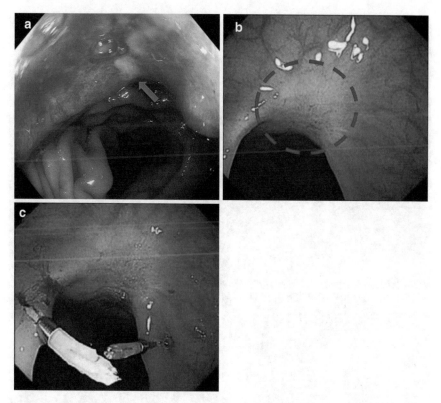

Fig. 25.1 Colonoscopy: (**a**) demonstrated one third annular tumor (arrow) with a margin of 6–8 cm from the anus before neoadjuvant therapy; (**b**) showed a scar-like formation about 1 cm in diameter on the posterior wall of the rectum at 7 cm from the anus; (**c**) biopsy indicated no tumor cells after neoadjuvant therapy

25.1   Introduction

In this surgical setting, the medical problem the stakeholders faced was whether to do the surgery for a cCR of low rectal cancer after neoadjuvant therapy. When an agent must choose between mutually exclusive options, to do or not to do a R0 resection, an ethical challenge occurs given that both have equal elements of right and wrong [5].

25.2   Search Strategy

The Web of Science (WOS) database was used to search related literature referable to this ethical dilemma presented. No restrictions were placed on the country or language. Published timeframe was the last ten years. The search terms and phrases

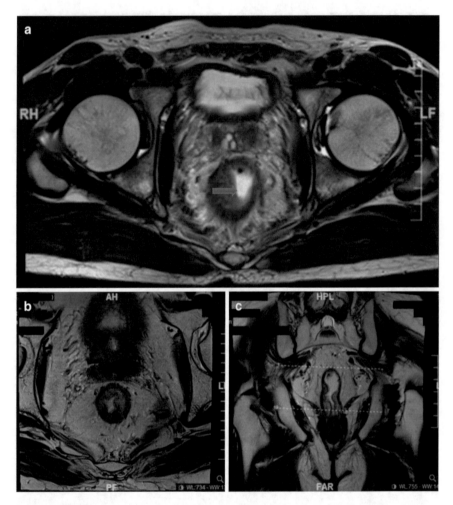

Fig. 25.2 Magnetic resonance (MR) images of an 81-year-old man with rectal adenocarcinoma before and after completion of chemoradiation therapy with possible clinical complete response: (**a**) demonstrated local thickening of the rectal wall with luminal stenosis, interruption of the continuous signal of the wall, and a rough serosal surface with a clear surrounding fat gap (arrow points to the tumor); (**b**) sagittal and (**c**) coronal images of the tumor following neoadjuvant therapy detailed tumor regression

were rectal cancer, wait and watch (W&W) strategy, neoadjuvant therapy. Then, further search was made via adding phrases as follows: autonomy or decision-making or ethics or challenge. PubMed and EndNote X9 were used to obtain the full texts and abstracts of articles available. Titles and abstracts were used to estimate the relevance to search categories.

25.3 Discussion

The central focus of Clinical Medical Ethics is how to reach medical and ethical decisions that are right for the patient. Through the search work, there are few reports in the literature that illustrate viewpoints from both the clinical and ethical perspectives. Arguments mainly concentrate on W&W strategy versus radical surgery approach in rectal cancer patients with a clinically complete response after neoadjuvant therapy which have tended to come from the long-term survival data.

The ultimate goal is to evaluate an ethical dilemma in a systemic fashion just as we would do in surgical problems. Therefore, the methodology described hereby focused on a structured approach to clinical and ethical decision-making via the Four-Box Model of Decision-Making [6]. The questions relating to this ethical problem are refined and listed in the Table 25.1.

Table 25.1 The four-box model of ethical questions in decision-making relating to the case

Elements of ethics	Questions to reflect on
Medical Indications *Beneficence* *Nonmaleficence*	1. What is the patient's medical problem? 2. What are the goals of treatment? 3. In what circumstances are R0 resection not indicated? 4. What are the probabilities of success of R0 resection and "Watch and Wait" treatment options? 5. In sum, how can this patient be benefited by each option of medical care, and how can harm be avoided?
Preferences of Patients *Respect for Autonomy*	1. Has the patient been informed of benefits and risks of R0 resection and "Watch and Wait" treatment recommendations, understood this information, and communicated consent? 2. Is the patient mentally capable and legally competent? 3. If mentally capable, what are the patient's preferences? 4. Is the patient unwilling or unable to cooperate with R0 resection? why?
Quality of Life *Beneficence* *Nonmaleficence* *Respect for Autonomy*	1. What are the prospects, with or without the resection, for a return to an acceptable quality of life and what physical, mental, and social deficits might the patient experience even if treatment succeeds? 2. Are there biases that might prejudice the provider's evaluation of the patient's quality of life? 3. What ethical issues arise concerning improving or enhancing a patient's quality of life? 4. Do quality of life assessment raise any questions that might contribute to a change of R0 resection to "Watch and Wait?"
Contextual Features *Justice*	1. Do decisions about treatment raise issues of fairness? 2. Are there professional, interprofessional, personal, interpersonal or business interests that might create conflicts of interest in the clinical treatment of patient? 3. Are there parties other than clinicians and patient, such as family members, who have a legitimate interest in clinical decisions? 4. Are there financial factors that create conflicts of interest in clinical decisions? 5. Are there problems of allocation of resources/religious factors/legal issues/considerations of clinical research and medical education that affect clinical decisions?

Adapted from Jonsen [6]

25.3.1 Medical Indications: The Principle of Beneficence

25.3.1.1 Why Does This Ethical Problem Occur?

Looking back on medical history, before the beginning of the nineteenth century, the local recurrence rate of rectal cancer after surgery was still the main bottleneck faced by colorectal surgeons, and the recurrence rate was as high as 40%. However, with the development of surgical techniques, especially the concept of total mesorectal resection, the local recurrence rate of rectal cancer has dramatically dropped to 5% since the 1990s [7]. In the current decade, neoadjuvant therapy was introduced with the goal of local recurrence control with additional value of increasing the proportion of anal sparing. Studies show that around 15% to 20% of patients with rectal cancer after neoadjuvant treatment have a pathological complete response (pCR) and good long-term follow-up [8]. Thus, a new clinical question arose: if neoadjuvant radiotherapy and chemotherapy could achieve pCR, is surgery still necessary for the patient?

Thinking about the essence of this question is also a surgical ethics issue, that is, due to the effectiveness of comprehensive treatment, will there be more possible choices for the patients? In addition to the survival rate that doctors most concentrated on in the past, can we now also switch some of our attention to quality of life and the preservation of organs? Various centers have accumulated valuable evidence through clinical research to try to answer this combined clinical and ethical challenge of how to further increase the ratio of pCR. Can patients avoid a series of injuries caused by surgery? Can the patient retain the anus and preserve the function of the rectum and anus through non-surgical comprehensive treatment? Therefore, the ethical challenge is whether the W&W strategy can be selected after nCRT for low rectal cancer. This is the question that both patients with low rectal cancer and their surgeons may face and the root cause comes from the historical evolution of rectal cancer treatment and the demand for stratified tailored management.

25.3.1.2 What is the Evidence for a Watch & Wait (W&W) Strategy?

The W&W strategy was first advocated by Habr-Gama in 2004 [9]. The study was of the long-term results of stage 0 distal rectal cancer following neoadjuvant chemoradiation with cCR. It demonstrated excellent long-term results irrespective of treatment strategy. In comparing operative with nonoperative treatment, the five-year overall survival (OS) was 100% vs 88% and the disease-free survival (DFS) was 92% vs 83%, respectively. Furthermore, surgical resection may not lead to improved outcomes in this situation and may be associated with high rates of temporary or permanent stoma construction and unnecessary morbidity and mortality rates, despite the early stage of this case series.

Subsequently, since cCR cannot be completely equivalent to pCR, multiple studies conducted from preliminary observations of efficacy compared cCR with pCR outcomes and proved those two were similar confirmed through long-term follow-up data [10, 11]. Accordingly, further studies were carried out to screen the potential benefit subgroups and optimize the strategy [12–16]. For instance, the cCR standard, the pCR standard evaluated through PET, treatment optimization to improve cCR, and the concept of near cCR was put forward [12–14]. On this basis, international registration systems were established in 2015 and promoted through multidisciplinary collaborations.

Between 2015 and 2017, the International Watch & Wait Database (IWWD)

> …identified 1009 patients who received neoadjuvant treatment and were managed by W&W in the database from 47 participating institutes (15 countries). We included 880 (87%) patients with a cCR. Median follow-up time was 3·3 years (95% CI 3·1–3·6). The 2-year cumulative incidence of local regrowth was 25·2% (95% CI 22·2–28·5%), …Distant metastasis were diagnosed in 71 (8%) of 880 patients. 5-year overall survival was 85% (95% CI 80·9–87·7%), and 5-year disease-specific survival was 94% (91–96%) [17].

Therefore, the large-sample registration database has confirmed the good oncology safety of the rectal cancer through W&W strategy in recent years, providing a new option for the treatment strategy of selected patients with rectal cancer [17–19].

In China, a randomized clinical trial of W&W was started in 2012 (ChiCTRTRC-12,002,488) and the results were published in 2017 [20]. Li et al. reported a group of 122 patients with cCR after nCRT in a multicenter fashion in 2015 [21]. In 2019, Chinese Wait & Watch Database (CWWD) was built in order to standardize RCTs of W&W treatment in China. The Chinese Medical Doctor Association (CMDA) issued an expert consensus which included aspects such as how to perform informed consent, what inclusion criteria to use, patient and doctor education and discussed hidden ethical challenges.

Despite certain contrary study results, until now, the evidence available is frequently based on small-to-moderate sized series from specialized centers and comes mostly from retrospective cohort studies [22]. As compared with randomized studies, retrospective studies may be biased in the selection of treatment options. For example, patients who decided to have surgical resection may have enrollment bias. Most articles did not collect the reasons for the selection of resection or observation due to the retrospective nature of the analysis, hence the potential bias may weigh the prognosis of one of the two groups more advantageously. In terms of data homogeneity, the quality of multi-center studies is more difficult to be consistent, such as the standard and definition of cCR, the consistency of surgical quality and the standardization of nCRT. For prospective randomized trials, there may be bottlenecks such as patient concerns and surgeon's preferences which may lead to difficulties in enrollment and adhering to the protocol.

In general, when analyzing the principle of patient's beneficence, special attention should be paid to critical thinking considering the amount of evidence available. In this scenario, although there is currently no robust evidence to support the W&W strategy as a standard approach, the results we have so far are promising and there is still space for a further discussion of the patient's demand of quality of life. Owing to the above factors, it is recommended to fully disclose all the options and ramifications with the patient when obtaining informed consent and strongly consider enrollment into a randomized controlled trial (RCT) of W&W strategy.

25.3.2 Patient Preferences: Autonomy

From the principle of respect for autonomy, this patient is an adult who was evaluated as mentally capable and legally competent. Therefore, respect for autonomy would require the surgeon to accept the patients' preference that he would rather not undergo surgery and has a strong will to preserve the function of his anus. The patient may refuse radical resection, but then must be prepared to bear the consequences. The patient must be fully informed of the benefits and risks between the standard treatment plan and the W&W strategy, understand this information, and communicate consent and understanding of the consequences of this decision. The surgeon should consider an alternate management plan when the patient rejects the recommendations of treatment that the surgeon judges to be in the patient's best medical interests. In addition, if the patient is unwilling to cooperate with medical treatment, ask why and find deep reasons that would help to jump out of the dilemma.

25.3.3 Quality of Life

The goals of the patient and the surgeon include increased length and quality of life. Patients with low rectal cancer undergoing neoadjuvant therapy and followed by radical surgery may develop surgery-related postoperative complications and long-term impairment of functions, such as fecal incontinence or urgency, frequent or fragmented bowel movements, emptying difficulties, and increased intestinal gas, known as low anterior resection syndrome. Urinary and/or sexual function may also be affected by sphincter-sparing procedures such as low anterior resection (LAR). For this patient, he may experience some of these functional impairments and suffer from concordant mental and social pressures. If a change from a R0 resection to a W&W strategy was chosen, the biggest challenge would be how to achieve the goal of increasing length of life for the patient while also improving their quality of life.

25.3.4 "External" Considerations

The major obstacle to implementing the W&W strategy is whether it can be remedied in a timely manner after failure and the determination of the follow-up interval. IWWD showed local regrowth occurred mostly in the first 2 years and in the bowel wall, emphasizing the importance of endoscopic surveillance to ensure the option of deferred curative surgery [17]. A study in 2019 included one hundred ninety-seven cT2-4 N0-2 M0 patients with cCR after nCRT and its conditional survival suggested that patients had significantly lower risks ($\leq$10%) of developing recurrences after 2 years of achieving cCR following nCRT [23]. These studies showed that if remedy procedure was performed immediately after local tumor recurrence was detected in time, W&W strategy may not have a significant impact on survival [9, 17, 23]. Therefore, a reasonable and close follow-up and timely remedial surgery are particularly critical to W&W strategy.

However, contextual features, such as psychological pressure and financial burden of patients arising from close follow-up are equal issues worthy of attention. A study from Netherlands assessed six hypothetical treatment-outcome scenarios. Wait-and-see was most often ranked highest by patients and volunteers (36% and 50%) among all scenarios while a substantial proportion also ranked wait-and-see as their lowest preference (38% in patients and 35% in volunteers). This gave insights into how patients may value the current rectal cancer treatment options based on their different psychological and social state [24].

Therefore, for this patient who meets cCR criteria, W&W strategy could be considered as the treatment option. For the early detection of tumor recurrence and patient's safety, a well-planned close follow-up focusing on physical examination, colonoscopy and MR to fully evaluate the local recurrence especially in the front two years is in great demand. However, even if the patient meets the inclusion criteria of a RCT, one still needs to carefully evaluate the "external" considerations to ensure that the patient has the ability to follow the protocol during the whole timeline of a RCT.

25.4 Case Conclusion

In this case, to address the ethical problems of surgery, we propose the tailored questions that should be asked based on the four-box model (Table 25.1) [6]. The next step is to determine the available options: R0 resection vs. W&W strategy; their goals; the values and norms to identify whether the W&W strategy is acceptable. For example, a fully understandable informed consent should be given to the patient. Has the center developed good inclusion criterion for a RCT and joined a WWD for the observation of patients? Will there be an appropriate multidisciplinary team to support a clinical trial? Will the patient have socio-psychological factors or problems with access to resources that may affect a close follow-up and so bias the clinical decision? At the conclusion of this process, after appropriate identification of all the above factors and fully ethically consent with the patient, the surgeon and patient are able to come to a consensus about the choice of W&W strategy or surgical intervention.

In this particular case, the 81-year-old man chose to return to his hometown and entered a trial of W&W in a colorectal center to do the observation. Now, in his fourth year of follow-up, he has shown no signs of local recurrence or distal metastasis.

25.5 More Scenarios

The following scenarios also illustrate other difficulties with the surgical practice in CRC anal preserving process. For example, for rectal cancer patients with a stage of T2 and without any high-risk factors for relapse, if the patient asks for neoadjuvant therapy because of a strong intention of saving the anus, how can we make the decision? For lower rectal cancer patients who undergo local excision by TME or colonoscopy but have high-risk independent factors for recurrent disease, should we do APR or follow the patient's intention not to do it? For colorectal cancer patients who have an indication for a Hartmann or APR but strongly do not agree with a colostomy or ileostomy, how can we make the decision? In general, we believe following a standardized ethical method to address and solve the clinical problems in each of these settings would add another dimension to increase the interrelationship between solutions and problems during the surgical practice and be helpful to the surgeons to strike a balance among different factors when they are taken into considerations.

25.6 Conclusion

The patient autonomy encounters dramatic changes with the development of medicine and science, such as more successful organ preservation and demanding better quality of life. As radiotherapy, internal medicine, imaging, artificial intelligence, etc. becomes more integrated into surgery, quality of life will become an increasingly important focus of both patients and medical providers in the future. Surgeons must learn to be fully aware of the ethical challenges among these surgical dilemmas and apply ethical principles of respect for patient autonomy, beneficence and non-maleficence, justice throughout the whole process of approaching and thinking through the issue in a systemic fashion. These ethical principles should be integrated into their daily surgical practice.

25.7 Selected References

- Habr-Gama A, Perez RO, Nadalin W, et al. Operative versus nonoperative treatment for stage 0 distal rectal cancer following chemoradiation therapy: long-term results. Ann Surg. 2004;24(4):711–8. https://doi.org/10.1097/01.sla.0000141194.27992.32

  – The W&W strategy, first put forward by Professor Habr-Gama with this study, provided a new option for the treatment strategy of selected cCR patients with rectal cancer.

- van der Valk MJM, Hilling DE, Bastiaannet E, et al. Long-term outcomes of clinical complete responders after neoadjuvant treatment for rectal cancer in the International Watch & Wait Database (IWWD): an international multicentre registry study. Lancet. 2018;391(10139):2537–45. https://doi.org/10.1016/s0140-6736(18)31078-x

  – This multi-center clinical study of cCR patients with long-term follow-up results is an important reference for clinical decision making.

References

1. Benson AB, Venook AP, Al-Hawary MM, et al. NCCN guidelines insights: rectal cancer, version 6.2020. J Natl Compr Cancer Netw. 2020;18(7):806–15. https://doi.org/10.6004/jnccn.2020.0032.
2. Edge SB, Compton CC. The American Joint Committee on Cancer: the 7th edition of the AJCC cancer staging manual and the future of TNM. Ann Surg Oncol. 2010;17(6):1471–4. https://doi.org/10.1245/s10434-010-0985-4.
3. Mace AG, Pai RK, Stocchi L, Kalady MF. American Joint Committee on Cancer and College of American Pathologists regression grade: a new prognostic factor in rectal cancer. Dis Colon Rectum. 2015;58(1):32–44. https://doi.org/10.1097/DCR.0000000000000266.
4. Glynne-Jones R, Wyrwicz L, Tiret E, et al.; for the ESMO Guidelines Committee. Rectal cancer: ESMO clinical practice guidelines for diagnosis, treatment and follow-up. Ann Oncol. 2017;28(Suppl 4):iv22–40. https://doi.org/10.1093/annonc/mdx224
5. Wall A, Angelos P, Brown D, Kodner IJ, Keune JD. Ethics in surgery. Curr Probl Surg. 2013;50(3):99–134. https://doi.org/10.1067/j.cpsurg.2012.11.004.
6. Jonsen AR, Sieger M, Winslade WJ. Clinical ethics: a practical approach to ethical decisions in clinical medicine. 8th ed. McGraw-Hill; 2015.
7. Heald RJ, Husband EM, Ryall RDH. The mesorectum in rectal cancer surgery-the clue to pelvic recurrence? Br J Surg. 1982;69(10):613–6. https://doi.org/10.1002/bjs.1800691019.
8. Tulchinsky H, Rabau M, Shacham-Shemueli E, et al. Can rectal cancers with pathologic T0 after neoadjuvant chemoradiation (ypT0) be treated by transanal excision alone? Ann Surg Oncol. 2006;13(3):347–52. https://doi.org/10.1245/aso.2006.03.029.
9. Habr-Gama A, Perez RO, Nadalin W, et al. Operative versus nonoperative treatment for stage 0 distal rectal cancer following chemoradiation therapy: long-term results. Ann Surg. 2004;24(4):711–8. https://doi.org/10.1097/01.sla.0000141194.27992.32.

10. Maas M, Beets-Tan RGH, Lambregts DMJ, et al. Wait-and-see policy for clinical complete responders after chemoradiation for rectal cancer. J Clin Oncol. 2011;29(35):4633–40. https://doi.org/10.1200/jco.2011.38.1335.
11. Pang K, Rao Q, Qin S, Jin L, Yao H, Zhang Z. Prognosis comparison between wait and watch and surgical strategy on rectal cancer patients after treatment with neoadjuvant chemoradiotherapy: a meta-analysis. Ther Adv Gastroenterol. 2019;12:1–12. https://doi.org/10.1177/1756284819892477.
12. Habr-Gama A, Perez RO, Wynn G, Marks J, Kessler H, Gama-Rodriques J. Complete clinical response after neoadjuvant chemoradiation therapy for distal rectal cancer: characterization of clinical and endoscopic findings for standardization. Dis Colon Rectum. 2010;53(12):1692–8. https://doi.org/10.1007/dcr.0b013e3181f42b89.
13. Habr-Gama A, Gama-Rodrigues J, Perez RO, et al. Late assessment of local control by PET in patients with distal rectal cancer managed non-operatively after complete tumor regression following neoadjuvant chemoradiation. Tech Coloproctol. 2008;12(1):74–6. PMID: 18524026.
14. Habr-Gama A, Perez RO, Proscurshim I, et al. Interval between surgery and neoadjuvant chemoradiation therapy for distal rectal cancer: does delayed surgery have an impact on outcome? Int J Radiat Oncol Biol Phys. 2008;71(4):1181–8. https://doi.org/10.1016/j.ijrobp.2007.11.035.
15. Asoglu O, Tokmak H, Bakir B, et al. The impact of total neo-adjuvant treatment on nonoperative management in patients with locally advanced rectal cancer: the evaluation of 66 cases. Eur J Surg Oncol. 2020;46(3):402–9. https://doi.org/10.1016/j.ejso.2019.07.012.
16. He F, Ju HQ, Ding Y, et al. Association between adjuvant chemotherapy and survival in patients with rectal cancer and pathological complete response after neoadjuvant chemoradiotherapy and resection. Br J Cancer. 2020;123(8):1244–52. https://doi.org/10.1038/s41416-020-0989-1.
17. van der Valk MJM, Hilling DE, Bastiaannet E, et al. Long-term outcomes of clinical complete responders after neoadjuvant treatment for rectal cancer in the International Watch & Wait Database (IWWD): an international multicentre registry study. Lancet. 2018;391(10139):2537–45. https://doi.org/10.1016/s0140-6736(18)31078-x.
18. Chadi SA, Malcomson L, Ensor J, et al. Factors affecting local regrowth after watch and wait for patients with a clinical complete response following chemoradiotherapy in rectal cancer (InterCoRe consortium): an individual participant data meta-analysis. Lancet Gastroenterol Hepatol. 2018;3(12):825–36. https://doi.org/10.1016/s2468-1253(18)30301-7.
19. Smith JJ, Strombom P, Chow OS, et al. Assessment of a watch-and-wait strategy for rectal cancer in patients with a complete response after neoadjuvant therapy. JAMA Oncol. 2019;5(4):e185896. https://doi.org/10.1001/jamaoncol.2018.5896.
20. Gu J, Du C, Li M, et al. The feasibility and efficiency of wait and see policy for patients with complete clinical response following neoadjuvant therapy in rectal cancer: a prospective cohort study from China [ASCO abstract 3610]. J Clin Oncol. 2017;35(15 suppl):3610. https://doi.org/10.1200.jco.2017.35.15_suppl.3610
21. Li J, Liu H, Yin J, et al. Wait-and-see or radical surgery for rectal cancer patients with a clinical complete response after neoadjuvant chemoradiotherapy: a cohort study. Oncotarget. 2015;6(39):42354–61. https://doi.org/10.18632/oncotarget.6093.
22. Bernier L, Balyasnikova S, Tait D, Brown T. Watch-and-wait as a therapeutic strategy in rectal cancer. Curr Colorectal Cancer Rep. 2018;14(2):37–55. https://doi.org/10.1007/s11888-018-0398-5.
23. São Julião GP, Karagkounis G, Fernandez LM, et al. Conditional survival in patients with rectal cancer and complete clinical response managed by watch and wait after chemoradiation: recurrence risk over time. Ann Surg. 2020;272(1):138–44. https://doi.org/10.1097/sla.0000000000003286.
24. Couwenberg AM, Intven MPW, Burbach JPM, et al. Utility scores and preferences for surgical and organ-sparing approaches for treatment of intermediate and high-risk rectal cancer. Dis Colon Rectum. 2018;61(8):911–9. https://doi.org/10.1097/dcr.0000000000001029.

Chapter 26
Invited Commentary for Anal Sparing Surgery: Pushing the Limits of Patient Autonomy

Kinga B. Skowron Olortegui ⓘ

Abstract The colorectal surgeon must decide whether to provide patients with the "tried and true" therapy for rectal cancer, or to recommend a novel, but not entirely proven non-operative option. Advancements in imaging have allowed for much more accurate identification of advanced-stage disease. Stage-specific treatment regimens and neoadjuvant therapy are currently employed. The question now to consider is the safety of organ preservation or "watch-and-wait" (W&W) treatment strategies after clinical complete response following neoadjuvant therapy. This approach has shown promise in various regions of the world.

Keywords Anal sparing surgery · Total neoadjuvant therapy · Watch and wait strategy · Advanced imaging · Moral distress

It is a dilemma of the modern colorectal surgeon, whether to provide patients with the "tried and true" therapy for rectal cancer, or to recommend a novel, not entirely proven non-operative option. We are fortunate to care for patients in a time when dramatic improvements in care have allowed for this choice. With the development of more advanced imaging, namely MRI, we have a much better understanding of clinical stage [1]. These advancements allowed for much more accurate identification of advanced-stage disease, and paved the way for stage-specific treatment regimens and neoadjuvant therapy. As neoadjuvant regimens have evolved, we have further made the leap to total neoadjuvant therapy (TNT), in which both full-dose chemotherapy and radiation are delivered in the neoadjuvant setting [2, 3]. This modality has resulted in a dramatic increase in the rate of pathologic complete response, and caused us to question whether some patients need surgery at all.

K. B. Skowron Olortegui (✉)
Section of Colon & Rectal Surgery, Department of Surgery, MacLean Center for Clinical Medical Ethics, University of Chicago, Chicago, IL, USA
e-mail: kskowron@bsd.uchicago.edu

© The Author(s), under exclusive license to Springer Nature Switzerland AG 2022
V. A. Lonchyna et al. (eds.), *Difficult Decisions in Surgical Ethics*, Difficult Decisions in Surgery: An Evidence-Based Approach, https://doi.org/10.1007/978-3-030-84625-1_26

371

When the medical community is buzzing with the potential of a novel therapy, it is only natural that patients ask to be a part of this movement. TME is not without drawbacks, as the authors outlined. Often, sphincter preservation cannot be achieved, and patients are faced with the possibility of a permanent ostomy. If the sphincter is preserved, function will likely not be the same. If the rectum can be *safely* saved, why not save it? There is quite a bit of data from Brazil regarding the safety of organ preservation or "watch-and-wait" (W&W) treatment strategies after clinical complete response following neoadjuvant therapy [4, 5]. While this is certainly feasible, there is not a consensus on appropriate patient selection [6, 7]. In the United States, W&W strategies are very much considered experimental, and clinical trials are ongoing in an effort to shed light on a the ideal treatment and follow up strategies [8].

While the authors point to moral distress on the part of the treating physicians with regard to lack of trust in the W&W strategies, we must ask ourselves, "what is our goal?" The goal of the doctor patient relationship is to be able to help patients come to an informed decision for what is best for them as an individual. It is ultimately the patient who must be comfortable with the level of risk that their choice incurs. The role of the ongoing research studies is to provide the patient with data, such that they can make that informed decision [9]. Armed with more specific data regarding risk of recurrence in *their* particular tumor after TNT, patients can make an educated decision regarding whether they are more averse to this level of risk, or to the prospect of post-operative complications or a stoma.

In this setting, perhaps the most comfortable solution ethically for the physician is to refer the patient for enrollment in a trial. This resolves our feeling of guilt at "allowing" the patient to choose an unproven treatment course. Trials often provide follow up care free of charge, including surveillance MRIs, which may be costly for the patient should their insurance provider disagree with an off-protocol W&W strategy. There is greater oversight, so that patients will be less likely to be simply "lost to follow up." The goal of strict follow up is to capture a recurrence early, such that they may be a candidate for salvage surgery. And, by recording their participation, we learn from their experience so that in the future, we may be able to provide more precise information to other patients.

It is our hope that in the near future, we will have a clear recommendation regarding W&W treatment strategies for rectal cancer. Until such a time, we encourage patients who are interested in W&W to enroll in a clinical trial.

References

1. Keller DS, Berho M, Perez RO, Wexner SD, Chand M. The multidisciplinary management of rectal cancer. Nat Rev Gastroenterol Hepatol. 2020;17:414–29. https://doi.org/10.1038/s41575-020-0275-y.
2. Cercek A, Roxburgh CSD, Strombom P, et al. Adoption of Total neoadjuvant therapy for locally advanced rectal Cancer. JAMA Oncol. 2018;4:e180071. https://doi.org/10.1001/jamaoncol.2018.0071.

3. Ludmir EB, Palta M, Willett CG, Czito BG. Total neoadjuvant therapy for rectal cancer: an emerging option: TNT for rectal Cancer. Cancer. 2017;123:1497–506. https://doi.org/10.1002/cncr.30600.
4. Habr-Gama A, Perez RO, Nadalin W, et al. Operative versus nonoperative treatment for stage 0 distal rectal cancer following chemoradiation therapy: long-term results. Ann Surg 2004;240:711–717; discussion 717–718. https://doi.org/10.1097/01.sla.0000141194.27992.32.
5. Habr-Gama A, São Julião GP, Vailati BB, et al. Organ preservation in cT2N0 rectal Cancer after neoadjuvant Chemoradiation therapy: the impact of radiation therapy dose-escalation and consolidation chemotherapy. Ann Surg. 2019;269:102–7. https://doi.org/10.1097/sla.0000000000002447.
6. Maas M, Lambregts DMJ, Nelemans PJ, et al. Assessment of clinical complete response after Chemoradiation for rectal Cancer with digital rectal examination, endoscopy, and MRI: selection for organ-saving treatment. Ann Surg Oncol. 2015;22:3873–80. https://doi.org/10.1245/s10434-0154687-9.
7. Sammour T, Price BA, Krause KJ, Chang GJ. Nonoperative management or "watch and wait" for rectal Cancer with complete clinical response after neoadjuvant Chemoradiotherapy: a critical appraisal. Ann Surg Oncol. 2017;24:1904–15. https://doi.org/10.1245/s10434-017-5841-3.
8. López-Campos F, Martín-Martín M, Fornell-Pérez R, et al. Watch and wait approach in rectal cancer: current controversies and future directions. W J Gastroenterol. 2020;26:4218–39. https://doi.org/10.3748/wjg.v26.i29.4218.
9. Chadi SA, Malcomson L, Ensor J, et al. Factors affecting local regrowth after watch and wait for patients with a clinical complete response following chemoradiotherapy in rectal cancer (InterCoRe consortium): an individual participant data meta-analysis. Lancet Gastroenterol Hepatol. 2018;3:825–36. https://doi.org/10.1016/s2468-1253(18)30301-7.

Chapter 27
Ethical Decision-Making of Treatment of Aortic Aneurysm, Elective or Emergent (Ruptured)

Ross Milner ⓘ and Rolla Zarifa

Abstract Vascular surgeons are frequently faced with difficult ethical decisions. One of the most common these surgeons are confronted with are the treatment of abdominal aortic aneurysms (AAA) not just in the emergent setting but also electively. This chapter will present two common complex cases and discuss the important ethical components on treating AAA. This chapter will touch on a patient's capacity, appointing a surrogate, the informed consent process, and the surgeon's role in the shared decision-making process.

Keywords Abdominal aortic aneurysms · Ruptured abdominal aortic aneurysms Vascular surgery ethics · Shared decision-making · Patient capacity Informed consent

27.1 Cases

Case 1

An 85-year-old male with a complex medical history, including coronary artery disease for which he had multiple cardiac stents placed and a recent stroke with no residual deficits, presents to the emergency department with new onset abdominal and back pain. He undergoes a CT angiogram showing a 7 cm infrarenal abdominal aortic aneurysm with significant fat stranding suggestive of a contained ruptured abdominal aortic aneurysm (rAAA). He is currently hemodynamically stable.

R. Milner (✉) · R. Zarifa
Division of Vascular Surgery, Department of Surgery, The University of Chicago Medicine & Biological Sciences, Chicago, IL, USA
e-mail: rmilner@surgery.bsd.uchicago.edu; rolla.zarifa@uchospitals.edu

© The Author(s), under exclusive license to Springer Nature Switzerland AG 2022
V. A. Lonchyna et al. (eds.), *Difficult Decisions in Surgical Ethics*, Difficult Decisions in Surgery: An Evidence-Based Approach,
https://doi.org/10.1007/978-3-030-84625-1_27

Case 2
A 70-year-old male with multiple comorbidities, including recent four vessel coronary artery bypass surgery, early end stage renal disease, hypertension, and chronic obstructive pulmonary disease, presents with a complex juxtarenal 6 cm AAA for elective repair.

27.2   Introduction

Treatment of abdominal aortic aneurysms (AAA) has dramatically changed in the last 40 years with improving mortality rates of patients with ruptured abdominal aortic aneurysms (rAAA). The history of AAA treatment was minimal before the twentieth century. We advanced from ligation to extra-arterial wrapping to, finally in 1952, direct reconstruction of the abdominal aorta with synthetic material [1]. From that time, the open repair technique was perfected, but mortality did not improve dramatically until Parodi's first endovascular stenting of an infrarenal AAA [2].

Now patients with rAAA who make it to the hospital alive and qualify for an endovascular aneurysm repair (EVAR) have a reported mortality as low as 30% [3].

It is important to first discuss the factors from a clinical perspective that go into a surgeon's decision-making. Surgeons operate using guidelines and evidence-based outcomes of treatments and then apply this information to patients individually. Most AAA are detected incidentally on imaging, but screening guidelines do exist. These guidelines are summarized in Table 27.1 and show how they differ between each organization [4, 5].

Table 27.1 Screening and surveillance guidelines for abdominal aortic aneurysms

	US Preventive Services Task Force (2019) [4]	Society for Vascular Surgery (2017) [5]
First Screening Ultrasound	• Men ages 65–75 years who have ever smoked • Selective screening for men ages 65–75 years who have never smoked • Women: no recommendation for screening	• Men and women ages 65–75 years who have ever smoked (strong) • First-degree relatives of patients who present with an AAA: between 65–75 years or older than 75 years and in good health (weak)
AAA 3.0–3.9 cm. seen on first US	N/A	Imaging needed every 3 years (weak)
AAA ≥ 4.0 cm. seen on first US	N/A	Imaging needed every 6–12 months (weak)

AAA: abdominal aortic aneurysm; N/A: not available; US: ultrasound

Table 27.2 Indications for Treatment of Abdominal Aortic Aneurysms [6–8]

Recommendations for elective repair
Men with a fusiform aneurysm greater than or equal to 5.5 cm in diameter
Women with a fusiform aneurysm greater than or equal to 5.0 cm in diameter
Aneurysm growth rate of 10 mm in 1 year in both genders
Aneurysms saccular in nature, dissections with mural thrombus, or fractures in saccular calcifications

Unlike screening guidelines, indications for treatment of AAA are clearer. The decision to treat a diagnosed AAA is based on anatomy and stems from the ADAM (The Veterans Affairs Aneurysm Detection And Management) trial and the UK Small Aneurysm Trial [6, 7]. Table 27.2 outlines the guidelines and indications for elective repair of AAA. These guidelines are established on the yearly risk of rupture of a AAA, based on its diameter. The yearly rupture risk is 0.3% for patients with a AAA between 3.0–3.9 cm., 1–11% for 5.0–5.9 cm, 11–22% for 6.0–6.9 cm and > 30% for aneurysms greater than 7 cm [6–8]. Patients who are symptomatic or present with a rAAA require immediate repair and do not fall into the size criteria for repair [8].

The difficulty with treating these aneurysms is deciding when surgical intervention will provide an overall benefit and what specific intervention (open vs. endovascular repair) will decrease their morbidity and mortality. It is important, in the elective repairs, to consider overall operative mortality risk, comorbidities, life expectancy, and patient preferences. There are multiple scoring systems that have been developed to help guide a surgeon's decision when to operate on rAAA, but not all are accurate. Table 27.3 summarizes some of these predictive risk models. The Glasgow Aneurysm Score and Hardman Index were derived almost 30 years ago and are not as applicable to an endovascular repair. These studies have been shown to be poor predictors of mortality in higher risk patients [9–11]. The Vascular Study Group of New England rAAA risk score requires intraoperative variables making its use impractical preoperatively for rAAA but is a great tool for elective AAA repairs [11]. The Harborview Medical Center (HMC) rAAA mortality risk scoring system (most recent and maybe most promising) is a tool that can be quickly used preoperatively in an emergent case [10]. Wang et al. conducted a retrospective study showing HMC risk scores and their associated mortality as: scores of 3 and 4 points—100%, 2 points—60.0%, 1 point—41.2% and 0 was 7.7% mortality ($p = 0.001$) [12]. On multivariate regression analysis, only the patient's pH and BP were determined to be independent predictors for mortality. A creatinine >2 mg/dL ($p = 0.080$) and age ($p = 0.459$) were not independent risk factors. In their study, patients with a free rupture had a 75% mortality [12]. The HMC scoring system along with CT scan findings of free rupture can be used as prognostic tools in discussing treatment options.

Surgeons use all of this information to help present the best treatment options to patients, but it is important to highlight those decisions are patient centered. Not only scientific evidence but specific circumstances of the patient's presentation,

Table 27.3 Risk predictive models

Scoring System	Variables Points		Interpretation and 30-Day Mortality
Glasgow Aneurysm Score [9]	• Age • Coronary artery disease • Cerebrovascular disease • Renal failure • Shock	age (years) 7 10 14 17	Score > 95% Indicates high mortality (> 80%)
Hardman Index [9]	• Age > 76 • Creatinine > 2.15 mg/dL • Hb < 9 mg • Ischemic changes on EKG • Loss of Consciousness	1 1 1 1 1	Score ≥ 3 Indicates high mortality (80–100%)
The Vascular Study Group of New England rAAA risk score [11]	• Age > 76 • Cardiac Arrest • Loss of Consciousness • Suprarenal Clamp	2 2 1 1	Score and mortality: 0 8% 1 25% 2 37% 3 60% 4 80% ≥ 5 87%
The Harborview Medical Center [10]	• Age > 76 • Creatinine > 2.0 mg/dL • Systolic BP ever < 70 mm Hg • pH < 7.2	1 1 1 1	Score and mortality (% EVAR vs. OR) 1 (7% vs. 30%) 2 (37% vs 80%) 3 (70% vs 82%) 4 (− vs. 100%)

rAAA: ruptured abdominal aortic aneurysm

Table 27.4 Ethical pillars to consider in evaluating patients with AAA

Beneficence	Choose the type of AAA repair and the timing of such to minimize mortality and morbidity
Nonmaleficence	Know that operating on asymptomatic patients with small aneurysms may cause immediate harm
Autonomy	Guide patients in their decision treatment using the shared decision making process and helping managing expectations in the post-operative phase
Justice	Offer all types of highly technical procedures for AAA repairs equally to all patients

overall health and functional status, expectations and perspective must be considered. Every step during this process involves an ethical choice by the surgeon (see Table 27.4). How a surgeon translates these guidelines, risk of rupture, and scoring systems to a patient is an ethical choice. How honest and detailed a surgeon is during the consent can be an ethical dilemma. The idea of shared decision-making is based on the ethical choices of what we define as "right and best" for our patients must blend with what the patient defines as "right and best" for them. Our two cases will serve as the focus for discussing these components of ethical decision-making in treating AAA, both elective and ruptured.

27.3   Search Strategy

Electronic searches were conducted in the PubMed database, Google Scholar, University of Chicago Library database, and Scott Memorial Library at Thomas Jefferson University database. The main search strategy used a combination of keywords including decision making OR ethics OR shared decision making OR utilization OR outcomes OR Screening guidelines OR AAA OR rAAA or open aortic aneurysm repair OR endovascular aortic aneurysm repair OR preoperative risk score OR prediction of mortality. We searched the years 1980 to 2020. We had about 1600 hits. We cross referenced the search with articles cited in multiple reviews and searched references of articles reviewed. The search was conducted by the author. 30 articles were reviewed for pertinence, sorted and selected for inclusion by the author.

27.4   Discussion

One of the hardest clinical problems a vascular surgeon is confronted with is highlighted in both cases presented. The principle of beneficence can be challenging in these specific vascular patients; specifically, how to devise a personalized treatment option with maximal benefits and minimal costs. The benefits in vascular surgery may be substantial to the patient but the risk can be equally detrimental. The idea of nonmaleficence is also not straightforward. What we see as harm to a patient might not be viewed by them as such. For example, we might value a patient requiring dialysis as significant harm, but a patient may be accepting of that. Weaving in these two ethical principles, we will discuss these cases separately since they can be handled slightly differently from a surgeon and patient shared treatment decision-making standpoint.

We will first analyze the important aspects that need to be taken into account when confronted with the 85-year-old with a rAAA who is hemodynamically stable. The surgeon initially needs to assess the urgency of the situation to decide how much time there is to discuss what the patient or family would want in regard to treatment options. If this patient was hemodynamically unstable, unconscious, or unable to participate in his treatment plan the surgeon has the power to assume they would want to live and move forward to the operating room. Caution needs to be taken when making these decisions as there are times when this assumption might be against the patient's wishes. Studies have shown that 74–94% of elderly would forgo any invasive procedure if it leads to a significant decline in their functional and cognitive status [13]. It would be ideal to assign this task to one of the team clinicians to call family, doctors, or other institutions to find out information on the medical state, quality of life, or documented verbal wishes of the patient. It is important but can be difficult and time consuming in an emergency setting to find this information. In this case, because the patient is hemodynamically stable, the surgeon has time to discuss the patient's preferences and treatment goals.

To involve the patient in the decision-making process, the patient needs to have capacity. The definition of capacity depends on the situation and can change from day to day. There are multiple models of what defines medical capacity, but they all generally have the same criteria. The patient must (1) understand the information presented to them, (2) be able to appreciate the significance of the situation, (3) reason through the information presented, and (4) express an opinion or choice [14]. It is important to understand that even though patients can make decisions in day-to-day tasks it does not always mean they have the capacity to understand the risk of an open AAA repair. A quick way to check if a patient has capacity is by having them repeat the information back to you after you give them some time to process the information [14]. If you deem the patient does not have capacity, you must extend the patient's decision-making authority to a healthcare power of attorney or surrogate decision maker. If there is no documentation of this information, there are state laws as to who is designated with this task, be it a parent, spouse or child or other. If the patient does have capacity at the beginning of their care, it is important to discuss and document who they appoint as their surrogate should they lose capacity. It is difficult being a designated surrogate and they may need to be reminded to put their own interests aside and make decisions by prioritizing the patient's values. Even with preoperative discussions, Shalowitz et al. showed that surrogates were only 68% accurate at predicting the patient's own decisions [15].

In an emergency setting, the surgeon may not have time to describe in great detail the risks and benefits of all treatment options with the patient during the informed consent process. The surgeon must highlight some of the most common and most life-changing risks. Whether an endovascular repair or open repair is performed in the emergency setting, the risks are relatively the same. These include bleeding (15–30%), renal failure requiring dialysis (23%), MI (6%), stroke (2%), multiple organ failure (1–3%), intestinal ischemia (23–40%), and ICU stays >5 days (27–32%) [5]. There is a higher risk of intra-operative or post-operative mortality with an open repair. When discussing these risks, the surgeon will also take into account the patient's comorbidities, as they can increase these risks. The patient needs to verbalize not only that they understand these risks, but that it could actually happen to them. The surgeon thus continues evaluating the level of capacity the patient has in making difficult decisions.

The surgeon also sets the patient's and family members' expectations of the post-operative care. They will need to know that the patient may require a ventilator, feeding tube, or other rescue therapies/procedures throughout their care. One way to preemptively manage the potential for prolonged postoperative care is by having a patient and family decide on a time-limited trial of care [14]. This is an agreement between the patient and the physician of how the patient's prognosis will dictate what specific therapies will occur over a specific period of time. These discussions give patients and family members clear expectations of what will happen after surgery. Giving best- and worst-case scenarios will also help manage their expectations. The discussion of whether to approach a rAAA in an endovascular fashion versus open surgery is not usually had with patients preoperatively. This decision is usually left to the surgeon's discretion and what is technically appropriate, based on their level of skill, and what will increase the patient's survival. SVS recommends that, if it is anatomically feasible, to treat a rAAA with EVAR. The Immediate Management of Patients with Rupture: Open Versus Endovascular Repair (IMPROVE) trial was a multicenter randomized trial of EVAR and open repair for patients presenting with a rAAA. There was no statistical significance in 30-day mortality for rAAA treated with EVAR (35.4%) compared to open repair (37.4%) [4]. We continue to favor EVAR for rAAA because IMPROVE does show that is offers patients a shorter length of stay in the hospital and higher chance to be dis-charged to home versus a facility. Follow-up after 1-year demonstrated that in rAAA EVAR showed no survival benefit compared to open repair [4].

Surgeons are often quick to offer surgical treatment but the option of comfort care in the elderly can also be a reasonable decision. It is the surgeon's obligation to present all of the options to the patient and family members. If they decide against aggressive treatment, they must understand that the outcome may be death. These discussions are very difficult to have and consulting with a palliative care team may be beneficial to all parties.

In the second case, elective discussions can be more in depth than in an emer-gency setting. This 70-year-old male with an incidental finding of a complex AAA was referred to the aortic clinic for treatment options. The first step is to determine the patient's understanding of the diagnosis of a AAA. This will give the surgeon a foundation from which to start the visit and discussion helping with the assessment of the patient's capacity. It is common to hear patients say" it's an enlarged artery that is like a bomb waiting to go off". This is also a good time to discuss the anat-omy of the aorta, where their aneurysm is specifically from an anatomic standpoint and the rupture risk based on the size and morphology of their aneurysm and what the recommendations are for treatment.

Surgeons do not always follow published guidelines and recommendations. A study by Dale et al. used a simulation center encounter to have physicians weigh the risk of a rAAA against the risk of a perioperative death with an elective repair of the AAA [15]. Of this group of surgeons, 77% chose to operate on the AAA at a time when the risk of rupture was lower than the risk of perioperative mortality. Surgeons who in a "practice" simulation which had a patient spontaneously rAAA after they chose to monitor the AAA were choosing surgery even earlier in the next patient simulation [16]. This demonstrates how surgeon's previous experiences influence what treatment options they discuss with patients. It is important for surgeons to recognize previous experience as a potential source of bias. Certain characteristics of some surgeons lead them to operate sooner than guidelines recommend: aversion to uncertainty, preference for action over inaction, assessing their operative skills as above average [16]. While guidelines are not set in stone, they are important and useful tools when guiding patients towards treatment. Surgeons must recognize that their personal characteristics may bias their recommendations.

Recent publications compared elective EVAR versus open repair and their long-term outcomes [3, 17]. EVAR's short-term benefits of fewer perioperative deaths and shorter hospital stays did not outweigh long-term survival. Also, long-term complications lead to further procedures [4, 17]. These results led to a wave of change in recommendations in the vascular world. In 2018, the UK National Institute for Health and Care Excellence (NICE) released recommendations favoring open repair over endovascular repair for unruptured aneurysms. This created significant debate because of the UK universal healthcare system. The controversy of only offering one treatment option to all patients highlights the importance of justice in medical ethics. Many surgeons did not agree with these recommendations because if they only offered an open repair it had the potential of significant harm in some patients. This led to a quick and interesting change in the 2020 NICE recommendations. Instead of stating open repair versus EVAR they ask the physicians to have a discussion of all risks and benefits of conservative therapy, EVAR and open repair [18]. The responsibility is left to the surgeon to discuss why open repair is recommended over EVAR in patients without abdominal pathologies and/or medical comorbidities, and notwithstanding the added anesthetic risks. If the discussion leads to EVAR it is important the surgeon inform the patient of the uncertainties around how complex EVAR improves perioperative survival or long-term outcomes, when compared with open surgical repair [18]. Most importantly they state that decisions should be made jointly between the surgeon and patient showing the value of the patient's autonomy.

The idea of shared decision making (SDM) (see Chap. 7) is valuable in determining the best treatment option for AAA. Shared decision making is not simply listing treatment options and risk and waiting for the patient to decide, but is an open discussion with the surgeon, patient, and family members. It is based on building trust and a solid relationship with the patient, which is not easily done in an emergent case [19]. Many vascular patients have multiple vascular issues thereby giving vascular surgeons the opportunity for longitudinal care. This fosters the development of a partnership between the patient and the surgeon. It is the surgeon's goal to offer their expertise and knowledge to best achieve the patient's goal or goals. Leading to an important element of SDM, it is important to know what the patient's specific goals are.

Not all patients have the same goals. A 60-year-old female who is relatively healthy and active with a AAA may not want yearly follow-up and imaging for the rest of her life. An 80-year-old might tell you "I just don't want to worry about this ticking time bomb" or "I just want to live to see my grandchildren." These goals are very different and will help guide the surgeon's wisdom in recommending treatment options. A lot of surgical data is based on mortality and morbidity and this is what drive's a surgeon's therapy [14]. Yes, patients want to survive but at what expense? It is the surgeon's job to learn what a patient is willing to trade off to survive, for example: loss of independence, living in a nursing home, dialysis, short- or long-term ventilator dependence. Knowing this information preoperatively will also help guide expectations of post-operative care.

A surgeon should not shy away from recommending a treatment plan when asked for their opinion, as some patients put it "If I was your father what would you tell me to do?" Just as important as the recommendation itself is the reasoning why a surgeon makes a recommendation. The surgeon also needs to be ready and accepting when patients do not agree with their recommendations. It is appropriate to give a patient time and space to discuss their options with their family without pressuring them for an immediate answer. SDM is a negotiating method that allows the surgeon to use his knowledge and experience to assist the patient in reaching their goal.

27.5 Conclusion

In our first case, after reviewing all the information, we had a long discussion with the patient and his two daughters who luckily made it to the hospital. We explained that if he did not have an operation that this rupture would progress and would be deadly, but surgery would have its own risks of complications. We discussed their goals and fears moving forward, such as the realistic possibility of not returning home, where he lived with his daughter, and the loss of independence. He stated his biggest fear was ending up with a stroke, leaving him significantly impaired, dialysis, or requiring a ventilator. If they did not pursue surgery, we would make sure the patient would be comfortable and his pain controlled. The patient requested to talk to his daughters in private and after some time they all agreed to move forward with surgery. The oldest daughter was already appointed his healthcare power of attorney. All agreed, that if the patient required ICU care including a ventilator, acute dialysis, or other extensive measures, that we would be allowed to push forward for 14 days and reassess at that time. We took the patient to the operating room for an EVAR. He was extubated the next day and was stable over the week in the ICU. Unfortunately, he aspirated, became septic requiring reintubation and IV antibiotics. He then developed acute kidney injury requiring dialysis and on hospital day 12 suffered a major stroke. At this point the daughters did not want to prolong his suffering and, as a team, we decided on hospice care. We waited to withdrawal treatment until his whole family gathered. He died surrounded by loved ones and with his daughters holding his hands. Even though we were not able to restore this patient's health, the family was very grateful and appreciative during every decision that we made together.

The conclusion of our second case was quite different. The patient initially presented to the clinic with a known complex AAA. Due to his recent prolonged hospitalization for his coronary bypass surgery, he was well versed on what complications and risks might arise. We discussed at length the complexity of his anatomy and what surgical options he had. He had a singular goal: to attend his only son's wedding in 6 months. He was presented with the options of open repair, complex EVAR, or conservative therapy. We presented all the risks and benefits at length and because of his comorbidities and the shorter recovery time (allowing him to make his son's wedding) we agreed to pursue the complex EVAR option. After reviewing his imaging, we decided to tackle this complex AAA with a fenestrated EVAR repair. When we started the operation, it became quickly apparent that his anatomy for multiple different reasons did not lend itself to making a fenestrated EVAR possible. We then attempted other options but were not successful. If continued, he would lose flow to a renal artery, most likely requiring dialysis. He also risked failure of the repair with a large type 1A endoleak due to a short neck. These options were discussed intraoperatively with his wife and we decided to abort the case and reevaluate his options with him. He was discharged and at the clinic visit we presented the possibility of another attempt at endovascular repair. We also discussed the open repair option and its increased risks due to his comorbidities. The patient's decision surprised the surgical team. He wished a more definitive repair and chose open repair regardless of the higher risk of complications. With the experience of a prolonged recovery after his previous surgery, he agreed to a more aggressive post-operative care including dialysis, ventilator use, and feeding tubes if needed. Two weeks later, he underwent a retroperitoneal open AAA repair. He tolerated the operation well, was extubated the next day, but his hospital stay was prolonged and complicated with ileus, urinary tract infection, poor nutritional intake requiring a feeding tube. He eventually was discharged to a nursing facility and eventually made it home. His son's wedding had to be postponed due to the COVID-19 pandemic, but he will be there when it is rescheduled.

In summary, surgeons possess significant insight from their medical knowledge, training, and personal experiences. It is a surgeon's duty to share this insight and wisdom when faced with a patient that has a AAA. Every patient and every circumstance is unique requiring us to approach every patient with a AAA with an open discussion. Throughout our experience, implementing a shared decision-making approach has empowered patients and improved the overall patient's perspective throughout the clinical course. The end goal for a vascular surgeon is to give patients autonomy in decisions about their health and optimize their quality of life. This is a skill all vascular surgeons need to develop and navigate throughout their career.

27.6   Selected References

- Xu J, Hall DE. Ethical Considerations. In: Chaer R., ed. *Vascular Disease in Older Adults: A Comprehensive Clinical Guide*. Springer; 2017:179–194. https://doi.org/10.1007/978-3-319-29285-4.

  – Discusses important ethical considerations and how to tackle difficult situations in the elderly vascular patient.

- Dale W, Hemmerich J, Moliski E, Schwarze ML, Tung A. Effect of Specialty and Recent Experience on Perioperative Decision-Making for Abdominal Aortic Aneurysm Repair. JAm Geriatr Soc. 2012;60(10):1889–1894. https://doi.org/10.1111/j.1532-5415.2012.04157.x

  – An interesting experiment that shows how past experiences affects geriatricians, anesthesiologists, and surgeons in making future recommendations to patients and how this advice can go against guidelines. This bias affects future patient outcomes

References

1. De Bakey ME, Cooley DA. Surgical treatment of aneurysm of abdominal aorta by resection and restoration of continuity with homograft. Surg Gynec Obstet. 1953;97:257–66.
2. Parodi JC, Palmaz JC, Barone HD. Transfemoral intraluminal graft implantation for abdominal aortic aneurysms. Ann Vasc Surg. 1991;5:491–9. https://doi.org/10.1007/BF02015271.
3. Desgranges P, Kobeiter H, Katsahian S, et al. Editor's choice—ECAR (Endovasculaire ou Chirurgie dans les Anévrysmes aorto-iliaques Rompus): a French randomized controlled trial of endovascular versus open surgical repair of ruptured Aorto-iliac aneurysms. Eur J Vasc Endovasc Surg. 2015;50:303–10. https://doi.org/10.1016/j.ejvs.2015.03.028.
4. Preventive Services Task Force US. Screening for abdominal aortic aneurysm: US Preventive Services Task Force recommendation statement. JAMA. 2019;322(22):2211–8. https://doi.org/10.1001/jama.2019.18928.
5. Chaikof EL, Dalman RL, Eskandari MK, et al. The Society for Vascular Surgery practice guidelines on the care of patients with an abdominal aortic aneurysm. J Vasc Surg. 2018;67(1):2–77. e2. https://doi.org/10.1016/j.jvs.2017.10.044.
6. Lederle FA, Johnson GR, Wilson SE, et al. Aneurysm detection and management veterans affairs cooperative study investigators. The aneurysm detection and management study screening program: validation cohort and final results. Arch Intern Med. 2000;160(10):1425–30. https://doi.org/10.1001/archinte.160.10.1425.
7. The UK Small Aneurysm Trial Participants. Mortality results for randomised controlled trial of early elective surgery or ultrasonographic surveillance for small abdominal aortic aneurysms. Lancet. 1998;352(9141):1649–55. https://doi.org/10.1016/S0140-6736(98)10137-X.
8. Tracci MC, Roy RA, Upchurch GR. Aortoiliac aneurysms: evaluation, decision making, and medical management. In: Sidawy AN, Perler BA, editors. Rutherford's vascular surgery and endovascular therapy. 9th ed. Elsevier; 2019. p. 1928–48.
9. Vos CG, de Vries J-PPM, Werson DAB, van Dongen EPA, Schreve MA, Ünlü Ç. Evaluation of five different aneurysm scoring systems to predict mortality in ruptured abdominal aortic aneurysm patients. J Vasc Surg. 2016;64(6):1609–16. https://doi.org/10.1016/j.jvs.2016.05.099.
10. Garland BT, Danaher PJ, Desikan S, et al. Preoperative risk score for the prediction of mortality after repair of ruptured abdominal aortic aneurysms. J Vasc Surg. 2018;68(4):991–7. https://doi.org/10.1016/j.jvs.2017.12.075.
11. Robinson WP, Schanzer A, Li Y, et al. Derivation and validation of a practical risk score for prediction of mortality after open repair of ruptured abdominal aortic aneurysms in a U.S. regional cohort and comparison to existing scoring systems. J Vasc Surg. 2013;57(2):354–61. https://doi.org/10.1016/j.jvs.2012.08.120.
12. Wang B, Rao A, Talathi S. Free rupture is the strongest predictor for mortality in ruptured abdominal aortic aneurysm. Poster presented at: 48th Society for Clinical Vascular Surgery Annual Symposium. March 14–18, 2020; Miami, FL. July 29, 2020. https://symposium.scvs.org/abstracts/2020/KC6.cgi
13. Fried TR, Bradley EH, Towle VR, Allore H. Understanding the treatment preferences of seriously ill patients. N Engl J Med. 2002;346(14):1061–6. https://doi.org/10.1056/NEJMsa012528.
14. Xu J, Hall DE. Ethical considerations. In: Chaer R, editor. Vascular disease in older adults: a comprehensive clinical guide. Springer; 2017. p. 179–94. https://doi.org/10.1007/978-3-319-29285-4.
15. Shalowitz DI, Garrett-Mayer E, Wendler D. The accuracy of surrogate decision makers: a systematic review. Arch Intern Med. 2006;166(5):493–7. https://doi.org/10.1001/archinte.166.5.493.
16. Dale W, Hemmerich J, Moliski E, Schwarze ML, Tung A. Effect of specialty and recent experience on perioperative decision-making for abdominal aortic aneurysm repair. J Am Geriatr Soc. 2012;60(10):1889–94. https://doi.org/10.1111/j.1532-5415.2012.04157.x.

17. Patel R, Sweeting MJ, Powell JT, Greenhalgh RM. Endovascular versus open repair of abdominal aortic aneurysm in 15-years' follow-up of the UK endovascular aneurysm repair trial 1 (EVAR trial 1): a randomised controlled trial. Lancet. 2016;388(10058):2366–74. https://doi.org/10.1016/S0140-6736(16)31135-7.
18. National Institute for Health and Care Excellence. Abdominal aortic aneurysm: diagnosis and management. NG156. NICE guidelines; 2020. Accessed July 20, 2020. https://www.nice.org.uk/guidance/NG156.
19. Elwyn G, Frosch D, Thomson R, et al. Shared decision making: a model for clinical practice. J Gen Intern Med. 2012;27(10):1361–7. https://doi.org/10.1007/s11606-012-2077-6.

Chapter 28
Denial of Life Support in Disabled Patients

Jaishankar Raman (iD)

Abstract Ventricular assist devices (VADs) and transplantation are the pillars of surgical treatment of end stage heart failure. A VAD is often implanted to temporize very sick patients with heart failure. This allows their circulation to improve and make heart transplantation less risky. VADs are complex machines that have alarms that are auditory. This chapter highlights the denial of lifesaving mechanical circulatory assistance in patients who are impaired in terms of hearing, sight or neurological state. This lack of the VAD option in some disabled patients may go against some fundamental tenets of medical ethics. We describe a deaf patient who ended up with a high-risk heart transplant due to the lack of the VAD option. We discuss the possibility of greater involvement of Clinical Ethicists in these complex decisions.

Keywords Denial of care · Ventricular assist device (VAD) · Heart transplant Disablities · Deafness

> **Case**
> Animated fist bumps characterized my first encounter with JAL. He was a very smiley and excitable young man in his 20s—but strangely silent. We then worked out that he was profoundly deaf and could understand American Sign

J. Raman (✉)
University of Melbourne, Fitzroy North, VIC, Australia

Deakin University, Melbourne, VIC, Australia

Deakin University, Geelong, VIC, Australia

University of Illinois at Urbana-Champaign, Champaign, IL, USA

Oregon Health & Science University, Portland, OR, USA

James Cook University, Townsville, Queensland, Australia

St Vincent's Hospital, Melbourne, VIC, Australia
e-mail: jraman@unimelb.edu.au

© The Author(s), under exclusive license to Springer Nature
Switzerland AG 2022
V. A. Lonchyna et al. (eds.), *Difficult Decisions in Surgical Ethics*, Difficult
Decisions in Surgery: An Evidence-Based Approach,
https://doi.org/10.1007/978-3-030-84625-1_28

Language (ASL) at a third grade level, despite being Hispanic. His mother who was constantly at his side, spoke no English and would translate rather poorly into ASL. We saw his father on very rare occasions; he was known to be abusive, angry and unreachable. Also, he found the difficulties in communication extremely frustrating and on more than one occasion had tried to get JAL sent to foster care. JAL had advanced heart failure with a dilated cardiomyopathy and had multiple hospital admissions due to heart failure. He was on Medicaid. The family struggled financially. Remarkably, they had cared for him all these years and he seemed to have had a reasonably normal life so far, except for the progressive heart failure symptoms.

He was evaluated for advanced heart failure therapy (a euphemism for transplant or ventricular assist device implantation) and was considered very high risk for any kind of intervention. In addition to his physical and medical limitations, his family situation and lack of a definite path of reimbursement presented insurmountable obstacles. We discussed his case in the multidisciplinary heart failure and transplant meeting. JAL was congenitally deaf, and his parents were undocumented immigrants from Central America. There was no mechanism for teaching sign language in Spanish in our community– the only option is American Sign Language (based on American English). This posed a major problem for his parents, who spoke very little English and no Spanish sign language. Now, that he was being evaluated for advanced heart failure therapy which required ongoing follow up and compliance with multiple medications, the task seemed almost insurmountable. His candidacy for implantation of a Ventricular Assist Device (VAD) was seriously considered. This would have allowed him to recover from decompensated heart failure and stabilize him for a heart transplant.

He had significant pulmonary hypertension, a marker of increased complications after heart transplantation. Typically, most patients with elevated pulmonary artery pressures are supported with a VAD for a few months, while the pressure within their lungs slowly abate. As we discussed his suitability for a VAD, a practical problem arose—all alarms on VADS are auditory with no visual or vibratory components. VADs are electrical pumps that pump blood continuously and require a power supply and a sophisticated software controller and interphase. Since these are complex pumps that can malfunction, there are a variety of safety alarms built into them—to reduce the likelihood of major complications, such as loss of battery charge, inadequate pumping, etc. Implanting a sophisticated piece of machinery in this young man, with no availability of reliable safety monitoring was deemed too risky.

28.1   Introduction

Ventricular Assist Devices (VAD) have been a major step forward in the management of end-stage heart failure, providing mechanical support to the failing heart
[1]. Implantation of these devices in sick patients makes their journey through heart
transplantation smoother while reducing risk of major circulatory complications.
These devices have auditory alarms and our attempts to find alternatives to the
alarms were unsuccessful. We describe a case of a young man who was deaf from a
young age, with severely impaired heart function—who could not receive a VAD
because the alarms were all auditory- and who went on to receive a high-risk heart
transplant.

In the lead up to the transplant, and as a follow up, we contacted all three major
companies that built durable or long-term VADs. None of them had ever considered
customizing alarms for physically disabled or disadvantaged people. Their standard
response was this was a sophisticated piece of machinery that cost upwards of $
85,000 (batteries not included!) and could not be modified for special disabilities
such as deafness, blindness, stroke, etc.

Rationing of care may be due to a variety of causes—most often due to financial
constraints or inability to pay [2]. This is especially true in the US where a significant sector of the population is not covered for medical care or expenses [3]. Of
course, if an uninsured patient presents as an emergency to a hospital, by law the
hospital is obliged to treat them [4].

28.2   Search Strategy

We searched for articles that mentioned the use of VADs and mechanical support in
patients with auditory and visual impairment. There was one contemporaneous article on visually impaired patients and VADs. There is only one recorded instance of
a deaf individual receiving a VAD and that was published well after we had dealt
with our index patient [5].

28.3   Discussion

Care of advanced heart failure patients is expensive and can be laden with many
emergencies and some periods of stability. This oscillating clinical course is not
well suited to cost containment. In instances where insurance is an issue, the care
can be fragmented, patchy or non-existent. The consistent ways of managing care
are through coordination with primary care physicians and/or community liaison
health workers.

Disabilities are, in themselves, expensive to manage. When this is laid on top of advanced heart failure, a convenient excuse and fallback is that the disability makes the patient ineligible for advanced therapies. This is despite good evidence to the contrary [6]. The American Disability Association does not have a specific stance on advanced heart failure therapies, except to say that patients with disabilities should not be denied treatment that is standard of care. As we go through the literature, there is a paucity of data on blind and deaf patients requiring implantation of advanced heart support, implantable cardiac devices and VADs. Of note, most public performances ranging from speeches to music events have sign language interpreters.

Does that mean that some disabilities are easier to manage and hence, get a pass? Certainly, there are examples of patients with intellectual impairment or disability, who have successfully had support with advanced mechanical devices and then progressed to transplantation, to return to a good level of activity [7].

What are the ethical guidelines we can set out? If these are clearly enunciated, is there hope that the medical fraternity will have access to it, and then follow those guidelines? Mechanical support of the circulation or the failing heart gets instituted in life-threatening situations. A common excuse is that there is usually not enough time to engage in discussions or moral arguments about the right decisions.

The four principles of bioethics were set out in the 1970s by Beauchamp and Childress [8]. They are autonomy, beneficence, nonmaleficence, and justice. Entwistle in a well thought article suggested that each of the principles of bioethics carry equal weight when one assesses the ethical course of action [9]. The appropriateness of an action is determined from the relative good and harm of individual principles are in question. When two or more principles are in conflict, the case can be difficult to navigate. The distribution of LVAD therapy often require complex ethical decision. A closer analysis of these principles is therefore important in every patient who is evaluated for VAD therapy.

Nonmaleficence is the principle of doing no harm and this would imply a low risk of complications, which could not be guaranteed in JAL specifically. Equal treatment of all patients underpins the concept of justice. However, this concept also applies to the larger community in terms of scarce resources being utilized with care taken to ensure optimum deployment of funds.

Justice may be viewed differently when therapies are very expensive. Limited and expensive therapies such as LVADs often pose ethical problems. Ethical principles suggest that all persons have an equal opportunity to receive adequate healthcare and that may not be the case in the USA, considering what has happened with Covid 19. However, we are discussing medical ethics as they would apply to an ideal or a more equitable healthcare scenario than we have at the moment. That would mean that all patients, regardless of underlying disability, should receive VAD implants for the treatment of end-stage heart failure. These are expensive devices that cost over US $ 90,000 just for the implant. Frequently, the hospitalization and associated procedures end up costing upwards of $500,000 and frequently over $ 1 million per patient.

Ideally, we should be able to deliver all therapies to all sections of humanity. Reality is different. The resources necessary to treat all patients may constrain the amount spent on individual patients who might need very expensive therapies. From a societal perspective, justice is served when the implantation of an LVAD does not drain the resource pool. There is also the emotional component of dealing with a young patient, with his/her adult life in front of them—and denial of a life-saving therapy based on the utilitarian argument of risk-benefits to society may seem mercenary.

The principles of autonomy and beneficence may govern LVAD implantation. Nonmaleficence favors implantation of a left ventricular assist device, in the absence of elevated risk. When the chance of benefit is low but the risk is high, the principles of justice may help with better ethical choices. The principle of beneficence may not be as clear in such cases.

Implanting a pump to supplant one's circulation is a very major step and one with many consequences, potential complications and management issues. This has promoted the need for VAD coordinators, VAD clinics, remote monitoring of VADs and shared care models to ensure prompt attention when a complication or management issue occurs. Increasingly, there is a move to involve palliative care teams to discuss options if there are major complications that threaten life or cause serious morbidity [10]. Consensus prior to implantation of these devices is key. Denial of mechanical support or implant of devices can be a fraught decision, even when made as part of a multi-disciplinary meeting [11]. Many multi-disciplinary groups, whether in the care of cancer patients or terminal heart failure patients, may not have a Medical Ethics component or member. Ethical conundrums and dilemmas therefore often get tabled. In some institutions, an Ethics consult is requested and the decision to proceed with implantation or to deny the implant is often delayed. This makes utilization of the Ethics Consultation less common.

This ethical dilemma also has connotations for blind patients, who may be at a significant disadvantage [12]. While the alarms are auditory, the mechanisms of dealing with them are all visual and require manual coordination. Some of these issues do not trigger design modifications, unless the population served is significant in number. Since VAD implants are still niche procedures in very sick patients, the companies that manufacture these expensive devices have not specifically designed modifications for patients with specific disabilities such as auditory and visual impairment [5]. There were no publications about the use of VAD implants in deaf patients at the time of JAL's evaluation. How about patients with a physical or cognitive disability resulting from a major neurological impairment such as stroke? There may be many issues with human-machine interface that make implants such as these even more problematic in terms of ongoing management [11]. The cognitive ability to manage alarms is an important element in ensuring safety. Physical disabilities affecting the regular care of the VADs, such as transport and care of batteries, the mechanics of connecting to the backup power supply, attention to alarms with prompt response, may also impact the clinical outcome. Does that mean we deny these disabled patients the opportunity of availing themselves of lifesaving or life-prolonging mechanical support devices?

Table 28.1 Ethical principles as applied to use of life support devices

Principles	Meaning	Relevance to case
Non-maleficence	by minimizing pain and suffering	Minimizing morbidity of transplant, by selecting LVAD implant as an option
Beneficence	a desired difference to the patient's well being	Implantation of LVAD
Self Determination	The goals and values of the patient and their family.	Proceeding with implant if patient & family wishes it
Justice	Fairness in the use of limited resources	Avoiding expensive therapies in high-risk situations

There are no specific guidelines or ethical directives in the management of patients with disabilities. The principles of medical ethics should serve as a guiding beacon (Table 28.1). Elements of trust between patients and their caring teams then come into place and make decisions complex. Multi-disciplinary heart failure teams have been meeting for well over two decades as a standard means of assessing patients for heart transplantation and associated procedures. Indeed, this is a standard mandated by the Centers for Medicare & Medicaid Services (CMS). Addition of Palliative Care physicians to these teams or multi-disciplinary discussions have been patchy but welcome. The low but steady rate of complications that can seriously impair or impinge on recovery has made it logical to include palliative care in the discussion of these patients. The same sentiment should be expanded to the inclusion of Clinical Ethicists. This particularly becomes important in the application and use of mechanical support devices, be they ECMO or VADs for support of the heart & circulatory system, dialysis for kidney support or ventilators for lung support. Denial of the use of any of these mechanical support modalities, when agreed upon following a multi-disciplinary discussion, seems logical and may be more palatable to the patient and their families. Detailed discussions about end-of-life care, alternative treatment options, family engagement and advanced care directives are all part of the course. The same could be true for withdrawal of care and/or deactivation of the device in some of these complex patients.

While many of these aspects are strongly recommended or even mandated, the use of these multiple facets of the specific disciplines, such as palliative care and medical ethics are not consistent. While some of these important components of patient involvement, family engagement and holistic care are not strictly medical, they are vital planks in steering our patients to good outcomes. They are often considered "soft" social aspects of decision making. There is also a perception that hard clinical data is the basis of scientific evidence, whereas the social sciences rely on nuanced and subjective assessments. The roles of social workers in these care teams are often consumed by coordinating logistics, travel arrangements and stays in the hospital! Social supports are usually evaluated quite rigorously as part of transplant and VAD workups, but always qualitatively. Qualitative data is very rarely capable of quantitation or statistical analysis. There is a tendency for many other social aspects to be largely glossed over. Disabilities fall under that category. The nuances of the kinds of disability get lost in the decision-making discourses.

28.4   Case Continued

In the case of our illustrative patient, the multi-disciplinary team with the data available to them decided that VAD implant was not safe under the circumstances. In an attempt to provide some modicum of support, we did insert an intra-aortic balloon counter pulsation pump which helped to unload his left ventricle and provided diastolic augmentation of the blood pressure. In order to allow him to move around, the device was inserted through a modified approach through the subclavian artery [13]. He then underwent a high-risk heart transplant procedure. The transplant procedure went very smoothly. However, immediately after the new heart started working, high pressures in the pulmonary artery were evident and this placed a significant strain on the right side of the heart. After waiting for about for about an hour, we decided to place JAL on a temporary right ventricular support device. His post-operative course was complicated and prolonged. He had to make a few additional trips back to the operating room for a variety of related complications. Eventually, we were able to wean him off the right ventricular assist device and get his chest closed. He stayed for a month in the ICU thereafter and made a full recovery. We saw him many times thereafter in follow up. His good cheer was unfailing and he was always very grateful. We knew that we had sailed very close to the wind, and there were many instances when he could have succumbed to a complication.

Peri-operatively, just before he was anesthetized for his first procedure, a very pro-active OR nurse realized that his deafness would be a significant barrier to communication. She made multiple placards with various words that would be used to convey messages to him visually, while he was being prepared for anesthesia. She also got his mother familiar with some of those words by attaching simple pictures alongside. This amazing local innovation made his care in the Operating Room and the ICU relatively smooth. We were able to modify these cards and make more of them. The staff then used these to communicate with the patient till he was ambulating in the ward.

Since he was not a candidate for a durable VAD implant, the other options offered were transplantation, medical therapy or hospice care. He and his family were adamant that they were not "giving up". He failed medical therapy spectacularly and came into the hospital in a decompensated state. We were able to tide him over for a few days with a balloon pump inserted through the subclavian artery, as an alternative to a conventional VAD, albeit less effective.

In cases like this, patient autonomy often comes sharply into focus. We were able to explain things quite well to his mother and to him. The senior heart failure cardiologist was a native Spanish speaker and had great rapport with both the patient and his mother. Multiple conversations were held with him and his family, before the consent was finally obtained. The patient was in hospital on medications supporting his heart function (inotropes) for at least 2 weeks before his transplant. The heart failure social workers and the nurse coordinators were also involved very closely with his care. He was also evaluated by the clinical psychologist associated with the heart failure team to ensure that he was of sound mental capacity and his sense of autonomy was preserved. Every opportunity was given for open disclosure and informed decision making.

28.5 Conclusion

Clinicians and allied health workers in these circumstances are constrained by the limitations of the available technologies. If there were an interest group or lobby that promoted the needs of specific disabilities, they would have their work cut for them in navigating the regulatory hurdles that many of the device makers use as excuses.

Regardless of the intangible obstacles that people of disabilities face, these become very important when clinical decisions need to be made. Many of them impact the patients themselves. The lack of good evidence is obvious, since most patients with disabilities get excluded from the Gold Standard in clinical trials—Randomized Controlled Trials (RCT). Furthermore, disabilities are heterogenous and the numbers are fortunately small. Guidelines therefore have to be developed, based on evidence for the general population and special circumstances related to each disability evaluated on its own merits. This is another case of customizing therapy to the patient. Adaptation of assistive technology was deployed in a deaf patient to a successful outcome [5] and may be a template for other possible innovations. Indeed, Crestanello in a timely editorial in the Journal of Thoracic and Cardiovascular Surgery suggested the use of adaptive and innovative technologies to cope with specific disabilities such as deafness, blindness, and other physical disabilities [14]. However, these would be dependent on the local surgical teams and their support infrastructure. Finally, the local circumstances, in terms of finances and regulatory framework often dictate the use of these advanced and cost-intensive therapies.

Denial of specific interventions such as insertion of a VAD or listing for a heart transplant may be difficult to justify, unless they are seen as part of the ethical framework that aligns with the Principles of Justice. This is specifically related to the fairness in the deployment of limited resources. However, these decisions may go against the other three, namely—Non-maleficence—based on minimizing pain and suffering; Beneficence—based on a desired difference to the patient's well-being; and Self Determination—based on the wishes of the patient and their family. Most multi-disciplinary panels should include ethicists for precisely these reasons where appropriate guidance on and practical interpretation of the principles of Medical Ethics are utilized.

28.6 Selected References

- Entwistle J III. The American Association for Thoracic Surgery 2016 Ethics Forum: Cost-effectiveness and the ethics of left ventricular assist device therapy. J Thorac Cardiovasc Surg. 2017;154(4):1315–1318. doi:https://doi.org/10.1016/j.jtcvs.2017.03.121

- This frames the ethics of LVAD therapy with the background of cost-effectiveness in a technology that is still expensive and evolving. The fundamentals of clinical ethics are emphasized within the context of mechanical circulatory support and VAD therapy.

- Teuteberg W, Maurer M. Palliative Care Throughout the Journey of Life With a Left Ventricular Assist Device. Circ Heart Fail. 2016;9:e003564. doi:https://doi.org/10.1161/circheartfailure.116.003564

  - Palliative care discussions in patients with LVAD and other life-extending therapies are an important cornerstone of the deployment of these technologies, should patients suffer debilitating complications. These are much better performed before the implant.

- Crestanello JA. Expanding left ventricular assist device use to patients with disabilities: The role of assistive technology. J Thorac Cardiovasc Surg. 2018;157:e3–4. doi:https://doi.org/10.1016/j.jtcvs.2018.07.079

  - The author makes a case for the innovative use of assistive technologies in patietns with disabilities.

References

1. Goldstein DJ, Naka Y, Hosrtmanshof D, et al. Association of Clinical Outcomes with left ventricular assist device use by bridge to transplant or destination therapy intent. The Multicenter study of MagLev Technology in Patients Undergoing Mechanical Circulatory Support Therapy with HeartMate 3 (MOMENTUM 3) randomized clinical trial. JAMA Cardiol. 2020;5(4):411–9. https://doi.org/10.1001/jamacardio.2019.5323.
2. Scheunemann LP, White DB. The ethics and reality of rationing in medicine. Chest. 2011;140(6):1625–32. https://doi.org/10.1378/chest.11-0622.
3. Berchick ER, Barnett JC, Upton RD. Health insurance coverage in the United States: 2018. Current population reports. US Census Bureau. US Dept Commerce; 2019. https://www.census.gov/library/publications/2019/demo/p60-267.html. Accessed 22 Nov 2020.
4. Zibulewsky J. The emergency medical treatment and active labor act (EMTALA): what it is and what it means for physicians. Baylor Univ Med Cent Proceed. 2001;14(4):339–46. https://doi.org/10.1080/08998280.2001.11927785.
5. Spiliopolous S, Hargesell V, Daupunt O. Left ventricular assist device therapy in a patient with hearing and speech disabilities. J Thorac Cardiovasc Surg. 2018;157(1):e1–2. https://doi.org/10.1016/j.jtcvs.2018.05.048.
6. Schumer EM, Black MC, Monreal G, Slaughter MS. Left ventricular assist devices: current controversies and future directions. Eur Heart J. 2016;37:3434–9. https://doi.org/10.1093/eyrheart/ehv590.
7. Samelson-Jones E, Mancini DM, Shapiro PA. Cardiac transplantation in adult patients with mental retardation: do outcomes support consensus guidelines? Psychosom. 2012;53(2):133–8.
8. Beauchamp TL, Childress JF. Principles of biomedical ethics. 8th ed. Oxford University Press; 2019.
9. Entwistle J III. The American Association for Thoracic Surgery 2016 ethics forum: cost-effectiveness and the ethics of left ventricular assist device therapy. J Thorac Cardiovasc Surg. 2017;154(4):1315–8. https://doi.org/10.1016/j.jtcvs.2017.03.121.

10. Teuteberg W, Maurer M. Palliative care throughout the journey of life with a left ven-
    tricular assist device. Circ Heart Fail. 2016;9:e003564. https://doi.org/10.1161/
    circheartfailure.116.003564.
11. Flint KM, Matlock DD, Lindenfeld J, Allen LA. Frailty and the selection of patients for des-
    tination therapy left ventricular assist device. Circ Heart Fail. 2012;5:286–93. https://doi.
    org/10.1161/circheartfailure.111.963215.
12. Ravi Y, Firstenberg M, Crestanello J, Sai Sudhakar CB. Mechanical circulatory support for the
    visually impaired: is it appropriate? Expert Rev Med Devices. 2011;8(2):155–7. https://doi.
    org/10.1586/erd.10.85.
13. Russo MJ, Jeevanandam V, Stepney J, et al. Intra-aortic balloon pump inserted through
    the subclavian artery: a minimally invasive approach to mechanical support in the ambula-
    tory end-stage heart failure patient. J Thorac Cardiovasc Surg. 2012;144:951–5. https://doi.
    org/10.1016/j.jtcvs.2012.03.007.
14. Crestanello JA. Expanding left ventricular assist device use to patients with disabilities: the role
    of assistive technology. J Thorac Cardiovasc Surg. 2018;157:e3–4. https://doi.org/10.1016/j.
    jtcvs.2018.07.079.

Part VII
Surgical Dilemmas in the Pediatric Patient/Family

Chapter 29
Changing Landscape of What Is Ethical and Appropriate

Eric Grossman ⓘ and Hannah Kornfeld ⓘ

Abstract This chapter examines medical ethics as it relates to pediatric surgical patients and their families. The changing landscape of medical ethics is reviewed and analyzed. Special consideration is given to how the dynamic factors of geography, resources, finances, and current events shape our collective view of medical ethics relative to pediatric patients.

Keywords Pediatric surgery · Pediatric ethics · Ethics and covid-19 · Appropriate care · Autonomy · Distributive justice · Surgical ethics · Ethical considerations Ethical relativism · Implicit bias

> **Case**
> Consider the case of a child born with closed gastroschisis to a 22-year-old, unemployed woman who smokes a pack of cigarettes a day. The mother received minimal prenatal care and only had a first trimester ultrasound given lack of access and education. The diagnosis of gastroschisis was not made until birth. The baby was born via vaginal delivery and APGARS were 7 and 9 at 0 and 5 minutes.
>
> Gastroschisis is an abdominal wall defect commonly cared for by pediatric surgeons and neonatologists. With the advent of self-expanding plastic ring silos as well as advancements in parenteral nutrition, gastroschisis is an extremely well-managed condition that carries with it a high rate of survival and treatment success. Unfortunately, closed gastroschisis, a variant of gastroschisis, results in strangulation of the extra-abdominal bowel. This can lead to small bowel ischemia, and potentially necrosis of nearly the entire small

E. Grossman (✉) · H. Kornfeld
Cottage Hospital, Santa Barbara, CA, USA
e-mail: egrossman@sbch.org; hkornfel@sbch.org

© The Author(s), under exclusive license to Springer Nature
Switzerland AG 2022
V. A. Lonchyna et al. (eds.), *Difficult Decisions in Surgical Ethics*, Difficult
Decisions in Surgery: An Evidence-Based Approach,
https://doi.org/10.1007/978-3-030-84625-1_29

bowel. If this condition is discovered at birth, the practitioners and the family are faced with a very difficult decision. One treatment option is to remove the non-viable bowel; which may result in short gut syndrome and intestinal failure. Such patients are managed with parenteral nutrition and potentially a small bowel transplant in the future. This pathway is fraught with difficulties including bacterial overgrowth, catheter associated sepsis, failure to thrive, and sometimes death. Alternatively, comfort care measures can be initiated upon recognition of this condition, and the baby will expire.

29.1 Introduction

The Greek philosopher, Heraclitus, is credited as saying "No man ever steps in the same river twice, for it's not the same river and he's not the same man" [1]. Such an homage to the permeance of change is readily apparent in the field of medical ethics. The variables that shape our collective view of medical ethics are numerous and constantly evolving. Notably, the ethical principles of individual autonomy, patients' rights, distributive justice and beneficence (Table 29.1) are often affected by geography, resources, finances, and current events. This chapter details the effects of such variables. Additionally, this chapter focuses on the importance of individual education, introspection, and the provider's awareness of potential inherent biases within one's own practice. Like Heraclitus's description of a river, medical ethics has evolved historically. Changes in our society may potentially lead providers, who are also influenced by these variables, to surprisingly different ethical conclusions than their predecessors. We will also explore evolving attitudes among providers who care for children and their families beyond the surgical setting. Lastly, we will discuss how the Coronavirus pandemic of 2020 is already influencing medical ethics within the pediatric surgical community [2].

Table 29.1 Ethical Principles Highlighted [2]

Ethical principles	Clinical manifestation
Autonomy	*Respect for an individual's decisions as they pertain to their own lives*
Distributive justice	*The socially just allocation of resources*
Ethical relativism	*The view that moral (or normative) statements are not objectively true, but "true" relative to a particular individual or society that happens to hold the belief*
Implicit bias	*People can act on the basis of prejudice and stereotypes without intending to do so*

29.2   Search Strategy

Literature search strategy included a database search of Stanford Encyclopedia of Philosophy, Google Scholar, Wikipedia, and PubMed with MESH term search of pediatric surgery, pediatric ethics, ethics and covid-19, appropriate care, autonomy, distributive justice, surgical ethics, ethical considerations, rural ethics, and ethical relativism. Results were limited to publications in English and preference was given to works published after 2000.

29.3   Discussion

29.3.1   Section 1. The Effect of Geography on Medical Ethics

Former Speaker of the House, Thomas O'Neill Jr. is credited with the phrase, 'All politics are local' [3]. The longevity of this adage is rooted in its succinct summary of the many complexities associated with politics, governance and human nature. Although many consider that medical and surgical ethics are founded upon universal truths and mores, these belief systems must also evolve and change. The patients, providers, and resources available at any given institution greatly affect and influence what is considered to be ethically appropriate medical care.

To illustrate geographic variations, consider the above case. The decision to operate or move to comfort care is extremely nuanced with multiple complexities and facets. The resources available to the institution, the unique qualities of the surrounding community, and the patient's family, especially the family's ability to assess the situation and make an informed decision, are all variables that play a large role in decision making.

Given these complexities, it is worth considering three specific geographical variations to illustrate how geography affects ethical decision making:

1. In rural America
2. In urban America
3. In Non-Western nations or cultures

Let us begin by examining the complex ethical questions at hand with special consideration to how they are affected by geography. Notably, the ethical concepts of patient autonomy, physician paternalism, and distributive justice are all captured in this scenario.

First, it is important to note that Western ethics are not monolithic. There are great differences between urban and rural communities. William Nelson [4] highlights some of the principles behind rural ethics. Specifically, he notes that, "Rural communities are unique not just because of their small population density or distance from an urban setting, but also because of the combination of their social, economic and geographical characteristics as well as their residents' cultural, religious and personal values." Shared decision-making and community values play a large role in rural ethics. Often patients rely on their clergy leaders or community Elders to help in their decision-making. Additionally, the strength of the community carries great importance in rural settings. This may manifest itself such that costly and long-term treatments may not be desirable as they are viewed to be overly burdensome on the group; conversely, a strong social fabric and community support may also lead to better aftercare and home-health assistance [4, 5]. The resources and efforts of the community are often prioritized over any individual, particularly in times of resource scarcity. In contrast, in communities with abundant resources, the burden of an individual's medical care can sometimes be shouldered among many. In such scenarios, the African proverb 'it takes a village to raise a child,' takes true shape [6].

Furthermore, authors Rice and Smith [7] from the University of York highlight how geography affects health, and in turn, affects ethics related concerns. On a very fundamental level, healthcare resources and finances are variably distributed amongst social, economic, and geographic distinctions; however, the difference extends beyond the physical limitations of medical resources. For example, "wide cultural influences on the use of health services might influence a threshold of ill health below which individuals choose not to seek medical intervention" [8]. For example, in tight knit communities with strong social connections, care may be avoided prior to medical emergencies, in order to maintain resource viability out of perceived responsibility to the community. It is estimated that 13% of all healthcare costs in the United States is dedicated to the last year of an individual's life, and in some geographic locations this is simply too high a price for minimal person-year return [8]. In urban locations and academic medical centers, a 'do everything' mentality is often more pervasive. Individual longevity, cost and the extent of heroic measures are often justified by the potential for medical advancements and supported by a plethora of resources and funding. Additionally, the underlying ethical principles and attitudes toward healthcare vary tremendously relative to a patient's location. Such cultural differences have great consequences during the extremes of life when providers determine the goals of care and undertake life-saving measures [7].

In contrast to Western cultures, some developing nations and middle eastern cultures have unique ethical frameworks. One well documented example herald from the Islamic Republic of Iran. Although the fundamentals of biomedical ethics in Iran largely mirror Western Ethics, one striking difference is the emphasis on life preservation. In Western culture, patient autonomy and even societal needs often run counter to the concept of preserving life. Examples include elective abortions, withdrawal of care, physician-assisted suicide, and—as in our case scenario—the cessation of medical intervention to allow a patient with closed gastroschisis to expire. Furthermore, religion can play a very large role in such societies, and some believe that all life is owned by God (see Chap. 19). This tenant greatly impacts all end-of-life and goals-of-care decisions. There is minimal debate in the Islamic

Republic as to whether to pursue all medical options available. In contrast to Western cultures, the concepts of distributive justice and patient autonomy are arguably less fundamental in comparison to the preservation of life [9, 10].

Given these nuances associated with geography, more or less emphasis can be placed upon either tenet of paternalism, patient autonomy, distributive justice, or sanctity of life. Therefore, let us now return to our case scenarios.

1. In rural America

   In this situation, it is common for physician paternalism and patient auton-omy to coexist in matters that differ from larger urban institutions. Resources might be restricted in rural America and limited in quantity, quality and availability. Additionally, the principles of distributive justice often weigh heavily in such environments, and individuals can be reluctant to become overly burdensome to their community. The contrary to this can also be true, and communities with a surplus of resources and caregivers can sometimes agree to pursue medical care despite all odds.

   Given these unique realities of Rural America, in some communities—for example the Amish—it might be ethically appropriate to ensure that the com-munity Elders are involved in the decision-making as well as considering the strains on the community that a baby with intestinal failure will impose. In this situation, conversations may be more often geared towards comfort care measures with the understanding that pursuing aggressive medical care may be prohibitively difficult.

2. In urban America

   In this situation, the principles of patient autonomy and respect for persons will likely be in the foreground. The patient and their family may be presented with treatment options and based upon their personal and individual set of beliefs, a treatment course will be charted

3. In Non-Western nations or cultures.

   Given the high value of life and the reluctance to perform any interventions that may be seen as counter to the preservation of life, it is likely for non-westerns cultures, particularly cultures adherent to Islamic law, to pursue aggressive medical measures regardless of resources available and individ-ual preferences. Alternatively, in sub-Sahara Africa, there may be villages and communities with limited medical resources, access to care or cultural beliefs that would drive them to obtain less intervention in cases that require complex, or prolonged medical attention.

Let us now return to our clinical case scenario. Shortly after birth, an honest and forthright discussion regarding the baby's condition and prognosis was had with the pediatric surgeons, neonatologists, and the baby's mother and grandmother. The mother was understandably confused and scared, although she appreciated the hon-esty of the medical professionals involved in her care as well as the love and support from her mother. As a devoted Christian, she relied heavily upon her faith; and when presented with the options of withdrawing care and pursing comfort measures as opposed to pursing bowel resection and potential intestinal failure, she elected for the latter. The baby underwent resection of the nonviable bowel and eventually developed short-gut syndrome. Nonetheless, despite being dependent on both parenteral and enteral nutrition, over the next five years, the baby continued to grow and develop. The family was forever grateful for the respect and care they received.

Overall, this case example highlights the absence of universal ethical truths, and the importance of respecting the ethical norms of a certain geography and culture (see Chap. 20).

29.3.2   Section 2. The Effect of Socioeconomic Status on Medical Ethics

29.3.2.1   Case Scenario

A full-term 3.2 kg baby boy with a prenatally diagnosed diaphragmatic hernia was born at a major medical institution in the United States. Both mom and dad were present during the prenatal visits and met with the Pediatric Surgeon as well as the Neonatologist in preparation for the delivery. Prenatal imaging was obtained, demonstrating a large diaphragmatic defect with the liver and stomach present in the chest. The family was counseled that although it is difficult to discern the severity of the underlying pulmonary pathology associated with a diaphragmatic hernia, there were signs portending a poor prognosis. Immediately after birth, the patient was persistently hypoxic, hypercapnic, and acidotic. Due to the severity of the disease, the patient was placed on ECMO.

Pediatric ECMO is a life saving measure utilized in the direst of circumstances. Due to the risks associated with the procedure, the potential for failure, and the scarcity of resources associated with its use, ECMO is fraught with ethically challenging decisions. The wide breadth of ethically difficult questions related to ECMO is beyond the scope of this chapter (see Chap. 30); however, this section focuses on one simple and fundamental question—.

29.3.2.2   For Whom Is ECMO Indicated?

This simple query transcends multiple pillars of medical ethics including, distributive justice, utilitarianism, beneficence, nonmaleficence, and respect for persons. In regard to distributive justice, the decision for whom ECMO is indicated is made by the involved medical teams taking into account the medical condition of the patient as well as the overall resources and limitations of the hospital at that given time. Furthermore, when this scarce resource no longer benefits the patient, conversations regarding its utility and futility are undertaken in preparation for decannulation. In extreme circumstances, the possibility exists for patients to be taken off ECMO unilaterally and against families wishes [11]. In a survey that assessed physician and resident attitude toward ECMO, 56% of respondents felt that physicians should have the right to discontinue ECMO over surrogates objection in the interest of resource stewardship and the complexity of knowledge necessary to fully grasp the concept of a 'Road to Nowhere' clinical situation [12].

To further explore this interaction, a deeper examination of the doctor-patient relationship must be explored. And although the doctor-patient relationship is a valued and sacred bond, it often exists between members of very different socioeconomic classes. Interestingly, this inequity is often punctuated by very different viewpoints and inherent ethical biases.

The association between social class and moral reasoning has been a topic of debate for centuries. Plato put forth the concept that elite individuals possess superior capacity for moral reasoning which thereby qualifies them for positions in leadership in government, laying the groundwork for his commitment to an epistocracy. In contrast, Karl Marx stressed that class hierarchy and arisotocracy corrupts individuals [13, 14].

Therefore, let us now examine how financial well-being and socioeconomic status might affect medical decision making in an attempt to potentially shed light on the challenging discussions surrounding ECMO allocation. Sociologists, Côté, Piff and Willer conducted a series of experiments revealing how members of higher socioeconomic classes display less empathy and increased emphasis upon utilitarian principle when compared to other members of society. Specifically, their experiments focused on hypothetical moral dilemmas where participants were forced to assess ethically challenging constructs designed to highlight their tendencies towards empathy and utilitarianism. The results of their studies demonstrated that individuals from higher socioeconomic classes are more likely to engage in utilitarian behavior, display less empathy and are more willing to take resources away from one individual if there was potential to benefit multiple others [15].

Given the results of these sociology experiments, pediatric surgeons, and those that care for critically ill children, (who often are members of a higher socioeconomic class) must reflect on their own practices to determine if such inherent biases are present.

The ethical difficulties associated with cannulation and decannulation are explored in a recent publication from the Seminars of Perinatology [11]. Drs. Kirsch and Munson, discuss the following relevant ethical principles including, respect for persons, autonomy, informed consent, non-malfeasance, best interests and distributive justice as they pertain to ECMO. Kirsch and Munson examine how each of these principles can be relied upon to help navigate complex and morally challenging questions regarding neonatal ECMO. When it appears that treatments have become futile, the authors recommend utilizing palliative care consultation, as well as shared decision-making, in an attempt to help the families, understand the gravity of the situation and agree to cessation of ECMO. However, the authors acknowledge that there will likely be variations in practice patterns and standards, depending upon geography, resource availability and institutional style. And although the authors recommend focusing on shared-decision making and conflict avoidance, they acknowledge that this does not address the potential for inherent provider biases to favor utilitarian principles over patient autonomy and respect for persons.

Presently, multiple consortiums are dedicated to collecting and aggregating data in efforts to help provide guidance for ECMO practitioners in their decision making. Nonetheless, ECMO encompasses nearly all of the complexities of medical ethics, and it is important that all practitioners remain diligent in their honest self-reflection to identify inherent biases and willingness to utilize ancillary services such as ethics consultations services and palliative care to help navigate these complex patients.

29.3.3   Section 3. Childhood Vaccines

29.3.3.1   Case Scenario

Dr. and Dr. Schmidt are professors at the local University of California College. One is a professor of Epidemiology and the other Political Science. They have three children ages 11, 9 and 6. The two older children are healthy boys; however, the six-year-old girl suffers from severe developmental delay. The etiology of this condition is unknown although believed to be from asphyxiation from complications during delivery. The Schmidt's are adamant that their children practice safe behaviors such as wearing helmets while on their bicycle, utilizing the appropriate car seat, and avoiding harmful toxins or chemicals in their foods.

Nonetheless, despite their insistence on safety and safe behavior, they are opposed to vaccinating their children. Their rationale is that given the low incidence of these preventable diseases, the risk of vaccination outweighs the benefit that is already provided by herd immunity.

Medical ethics have evolved considerably over the last century. The paradigm has shifted from a pedagogical and authoritative style of doctoring to one of patient autonomy and informed decision making. No medical quandary highlights this shift better than childhood vaccinations. Childhood immunization represents a balance between parents' autonomy in deciding whether to immunize their children and the benefits to public health from mandating vaccines. Additionally, the questions surrounding vaccinations highlight the concept of distributive justice insofar as benefits and burdens are allocated to those who vaccinate and those who do not.

The most frequently cited rationales for electing not to vaccinate one's children is based upon the concepts of herd immunity and Economic Game Theory. The theory is that if a certain threshold of the population is immunized against a certain disease, the likelihood that any given individual (either vaccinated or not vaccinated) will contract the disease is exceedingly low. Furthermore, as the incidence of contracting the disease declines, the relative risk of a complication from the vaccine appears more profound.

When evaluated from this perspective, vaccination decisions are not simply selfish or selfless but involve complex relationships between these motivations [16].

Critics of such behavior offer the counter point, should individuals who do not assume any level of risk be allowed to benefit from vaccination?

The principles of distributive justice imply that all who are able to bear the burden of a risk should do so in order to reap the benefits of such. Furthermore, the principle of beneficence guides us to vaccinate those who are able to in order to prevent disease in those who are not able to receive the vaccine.

The collective response from medical professionals to families who refuse to vaccinate their children is varied. Some argue that there should be financial or punitive penalties imposed upon families that do not vaccinate. Others have proposed that families who do not vaccinate their children be ineligible to receive certain social benefits. In an attempt to promote public health, the State of California recently passed legislation removing the option of personal belief exemptions for parents to withhold vaccines from their children [17]. In contrast, the American Academy of Pediatrics stresses that healthcare providers address vaccine refusal through hearing the family's concerns and discussing the risks that accompany not vaccinating one's child, rather than instituting penalties to nonconformists [18].

Complicating the question regarding childhood vaccinations, is how the state could impose universal vaccines and enforce such a policy even if herd immunity is consistent with distributive justice, and vaccinations are in accordance with the principles of beneficence. The US Supreme Court has upheld the constitutionality of state vaccination laws; however, all states allow medical exemptions, 48 states offer religious exemptions, and 17 states offer philosophical or personal exemptions [19]. Therefore, despite an overwhelming majority of individuals in favor of vaccination, there exists innumerable loopholes enabling those who wish to forgo vaccination as well as a paucity of legal avenues, to enforce any such pro-vaccination regulation.

In an attempt to disincentivize the of refusal vaccinations, some have argued that withholding childhood vaccination is a form of neglect and child abuse and therefore punishable by the state. Unfortunately, even if vaccine refusal amounts to medical neglect, it is not clear that this finding mandates state intervention [20]. Furthermore, the American Academy of Pediatrics states that it "does not support the stringent application of medical neglect laws when children do not receive recommended immunizations" [21, 22].

Authors Williamson and Glaab propose the following measures to delicately navigate this ethically challenging quagmire. First and foremost, they stress the importance of establishing rapport and trust between the provider and patient. Additionally, taking time to understand the family's reluctance to obtain vaccinations is paramount. Finally, they emphasize the importance of a consistent message among Healthcare professionals. This clarity of message streamlines the conversations and decreases potential areas of ambiguity [23].

In conclusion, childhood vaccinations encompass how medical ethics have evolved over the last few decades. Our collective appreciation of patient autonomy and respect for persons has grown tremendously as our paternalistic and utilitarian principles have lessened. Nonetheless, public health officials and medical professionals must find a balance between respecting parental rights and autonomy while maximizing the greater good of herd immunity in order to successfully navigate this ever-changing dilemma [20].

29.3.4 Section 4. How the Coronavirus Pandemic Has Affected Medical Ethics

29.3.4.1 Case Scenario

Elizabeth Lake is a single mom who works full-time as a financial advisor and cares for her 11-year-old son, Alex. During the coronavirus pandemic, Ms. Lake has been working from home based upon the recommendations of her boss and local public health officials. Last week, Alex developed abdominal pain, fever and nausea. Ms. Lake contacted her pediatrician and was offered a virtual visit. During the visit, Alex was tired and did not participate much in the Zoom-exam. The pediatrician thought this might represent a viral gastroenteritis that has been going around in Alex's "Pod-learning school" and told them to contact the office if the symptoms did not resolve in the next few days. Over the next forty-eight hours, Alex's symptoms worsened with high fevers and persistent abdominal pain. When Ms. Lake took Alex to the emergency department, his WBC was 19 and a CT scan demonstrated perforated appendicitis with phlegmonous changes and a 4 cm abscess in the pelvis.

The full effects from the pandemic of COVID-19 have yet to be realized; however, it has brought to the global forefront ethical questions that recently have been confined to resource poor populations and academic exercises (see Chap. 40). This section will use case scenarios and hospital policies to examine the themes of beneficence and distributive justice in times of crisis. Additionally, we will examine what specific 'carve-outs' and considerations are made for children.

COVID-19 has forced a shift from patient-centered ethics to distributive and public health centered decision making. Physicians are trained to be advocates for their patients, but in the setting of a pandemic, attention has shifted from the individual, to the collective. Surgeons cancelled their elective cases to preserve resources and minimize exposure [24]. Questions then began to arise on the definition of 'elective.' Certainly, most can agree that minimally symptomatic hernias and pectus repairs can wait, but what about cancers, appendicitis, and biliary disease? The American College of Surgeons (ACS) and the American Pediatric Surgical Association (APSA) put forth guidelines that prioritize timely surgical care for necessary pediatric cases, while optimizing resources [25, 26].

However, despite these efforts for clarity, the management of pediatric appendicitis during the coronavirus pandemic has been challenging. Authors Snapiri and colleagues present seven cases detailing the rising incidence of complicated pediatric appendicitis [27]. They report that the appendicitis complication rate in the COVID-19 period was roughly twice as high as complication rates during the same period in the previous year. The rationale for the delay in diagnosis is twofold. First, families were reluctant to seek medical attention; and second, providers have adjusted their practice patterns to avoid in-person encounters and physical examination. In response to this unexpected rise in complications, the authors counter that physicians should be diligent in their efforts to examine and evaluate pediatric patients, and slow to adapt telehealth, when there is a concern for appendicitis [27].

In Italy, where the effects from the coronavirus were devastating, Ciacchini and colleagues reported similar findings in a letter to the editor [28]. Specifically, they report four pediatric patients in which there was delay in presentation due to the fears surrounding Coronavirus. The authors concluded that the diagnostic delay was caused by the widespread tendency of parents to avoid hospitals and pediatricians. They concluded that modalities of virtual visits and telehealth should be employed with extreme care, as the physical examination remains crucial for a correct and timely evaluation. Furthermore, they highlight that due to the relatively benign course of Covid-19 in pediatric patients, the risk of delayed diagnosis and potential for missed opportunities for intervention may be greater than the risk of coronavirus infection [28].

The recommendation for biliary disease differed between adults and children. In adults the ACS recommends pain management and deferred surgery for symptomatic cholelithiasis and antibiotics for cholecystitis with any comorbidities, while in children it is acceptable to manage both with upfront surgery. Presumably this recommendation stems from prioritization of opioid minimization in children, but one must weigh the risk of exposure, and the need for extra resources, both in equipment and personnel.

In a recent publication from China, Tang and colleagues describe classifications and preventative strategies to be implemented for children undergoing surgical procedures in the era of Coronavirus. They describe both the preoperative intraoperative and postoperative techniques recommended to decrease transmission as well as classifying surgeries as emergency or elective in an attempt to minimize utilization of scarce resources [29].

The collective response from children's hospitals across North America has been catalogued; and most hospitals reported significant staffing changes to minimize exposure of healthcare workers as well as canceling elective operations. The risk of COVID-19 transmission has also influenced hospitals to consider reducing use of laparoscopy for operations, and in some cases, to restructure management of pediatric appendicitis. Finally, 13% of surveyed children's hospitals report that they were uniformly treating acute appendicitis nonoperatively, which is a change from their prior practice. It remains to be seen if this emphasis on the collective good and distributive justice, in opposition to maximizing the good for any given individual patient will prove to be beneficial [30].

In addition, to restructuring treatment patterns for pediatric surgical diseases, there has been much attention devoted to just resource allocation. The concern for resource scarcity in terms of PPE, ventilators and medications has been covered extensively in the news; (see Chap. 36) however, this concept is not foreign to medical professionals. Resource allocation plagues much of the decision making in geographically isolated and financially constrained locations. During COVID-19, most hospitals developed a triage system that typically put extensive prioritization on age. In parts of Italy, all patients above 80 years old, regardless of health, were ineligible for mechanical ventilation. In many hospitals, comorbid conditions such as a history of an MI, active cancer (regardless of stage), cerebral vascular disease, poorly controlled diabetes and various neurodegenerative disorders precluded the use of a ventilator should resources become scarce and prioritization measures enacted. Many hospitals explicitly state that prioritization of ventilators was based on potential 'life-years' remaining, by which children are prioritized. The near universal decision to prioritize the otherwise young and healthy during COVID-19 might seem magnanimous; however, it is arguably different than the goals of our current healthcare system. Presently, in the United States, tremendous resources are spent to preserve the lives of the aged. Elderly Americans are eligible for free and universal coverage, and a disproportionately large amount of spending is directed to the aged population. In contrast, a COVID-19 prioritization system that values pediatric life over the aged, may not be consistent with our collective societal goals, and is worthy of conversation and examination.

In conclusion, COVID-19 has stressed our medical system unlike any crisis in recent memory. In response, physicians and medical ethicists have responded wholeheartedly to promote social health, patient safety, and preservation of life. However, the scarcity of reliable data, the restructuring of current medical practices, the emphasis on non-operative management of common surgical diseases, and prioritization of scarce resources, has resulted in unintended consequences worthy of further analysis.

29.4 Conclusion

At the Institute for Advanced Study in Princeton University, a student of Albert Einstein's noticed that the examination was the same as the year prior. When asked why Einstein was presenting the class with an identical exam, he replied that although questions were the same, the answers have changed [31]. This wonderful anecdote beautifully captures Einstein's understanding of human nature, as well as the nature of science, knowledge and even medical ethics. This chapter has highlighted that physicians and ethicists have grappled with the same morally complex questions for years; however, the answers are continually changing based upon geography, social resources, the practitioner's inherent biases, and even international global pandemics. As responsible and ethical practitioners, it is our responsibility to objectively assess each situation, as well be willing to undergo honest self-reflection, in an attempt to navigate the ever-changing landscape of what is ethical and appropriate care in pediatric patients.

29.5   Selected References

- Nelson WA, Barr PJ, Castaldo MG. The opportunities and challenges for shared decision-making in the rural United States. HEC Forum. 2015;27 [2]:157–170. doi:https://doi.org/10.1007/S10730-015-9283-7

  - A discussion on the impact of the rural setting on shared decision making.

- Kirsch R, Munson D. Ethical and end of life considerations for neonates requiring ECMO support. Semin Perinatol. 2018;42(2):129–137. doi:https://doi.org/10.1053/j.semperi.2017.12.009

  - An exploration of the range of ethical considerations encountered when caring for a patient on ECMO.

- Piff PK, Stancato DM, Cote S, Mendoza-Denton R, Keltner D. Higher social class predicts increased unethical behavior. Proc Natl Acad Sci U S A. 2012;109(11):4086–4091. doi:https://doi.org/10.1073/pnas.1118373109

  - A series of clever and provocative sociology experiments examining how higher social class predicts increased unethical behavior.

- Ingram ME, Raval MV, Newton C, Lopez ME, Berman L. Characterization of initial North American pediatric surgical response to the COVID-19 pandemic. J Pediatr Surg. 2020;55(8):1431–1435. doi:https://doi.org/10.1016/j.jpedsurg.2020.06.001

  - An initial evaluation on how the COVID-19 pandemic effected pediatric surgical policy across North America hospitals.

References

1. Powell SK. Nothing is permanent but change (Heraclitus). Prof Case Manag. 2011;16(4):165–6.
2. Beauchamp TL, Childress JF. Principles of biomedical ethics. 8th ed. Oxford University Press; 2019.
3. Tip O'Neill. *Wikipedia Encyclopedia*. Accessed December 7, 2020. https://en.wikipedia.org/wiki/Tip_O%27Neill#:~:text=Four%20years%20later%2C%20he%20helped,%22All%20politics%20is%20local.%22.
4. Nelson W, Pomerantz A, Howard K, Bushy A. A proposed rural healthcare ethics agenda. J Med Ethics. 2007;33(3):136–9. https://doi.org/10.1136/jme.2006.015966.
5. Nelson WA, Barr PJ, Castaldo MG. The opportunities and challenges for shared decision-making in the rural United States. HEC Forum. 2015;27(2):157–70. https://doi.org/10.1007/S10730-015-9283-7.
6. It takes a village. *Wikipedia Encyclopedia*. Accessed December 7, 2020. https://en.wikipedia.org/wiki/It_takes_a_village.

7. Rice N, Smith PC. Ethics and geographical equity in health care. J Med Ethics. 2001;27(4):256–61.
8. Aldridge MD, Kelley AS. The myth regarding the high cost of end-of-life care. Am J Public Health. 2015;105(12):2411–5. https://doi.org/10.2105/ajph.2015.302889.
9. Aramesh K. A brief history of biomedical research ethics in Iran: conflict of paradigms. Dev World Bioeth. 2015;15(2):107–12. https://doi.org/10.1111/dewb.12053.
10. Larijani B, Zahedi F, Malek-Afzali H. Medical ethics in the Islamic Republic of Iran. East Mediterr Health J. 2005;11(5–6):1061–72.
11. Kirsch R, Munson D. Ethical and end of life considerations for neonates requiring ECMO support. Semin Perinatol. 2018;42(2):129–37. https://doi.org/10.1053/j.semperi.2017.12.009.
12. Meltzer EC, Ivascu NS, Stark M, Orfanos AV, Acres CA, Christos PJ, et al. A survey of physicians' attitudes toward decision-making Authority for Initiating and Withdrawing VA-ECMO: results and ethical implications for shared decision making. J Clin Ethics. 2016;27(4):281–9.
13. Piff PK, Stancato DM, Cote S, Mendoza-Denton R, Keltner D. Higher social class predicts increased unethical behavior. Proc Natl Acad Sci U S A. 2012;109(11):4086–91. https://doi.org/10.1073/pnas.1118373109.
14. Marxian Class Theory. *Wikipedia Encyclopedia*. Accessed December 7, 2020. https://en.wikipedia.org/wiki/Marxian_class_theory.
15. Cote S, Piff PK, Willer R. For whom do the ends justify the means? Social class and utilitarian moral judgment. J Pers Soc Psychol. 2013;104(3):490–503. https://doi.org/10.1037/a0030931.
16. Shim E, Chapman GB, Townsend JP, Galvani AP. The influence of altruism on influenza vaccination decisions. J R Soc Interface. 2012;9(74):2234–43. https://doi.org/10.1098/rsif.2012.0115.
17. Mello MM, Studdert DM, Parmet WE. Shifting vaccination politics – the end of personal-belief exemptions in California. N Engl J Med. 2015;373(9):785–7. https://doi.org/10.1056/nejmp1508701.
18. Diekema DS. American academy of Pediatrics committee on B. responding to parental refusals of immunization of children. Pediatrics. 2005;115(5):1428–31. https://doi.org/10.1542/peds.2005-0316.
19. Jackson CL. State laws on compulsory immunization in the United States. Public Health Rep. 1969;84(9):787–95.
20. Hendrix KS, Sturm LA, Zimet GD, Meslin EM. Ethics and childhood vaccination policy in the United States. Am J Public Health. 2016;106(2):273–8. https://doi.org/10.2105/ajph.2015.302952.
21. Religious objections to medical care. American Academy of Pediatrics Committee on bioethics. Pediatrics. 1997;99(2):279–81. https://doi.org/10.1542/peds.99.2.279.
22. Parasidis E, Opel DJ. Parental refusal of childhood vaccines and medical neglect Laws. Am J Public Health. 2017;107(1):68–71. https://doi.org/10.2105/ajph.2016.303500.
23. Williamson L, Glaab H. Addressing vaccine hesitancy requires an ethically consistent health strategy. BMC Med Ethics. 2018;19(1):84. https://doi.org/10.1186/s12910-018-0322-1.
24. Angelos P. Surgeons, ethics, and COVID-19: early lessons learned. J Am Coll Surg. 2020;230(6):1119–20. https://doi.org/10.1016/j.jamcollsurg.2020.03.028.
25. COVID-19 for Pediatric Surgery Library. American Pediatric Surgical Association. Accessed December 7, 2020. https://www.pedsurglibrary.com/apsa/view/PedSurg%20Resource/1884034/all/COVID_19_for_Pediatric_Surgeons.
26. COVID-19: Guidance for Triage of Non-Emergent Surgical Procedures. American College of Surgeons. Accessed December 7, 2020. https://www.facs.org/covid-19/clinical-guidance/triage.
27. Snapiri O, Rosenberg Danziger C, Krause I, Kravarusic D, Yulevich A, Balla U, et al. Delayed diagnosis of paediatric appendicitis during the COVID-19 pandemic. Acta Paediatr. 2020;109(8):1672–6. https://doi.org/10.1111/apa.15376.

28. Ciacchini B, Tonioli F, Marciano C, Faticato MG, Borali E, Pini Prato A, et al. Reluctance to seek pediatric care during the COVID-19 pandemic and the risks of delayed diagnosis [letter]. Ital J Pediatr. 2020;46(1):87. https://doi.org/10.1186/s13052-020-00849-w.
29. Daxing Tang JT, Wang J, Chen Q, et al. Prevention and control strategies for emergency, limited-term, and elective operations in pediatric surgery during the epidemic period of COVID-19. W. J Pediatr Surg. 2020;3:e000122. https://doi.org/10.1136/wjps-2020-000122.
30. Ingram ME, Raval MV, Newton C, Lopez ME, Berman L. Characterization of initial north American pediatric surgical response to the COVID-19 pandemic. J Pediatr Surg. 2020;55(8):1431–5. https://doi.org/10.1016/j.jpedsurg.2020.06.001.
31. Albert Einstein Quotes. Good Reads. Accessed December 7, 2020. https://www.goodreads.com/quotes/226558-student-dr-einstein-aren-t-these-the-same-questions-as-last.

Chapter 30
A Careful Balance of the Benefits and Burdens of Pediatric ECMO

Samara Lewis ⓘ, Maria Urdaneta Perez, Catherine Hunter ⓘ, and Erica M. Carlisle ⓘ

Abstract Over the past several decades, extracorporeal membrane oxygenation (ECMO) has been utilized for an increasingly diverse range of pediatric pathologies. While this expansion has allowed pediatric patients to survive physiologic insults previously deemed lethal, it has also generated complex clinical scenarios and rich ethical discussions. As providers work to better understand the circumstances in which ECMO benefits pediatric patients, they must consider the limitations of this invasive, physiologically demanding technology and the potential moral distress and emotional burden it's use may create for patients, families, and healthcare providers. In this chapter, we first highlight benefits experienced by pediatric patients when ECMO is used as a bridge to recovery, corrective surgery, transplant, or decision making. We then discuss the ethical challenges inherent to the expansion of ECMO: withholding or withdrawing care, informed consent in emergent settings, exposure of children to significant morbidity, and equitable distribution of this relatively scarce and resource intensive technology. We suggest that a balance must be found between the benefits and burdens of pediatric ECMO.

Keywords Pediatrics · ECMO · Ethics · Moral distress · Futility · Possibly inappropriate intervention

S. Lewis · M. U. Perez · C. Hunter
Division of Pediatric Surgery, Department of Surgery, University of Oklahoma, Norman, OK, USA

E. M. Carlisle (✉)
Division of Pediatric Surgery, Department of Surgery, University of Iowa Carver College of Medicine, University of Iowa Hospitals and Clinics, Iowa City, IA, USA
e-mail: erica-carlisle@uiowa.edu

© The Author(s), under exclusive license to Springer Nature Switzerland AG 2022

415

V. A. Lonchyna et al. (eds.), *Difficult Decisions in Surgical Ethics*, Difficult Decisions in Surgery: An Evidence-Based Approach,
https://doi.org/10.1007/978-3-030-84625-1_30

Case Presentation

A 13-year-old boy, six months status post bone marrow transplant for relapsed AML currently in remission, presents to the hospital with pulmonary graft versus host disease and hemophagocytic lymphohistiocytosis complicated by adenovirus infection. The patient is intubated and undergoes aggressive treatment with slow improvement. On hospital day 32, he acutely decompensates due to pulmonary hemorrhage and Gram-negative bacteremia. Despite maximum support, he remains hemodynamically unstable. The Pediatric Intensive Care team informs the patient's family that ECMO offers the only chance of survival and consults Pediatric Surgery for ECMO cannulation. Due to prolonged ventilation with its increased risk of barotrauma, active pulmonary hemorrhage, and the patients' co-morbidities, the surgery team considers ECMO inappropriate. The disagreement between the intensivists and the surgeons leaves the family confused about the best option for their child (see Table 30.1).

30.1 Introduction

Extracorporeal membrane oxygenation (ECMO) is a life-sustaining technology that supports patients while they recover from, or undergo treatment for, a wide range of physiologic insults [1]. At its inception, slightly modified heart-lung bypass machines used in cardiac surgery were adapted for ECMO [2]. Over time, ECMO circuits have become increasingly refined, allowing their use in even the most delicate pediatric patients [2]. Neonates with respiratory failure due to meconium aspiration, infant respiratory distress syndrome, and persistent fetal circulation were some of the first patients to be supported with ECMO with a nearly 50% survival

Table 30.1 Ethical dilemmas influencing this case

Conflict between beneficence and maleficence
PICU providers considered ECMO cannulation to be a beneficent act. Conversely, the surgery providers were concerned that ECMO was potentially inappropriate (futile) for this patient thus rendering it a maleficent act.
Autonomy
The immediacy of the patient's clinical decompensation required an urgent decision be made regarding ECMO cannulation. In this relatively pressured setting, the informed consent process may have been rushed thus potentially impacting the patient's family ability to make a truly informed decision regarding cannulation.
Justice
Malignancy, pulmonary barotrauma, and pulmonary hemorrhage have historically been deemed contraindications to ECMO. Consideration of ECMO for this patient thus expands is traditional use. Some may argue that utilization of this limited, costly, resource intensive intervention in this manner is an unjust distribution of healthcare resources.

rate [2]. Impressive neonatal outcomes prompted expansion of ECMO to increasingly diverse populations of pediatric patients, and recently we have seen ECMO successfully used to support pediatric patients with pathology previously deemed lethal [1].

Named in relation to cannula position, there are two approaches to ECMO: venous-arterial (VA) and venous-venous (VV). VA ECMO removes blood from the body through venous access, cycles it through an oxygenator, and re-perfuses it into the patient through arterial access. This perpetuates the flow of oxygenated blood without reliance on the heart and is thus used when cardiac function is impaired. In VV ECMO, deoxygenated blood is removed from the body via one venous cannula, cycled through an oxygenator, and returned via a second venous cannula (or a second port in a dual lumen venous cannula). Given dependence on cardiac function for forward flow, VV ECMO is used in patients with preserved cardiac function. In short, ECMO oxygenates and ventilates patients without reliance on cardiopulmonary function, thus allowing patients the physiologic support necessary to recover from or undergo treatment for insults that would otherwise be fatal. In this sense, ECMO can be considered a bridge to recovery, transplant, or corrective surgery [3, 4]. It may also be considered a bridge to decision making in clinical settings that require time to gather more information about the patients' clinical trajectory [3, 4]. When used appropriately, ECMO is associated with improved patient outcomes, however, use of ECMO in clinical settings in which it is less well indicated may result in increased morbidity, increased cost, and increased moral distress for families and providers without an associated increase in survival [4]. EMCO utilization in such settings exposes ethical challenges such as assuring adequate informed consent in emergent settings and equitable distribution of this relatively scarce and resource intensive technology. In this chapter, we discuss the benefits and burdens of pediatric ECMO to highlight the importance of balancing beneficence and non-maleficence in pediatric ECMO.

30.2   Search Strategies

We searched databases including PubMed, Google Scholar, Medline, and OVID. MeSH search terms included: pediatric; neonatal; ECMO; extracorporeal life support; ethical life support organization (ELSO); ethical dilemma; ethics; Futile Care; Fantasy Care; potentially inappropriate intervention; ethical consent; informed consent; longshot; last-ditch; bridge to transplant, decision, recovery, and surgery. Exclusion criteria included abstracts and patient's > 18 years old.

30.3 Discussion

30.3.1 Benefits of ECMO in Pediatrics

ECMO has been increasingly relied upon to support pediatric patients as they recover from, or undergo treatment for, physiologic insults previously deemed lethal [1]. In this capacity, ECMO may be considered a bridge to recovery, a bridge to transplant, a bridge to curative surgery, or a bridge to a decision [3, 4]. Review of the successful implementation of ECMO each of these arenas illustrates the benefits of ECMO in pediatrics.

30.3.2 ECMO as a Bridge to Recovery

Utilization of ECMO as a Bridge to Recovery is more prominent in pediatrics than in adult medicine [1]. In these settings, ECMO is utilized to support patients while they recover from a given insult. For example, for patients with acquired pulmonary and cardiac pathologies, such as pneumonia, pertussis, drowning, and fulminant myocarditis, ECMO is utilized as Bridge to Recovery. ECMO is also utilized as a bridge to recovery in some congenital pulmonary conditions such as congenital diaphragmatic hernia.

The role of ECMO as a Bridge to Recovery has perhaps been most impressive in neonates with meconium aspiration syndrome (MAS). Inclusion of ECMO in the care of these babies has improved overall survival rates from 57% to 93% [5]. While ECMO is typically considered an "optional" adjunct to standard care, the impressive survival rate of neonates that receive ECMO support while they recover from MAS and the relatively low rate of morbidity for these babies, has prompted some to question whether it should be considered standard care as opposed to an "optional" or "heroic" adjunct [5]. Specifically, some wonder if parents should be able to refuse ECMO cannulation for neonates with MAS given the high survival rates and low morbidity [5]. While the risks of hemorrhage, infection, and long-term neurologic impairment do exist, some suggest that the drastic improvement in survival offsets these risks [5].

ECMO has also been found to provide meaningful physiologic support for the significant number of pediatric patients with acquired infections, such as pneumonia, influenza, and myocarditis [1, 6–8]. Reported overall survival for pediatric patients who undergo ECMO cannulation for acquired pulmonary infections is estimated between 52% [7] and 62% [9]. Although used more frequently to support patients with pulmonary infections, the use of ECMO to support pediatric patients with infectious myocarditis has resulted in survival rates between 52% [7] and 70% [1, 8, 10, 11]. Notably, during the 2015–2016 influenza outbreak, 14% of pediatric patients in the United States with influenza underwent ECMO cannulation with a survival rate of 100% [12]. Recently, successful use of ECMO to support patients with pertussis has been observed noting a 28% survival rate in these children [13]. While these survival rates are less striking than those for neonates who undergo ECMO cannulation for MAS [5], improved survival in otherwise dismal settings highlights the benefit of ECMO for children with acquired infections.

ECMO has also been used as a Bridge to Recovery for neonates with congenital diaphragmatic hernias (CDH). Due to the defect in their diaphragm, these babies suffer from impaired lung development resulting in varying degrees of pulmonary hypoplasia and pulmonary hypertension [14]. For some, the pulmonary hypoplasia and pulmonary hypertension are so severe, that survival without ECMO is not possible [15]. ECMO allows time for treatment of the pulmonary hypertension and lung development such that these infants may survive [14]. Timing of surgical repair of the diaphragm following initiation of ECMO is controversial. Early repair (< 72 hours after ECMO initiation), late repair (> 72 hours), and post-cannulation repair have all been suggested [16–18]. Initial review of early surgical repair (< 25 hrs) suggested survival rates as high as 75% [19, 20], however the increased rate of complications from bleeding following early repair tempered enthusiasm about this apparent success [21]. Subsequent studies identified a high risk of bleeding and relatively low survival rates for infants repaired while on ECMO [21–23], shifting focus to whether post-cannulation repair might improve survival. A large database review in 2009 identified 77% survival in post-cannulation repair as compared to 48% survival if repaired while on ECMO [17]. These results were contrasted by a 2014 single center, retrospective study that identified 100% survival in infants repaired post-cannulation and 44% survival for repair while on ECMO [14]. The recent introduction of anti-fibrinolytic therapy and anticoagulation protocols has resulted in an overall decrease in bleeding complications which may minimize some of the risk of repair while on ECMO [24]. This is supported by a 2015 systematic review that identified that early repair on ECMO therapy may be associated with improved survival [24]. The marked variation in survival rates across the literature highlights the complexity of caring for neonates with CDH. This complexity creates challenges in assessing an individual babies' prognosis thereby impacting prenatal and postnatal counseling for families and inciting various ethical challenges.

30.3.3   Bridge to Corrective Surgery

ECMO is also used as a bridge to a temporary device or corrective surgery in children with cardiac disease. For some children with heart failure, temporary ECMO support allows improvements in cardiac function that make these children candidates for ventricle assist device (VAD) placement. VAD can then be used as a bridge to transplantation. Interestingly, for some children with primary myocardial disease, continued cardiac improvement with VAD alone has resulted in cardiac recovery with no further need for mechanical support or surgical intervention [6]. This intervention strategy can be used across a wide breadth of cardiac pathologies including congenital abnormalities with single or double ventricle abnormalities, primary myocardial disease, and primary pulmonary hypertension. Estimated survival in this patient population is between 38–55% [25–31] when ECMO is used alone, but with ECMO weaning protocols and VAD use after cardiac function has improved, survival rates as high as 73% have been observed [6]. This increase in survival may offset the burdens that ECMO cannulation may place on family, health care workers, and patients.

ECMO can also be a bridge to corrective surgery for pediatric patients with congenital cardiac anomalies. ECMO cannulation may occur prior to or after surgical repair. Although, many different structural abnormalities exist in congenital heart disease, patients are generally grouped into one of two common categorical classifications; single versus double ventricle pathologies or by Risk Adjustment in Congenital Heart Surgery (RACHS)-1 categories [32], a scoring system that groups patients according to mortality risk. Categorization of patients is important, as it allows calculation of overall survival rates in this population. Overall survival in patients with any form of congenital heart defect requiring ECMO support ranges from 48% [33] to 62% [34, 35], with ECMO support prior to or following repair being 73% [35] and 41% [36]-49% [35], respectively. This suggests that those patients who are able to be weaned from ECMO prior to repair have improved survival rates. One specific structural abnormality that has been well investigated is hypoplastic left heart syndrome (HLHS), which requires staged operative repair [37, 38]. Patients with HLHS have overall survival rates of about 16% [10] following stage 1 repair and 31% [37]–36% [38] following stage 2 repair. Duration of ECMO support is negatively associated with survival rates for these children, with mortality rates of 45% [33] at 2–6 days, 69% [33] at greater than 7 days, and overall survival rates of 23% with ECMO runs greater than 14 days [33]. Although clearly not a panacea, ECMO support for these children provides a temporary bridge to the possibility of surgical repair [33].

30.3.4 Bridge to Transplant

ECMO is used as a bridge to pediatric cardiac transplant, in situations when congenital abnormalities are too severe for repair, surgical repair is unsuccessful or in severe cases of myocarditis or cardiomyopathy [10, 11, 35, 38–41]. Patients with high risk [4–6] RACHS-1 category abnormalities, such as transposition of the great vessel, truncus arteriosus, Tetralogy of Fallot, Ebstein's abnormality, tricuspid atresia, and hypoplastic left heart, may benefit from ECMO in such settings [32–33]. In a retrospective review of the Organ Procurement and Transplantation Network, 11% of pediatric cardiac transplant patients required preoperative ECMO support [42]. Reported overall survival for children supported with ECMO prior to transplant is between 33% [41] and 64% [39–40, 42, 43], and survival after transplant increases to 96% [42]. Without ECMO, these children may not survive while awaiting organ allocation or while their newly transplanted heart recovers [6, 41].

30.3.5   *Bridge to Decision Making*

For many patients, ECMO offers a Bridge to Decision. In this capacity, ECMO is typically initiated urgently to allow initial stabilization of the patient with time for providers to gather the information needed to determine if the insult suffered is survivable. Utilization of ECMO for this purpose prompts consideration of numerous ethical issues. For example, delay of impending death by ECMO cannulation may reveal that the patient has suffered a non-survivable insult. Surrogate decision makers and health care providers are then tasked with the potentially distressing decision to withdraw care. This highlights the need to make careful decisions about the clinical settings in which utilization of ECMO as a bridge to decision is appropriate. Further research time-limited trials are necessary to delineate the subgroups of patients that will be well served by ECMO cannulation with this intent.

Initial efforts have been made to evaluate the use of ECMO cannulation during active CPR. In children, the survival rates in this setting are surprisingly high, ranging from 38% [28] overall to 46% [27] to 77% [6] for children with certain cardiac conditions. Such findings suggest that it may be reasonable to cannulate during active CPR. The importance of using well-defined guidelines, when ECMO is used as a Bridge to Decision, must be emphasized to minimize undue harm to the patient and assure upfront, transparent discussions with families and medical team members about the limitations of ECMO support in these settings [3].

30.3.6   *Burdens of ECMO in Pediatrics*

The benefits and versatility of ECMO support has prompted its expansion in pediatrics. However, far from a simple rescue intervention, ECMO is a resource intensive technology that is associated with, multiple risks and significant short and long-term complications. Its use may thus be associated with multiple ethical issues for patients, families, and health care providers. Here, we highlight ethical challenges with withdrawing care, futility, equitable distribution of resource intensive care, and challenges with assuring informed consent in urgent settings.

30.3.7   *Challenges with Withdrawing*
and Withholding Treatment

As we expand the patient populations and pathologies for which we deem ECMO an appropriate intervention, we will undoubtably encounter settings in which patients do not improve despite a trial of ECMO. It is thus critically important to assure frank discussion of the clinical markers of progress as well as a defined time period in which progress should be demonstrated to help families and health care team members understand what constitutes a reasonable trial of ECMO. In prior sections, we discussed using ECMO as a bridge to recovery, a bridge to corrective surgery, a bridge to transplant, or a bridge to decision. When it becomes evident that a patient will not survive to recovery, surgery, or transplant, one may presume that the physiologic insult suffered by the patient is not survivable. In this setting, some suggest that ECMO has become a "bridge to nowhere" and withdrawal of support is indicated [44].

The precise timeframe for how long an individual patient should remain with ECMO support is ill-defined, however recent work suggests that ECMO trials longer than 21 days are not associated with favorable outcomes for children [9]. Some suggest that there should be no arbitrary cutoff point for duration of ECMO support. Rather, they suggest that ECMO should be continued in the absence of devastating complications or other clinical issues that preclude subsequent transplantation, surgery, or recovery [45]. This argument highlights the extreme importance of clear, early communication regarding the clinical changes or complications that would render decannulation appropriate. Organized, transparent, and repeated communication regarding the risks and benefits of ECMO as well as the signs of clinical improvement/compromise must be had with families and other health care providers [3]. Constant analysis of the achievement or failure to reach the clinical goals may prevent misunderstandings and distress surrounding discussion of withdrawal of support [46].

Although there are no ethically relevant differences between the decision to withdrawal or withholding a given intervention, these actions tend to *feel* very different to health care providers [47]. Overall, withdrawal of support is typically perceived as more distressing, as it is considered an active decision [48]. Conversely, withholding support is typically considered a passive omission that allows the patient to deteriorate in a way that is not related to a specific action [48]. This passive omission tends to garner less moral distress to providers and parents. This challenge highlights the importance of careful patient selection and clearly defined goals prior to initiation of ECMO.

Consideration of futility is inherent to discussions regarding decisions to withhold or withdraw care. Medical futility can be broadly defined as any intervention that will not provide any substantial benefit to the patient [47]. Arguably, a definition such as this can lead to ambiguity in what constitutes substantial benefit, and such decisions may thus invoke value judgments. This ambiguity and need for value-based decision making may result in conflicts between patients, families, and providers. Given the challenges that arise in discussions of futility, The American Thoracic Society ad hoc Committee on Futile and Potentially Inappropriate Treatment has put forth a statement endorsing a change in terminology from "futile" to "potentially inappropriate care." [49] The group asserts that "potentially inappropriate" is a less polarizing term that may facilitate discussion rather than opposition when determining whether proposed interventions will benefit a given patient. Recognizing that conflict over potentially inappropriate interventions may ensue, the committee outlines a systematic approach to conflict resolution that includes obtaining expert consultation, written notification to surrogates upon initiation of the conflict-resolution process, development of a timeline for expected decision making, obtaining a second medical opinion regarding the appropriateness of the proposed intervention, and case review by an interdisciplinary institutional committee [49].

Should conflict arise, engagement of the hospital ethics committee, social workers, and lawyers may help facilitate resolution. Some have argued that any program that involves invasive, resource-intensive interventions and end-of-life discussions as part of patient care should require routine ethics consultation [50–51]. Focus on the best interest of the patient as well as acceptance of the limitations of our ability to accurately prognosticate for a given patient may help focus these discussions [52]. Interestingly, Courtwright et al. performed a retrospective chart review of all ECMO ethics consultations in the cardiothoracic surgery intensive care unit at the Massachusetts General Hospital from 2013–2017. The authors describe that 39% of the 113 patients who underwent ECMO cannulation were seen by the ethics consultation service. Disagreement about continued use of ECMO was the most frequent ethical issue described. Within this, disagreement among health care providers, disagreement among surrogates, and disagreement between providers and surrogates were all expressed. This investigation demonstrates that the majority of disagreements centered upon whether enough time had elapsed to consider a reasonable trial of ECMO [53]. When two health care providers do not agree, moral distress can result. Moral distress is defined as distress regarding external factors that prevent one from behaving in a way that he/she deems ethically appropriate [47]. Frequent team communication and transparent time limited trials can help to minimize this burden [3, 47].

30.3.8   Equitable Distribution of Costly, Resource Intensive Care

Some argue that discussion of the cost of care ought not be considered at the bedside of an individual patient but rather at the community or society level. However, discussions regarding the potential cost of ECMO do seem to ensue when discussing the appropriateness of cannulation of individual patients. Evidence-based protocols regarding appropriate cost-effective cannulation may help alleviate some of this bedside based decision-making, however limited data currently exists to drive protocol development. Outcome analysis, cost analysis, and quality of life studies across diverse patient populations are required for thoughtful development of these guidelines. Most currently available discussions focus upon the cost of the ECMO run itself including intensive care days, staffing costs, etc. [54] However, equally important to a complete discussion about the ethical appropriateness of ECMO is a discussion of post-cannulation quality of life as well as the cost of continued care for the patient should he or she survive the insult that resulted in needing ECMO. One may question whether it is an appropriate use of resources to initiate ECMO if the patient's expected survival will encompass debilitating chronic illnesses requiring significant reliance on artificial support or aggressive medical technology for long-term survival (stroke, amputation secondary to ischemia, etc.) Data evaluating such costs is emerging, and refinement of these investigations may aid in determining the relative societal value of ECMO for certain medical indications.

Much of the work in this area queries two specific questions: (1) Do patients have improved outcomes with ECMO as compared to conventional care? (2) How does ECMO impact the cost of care? Identification of distinct subgroups of pediatric patients that could cost-effectively benefit from inclusion of ECMO in their care would help establish appropriate patient selection for ECMO, identify reasonable treatment courses, and offer guidance on appropriate indications for withdrawal of ECMO support [55]. For example, in 2013, Lowry et al. performed a retrospective analysis of the Health Care Cost and Use Project Kids' Inpatient Database to evaluate the use of ECMO as an adjunct to cardiopulmonary resuscitation after cardiac arrest compared with conventional cardiopulmonary resuscitation among hospitalized infants and children in the United States. Neither multivariable analysis or propensity-matched analysis identified a significant difference in survival between groups, and the median length of stay and charges were considerably greater for ECMO-CPR survivors [54]. However, other groups have demonstrated that ECMO can be a cost-effective technology. For example, Petrou et al. conducted a randomized controlled trial of newborn infants with severe respiratory failure who underwent ECMO cannulation at centers throughout the United Kingdom. They concluded ECMO was cost-effective at four years after looking at cost per additional life-year and per disability-free life-year gained [56]. Other studies have demonstrated shorter hospitalization and lower morbidity rates without increased hospital costs after looking at outcomes in infants older than 24 weeks estimated gestational age (age 24–72 hours), that underwent ECMO cannulation early in the course of severe respiratory failure [57].

Further work must be dedicated to increasing our understanding of the long-term costs associated with pediatric ECMO. In initial efforts to examine post-discharge costs for pediatric patients who undergo ECMO, Fernando et al. reviewed population-level data regarding the short and long-term outcomes and costs among critically ill pediatric patients receiving ECMO in Ontario, Canada [58]. Specifically, they evaluated the total direct healthcare costs in the year following hospital discharge for these patients. The group found that while pediatric patients who receive ECMO support garner significant hospital-related costs, the majority of costs were incurred during the inpatient hospitalization, with few costs incurred following discharge [58]. Further efforts to identify the care needed and costs incurred following ECMO will help frame the discussion around its appropriate integration into pediatric medicine.

30.3.9 Risk of Morbidity Associated with ECMO Support

In addition to being a costly, resource intensive intervention, ECMO is an invasive intervention that is associated with significant morbidity [9, 57, 58]. Cannulas must be surgically placed into critical arteries and veins, and the circuit involves a series of devices and tubing prone to clotting and typically dependent on full anticoagulation of the patient to maintain patency. Common complications thus include bleeding from the cannula site, surgical site, or brain, embolism, infection at the cannula insertion site, membrane lung failure, tubbing rupture, and pump malfunction [9, 57–58]. Mechanical and catheter-related complications are commonly associated with cannula placement and are strongly associated with the cannulation approach utilized. Higher rates of cannula site bleeding, hemorrhage, hemolysis, mechanical cannula problems, and renal complications have been observed in dual-lumen VV ECMO compared to the more traditional multisite VV ECMO [59]. Additionally, imprecise placement (required to ensure the direction of the infusion jet) and instability of catheter after the placement are associated with mechanical complications such as cardiac injuries or perforation [59].

Discussion of these risks highlights the challenges with consideration of ECMO for certain pediatric patients. As providers strive to balance beneficence and non-maleficence in their decisions regarding utilization of ECMO for a given patient, they must consider whether the patient is particularly vulnerable to any of the previously described risks. For example, should children with intraventricular hemorrhages (IVH) undergo ECMO? Due to the need for anticoagulation, this has been a relative contraindication, however guidelines are becoming more inclusive and children with Type 1 and 2 IVH may be considered for ECMO at some centers [60]. Additionally, the caliber of the blood vessels in pediatric patients may be too small to generate adequate ECMO flows [60]. Additionally, younger children have immature coagulation systems (lower concentrations of antithrombin) and fragile germinal matrices which increases their risk for developing intracranial hemorrhage [61]. Such risks must be transparently discussed during the informed consent process with patients' surrogate decision makers, and providers must recognize that for some patients, the risks may outweigh the benefits of a trial of ECMO.

30.3.10 Challenges with Informed Consent

The triangular relationship between patient, provider, and parent can render the informed consent process more challenging in pediatrics than it is in adult medicine. While debate exists about when it is appropriate to seek assent of children in the informed consent process [62], parents are generally tasked with making decisions for their children. Parents are expected to make decisions that are in the "best interest" of their children. Engaging parents in the informed consent process requires transparent and accurate communication of information to assure they understand the proposed treatment course, associated risks, and expected outcomes. Frank, honest discussion can help parents determine if ECMO is in their child's best interest [47].

Discussions surrounding ECMO, and the often-emergent setting in which such discussions occur, may make it difficult for parents to make truly informed decisions regarding ECMO. Although shared decision making is typically considered the preferred approach to clinical counseling [47], a qualitative study in pediatric traumatic brain injury patients, found unanimously that parents felt that in life-threatening scenarios, decision for intervention should be made by the providers [63]. Such provider-led decision making may offset the potential decisional conflict and regret parents may face with when engaging in shared decision making, however this responsibility may place a significant burden on health care providers. Weiss et al. suggest regularly scheduled team discussions involving all care providers about risk, benefits, and prognosis of the patient may help prevent a single individual from carrying the guilt associated with an unsuccessful outcome [47].

30.4   Case Resolution

The PICU team and family were both adamant about continuing with ECMO cannulation. The surgeons felt pressure to cannulate and eventually did cannulate the patient for VA ECMO. The patient suffered numerous complications—bleeding, leg ischemia, etc.—with limited physiologic improvement. After about 3 weeks, ECMO support was withdrawn, and the patient died.

This case highlights several of the ethical challenges that occur as we expand the pediatric pathologies for which we consider ECMO treatment appropriate. Previous studies have questioned the appropriateness of ECMO in pediatric oncology patients, due to poor survival rates [64]. Recent analysis of specific subsets of oncology patients have shown that ECMO support can benefit these patients, and ECMO is actually recommend for certain pediatric oncology patients in ARDS that is not responsive to medical treatment [65, 66]. This case also highlights the difficulty of offering accurate prognosis as well as the difficulties that arise when members of the healthcare team disagree about what constitutes potentially inappropriate care. Further, this case illustrates how providers may encounter moral distress, in that the PICU providers believed this patient required ECMO but were physically unable to provide it, and the surgeons believed ECMO would cause more harm to the patient with no increase in survival but felt pressured by the intensivists and family to provide it. The difficulty of the informed consent process is also notable in this case in that the immediacy of the patients decline and the urgency with which the patient needed ECMO likely prompted a rushed informed consent process.

30.5   Conclusion

Expansion of the indications for ECMO support has allowed pediatric patients to survive physiologic insults previously deemed lethal. We have highlighted the improved survival for patients when ECMO is used as a Bridge to Recovery, Corrective Surgery, Transplant, or Decision Making. However, ECMO use in pediatrics is fraught with multiple ethical challenges—withholding or withdrawing care, potentially inappropriate treatment, equitable distribution of a resource intensive intervention, relatively high risks of morbidity, and challenges with informed consent. We suggest that preemptive, transparent discussions regarding ECMO cannulation that include discussion of time limited trials and expectations for success as well as indications for decannulation be had by all providers. Engagement of hospital ethics committees is also advised as an adjunct resource to assure collegial interactions among patients, families, and providers. Such efforts are imperative to minimize the emotional burden and moral distress that can result when disagreement occurs. These efforts can help balance the benefits and burdens of pediatric ECMO.

30.6   Selected References

- Carlisle EM, Loeff DS. Emerging issues in the ethical utilization of pediatric extracorporeal membrane oxygenation. Curr Opin Pediatr. 2020;32(3):411–415. doi:https://doi.org/10.1097/MOP.0000000000000901

  - Over the past several decades, the patient population for whom ECMO is medically appropriate has expanded resulting in consideration of numerous ethical issues. In this review, authors explore whether clinic settings exist in which ECMO is ethically obligatory as well as how to navigate disagreements about decannulation. They also provide discussion of how to assure ethical expansion of pediatric ECMO by reviewing ethical challenges with integration of other disruptive healthcare modalities into patient care.

- Weiss EM, Fiester A. From "Longshot" to "Fantasy": Obligations to Pediatric Patients and Families When Last-Ditch Medical Efforts Fail. Am J Bioeth. 2018;18(1):3–11. doi:https://doi.org/10.1080/15265161.2017.1401157

  - In this paper, authors employ two pediatric cases to explore the transition from longshot to fantasy care. They subsequently provide a framework to guide discussion among providers and between providers and families regarding this challenging transition.

References

1. Barbaro RP, Paden ML, Guner YS, et al. Pediatric extracorporeal life support organization registry international report 2016. ASAIO J. 2017;63(4):456–63. https://doi.org/10.1097/mat.0000000000000603.
2. Featherstone PJ, Ball CM. The early history of extracorporeal membrane oxygenation. Anaesth Intensive Care. 2018;46(6):555–7.
3. Carlisle EM, Loeff DS. Emerging issues in the ethical utilization of pediatric extracorporeal membrane oxygenation. Curr Opin Pediatr. 2020;32(3):411–5. https://doi.org/10.1097/MOP.0000000000000901.
4. Di Nardo M, Dalle Ore A, Testa G, et al. Principlism and Personalism. Comparing two ethical models applied clinically in neonates undergoing extracorporeal membrane oxygenation support. Front Pediatr. 2019;7:312. https://doi.org/10.3389/fped.2019.00312.
5. Peterec SM, Bizzarro MJ, Mercurio MR. Is extracorporeal membrane oxygenation for a neonate ever ethically obligatory? J Pediatr. 2018;195:297–301. https://doi.org/10.1016/j.peds.2017.11.018.
6. Chrysostomou C, Morell VO, Kuch BA, O'Malley E, Munoz R, Wearden PD. Short- and intermediate-term survival after extracorporeal membrane oxygenation in children with cardiac disease. J Thorac Cardiovasc Surg. 2013;146(2):317–25. https://doi.org/10.1016/j.jtcvs.2012.11.014.
7. Merrill ED, Schoeneberg L, Sandesara P, et al. Outcomes after prolonged extracorporeal membrane oxygenation support in children with cardiac disease – extracorporeal life support organization registry study. J Thorac Cardiovasc Surg. 2014;148(2):582–8. https://doi.org/10.1016/j.jtcvs.2013.09.038.
8. Gonzalez DO, Sebastiao YV, Cooper JN, Minneci PC, Deans KJ. Pediatric extracorporeal membrane oxygenation mortality is related to extracorporeal membrane oxygenation volume in US hospitals. J Surg Res. 2019;236:159–65. https://doi.org/10.1016/j.jss.2018.11.043.
9. Ares GJ, Buonpane C, Helenowski I, Reynolds M, Hunter CJ. Outcomes and associated ethical considerations of long-run pediatric ECMO at a single center institution. Pediatr Surg Int. 2019;35(3):321–8. https://doi.org/10.1007/s00383-019-04443-y.
10. Rajagopal SK, Almond CS, Laussen PC, Rycus PT, Wypij D, Thiagarajan RR. Extracorporeal membrane oxygenation for the support of infants, children, and young adults with acute myocarditis: a review of the extracorporeal life support organization registry. Crit Care Med. 2010;38(2):382–7. https://doi.org/10.1097/ccm.0b013e3181bc8293.
11. Teele SA, Allan CK, Laussen PC, Newburger JW, Gauvreau K, Thiagarajan RR. Management and outcomes in pediatric patients presenting with acute fulminant myocarditis. J Pediatr. 2011;158(4):638–643.e1. https://doi.org/10.1016/j.peds.2010.10.015.
12. Uda K, Shoji K, Koyama-Wakai C, et al. Clinical characteristics of influenza virus-induced lower respiratory infection during the 2015 to 2016 season. J Infect Chemother. 2018;24(6):407–13. https://doi.org/10.1016/j.jiac.2018.01.002.
13. Domico M, Ridout D, MacLaren G, et al. Extracorporeal membrane oxygenation for pertussis: predictors of outcome including pulmonary hypertension and leukodepletion. Pediatr Crit Care Med. 2018;19(3):254–61. https://doi.org/10.1097/pcc.0000000000001454.
14. Partridge EA, Peranteau WH, Rintoul NE, et al. Timing of repair of congenital diaphragmatic hernia in patients supported by extracorporeal membrane oxygenation (ECMO). J Pediatr Surg. 2015;50(2):260–2. https://doi.org/10.1016/j.pedsurg.2014.11.013.
15. The Congenital Diaphragmatic Hernia Study Group. Estimating disease severity of congenital diaphragmatic hernia in the first 5 minutes of life. J Pediatr Surg. 2001;36(1):141–5. https://doi.org/10.1053/jpsu.2001.20032.
16. Fallon SC, Cass DL, Olutoye OO, et al. Repair of congenital diaphragmatic hernias on extracorporeal membrane oxygenation (ECMO): does early repair improve patient survival? J Pediatr Surg. 2013;48(6):1172–6. https://doi.org/10.1016/j.jpedsurg.2013.03.008.

17. Bryner BS, West BT, Hirschl RB, et al. Congenital diaphragmatic hernia requiring extracorporeal membrane oxygenation: does timing of repair matter? J Pediatr Surg. 2009;44(6):1165–71.; discussion 1171–1172. https://doi.org/10.1016/j.jpedsurg.2009.02.022.
18. Desai AA, Ostlie DJ, Juang D. Optimal timing of congenital diaphragmatic hernia repair in infants on extracorporeal membrane oxygenation. Semin Pediatr Surg. 2015;24(1):17–9. https://doi.org/10.1053/j.sempedsurg.2014.11.004.
19. Connors RH, Tracy T Jr, Bailey PV, Kountzman B, Weber TR. Congenital diaphragmatic hernia repair on ECMO. J Pediatr Surg. 1990;25(10):1043–6.; discussion 1046–1047. https://doi.org/10.1016/0022-3468(90)90215-u.
20. Sigalet DL, Tierney A, Adolph V, et al. Timing of repair of congenital diaphragmatic hernia requiring extracorporeal membrane oxygenation support. J Pediatr Surg. 1995;30(8):1183–7. https://doi.org/10.1016/0022-3468(95)90017-9.
21. Lally KP, Paranka MS, Roden J, et al. Congenital diaphragmatic hernia. Stabilization and repair on ECMO. Ann Surg. 1992;216(5):569–73. https://doi.org/10.1097/00000658-199211000-00008.
22. Khan AM, Lally KP. The role of extracorporeal membrane oxygenation in the management of infants with congenital diaphragmatic hernia. Semin Perinatol. 2005;29(2):118–22. https://doi.org/10.1053/j.semperi.2005.04.005.
23. Clark RH, Hardin WD Jr, Hirschl RB, et al. Congenital diaphragmatic hernia study group. Et al. current surgical management of congenital diaphragmatic hernia: a report from the congenital diaphragmatic hernia study group. J Pediatr Surg. 1998;33(7):1004–9. https://doi.org/10.1016/s0022-3468(98)90522-x.
24. Puligandla PS, Grabowski J, Austin M, et al. Management of congenital diaphragmatic hernia: a systematic review from the APSA outcomes and evidence based practice committee. J Pediatr Surg. 2015;50(11):1958–70. https://doi.org/10.1016/j.pedsurg.2015.09.010.
25. Morris MC, Ittenbach RF, Godinez RI, et al. Risk factors for mortality in 137 pediatric cardiac intensive care unit patients managed with extracorporeal membrane oxygenation. Crit Care Med. 2004;32(4):1061–9. https://doi.org/10.1097/01.ccm.0000119425.04364.cf.
26. Alsoufi B, Al-Radi OO, Gruenwald C, et al. Extra-corporeal life support following cardiac surgery in children: analysis of risk factors and survival in a single institution. Eur J Cardiothorac Surg. 2009;35(6):1004–11.; discussion 1011. https://doi.org/10.1016/j.ejcts.2009.02.015.
27. Kane DA, Thiagarajan RR, Wypij D, et al. Rapid-response extracorporeal membrane oxygenation to support cardiopulmonary resuscitation in children with cardiac disease. Circulation. 2010;122(11 Suppl):S241–8. https://doi.org/10.1161/circulationaha.109.928390.
28. Thiagarajan RR, Laussen PC, Rycus PT, Bartlett RH, Bratton SL. Extracorporeal membrane oxygenation to aid cardiopulmonary resuscitation in infants and children. Circulation. 2007;116(15):1693–700. https://doi.org/10.1161/circulationaha.106.680678.
29. Chan T, Thiagarajan RR, Frank D, Bratton SL. Survival after extracorporeal cardiopulmonary resuscitation in infants and children with heart disease. J Thorac Cardiovasc Surg. 2008;136(4):984–92. https://doi.org/10.1016/j.jtcvs.2008.03.007.
30. Loforte A, Delmo Walter EM, Stiller B, et al. Extracorporeal membrane oxygenation for intraoperative cardiac support in children with congenital heart disease. Interact Cardiovasc Thorac Surg. 2010;10(5):753–8. https://doi.org/10.1510/icvts.2009.220475.
31. Hannan RL, Ojito JW, Ybarra MA, O'Brien MC, Rossi AF, Burke RP. Rapid cardiopulmonary support in children with heart disease: a nine-year experience. Ann Thorac Surg. 2006;82(5):1637–41. https://doi.org/10.1016/j.athoracsur.2006.05.091.
32. Jenkins KJ. Risk adjustment for congenital heart surgery: the RACHS-1 method. Semin Thorac Cardiovasc Surg Pediatr Card Surg Annu. 2004;7:180–4. https://doi.org/10.1053/j.pcsu.2004.02.009.
33. Gupta P, Robertson MJ, Beam B, et al. Relationship of ECMO duration with outcomes after pediatric cardiac surgery: a multi-institutional analysis. Minerva Anestesiol. 2015;81(6):619–27.

34. Bautista-Hernandez V, Thiagarajan RR, Fynn-Thompson F, et al. Preoperative extracorporeal membrane oxygenation as a bridge to cardiac surgery in children with congenital heart disease. Ann Thorac Surg. 2009;88(4):1306–11. https://doi.org/10.1016/j.athorasur.2009.06.074.

35. Barrett CS, Chan TT, Wilkes J, Bratton SL, Thiagarajan RR. Association of Pediatric Cardiac Surgical Volume and Mortality after Cardiac ECMO. ASAIO J. 2017;63(6):802–9. https://doi.org/10.1097/mat.0000000000000558.

36. Kumar TK, Zurakowski D, Dalton H, et al. Extracorporeal membrane oxygenation in postcardiotomy patients: factors influencing outcome. J Thorac Cardiovasc Surg. 2010;140(2):330–336. e2. https://doi.org/10.1016/j.jtcvs.2010.02.034.

37. Roeleveld PP, Wilde R, Hazekamp M, Rycus PT, Thiagarajan RR. Extracorporeal membrane oxygenation in single ventricle lesions palliated via the hybrid approach. World J Pediatr Congenit Heart Surg. 2014;5(3):393–7. https://doi.org/10.1177/2150135114526420.

38. Jolley M, Yarlagadda VV, Rajagopal SK, Almodovar MC, Rycus PT, Thiagarajan RR. Extracorporeal membrane oxygenation-supported cardiopulmonary resuscitation following stage 1 palliation for hypoplastic left heart syndrome. Pediatr Crit Care Med. 2014;15(6):538–45. https://doi.org/10.1097/pcc.0000000000000159.

39. Miana LA, Silva G, Caneo LF, et al. Rational use of mechanical circulatory support as a bridge to Pediatric and congenital heart transplantation. Braz J Cardiovasc Surg. 2018;33(3):242–9. https://doi.org/10.21470/1678-9741-2018-0081.

40. Imamura M, Dossey AM, Prodhan P, et al. Bridge to cardiac transplant in children: Berlin heart versus extracorporeal membrane oxygenation. Ann Thorac Surg. 2009;87(6):1894–901.; discussion 1901. https://doi.org/10.1016/j.athoracsur.2009.03.049.

41. Gedik E, Atar F, Ozdemirkan A, et al. Perioperative Venoarterial extracorporeal membrane oxygenation support during heart transplant. Exp Clin Transplant. 2017;15(Suppl 1):224–30. https://doi.org/10.6002/ect.mesot2016.p100.

42. Yarlagadda VV, Maeda K, Zhang Y, et al. Temporary circulatory support in U.S. children awaiting heart transplantation. J Am Coll Cardiol. 2017;70(18):2250–60. https://doi.org/10.1016/j.jacc.2017.08.072.

43. Dipchand AI, Mahle WT, Tresler M, et al. Extracorporeal membrane oxygenation as a bridge to Pediatric heart transplantation: effect on post-listing and post-transplantation outcomes. Circ Heart Fail. 2015;8(5):960–9. https://doi.org/10.1161/circulationfailure.114.001553.

44. Jaramillo C, Braus N. How should ECMO initiation and withdrawal decisions be shared? AMA J Ethics. 2019;21(5):E387–93. https://doi.org/10.1001/amajethics.2019.387.

45. Kirshbom PM, Bridges ND, Myung RJ, Gaynor JW, Clark BJ, Spray TL. Use of extracorporeal membrane oxygenation in pediatric thoracic organ transplantation. J Thorac Cardiovasc Surg. 2002;123(1):130–6. https://doi.org/10.1067/mtc.2002.118504.

46. Kirsch R, Munson D. Ethical and end of life considerations for neonates requiring ECMO support. Semin Perinatol. 2018;42(2):129–37. https://doi.org/10.1053/j.semperi.2017.12.009.

47. Weiss EM, Fiester A. From "longshot" to "fantasy": obligations to Pediatric patients and families when last-ditch medical efforts fail. Am J Bioeth. 2018;18(1):3–11. https://doi.org/10.1080/15265161.2017.1401157.

48. Melltorp G, Nilstun T. The difference between withholding and withdrawing life-sustaining treatment. Intensive Care Med. 1997;23(12):1264–7. https://doi.org/10.1007/s001340050496.

49. Bosslet GT, Pope TM, Rubenfeld GD, et al. An official ATS/AACN/ACCP/ESICM/SCCM policy statement: responding to requests for potentially inappropriate treatments in intensive care units. Am J Respir Crit Care Med. 2015;191(11):1318–3013. https://doi.org/10.1164/rccm.201505-0924st.

50. Schneiderman LJ, Gilmer T, Teetzel HD. Impact of ethics consultations in the intensive care setting: a randomized, controlled trial. Crit Care Med. 2000;28(12):3920–4.

51. Schneiderman LJ, Gilmer T, Teetzel HD, et al. Effect of ethics consultations on nonbeneficial life-sustaining treatments in the intensive care setting: a randomized controlled trial. JAMA. 2003;290(9):1166–72. https://doi.org/10.1001/jama.290.9.1166.

52. Bester JC. The best interest standard is the best we have: why the harm principle and constrained parental autonomy cannot replace the best interest standard in Pediatric ethics. J Clin Ethics 2019;30(3):223–231. PMID: 31573966.
53. Courtwright AM, Robinson EM, Feins K, et al. Ethics committee consultation and extracorporeal membrane oxygenation. Ann Am Thorac Soc. 2016;13(9):1553–8. https://doi.org/10.1513/annalsats.201511-7570c.
54. Lowry AW, Morales DL, Graves DE, et al. Characterization of extracorporeal membrane oxygenation for pediatric cardiac arrest in the United States: analysis of the kids' inpatient database. Pediatr Cardiol. 2013;34(6):1422–30. https://doi.org/10.1007/s00246-013-0666-8.
55. Van Litsenburg R, De Mos N, Edgell D, Gruenwald C, Bohn DJ, Parshuram CS. Arch Dis Child Fetal Neonatal Ed. 2005;90(2):F176–7. https://doi.org/10.1136/adc.2003.047779.
56. Petrou S, Edwards L. Cost effectiveness analysis of neonatal extracorporeal membrane oxygenation based on four year results from the UK collaborative ECMO trial. Arch Dis Child Fetal Neonatal Ed. 2004;89(3):F263–8. https://doi.org/10.1136/adc.2002.025635.
57. Schumacher RE, Roloff DW, Chapman R, Snedecor S, Bartlett RH. Extracorporeal membrane oxygenation in term Newborns. A prospective cost-benefit analysis. ASAIO J. 1993;39(4):873–9.
58. Fernando SM, Qureshi D, Tanuseputro P, et al. Long-term survival and costs following extracorporeal membrane oxygenation in critically ill children-a population-based cohort study. Crit Care. 2020;24(1):131. https://doi.org/10.1186/s13054-020-02844-3.
59. Zamora IJ, Shekerdemian L, Fallon SC, et al. Outcomes comparing dual-lumen to multisite venovenous ECMO in the pediatric population: the extracorporeal life support registry experience. J Pediatr Surg. 2014;49(10):1452–7. https://doi.org/10.1016/j.jpedsurg.2014.05.027.
60. Thompson AF, Luan J, Al Aklabi MM, Cave DA, Ryerson LM, Noga ML. Pediatric extracorporeal membrane oxygenation (ECMO): a guide for radiologists. Pediatr Radiol. 2018;48(10):1488–502. https://doi.org/10.1007/s00247-018-4211-z.
61. Butt W, MacLaren G. Concepts from paediatric extracorporeal membrane oxygenation for adult intensivists. Ann Intensive Care. 2016;6(1):20. https://doi.org/10.1186/s13613-016-0121-0.
62. Katz AL, Webb SA. Informed consent in decision-making in Pediatric practice. Pediatrics. 2016;138(2):e20161485. https://doi.org/10.1542/peds.2016-1485.
63. Marsh R, Matlock DD, Maertens JA, et al. Parental involvement in decision making about intracranial pressure monitor placement in children with traumatic brain injury. J Neurosurg Pediatr. 2020;25:183–91. https://doi.org/10.3171/2019.8.peds19275.
64. Stecher SS, Beyer G, Goni E, et al. Extracorporeal membrane oxygenation in predominantly Leuco- and thrombocytopenic Haematologic/oncologic patients with acute respiratory distress syndrome – a single-Centre experience. Oncol Res Treat. 2018;41(9):539–43. https://doi.org/10.1159/000489718.
65. Al Ameri A, Koller C, Kantarjian H, et al. Acute pulmonary failure during remission induction chemotherapy in adults with acute myeloid leukemia or high-risk myelodysplastic syndrome. Cancer. 2010;116(1):93–7. https://doi.org/10.1002/cncr.24711.
66. Huprikar NA, Peterson MR, DellaVolpe JD, et al. Salvage extracorporeal membrane oxygenation in induction-associated acute respiratory distress syndrome in acute leukemia patients: a case series. Int J Artif Organs. 2019;42(1):49–54. https://doi.org/10.1177/0391398818799160.

Chapter 31
Ethics of Pediatric Bariatric Surgery

Annie Hess and Baddr A. Shakhsheer

Abstract Childhood obesity affects approximately 4.5 million children in the United States, increasing an individual's morbidity and mortality. Several ethical dilemmas arise when considering metabolic and bariatric surgery (MBS) as a treatment option for pediatric patients. The benefit-risk ratio must be determined for each individual patient. Though more research is needed to determine long-term consequences of MBS, obesity without surgical intervention poses a significant risk. A multi-disciplinary approach is needed to determine a patient's candidacy. Assent and consent from a patient and their surrogate decision maker is necessary. In situations where assent is not possible, such as in syndromic obesity, careful consideration is necessary. Psychosocial problems, finances, or insurance status should not be barriers to surgery. MBS centers have a moral imperative for a just allocation of resources.

Keywords Metabolic and bariatric surgery · Pediatric surgery · Childhood obesity
Ethics · Syndromic obesity

A. Hess
Washington University School of Medicine, St. Louis, MO, USA
e-mail: annie.hess@wustl.edu

B. A. Shakhsheer (✉)
Washington University School of Medicine, St. Louis, MO, USA

Division of Pediatric Surgery, Department of Surgery, Washington University School of Medicine, St. Louis, MO, USA
e-mail: baddr@wustl.edu

© The Author(s), under exclusive license to Springer Nature Switzerland AG 2022

V. A. Lonchyna et al. (eds.), *Difficult Decisions in Surgical Ethics*, Difficult Decisions in Surgery: An Evidence-Based Approach,
https://doi.org/10.1007/978-3-030-84625-1_31

433

Case Presentation
Ms. JY is a 15-year-old female who presents to clinic for evaluation of bariatric surgery. The patient has a BMI of 52 and multiple co-morbidities, including type 2 diabetes, on metformin and insulin, obstructive sleep apnea, and severe depression, managed with sertraline. She has tried multiple structured weight loss programs, including two inpatient stays, without improvement in her weight or co-morbidities. She notes severe anxiety as she has been bullied for years due to her weight. Her mother has undergone Roux-en-Y gastric bypass for morbid obesity and her father has undergone sleeve gastrectomy. Both had uncomplicated courses and have been happy with their results. They both encourage their daughter to proceed with bariatric surgery, though they are worried about the financial burden. The patient is hesitant to proceed because of the necessary lifestyle changes.

31.1   Introduction

Childhood obesity rates have reached epidemic proportions and continue to increase, with approximately 4.5 million children meeting criteria for obesity (BMI > 95th percentile for age and sex) or severe obesity (BMI > 120% of 95th percentile or BMI > 35 kg/m^2) in the United States [1]. Childhood obesity is associated with increased cardiovascular mortality of 3 to 5 times at age 50 compared to those children without obesity, increased risk of type 2 diabetes and its sequelae, obstructive sleep apnea, nonalcoholic fatty liver disease, and gastroesophageal reflux, amongst other co-morbidities [2]. Unfortunately, lifestyle interventions such has diet and exercise have had trouble with short term efficacy and demonstrated minimal long-term benefit [3]. Metabolic and bariatric surgery (MBS) has been shown to be the only efficacious long-term treatment for obesity in adults, not only reducing weight but improving co-morbidities [2]. As MBS becomes a more popular choice for treating pediatric patients, several ethical aspects must be considered. We will attempt to frame the dilemmas presented using the framework presented by Jonsen et al.: medical indications, patient preferences, quality of life, and contextual features (Table 31.1) [4].

31.2   Search Strategy

To search the literature, three topics were searched and reviewed. Databases used for all searches were PubMed and Embase. The search was limited to articles from 2008 and newer. The first topic was the ethics of treating childhood obesity. Terms used were "pediatric, child, or adolescent", "obesity", and "ethics." Results were narrowed down by searching for "treatment" or "intervention." The second topic

Table 31.1 Ethical framework regarding adolescent bariatric surgery

Ethical components	Questions to ask
Medical indications	1. What is this patient's benefit-risk ratio? 2. What is the likely outcome with surgery? Without surgery? 3. How can ethics research be conducted to improve our knowledge base of medical indications?
Patient preferences	1. What does the parent/guardian want? What does the child want? 2. Are there any barriers to assent? 3. Are all aspects of informed consent met by the patient, physician and surrogate decision maker? 4. Do any special circumstances exist?
Quality of life	1. What does the patient value regarding their lifestyle? 2. Are there any psychosocial barriers that must be optimized prior to surgery? 3. Do any biases need to be addressed regarding obesity?
Contextual features	1. Is there any provider or health care system issues that might influence treatment decision? 2. How can we optimize justice for regarding MBS for all obese adolescent patients?

Adapted from Jonsen et al. [4]

was pediatric bariatric surgery outcomes. Terms used were "pediatric, child or adolescent", "bariatric", "surgery", and "outcomes." Articles were narrowed by elevating those relating to complications, long term clinical trials, and fertility/pregnancy. The third topic was ethics regarding management of if disorders or sex development. Keywords were "ethics", "disorders of sex development" or "gender-affirming", "treatment" or "intervention."

31.3   Discussion

31.3.1   Medical Indications

Ethical practitioners must balance the principles of beneficence and non-maleficence to determine the benefit-risk ratio for the patient (Table 31.2). Practitioners must define the ultimate goals of treating obesity and what interventions lead to those goals, the probability of their successes, and the risks associated with such interventions. The medical problem of childhood obesity is well-defined, and it is well understood that childhood obesity increases an individual's morbidity and mortality [5]. There are many specific goals of treatment, but all must improve quality of life and reduce the risk of death and complications. However, an individual's goals take utmost precedence, and all treatments must be tailored to their specific goals. As bariatric surgery has emerged as a treatment for childhood obesity, several dilemmas have arisen when considering the benefit-risk ratio. Do we have enough data to ensure minimization of risks and long-term complications for MBS, especially

Table 31.2 Principles of ethics in pediatric bariatric surgery

Autonomy	• Both patient assent and parental/surrogate decision-maker consent is required • Surrogate decisions must act in the best interest of the patient • Patient preference must take precedence, and a multi-disciplinary approach is necessary for evaluating a patient's readiness • Goals of treatment should be tailored to a patient's goals
Beneficence	• MBS improves outcomes related to co-morbidities and quality of life • MBS centers must evaluate a patient's preferences and values, medical indications, and likelihood of obtaining desirable medical outcomes
Non-maleficence	• Obesity, without intervention, could impose harm to an individual • More research is needed to further elicit the long-term consequences of MBS
Justice	• MBS centers have a moral imperative to offer bariatric service to all individuals • Distributive justice must be applied to all aspects of MBS care

given the longevity of most pediatric patients? Given the lack of long-term efficacy of lifestyle changes and the possible mal effects of subjecting a pediatric patient to a therapy unlikely to succeed, is it ethical to offer stand-alone lifestyle changes as a sustainable and efficacious therapy for severe obesity [6]?

31.3.2 Treating Childhood and Adolescent Obesity

Structured weight loss programs are the current "gold standard" of treatment for obesity [7]. They consist of diet changes, increased activity, behavioral modification, and parental involvement [7]. Parental involvement has been shown to be crucial in addressing environmental factors when dealing with weight loss in pediatric patients. While they are the current mainstay of treatment, they have been shown to have limited sustained improvement in BMI and comorbidities in severely obese populations and older adolescents [6, 8]. The main argument for their use is that they are safe, non-invasive, with limited risk to the patient. The implementation of structured weight loss is varied and there is no consensus on "best" practices [9]. Benefits are minimal with an expected ~1–3 kg/m^2 reduction in BMI and with high rates of non-completion [9]. In a large meta-analysis of all structured weight loss programs, the effectiveness of these interventions was found to be small, with only a 0.25 BMI point reduction [10]. Additionally, these interventions are less likely to be effective in children with severe obesity and in older children [6]. This "gold standard" therapy is considered such because of its minimal direct negative consequences rather than its efficacy.

The American Society for Metabolic and Bariatric Surgery (ASMBS) has recommended that prior weight loss attempts should no longer be a barrier to the surgery [2]. Further, the minimal direct negative consequences are short sighted, as multiple studies have demonstrated the long-term sequelae of pediatric obesity. With the view that this is an "otherwise healthy population," the practitioner may choose less invasive interventions, which may be to the ultimate detriment of the patient.

31.3.3 Risks and Long-Term Complications of Metabolic Bariatric Surgery

MBS in pediatric patients has been shown to significantly improve cardiovascular disease (CVD) risk factors, insulin resistance, nonalcoholic fatty liver disease, and quality of life [2]. In studies with long term follow up, patients had a ~27% reduction of weight at 3 years [11]. There is a scarcity of studies analyzing the longer-term outcomes in pediatric patients. There are only 10 studies with follow up longer than five years, and only one at ~13 years [12]. However, there is promising data that adolescents, compared to adults, have similar weight loss with greater improvement of comorbidities [13]. Long term studies in adolescent patients, however, are still pending.

Consideration of the risks of MBS in pediatric patients is important, especially when comparing to lifestyle changes, where physiologic risk is minimal. A multi-center prospective study in this patient population shows that 8% of all pediatric MBS patients experience major perioperative complications, ~15% have minor complications, and ~5% suffer major morbidity in 3 years [14]. The major perioperative complications are reoperation (primarily for bleeding), anastomotic leak, and obstruction. Minor complications include readmission for dehydration, abdominal pain, and UTIs [14]. In the long term, 50% of adolescent bariatric patients experience anemia secondary to low levels of micronutrients (iron, folate, B6, or B12) and vitamin D deficiency [2, 15]. Following surgery, patients must be diligent with their medications, which includes vitamin and mineral supplementation, ursodiol, and acid reducing medications, and protein and fluid intake. Poor compliance to medical therapy in the pediatric population consistently leads to anemia.

Additional considerations must be given to the risk of fertility and pregnancy following MBS. Obesity increases infertility and pregnancy-related morbidity and mortality [2]. Following MBS and weight loss, fertility increase and health outcomes of both mother and child improve [16]. However, pregnancy during the rapid weight loss period following surgery (up to two years post-operatively) in adult patients has been shown to have increased complications including small for gestational age and nutritional deficiency [2, 16]. Most adolescent patients undergo sexual debut during their post-operative period and are thus at increased risk of pregnancy in the aforementioned period [17]. MBS centers must be able to provide ongoing education and counseling regarding these risks and benefits and post-operative contraception.

When evaluating the benefit-risk ratio for a patient, providers and caregivers might be reluctant to offer a drastic, permanent change to an otherwise healthy child. When the benefits are immediate, it is easier to conceptualize the benefit-risk ratio. For example, if a young child is doubled over in pain secondary to appendicitis, a parent will more readily agree to surgery for their unwell child. However, a patient with the disease of obesity may have risks and complications of their disease that are initially less debilitating but are nevertheless considerably harmful.

31.3.4   MBS Candidate Requirements

The ASMBS offers a comprehensive review of patient eligibility for MBS [2]. One of the requirements is that the potential patients and their support system undergo comprehensive psychologic evaluation. This evaluation is intensive and required regardless of pre-existing mental health issues. During this evaluation, a behavioral specialist evaluates the patient's ability to cope with surgery and adapt to the permanent lifestyle changes necessary for success. Not everyone who desires MBS and meets the medical indications for surgery will become a candidate following this evaluation. The impact of a patient's psychosocial support and its ethical implications are discussed in the next section.

The ideal age of surgery has also been debated. The terms "pediatric" and "adolescent" are both used when referring to metabolic and bariatric surgery programs related to children. The recent American Association of Pediatrics (AAP) statement defines "pediatric" as any person less than 18 years old and "adolescent" as any person from age 13 to 18 [18, 19]. The ASMBS has no age guidelines [2]. The minimum age for bariatric surgery is a matter of debate but, according to the AAP policy statement, there is no evidence to support age-based eligibility requirements [18, 19]. Further, evidence in the field shows that metabolic and bariatric surgery does not lead to any stunting of growth [15, 20]. Additional studies have shown continued growth after metabolic and bariatric surgery on patients younger than 14 years old, though long term studies are required [21]. Removing the age requirement increases the number of patients eligible for surgery but raises ethical concerns about the ability of a pediatric patient to express their desire for surgery. These are discussed in the next section.

31.3.5   Patient Preferences

In the case of pediatric bariatric surgery, one must consider the preferences of the patient and of the parent(s)/guardian(s). This is especially true given the behavioral consequences of these surgeries, such as altered eating habits and the need for lifelong vitamin and mineral supplementation. The majority of pediatric bariatric surgery patients are adolescents, who should provide assent to surgery to maximize outcomes.

31.3.6   Consent and Assent

Consent is the legal contract that a patient agrees to undergo a medical intervention following an in-depth discussion with the physician regarding details of the treatment options, benefits, risks, and alternatives. Practically it is the agreement that a physician and a patient enter, respecting a patient's autonomy to choose or express their preferences [4]. As pediatric patients are legally (in most cases) unable to provide consent, the AAP recommends obtaining assent from patients prior to interventions [22]. Assent is an expression of agreement to proceed, rather than a contractual consent [22]. Regarding MBS and pediatric patients, dilemmas arise when parents and patients are not in agreement regarding preferences. This may be magnified by the "elective" nature of MBS procedures. Further, lifestyle habits change dramatically after MBS and the changes are life-long. Though pediatric patients can only assent to the procedure, their preferences should be an essential component of the decision-making process as their motivation often determines success of the operation.

According to ASMBS, when a pediatric patient is capable of assenting, proceeding with surgery requires both positive patient assent and parental consent [2]. Assent requires decision-making capacity and understanding of risks and benefits of the procedure and long-term sequela. Similar frameworks for consent and assent occur in surgery for gender confirmation surgery and Disorders of Sexual Development (DSD).

Transgender and gender nonconforming adolescents often desire gender affirming care, which can include irreversible surgical care. Multiple organizations, including the World Professional Association for Transgender Health (WPATH), have recommended that irreversible procedures be delayed until the patient can legally consent at the age of 18 [23]. However, harm can result in delaying these operations. Guidelines suggest that gender dysphoria itself does not preclude a patient's decision-making capacity. Rather, an understanding of the risks, benefits, and long-term complications matter more than a patient's age alone [24]. Further, minors can legally consent to other treatments in certain conditions including treatment for drug abuse, contraception, and abortion.

Disorders of Sexual Development comprise a spectrum of disorders where external and internal genital are ambiguous or atypical. Surgery can be considered to optimize urogenital function, reduce cancer risk, and alter the appearance of external genitalia. These surgeries were formerly considered in an infant's development. However, as studies have illustrated harm resulting from parental decisions during infancy leading to external genitalia that may not match the patient's gender identity, new ethical guidelines were proposed. While these issues have not been definitively solved, six guiding principles have been proposed: (1) minimizing physical risk to child, (2) minimizing psycho-social risk to child, (3) preserving potential for fertility, (4) preserving or promoting capacity to have satisfying sexual relations, (5) leaving options open for the future, and (6) respecting the parents' wishes and beliefs [25].

Despite the obvious differences between DSD operations and MBS, a number of these basic principles overlap. The upmost importance is reducing risk, both current and future, to a child. Minimizing psycho-social risk continues to be a concern. The decision to intervene early via surgery can have positive and negative consequences and must be properly weighed against non-intervention.

31.3.7 Cognitive Disabilities

Pediatric obesity is higher in certain subpopulations, including youth with cognitive impairment or developmental disabilities [24]. Additionally, ~25 obesity syndromes exist in conjunction with cognitive impairment/developmental delay (CI/DD), most notably Prader-Willi Syndrome [26]. Children with CI/DD are 2–3 times more likely to suffer from obesity with less treatment options [27]. There is limited data that MBS does offer a hope of reducing their overall mortality and morbidity [27]. With a wide spectrum of cognitive abilities, undergoing psychologic testing during the pre-operative evaluation is challenging. It is likely that these patients will be unable to assent to the procedure. It is imperative that a multidisciplinary team, including psychologist, child life specialist, and social worker have an in-depth knowledge of the patient's cognitive abilities, their guardians' understanding of the procedure, and the patient's psychosocial support system [27]. There is concern that these patients will have limited ability to follow post-operative diet modifications predisposing them to greater complications. There is an imperative to continue to study the long-term effects of MBS on these patients.

The optimal age for MBS in the population of patients with CI/DD is as yet undetermined. As adolescents, these patients typically have a higher level of support system, compared to adult patients with CI/DD. These improved resources, in theory, could lead to improved outcomes.

31.3.8 Quality of Life and Psychosocial Barriers

The goal of MBS is to improve a patient's quality of life. Multiple studies have noted that physicians are notoriously poor at judging a patient's quality of life [28]. With pediatric patients, a common legal practice evoked is the best interest standard: clinicians and surrogate decision makers must act in the best interest of the child, maximizing benefits and minimizing harms [22]. Competent adults have the ability to express preferences about the future, while drawing on previous experiences to judge future values. Children have a diminished history of preferences and a long future in which to live with the results of these decisions. It is therefore imperative that an MBS committee understand the patient's current preferences, while accounting for the family's values and preferences.

31.3.9 Cultural Norms

Eating has a strong cultural significance. MBS threatens to alter a support system that is based on those cultural norms. Beyond food, obesity is related with high amount of bias and prejudice in society as well as in the medical field [29]. Patients with obesity can be perceived as lazy, having weak will power, and having poor adherence to treatments. Obesity can be seen as an individual's failure and lack of personal control with surgery offering a "short cut" that those with better self-control would not necessitate [30]. Although MBS offers an improvement in measurable outcomes, such as reduced cardiovascular incidence and improved glucose control, it can also be seen perpetuating the societal ideals of beauty rather than true health [30]. Ethical physicians must critically evaluate the end points of treatment and their biases. This is best done by evaluating a patient's preferences and values, medical indications, and likelihood of obtaining desirable medical outcomes.

31.3.10 Social Support Structure

Strong support has positive influence on an adult patient's success following bariatric surgery [31]. Pediatric treatment requires more intimately involved caregivers: encouragement for proper eating, purchasing of appropriate food choices and vitamin supplementation, post-operative visits and appointments. Ultimately, bariatric surgery can be a burden on the patient and the family as their lifestyle is permanently changed. This change is often more expensive and cumbersome, as the pediatric patient is dependent on others for success. This dependence, in addition, provides multiple avenues for potential failure and potential harm. The ASMBS recognizes the importance of social support, but also the increased higher likelihood of dysfunction if denied MBS. Thus, the lack of family support is no longer a barrier to surgery. The ethical question is, is it fair to jeopardize a patient's future wellbeing, due to their current socioeconomic circumstance?

The best interest principal mandates that clinicians proceed in a manner that maximizes benefits and minimizes harm, while keeping the entirety of a patient's interest in mind. In adult patients, lower socioeconomic status can be associated with a lesser weight loss [32]. Adult patients who are married also have better rates of success compared to single patients [33]. With studies like these and more, one could extrapolate that having a strong social and economic support system is imperative for success. However, MBS in an adolescent has the potential to significantly change the patient's trajectory from one of co-morbidities that alter quality of life early in adulthood to one of better health. The potential wellbeing of a child and future adult is in the best interest of the patient. As noted in the October 2019 AAP statement, despite socioeconomic status, race, or other factors, all pediatric patients should have access to MBS [18].

31.3.11 Contextual Features: Justice of Allocation of Resources

The decision to proceed with bariatric surgery for a patient exists in the context of a larger health care system with limited resources and a growing epidemic of obesity across the world. The principle of justice requires that each participant in a system receives an equal distribution of the benefits and burdens [4]. Regarding obesity, there exists an unequitable share of the burdens. There are significant health disparities, with higher rates of obesity in African American, Native American, and Hispanic adolescents. Disproportionately, these populations undergo a lower rate of MBS in their adults [2]. Pediatric obesity disproportionally affects the socially disadvantaged as well [34]. Pediatric obesity is more likely to represent a failure of the social structure, rather than the failure of an individual.

MBS surgery centers have a moral imperative to offer bariatric services to all individuals, regardless of their financial resources [18]. Pediatric hospitals and MBS centers must value distributive justice and work tiresomely to ensure distributive justice to all patients [5]. This extends to every aspect of the MBS program: preoperative weight loss programs, post-operative care and access to post-operative nutrition and medicines.

Case Conclusion

Ms. JY undergoes evaluation by a multi-disciplinary team. After thorough discussions with the surgeon, dietician, physiologist, and previous patients, JY feels like she understands what her life will entail should she proceed with surgery. She understands the risks of surgery and well as the risks of her current obesity should she not undergo surgery. The committee decides that she meets criteria for MBS and surgery is offered. She ultimately gives her assent. In preparation for surgery, her parents meet with a financial counselor and discuss options. The hospital has offered her parents help with both the costs of surgery and with prescriptions following.

31.4 Conclusion

There are several ethical issues in pediatric bariatric surgery to consider. The patient's benefit-risk ratio must be optimized. Ultimately more research is needed to further elicit the long-term consequences of MBS on adolescent patients. As it now stands, delaying bariatric surgery could provide more harm to a child compared to the risk of an operation. Patient preferences are of utmost concern and a multi-disciplinary approach is needed. Assent must be obtained from an adolescent, and surrogate decision maker must act in the best interest of the patient. Populations, such as syndromic obesity, exist that warrant careful consideration regarding surgery. Patients, family members, and healthcare providers need to recognize their own biases towards obesity and preferences of quality of life. Difficult psychosocial situations must be optimized prior to surgery but are not barriers that should prevent surgery. Lastly, MBS centers have a moral imperative to provide just allocation of resources to patients, regardless of financial or insurance status.

31.5 Selected References

- Pratt JSA, Browne A, Browne NT, et al. ASMBS pediatric metabolic and bariatric surgery guidelines, 2018. Surg Obes Relat Dis. 2018;14(7):882–901. https://doi.org/10.1016/j.soard.2018.03.019.

    - The ASMBS peformed a comprehensive literature search regarding pediatric bariatric surgery and updated their evidence-based guidelines in 2018. This reviews obesity related co-morbidities, including risks and outcomes following MBS, decision making and patient selection, and treatment options. It serves as the current standard of care regarding MBS in pediatric patients.

- Caniano DA. Ethical issues in pediatric bariatric surgery. Semin Pediatr Surg. 2009;18(3):186–92. https://doi.org/10.1053/j.sempedsurg.2009.04.009.

    - A concise review of current ethical issues in pediatric bariatric surgery. Addressed are the necessity of a favorable benefit/risk profile, extensive preoperative counseling to obtain informed consent and justice regarding allocation of resources. Importantly, the author addresses the need to conduct clinical research given that pediatric bariatric surgery is an innovative treatment. Although written prior to much of the literature surrounding pediatric MBS and its outcomes, it serves as the ethical framework upon which to develop the arguments presented in this chapter.

References

1. Skinner AC, Ravanbakht SN, Skelton JA, Perrin EM, Armstrong SC. Prevalence of obesity and severe obesity in US children, 1999–2016. Pediatrics. 2018;141(3):e20173459. https://doi.org/10.1542/peds.2017-3759.
2. Pratt JSA, Browne A, Browne NT, et al. ASMBS pediatric metabolic and bariatric surgery guidelines, 2018. Surg Obes Relat Dis. 2018;14(7):882–901. https://doi.org/10.1016/j.soard.2018.03.019.
3. Levine MD, Ringham RM, Kalarchian MA, Wisniewski L, Marcus MD. Is family-based behavioral weight control appropriate for severe pediatric obesity? Int J Eat Disord. 2001;30(3):318–28. https://doi.org/10.1002/eat.1091.
4. Jonsen AR, Siegler M, Winslade WJ. Clinical ethics: A practical approach to ethical decisions in clinical medicine. 8th ed. McGraw-Hill Education; 2015.
5. Caniano DA. Ethical issues in pediatric bariatric surgery. Semin Pediatr Surg. 2009;18(3):186–92. https://doi.org/10.1053/j.sempedsurg.2009.04.009.
6. Danielsson P, Kowalski J, Ekblom O, Marcus C. Response of severely obese children and adolescents to behavioral treatment. Arch Pediatr Adolesc Med. 2012;166(12):1103–8. https://doi.org/10.1001/2013.jamapediatrics.319.
7. Altman M, Wilfley DE. Evidence update on the treatment of overweight and obesity in children and adolescents. J Clin Child Adolesc Psychol. 2015;44(4):521–37. https://doi.org/10.1080/15374416.2014.963854.

8. Kalarchian MA, Levine MD, Arslanian SA, et al. Family-based treatment of severe pediatric obesity: randomized, controlled trial. Pediatrics. 2009;124(4):1060–8. https://doi.org/10.1542/peds.2008-3727.

9. Kumar S, Kelly AS. Review of childhood obesity: from epidemiology, etiology, and comorbidities to clinical assessment and treatment. Mayo Clin Proc. 2017;92(2):251–65. https://doi.org/10.1016/j.mayocp.2016.09.017.

10. Wang Y, Cai L, Wu Y, et al. What childhood obesity prevention programs work? A systematic review and meta-analysis. Obes Rev. 2015;16(7):547–65. https://doi.org/10.1111/obr.12277.

11. Coles N, Birken C, Hamilton J. Emerging treatments for severe obesity in children and adolescents. BMJ. 2016;354:i4116. https://doi.org/10.1136/bmj.i4116.

12. Ruiz-Cota P, Bacardí-Gascón M, Jiménez-Cruz A. Long-term outcomes of metabolic and bariatric surgery in adolescents with severe obesity with a follow-up of at least 5 years: a systematic review. Surg Obes Relat Dis. 2019;15(1):133–44. https://doi.org/10.1016/j.soard.2018.10.016.

13. Inge TH, Courcoulas AP, Jenkins TM, et al. Five-year outcomes of gastric bypass in adolescents as compared with adults. N Engl J Med. 2019;380(22):2136–45. https://doi.org/10.1056/nejmoa1813909.

14. Inge TH, Zeller MH, Jenkins TM, et al. Perioperative outcomes of adolescents undergoing bariatric surgery: the Teen-Longitudinal Assessment of Bariatric Surgery (Teen-LABS) study. JAMA Pediatr. 2014;168(1):47–53. https://doi.org/10.1001/jamapediatrics.2013.4296.

15. Inge TH, Jenkins TM, Xanthakos SA, et al. Long-term outcomes of bariatric surgery in adolescents with severe obesity (FABS-5+): a prospective follow-up analysis. Lancet Diabetes Endocrinol. 2017;5(3):165–73. https://doi.org/10.1016/s2213-8587(16)30315-1.

16. Johansson K, Cnattingius S, Näslund I, et al. Outcomes of pregnancy after bariatric surgery. N Engl J Med. 2015;372(9):814–24. https://doi.org/10.1056/nejmoa1405789.

17. Zeller MH, Brown JL, Reiter-Purtill J, et al. Sexual behaviors, risks, and sexual health outcomes for adolescent females following bariatric surgery. Surg Obes Relat Dis. 2019;15(6):969–78. https://doi.org/10.1016/j.soard.2019.03.001.

18. Armstrong SC, Bolling CF, Michalsky MP, et al. AAP Section on Obesity, Section on Surgery. Pediatric metabolic and bariatric surgery: evidence, barriers, and best practices. Pediatrics. 2019;144(6):e20193223. https://doi.org/10.1542/peds.2019-3223.

19. Bolling CF, Armstrong SC, Reichard KW, et al. AAP Section on Obesity, Section on Surgery. Metabolic and bariatric surgery for pediatric patients with severe obesity. Pediatrics. 2019;144(6):e20193224. https://doi.org/10.1542/peds.2019-3224.

20. Olbers T, Beamish AJ, Gronowitz E, et al. Laparoscopic Roux-en-Y gastric bypass in adolescents with severe obesity (AMOS): a prospective, 5-year, Swedish nationwide study. Lancet Diabetes Endocrinol. 2017;5(3):174–83. https://doi.org/10.1016/s2213-8587(16)30424-7.

21. Alqahtani A, Elahmedi M, Qahtani AR. Laparoscopic sleeve gastrectomy in children younger than 14 years: refuting the concerns. Ann Surg. 2016;263(2):312–9. https://doi.org/10.1097/sla.0000000000001278.

22. Katz AL, Webb SA, AAP Committee on Bioethics. Informed consent in decision-making in pediatric practice. Pediatrics. 2016;138(2):e20161485. https://doi.org/10.1542/peds.2016-1485.

23. Murphy TF. Adolescents and body modification for gender identity expression. Med Law Rev. 2019;27(4):623–39. https://doi.org/10.1093/medlaw/fwz006.

24. Kimberly LL, Folkers KM, Friesen P, et al. Ethical issues in gender-affirming care for youth. Pediatrics. 2018;142(6):e20181537. https://doi.org/10.1542/peds.2018-1537.

25. Gillam LH, Hewitt JK, Warne GL. Ethical principles for the management of infants with disorders of sex development. Horm Res Paediatr. 2010;74(6):412–8. https://doi.org/10.1159/000316940.

26. Chung WK. An overview of monogenic and syndromic obesities in humans. Pediatr Blood Cancer. 2012;58(1):122–8. https://doi.org/10.1002/pbc.23372.

27. Matheson BE, Colborn D, Bohon C. Bariatric surgery in children and adolescents with cognitive impairment and/or developmental delay: current knowledge and clinical recommendations. Obes Surg. 2019;29(12):4114–26. https://doi.org/10.1007/s11695-019-04219-2.
28. Sprangers MAG, Aaronson NK. The role of health care providers and significant others in evaluating the quality of life of patients with chronic disease: a review. J Clin Epidemiol. 1992;45(7):743–60. https://doi.org/10.1016/0895-4356(92)90052-O.
29. Ogden J, Flanagan Z. Beliefs about the causes and solutions to obesity: a comparison of GPs and lay people. Patient Educ Couns. 2008;71(1):72–8. https://doi.org/10.1016/j.pec.2007.11.022.
30. Saarni SI, Anttila H, Saarni SE, et al. Ethical issues of obesity surgery – a health technology assessment. Obes Surg. 2011;21(9):1469–76. https://doi.org/10.1007/s11695-011-0386-1.
31. Lent MR, Bailey-Davis L, Irving BA, et al. Bariatric surgery patients and their families: health, physical activity, and social support. Obes Surg. 2016;26(12):2981–8. https://doi.org/10.1007/s11695-016-2228-7.
32. Akkary E, Nerlinger A, Yu S, Dziura J, Duffy AJ, Bell RL. Socioeconomic predictors of weight loss after laparoscopic Roux-Y gastric bypass. Surg Endosc. 2009;23(6):1246–51. https://doi.org/10.1007/s00464-008-0138-z.
33. Carden A, Blum K, Arbaugh CJ, Trickey A, Eisenberg D. Low socioeconomic status is associated with lower weight-loss outcomes 10-years after Roux-en-Y gastric bypass. Surg Endosc. 2019;33(2):454–9. https://doi.org/10.1007/s00464-018-6318-6.
34. Blacksher E. Children's health inequalities: ethical and political challenges to seeking social justice. Hastings Cent Rep. 2008;38(4):28–35. PMID: 25165348

Chapter 32
Death by Neurologic Criteria in Neonatal and Pediatric Intensive Care Units

Robert M. MacGregor ⓘ **and Baddr A. Shakhsheer**

Abstract The diagnosis of death by neurologic criteria, sometimes referred to as "brain death," in pediatric patients is made when there is the absence of neurologic function with a known irreversible cause of coma. The process of declaring death by neurologic criteria in pediatric patients is complex and requires a multidisciplinary approach between members of the clinical team and family members. Navigating numerous factors that contribute to the diagnosis of death by neurologic criteria, including the parent's role in decision making, diverse cultural and ethnic family practices, variability in the diagnosis between societies and institutions, and unique ethical challenges ensures the medical team can effectively provide the guidance and support needed during this difficult process. More training is required for pediatric facilities and providers to effectively provide the care necessary during difficult end-of-life decisions.

Keywords Death by neurologic criteria · Brain death · Pediatric intensive care Coma · Organ donation · Donation after cardiac death · Guidelines

R. M. MacGregor
Department of Surgery, Washington University School of Medicine, Barnes Jewish Hospital, St. Louis, MO, USA
e-mail: m.macgregor@wustl.edu

B. A. Shakhsheer (✉)
Division of Pediatric Surgery, Department of Surgery, Washington University School of Medicine, St. Louis, MO, USA
e-mail: baddr@wustl.edu

© The Author(s), under exclusive license to Springer Nature Switzerland AG 2022
V. A. Lonchyna et al. (eds.), *Difficult Decisions in Surgical Ethics*, Difficult Decisions in Surgery: An Evidence-Based Approach,
https://doi.org/10.1007/978-3-030-84625-1_32

Case

An eight-year-old female presented to the hospital after being hit by a car. On arrival, her Glasgow Coma Scale (GCS) score was 3 and mechanical ventilation was instituted. She was found with numerous intra-abdominal solid organ injuries, all managed non-operatively, as well as a devastating traumatic brain injury. After resuscitation and correction of her metabolic disturbances in the pediatric ICU, the patient remained unresponsive with absent gag, cough, corneal, oculocephalic, and oculovestibular reflexes. Acknowledging the patient's poor neurologic status in the setting of a severe neurologic injury, the trauma surgery team consulted the pediatric ICU (PICU) team regarding the timing of death by neurologic criteria examination and testing. The PICU attending communicated to the trauma team that she does not believe in the diagnosis of "brain death" and therefore would not initiate further examination and testing. The child remained on ventilatory support for three more days, during which the PICU and trauma teams attempted to communicate to the grieving family the severity of the child's injuries and poor prognosis. The family expressed frustration and sadness regarding their child's poor clinical status without signs of improvement or changes in the medical treatment plan.

32.1 Introduction

Determination of death by neurologic criteria in pediatric patients is not an infrequent process in neonatal and pediatric intensive care units (ICU). Also known as brain death, death by neurologic criteria is declared after physical examination and neurologic testing determine there is an absence of neurologic function in the setting of a known irreversible cause of coma. Though difficult, it is important for health care providers to understand and guide the patient's family and care team through the process of death by neurologic criteria determination. This process is inherently complex, which is reflected by the fact there are no universally accepted guidelines for making this determination.

The improvement in resuscitation and transplant technology has facilitated the expansion of historical "cardiorespiratory criteria" of death to also include neurologic criteria. Knowing the definitions and prerequisite conditions that pediatric patients must meet prior to determination of death by neurologic criteria is important for pediatric surgeons for several reasons. First, the declaration of death by neurologic criteria is common in intensive care units, as a study of five U.S. teaching hospitals found 16% of all deaths in the PICU were attributed to death by neurologic criteria [1]. Second, the fair allocation of extensive resources required to maintain cardiorespiratory function in the setting of severe neurological injury should be considered and appropriately administered to patients with potential for

Table 32.1 Principles of medical ethics as applied to declaration of death

Autonomy	Patient families and clinicians play a significant role in ensuring that medical decisions made in the determination of death by neurologic criteria are in the patient's best interest.
Beneficence	Short-term extension of care following declaration of death by neurologic criteria may support grieving families or facilitate cultural/religious needs.
Non-maleficence	Principle of non-maleficence may limit the practice of donation after cardiac death, especially in pediatric patients.
Justice	Efficient diagnosis of death by neurologic criteria contributes to rationing critical hospital resources to those who will benefit the most.

recovery. Third, patients who have been declared dead by neurologic criteria may provide the gift of organ donation, especially given the chronic shortage of transplantable organs. Finally, prolonging the process of death by neurologic criteria determination adds stress to the families of patients in the ICU [2].

This chapter details a brief history of the determination of death by neurologic criteria, outlines specific guidelines and criteria for "brain death" in pediatric patients, and explores the ethical dimensions that this entity brings about in clinical settings (see Table 32.1).

32.2 Search Strategy

A literature search of English language publications was performed to identify cases and studies of death by neurologic criteria in neonatal and pediatric patients. The following databases were searched: PubMed, Embase, and Cochrane Evidence Based Medicine. The search terms used were the following: ["death by neurologic criteria" OR "brain death" OR "coma" OR "donation after cardiac death"] AND ["pediatric ICU" OR "neonatal ICU" OR "pediatric"].

32.3 History of the Determination of Death by Neurologic Criteria

The concept of death by neurologic criteria first emerged in 1959 after French neurophysiologists Mollaret and Goulon recognized a state beyond coma characterized by loss of consciousness, motor activity, sensation, and vegetative functions [3]. In the subsequent decade, it became more feasible to maintain respiratory function in patients without brainstem function with the advent of a mechanical ventilator. In 1968, the *Report of the Ad Hoc Committee of the Harvard Medical School to Examine the Definition of Brain Death* was published in JAMA and was the first definition of death using neurologic criteria [3]. It described certain clinical findings of a patient with a neurologically devastated brain to include absent corneal/pupillary reflexes, no movements or breathing, and no response to external stimuli.

Since then, numerous expert groups have published guidelines for the declaration of death by neurologic criteria and/or brain death, though it is important to note there are no universally accepted guidelines at this time. One of the first in the United States was the drafting of the Uniform Determination of Death Act in 1981 by the National Conference of Commissioners on Uniform State Laws and the American Medical and Bar Associations, which provided legal support for neurological determination of death [4]. The Act stated individuals who sustained irreversible cessation of circulatory and respiratory function or irreversible cessation of all functions of the entire brain (including brainstem) were dead. However, these guidelines were only applied to children older than five years-old due to perceived increased resilience and improved recovery of a child's brain after injury compared to adults.

Years later the American Academy of Pediatrics (AAP) published guidelines to assist physicians in diagnosing death by neurologic criteria in infants and children. These guidelines were subsequently updated and supported in 2011 by multiple societies, including the Child Neurology Society and Society of Critical Care Medicine [5]. The updates to the initial guidelines included details regarding the initial waiting period before first conducting the examination of death by neurologic criteria; the number of apnea tests; the number of examinations and inter-examination intervals; and the use of ancillary tests. To date, these guidelines are the most widely accepted throughout the pediatric medical community.

32.4   Determination of Death by Neurologic Criteria in Pediatrics

32.4.1   Epidemiology

The incidence of death by neurologic criteria in children has been relatively stable over the past few decades and its prevalence is approximately 15–20% of deaths in large academic US pediatric ICUs, as shown in a prospective case series including five geographically diverse, U.S. teaching hospitals [1]. As expected, the patients in the study were young and healthy prior to a new-onset illness or injury and the predominant mode of death was withholding or withdrawal of life-sustaining therapies. A more recent retrospective multicenter study found 21% of patient deaths in pediatric ICUs were declared dead by neurologic criteria, with 44% of patients between the ages of 2 and 12 years [6]. The most common causative mechanisms of death by neurologic criteria included hypoxic-ischemic injury (53%), traumatic brain injury, (20%), and shock and/or respiratory arrest without cardiac arrest (13%).

32.4.2   Prerequisites for Death by Neurologic Criteria Declaration

Prior to initiating a death by neurologic criteria evaluation, clinicians should perform a careful history, physical examination, and initial diagnostic studies to rule out reversible causes of coma in a child or infant. Per guidelines, the patient must have sustained a neurological injury capable of causing neurological death. Conditions that may mimic death by neurologic criteria must be treated, which include hypotension, hypothermia, and electrolyte and metabolic disturbances. Patients who are found hypothermic should be rewarmed to at least 35 °C and observed for a period of time prior to neurologic examination [5]. Analgesic and sedation medications should be discontinued prior to examination for death by neurologic criteria and use of a nerve stimulator can determine the necessity of neuromuscular blockade clearance. Examinations should also be delayed following cardiopulmonary resuscitation or severe acute brain injury for at least 24–48 hours or longer if there is variability in exams [5].

32.4.3   Clinical Exam

The clinical exam is used to elucidate brain and brainstem function. The first clinical exam in the determination of death by neurologic criteria may occur once the cause of the coma is identified, confounding factors have been corrected and the patient's condition is deemed irreversible. Two examinations must be performed by two separate physicians. The first examination establishes that the patient has met criteria for death by neurologic criteria and the second confirms the diagnosis. Each examination must include an apnea test. The examinations must be separated by an observation period of at least 12 hours for infants greater than 30 days old to children 18 years of age [5].

Neurologic examination includes testing of high neurologic function, presence of brain stem reflexes, and cranial nerve function. Complete loss of consciousness (GCS score of 3) is found when the patient is unresponsive to all stimulation mediated above the spinal cord, no spontaneous eye movement, and no motor response to noxious stimuli. Importantly, clinicians should be informed and educate the patient's family regarding spinal reflexes that may be present despite a diagnosis of death by neurologic criteria. These include myoclonus, plantar response, triple flexion reflex, and undulating toe reflex. Cranial nerve function is assessed for the presence of brain stem reflexes including gag, cough, pupillary light, corneal, oculocephalic, and oculovestibular reflexes. The pupils in death by neurologic criteria should be 4 to 9 mm and non-reactive to light and no blinking or eye movement should be seen after lightly touching the cornea of each eye [5]. Suction devices can assess gag reflex by stimulating the posterior pharynx or the cough reflex by advancing a catheter down the endotracheal tube to the carina.

32.4.4   Apnea Test

Once a neurological examination has been performed and is consistent with death by neurologic criteria, an apnea test should subsequently be completed to confirm loss of spontaneous respirations and neurologic drive to breathe. The patient must be normothermic, normotensive, and not have any contraindications to apnea testing including a high cervical spine injury and severe hypoxemia due to acute lung injury. Apnea testing is started when the patient has normal $PaCO_2$ and pH on arterial blood gas sample. The patient is preoxygenated for approximately 5 minutes, after which the patient is disconnected from the ventilator or placed in a mode without mechanical intermittent mandatory ventilation. During the 8 to 10-minute exam, the patient's chest and abdomen should be directly observed and heart rate, blood pressure, and oxygenation levels should be monitored. If no movement is witnessed, a second arterial blood gas is obtained. Death by neurologic criteria is diagnosed if the $PaCO_2$ rises 20 mmHg above baseline and is greater than 60 mmHg without any respiratory effort during the course of the apnea test [5]. If the patient becomes hemodynamically unstable or the oxygen saturations fall below 85%, the apnea test must be terminated.

32.4.5   Ancillary Testing

Ancillary testing is not required to make a diagnosis of death by neurologic criteria and is never a substitute for the neurological exam. Examples of ancillary testing include electroencephalogram (EEG), radionucleotide cerebral blood flow (CBF), and four-vessel cerebral angiography. These modalities are used in instances when the neurological exam or apnea test cannot be completed safely due to the patients underlying medical condition or if there is uncertainty with the validity of the testing [5]. Death by neurologic criteria cannot be declared if the ancillary study is equivocal or there is concern regarding the validity of the study. Children should be observed for at least 12 hours prior to repeat neurological exam and apnea testing or an additional ancillary study.

32.4.6   Determination of Death by Neurologic Criteria
in the Neonatal ICU

Determination of death by neurologic criteria in neonates is complex. The accepted medical standards for diagnosis of death by neurologic criteria for adults and children are not always applicable to neonatal patients. In fact, preterm and term neonates younger than 7 days of life were excluded from the 1987 Task Force Guidelines. The incidence of death by neurologic criteria in newborns remains largely unknown, though prior reports estimate approximately 3% of total newborn deaths are due to death by neurologic criteria [7]. The most common cause of death by neurologic criteria in neonates is due to hypoxic ischemic encephalopathy. Other causes in this age group include intracranial hemorrhage due to trauma, congenital malformation, central nervous system vascular injury, meningitis, sudden infant death syndrome, and meningitis [7]. The diagnosis of death by neurologic criteria cannot be made in preterm infants less than 37 weeks gestational age.

The neurological examination in neonates may be difficult due to the fact some brain stem reflexes may not be completely developed. The oculocephalic, oculovestibular, and gag reflexes are usually reliable. Other reflexes may not be as reliable in a compromised infant on ventilatory support and in infants with ancephaly due to physical abnormalities (including ocular and otic congenital defects). Apnea testing is the most critical test in the determination of death by neurologic criteria in the neonate, and can be performed in all infants greater than 32 weeks gestational age. Of note, ancillary tests such as EEG and cerebral blood flow measurements are not reliable in newborns because of the open fontanel and lack of increase in intracranial pressures as seen in adults.

There is a paucity of literature published regarding the diagnosis of death by neurologic criteria in the neonate. This can be attributed to the difficulty in obtaining a reliable neurological exam combined with lack of utility of certain ancillary studies in this patient population. Diagnosing death by neurologic criteria in neonates requires repeated neurological examinations in conjunction with apnea testing and an observational period of 24 hours between exams [5]. Though the 2011 AAP updates provided a framework for the diagnosis of death by neurologic criteria in neonates, it remains a challenge due to inherent clinical complexities as well as social, religious, and ethical factors.

32.4.7 Parental Role in Decision Making

The American Academy of Neurology argues that physicians have the "moral authority and professional responsibility" to perform evaluations to determine whether a patient is brain dead even if the family does not consent [8]. In fact, most pediatric neurologists and intensivists do not feel consent is necessary before testing for death by neurologic criteria, though laws vary from state to state. Further, disagreement exists between experts regarding how to proceed when parents refuse to allow testing to confirm death by neurologic criteria. This is important as parents have no legal right to demand therapies after a patient is declared dead. However, until the patient undergoes a formal death by neurologic criteria examination, they remain legally alive and the parents as legal guardians are allowed to make medical decisions [8].

Obtaining legal consent is based on the ethical principle of respect for persons, though in situations such as emergent care, consent may be assumed due to the principle of beneficence [9]. In this emergency setting, it is also reasonable to argue testing for death by neurologic criteria is premature and not in the patient's best interest. Therefore the ethical justification for overruling the parent's refusal for determination of death by neurologic criteria is unclear. Those who support that parental consent is unnecessary claim continued mechanical support for futile clinical status is inappropriate; providing appropriate medical care requires an accurate diagnosis; and limited intensive care resources should be allocated fairly. Those who oppose believe physicians should respect the parent's refusal and attempt to understand the reasoning for refusal instead of unilaterally performing testing for the determination of death by neurologic criteria [9].

The concept of brain death as death by neurologic criteria can be difficult to fully comprehend for both medical professionals and patient families [10]. Interestingly, in a survey of accredited pediatric training programs across the U.S., only 36% of residents and 39% of faculty members correctly defined the concept of brain death [11]. It should be no surprise that as the family works to accept the death of their child, understanding death by neurologic criteria may be particularly difficult. Modern medical technology can maintain vital signs that may insinuate a more optimistic picture than the true critical clinical condition. Further, it may prevent families from being able to shift their focus to making end-of-life decisions (i.e. organ donation, autopsy). A recent randomized-controlled study examined the impact of family presence during evaluation of adult patients for determination of death by neurologic criteria and found the family had an understanding of death by neurologic criteria without adversely impacting their psychological [12]. There are no such studies in pediatric patients and their families as of yet.

32.4.8   Societal Differences in Determination of Death by Neurologic Criteria

The complexity of the process in determining death by neurologic criteria is reflected in the fact that there are no universally accepted guidelines for making this determination. Cultural, religious, societal, and spiritual differences in patients and their families across the world make it challenging to provide a universal framework to define and accept death by neurologic criteria. Further, medical societies from countries around the world do not always agree on the criteria used to determine death by neurologic criteria.

The first successful organ transplantation performed in Japan was in 1999, years after an unfortunate outcome with the first heart transplant surgery in 1968 that resulted in decades of distrust with the medical community. As a consequence, a social consensus in Japan as to whether death by neurologic criteria should be accepted as a determination of death has yet to be reached. The Takeuchi criteria, were published in 2000, and provided the first framework for medically declaring death by neurologic criteria in children in Japan, but excluded infants under 12 weeks of age [13]. This was updated in 2009 and included guidelines such as

24-hour observation period between examinations in patients less than 6 years of age, use of magnetic resonance imaging to establish "definitive diagnosis of underlying disease," mandatory use of EEG to show isoelectric activity, and exclusion of abused children from organ donation. [13] The lack of acceptance of death by neurologic criteria determination by citizens of Japan has been attributed in part due to the overall perception that a death by neurologic criteria diagnosis is only performed for the purposes for organ donation, not what is best for the patient and family [13].

The 2006 recommendations from a Canadian forum outlined more specific guidelines for the determination of death by neurologic criteria in children [14]. Based on their guidelines, full-term newborns between 48 hours of life and less than 30 days old must have serial neurologic examinations separated by 24 hours, and include absent oculocephalic and suck reflexes. For infants and children 30 days and older, there are no specific regulations for interval duration between examinations. Ancillary tests are required if clinicians are unable to establish clinical criteria or if there is presence of confounders.

In addition to societal differences in the diagnosis of death by neurologic criteria around the world, faith-based differences also exist. The family's decision and eventual acceptance of examinations to determine death by neurologic criteria may be based on personal beliefs or interpretation of religious scripture, both which should be viewed as valid [10]. Open communication should be continued between the medical team and family to ensure the proper members of their religious community are available to assist in the discussion, should they so choose. For instance, members of the Jewish and Muslim faith typically inter the body within 24 hours of death. Those practicing Hinduism believe in reincarnation and the proper treatment of the body after demise [10]. For these reasons, it is important to ensure a family's faith traditions are considered to keep an effective relationship with family members.

32.4.9   Donation After Cardiac Death in Pediatrics

The availability of organs from brain-dead donors has not met the demand of patients across the U.S. who are in need of organ transplants. This has led to a resurgence of interest in the use of donation after cardiac death (DCD), with some success in increasing the number of organs available for donation. Numerous societies, including the Society of Critical Care Medicine, American Medical Association, and Institute of Medicine have all evaluated and supported DCD and the ethical treatment of patients at the end of life [15]. However, the implementation of DCD policies in children's hospitals have lagged behind those in adult hospitals. Initiating DCD policy requires collaboration between an organ procurement organization, physician liaison, and the hospital ethics committee.

Donation after cardiac death typically occurs in a patient with catastrophic brain injury who has not worsened to death by neurologic criteria. It is only after the family has made a decision to withdraw support that physicians may discuss the option of DCD. Donation after cardiac death is usually considered in instances where the patient's death is expected to occur rapidly, usually within one hour of withdrawal of support. It can be difficult to predict which patients will die within this hour. It is important to consider the emotional impact that it would have on the family to undergo a failed attempt at DCD. This may occur if the patient does not proceed to cardiac death within the defined period, which renders the organs not amenable to transplantation secondary to prolonged hypoxemia/ischemia. In addition, clear expectations must be communicated to the family, as the patient must be moved to be prepared for organ recovery within five to ten minutes of cardiac death [15]. This often causes further burden as the family is not allowed extensive time to grieve with their child at the time of death. Monitoring after terminal extubation should occur for 5 minutes to minimize the risk of autoresuscitation in younger and healthier children, after which organ recovery begins [15].

The total reported experience of DCD from children's hospitals remains sparse. Given the need for transplanted organs and the desire of some families to be able to provide the gift of organ donation, pediatric centers should continue to carefully explore donation after cardiac death. Pediatric providers may need greater familiarity with the concepts surrounding DCD in order to implement policies appropriately. **Most importantly, the care of the patient and his or her family should remain the focus during this donation process**.

32.4.10   *"Accepting" Death by Neurologic Criteria*

The diagnosis of death by neurologic criteria is a challenging process for both the patient family and medical team and can be filled with emotion, fear, frustration, and conflict. This stems from the compassion felt for the patient and the unfortunate reality of the clinical situation. Difficulty in accepting death by neurologic criteria is normal. Parents may wish to delay death by neurologic criteria testing in a desire to have more time with their child. In addition, cultural, religious, or spiritual beliefs provide optimism and hope the child will recover [16]. Family members see a beating heart and chest wall rising and falling with the ventilator and have difficulty accepting the death of their child. Frustration and conflict may ensue due to mistrust or a breakdown in communication with the clinical team regarding the child's prognosis. This often manifests through feelings that the medical team is "giving up" on the child [16].

Physicians have an obligation to help families navigate the complex process of determining and accepting death by neurologic criteria. Some techniques that may be useful are offering a "finite-goal accommodation" to allow additional family and friends to visit or establishing a "time-limited trial" to monitor for signs of neurologic recovery [16]. These practices are a compromise and can help the medical team build compassion for the patient and family, while at the same time allowing the parents more time to recognize their child will not recover neurologic function. Throughout the process, consistent, clear, and considerate communication is vital across all members of the medical team. Setting well-defined expectations early in the hospital course regarding neurologic recovery and explaining differences between purposeful neurologic function and spinal reflexes are important. Allowing family presence during consistent clinical testing practices can help to improve understanding of the severity of injury [12]. Finally, the medical and legal acceptance by the medical community that irreversible loss of brain function is death provides more certainty for family members as they grieve the loss of a child who is beyond recovery [17]. Pediatric facilities and pediatric providers may need greater training in these concepts, as the familiarity with definitions and processes surrounding death by neurologic criteria may be less familiar.

The need for further training and standardization of this process is reflected in the fact that there remains variability in the actual practices used to define death by neurologic criteria in NICUs and PICUs across the country [18]. Critically ill children are cared for at a variety of hospital settings across the country, including adult hospitals, academic centers, and community or county hospitals, by a variety of specialists. In addition, declaring death on the basis of cessation of brain function is controversial, and the AAP guidelines previously established have not been updated to include the wide variety of testing modalities currently available. These factors contribute to the potential for variability and confusion in determining death in children through neurologic criteria [19].

A multidisciplinary approach to assist family and friend acceptance of death by neurologic criteria is useful. Consulting services such as bioethics and palliative care teams can provide additional support and expertise for the medical team. Families needing religious or spiritual guidance should receive support from both the hospital Chaplain and community spiritual leaders. Social workers may assist in providing access to support services, counseling, and coordination based on the needs of the family. Giving families appropriate time, continuity of relationships, and a multidisciplinary approach can increase trust and provide support during the grieving process.

32.5   Case Conclusion

A goal-of-care meeting was held after three days, during which the family decided to redirect care and not pursue further life-support measures. The patient passed away peacefully that evening.

32.6   Conclusion

The diagnosis of death by neurologic criteria requires a conscientious and empathetic approach from all members of the medical team. Physicians and other team members have an obligation to ensure open communication with family members as they face difficult end-of-life decisions and attempt to comprehend their child's illness. Considerations for the pediatric patient include clear and concise communication regarding findings of physical examination and apnea testing, inclusion of the family in each step of the process, and facilitation of discussion with parents prior to the final declaration of death by neurologic criteria. Consideration of differences in societal, cultural, and religious practices improve the relationship and trust a family holds with the pediatric medical team. Finally, keeping the needs of the pediatric patient and the family at the center of the process of declaring death by neurologic criteria helps to navigate its complex ethical and emotional challenges.

32.7 Selected References

- Greer DM, Shemie SD, Lewis A, et al. Determination of Brain Death / Death by Neurologic Criteria–The World Brain Death Project. JAMA. 2020;324(11):1078–1097. doi:https://doi.org/10.1001/jama.2020.11586

  - A large multidisciplinary, international panel formulates a consensus statement of recommendations on determination of brain death / death by neurologic criteria based on literature review and expert opinion.

- Kirschen MP, Francoeur C, Murphy M, et al. Epidemiology of Brain Death in Pediatric Intensive Care Units in the United States. JAMA Pediatr. 2019;173(5):469–476. doi:https://doi.org/10.1001/jamapediatrics.2019.0249

  - A study using a national multicenter database to determine the epidemiology and clinical characteristics of pediatric patients declared brain dead in the United States.

- Magnus D, Wilfond B, Caplan A. Accepting Brain Death. N Engl J Med. 2014;370(10):891–894. doi:https://doi.org/10.1056/NEJMp1400930

  - Experienced physician reflections on patient family and medical team "acceptance" of death by neurologic criteria.

References

1. Burns JP, Sellers DE, Meyer EC, Lewis-Newby M, Truog RD. Epidemiology of death in the PICU at five U.S. teaching hospitals. Crit Care Med. 2014;42(9):2101–8. https://doi.org/10.1097/CCM.0000000000000498.
2. McAdam JL, Puntillo K. Symptoms experienced by family members of patients in intensive care units. Am J Crit Care. 2009;18(3):200–9. https://doi.org/10.4037/ajcc2009252.
3. Report of the ad hoc Committee of the Harvard Medical School to examine the definition of brain death. JAMA. 1968;205:337–40. https://doi.org/10.1001/jama.1968.03140320031009.
4. President's Commission on Ethical Problems in Medicine and Biomedical and Behavioral Research. Defining death: a report on the medical, legal, and ethical issues in definition of death. Government Printing Office; 1981.

5. Nakagawa T, Ashwal S, Mathur M, Mysore M. Clinical report-guidelines for the determination of brain death in infants and children: an update of the 1987 task force recommendation. Pediatrics. 2011;128(3):e720–40. https://doi.org/10.1542/peds.2011-1511.
6. Kirschen MP, Francoeur C, Murphy M, et al. Epidemiology of brain death in Pediatric intensive care units in the United States. JAMA Pediatr. 2019;173(5):469–76. https://doi.org/10.1001/jamapediatrics.2019.0249.
7. Ashwal S. Brain death in the newborn. Clin Perinatol. 1997;24:859–82. https://doi.org/10.1016/S0095-5108(18)30154-4.
8. Russell JA, Epstein LG, Greer DM, Kirschen M, Rubin MA. Lewis a; for the brain death working group. Brain death, the determination of brain death, and member guidance for brain death accommodation requests: AAN position statement. Neurology. 2019;92(6):228–32. https://doi.org/10.1212/WNL.0000000000006750.
9. Lee BM, Trowbridge A, McEvoy M, Wightman A, Kraft SA, Clark JD. Can a parent refuse the brain death examination? Pediatrics. 2020;145(4):e20192340. https://doi.org/10.1542/peds.2019-2340.
10. Randhawa G. Death and organ donation: meeting the needs of multiethnic and multifaith populations. Br J Anaesth. 2012;108(1):i88–91. https://doi.org/10.1093/bja/aer385.
11. Harrison AM, Botkin JR. Can Pediatricians define and apply the concept of brain death? Pediatrics. 1999;103(6):e82. https://doi.org/10.1542/peds.103.6.e82.
12. Tawil I, Brown LH, Comfort D, et al. Family presence during brain death evaluation: a randomized controlled trial. Crit Care Med. 2014;42(4):934–42. https://doi.org/10.1097/CCM.0000000000000102.
13. Araki T, Yokota H, Fuse A. Brain death in Pediatric patients in Japan: diagnosis and unresolved issues. Neurol Med Chir (Tokyo). 2016;56(1):1–8. https://doi.org/10.2176/nmc.ra.2015-0231.
14. Shemie SD, Doig C, Dickens B, et al. Pediatric reference group and the neonatal Referencwe group. Severe brain injury to neurological determination of death: Canadian forum recommendations. CMAJ. 2016;174(6):S1–12. https://doi.org/10.1503/cmaj.045142.
15. Recommendations for nonheartbeating donation. A position paper by the ethics committee, American College of Critical Care Medicine, Society of Critical Care Medicine. Crit Care Med. 2001;29:1826–31. https://doi.org/10.1097/00003246-200109000-00029.
16. Greer DM, Shemie SD, Lewis A, et al. Determination of brain death / death by neurologic criteria – the world brain death project. JAMA. 2020;324(11):1078–97. https://doi.org/10.1001/jama.2020.11586.
17. Magnus D, Wilfond B, Caplan A. Accepting brain death. N Engl J Med. 2014;370(10):891–4. https://doi.org/10.1056/NEJMp1400930.
18. Mathur M, Petersen L, Stadtler M, et al. Variability in Pediatric brain death determination and documentation in Southern California. Pediatrics. 2008;121(5):988–93. https://doi.org/10.1542/peds.2007-1871.
19. Shemie SD, Pollack MM, Morioka M, Bonner S. Diagnosis of brain death in children. Lancet Neurol. 2007;6(1):87–92. https://doi.org/10.1016/S1474-4422(06)70680-9.

Chapter 33
Ethical Issues Raised by Fetal Interventions for Lethal Anomalies

Vijaya Vemulakonda and Margret Bock

Abstract The evaluation and treatment of prenatally diagnosed complex genitourinary anomalies continues to evolve. The availability of novel fetal interventions has allowed for increased survivability of previously "lethal" fetal anomalies. However, the lack of clear evidence on the longer-term efficacy of these interventions has led to controversy about who should be eligible for treatment and how these treatments should be evaluated. We present a case of an infant with prenatally diagnosed bilateral renal agenesis treated with fetal amnioinfusion. We provide a discussion of the ethical issues surrounding use of novel treatments outside of the research setting as well as the secondary effects of intervention on longer-term survival and care.

Keywords Fetal intervention · Lethal anomalies · Renal agenesis · Neonatal renal replacement therapy · Amnioinfusion

V. Vemulakonda (✉)
Pediatric Urology, University of Colorado School of Medicine, Aurora, CO, USA

Congenital Anomalies of the Kidney and Urinary Tract Program, Fetal Genitourinary Anomalies Working Group, Children's Hospital Colorado, Aurora, CO, USA
e-mail: Vijaya.vemulakonda@childrenscolorado.org

M. Bock
Congenital Anomalies of the Kidney and Urinary Tract Program, Fetal Genitourinary Anomalies Working Group, Children's Hospital Colorado, Aurora, CO, USA

Pediatric Nephrology, University of Colorado School of Medicine, Aurora, CO, USA
e-mail: Margret.bock@childrenscolorado.org

© The Author(s), under exclusive license to Springer Nature
Switzerland AG 2022
V. A. Lonchyna et al. (eds.), *Difficult Decisions in Surgical Ethics*, Difficult
Decisions in Surgery: An Evidence-Based Approach,
https://doi.org/10.1007/978-3-030-84625-1_33

Case

MOC is a 35-year-old G3 P0 female who presented during her singleton pregnancy at 21 weeks and 6 days gestation. Fetal imaging revealed normal fetal growth, but also anhydramnios, bilateral renal agenesis with absence of a urinary bladder, cardiac hypertrophy with a pericardial effusion, and a single umbilical artery. Multidisciplinary care meetings with maternal fetal medicine, neonatology, pediatric surgery, transplant surgery, pediatric nephrology, pediatric urology, social work and psychology were held with MOC and her partner. The confirmed diagnosis of bilateral renal agenesis (a lethal outcome for a fetus without experimental treatment) was presented and possibilities for intervention and non-intervention were described, including potential risks, benefits and uncertainties associated with treatments for both MOC and the fetus. Detailed discussion with MOC and her partner about the option of fetal treatment intervention (amnioinfusions to restore the absence of amniotic fluid, allowing pulmonary development) focused on the high risk for significant morbidity and mortality at each step of the way. Beginning at fetal intervention and continuing through the neonatal period, the anticipated requirements for pulmonary survival, infant and chronic dialysis, and eventual possible kidney transplant surgery and bladder reconstruction, were discussed in great detail. They decided to proceed with serial amnioinfusions, of which the first of 7 weekly infusions of normal saline was completed at 23 weeks and 2 days gestation. The family elected to proceed with peritoneal dialysis if pulmonary survival was achieved.

At 35 weeks' gestation a female infant weighing 1.90 kg was born via cesarean section. The child was intubated shortly after delivery due to hypoxemia and respiratory distress. An echocardiogram (ECHO) revealed pulmonary valve stenosis and moderate bilateral ventricular hypertrophy. A peritoneal dialysis catheter was placed on day-of-life (DOL) 2 and allowed to rest for 72 hours prior to initiation of low volume manual PD. During the next 14 days she returned twice to the operating room due to PD catheter exit site leaks and catheter malfunction. Due to continuous leaks despite rest and intervention, after consultation with the multi-disciplinary team, the family elected to proceed with placement of a central venous catheter on DOL 20 for continuous renal replacement therapy (CRRT). Within 12 hours of CRRT initiation (citrate anticoagulation) a large gastrointestinal bleed resulted in significant blood product resuscitation. Over the following nine days the CRRT circuit clotted and was restarted a total of six times, and the CVC was replaced twice. Cardiopulmonary arrest occurred on DOL 25 in the setting of massive blood loss from the catheter site, requiring chest compression, multiple doses of epinephrine, as well as multiple blood products. After 14 days of PD catheter rest and nine days of CRRT with aggressive nutritional rehabilitation, options were presented to the family of pursuing comfort care or re-initiating low volume PD. Manual PD was re-initiated at very low volumes with an immediate leak at the tunnel exit site. The infant remained on high ventilator settings and a follow-up echocardiogram on DOL 33 revealed a dysplastic severely stenosed pulmonary valve with a new subvalvular obstruction and severe RV hypertrophy. Without viable dialysis options, in the setting of new ECHO findings, the option of comfort care discussed with the family and agreed to on DOL 35. Two days later the family changed their mind and sought second opinions at multiple large pediatric centers. Transfer of care was approved by only one center and initiated on DOL 40.

33.1   Introduction

Evolution of sophisticated prenatal imaging and genetic screening has aided in diagnosis of complex fetal conditions, often times weeks to months before birth. In turn, progress in fetal and pediatric surgery have introduced potential for prenatal intervention, adding potential benefits as well as risks to fetal health. The possibility of invasive fetal therapy introduces complicated ethical issues including: (1) concerns around definitions of fetal autonomy in the decision making and consent process; (2) uncertainty of potential benefit to the fetus of planned intervention; (3) introduction of potential risk to the pregnant mother, without possibility of true personal benefit; and (4) definitions of surgical innovation (see Chap. 50) versus medical research in fetal procedures. Within the framework of core ethical principles (specifically including autonomy, beneficence, non-maleficence, and justice) we evaluate key related issues brought forward by fetal intervention for lethal anomalies (see Table 33.1).

33.2   Search Strategy

A search was conducted in PubMed using the following terms, singularly and in various combinations: renal anhydramnios, amnioinfusion, renal agenesis, fetal bladder outlet obstruction, neonatal dialysis, neonatal renal replacement therapy, living donor advocate, ethics of neonatal dialysis, autonomy, periviability, maternal informed consent, fetal research, surgical innovation, moral distress. Research work was divided between the authors to capture as many relevant articles as possible.

Table 33.1 Ethical principles in intervention for lethal fetal anomalies

Core ethical principles	Application to intervention for lethal fetal anomalies
Autonomy	Maternal and fetal autonomy are closely linked but need to be addressed individually. As a patient, the mother's autonomy is well-defined. Fetal autonomy, however, is dependent on viability and ability to survive ex-vivo. While this typically occurs at about 24 weeks gestation, the definition and timing of viability is complicated in fetuses with lethal diagnoses, such as BRA.
Beneficence	Once a fetus with BRA is considered a patient, its life and well-being should be protected. Protecting fetal well-being in this case may well complicate the very same efforts directed toward the mother as a patient.
Non-maleficence	Any interventions considered or carried out on behalf of the fetus, must be weighed against potential harm to the mother. Potential for long-term harm to the fetus and infant/child from short-term benefits of fetal intervention (such as loss of dialysis access, non-eligibility for kidney transplantation) also need to be considered carefully.
Justice	Fetal intervention and its long-term sequalae are limited, costly healthcare resources for a very small population. Equity in access to these interventions, as well as financial effects on the patient, family, healthcare system and society long-term play into the ethical decision-making framework.

BRA = bilateral renal agenesis

33.3   Discussion

While there is no question of the mother's status as a patient with *autonomy* under this rubric, the ethical status of the fetus as a patient is less clear. Clinically, the fetus is considered a patient when making decisions about fetal intervention. However, this does not translate to consideration of the fetus as a person independent of the mother and consideration of the fetus in ethical decisions is dependent on the likelihood of the fetus becoming a child and a person [1, 2]. The fetus's moral status is dependent upon viability based on ability to survive ex vivo. Once viability is achieved, it is then considered a patient [2]. While in general, 24 weeks gestation is considered to be the threshold for viability, this may not hold true in the setting of bilateral renal agenesis, where lung development is often significantly impaired in the absence of intervention. As a result, viability and consideration of the fetus as a separate patient should be tailored to each individual case, with recognition of the mother's ability to withdraw the status of patient from her fetus prior to the establishment of viability. Once the fetus is considered a patient, the physician is required by the principle of *beneficence* to not only protect the life and well-being of the fetus but must also balance this within the framework of beneficence and *non-maleficence* to the mother. As a result, any potential benefit to the fetus must be weighed against the potential harm to the mother when considering the appropriateness of any fetal intervention. Additionally, short-term benefits to the fetus must also be weighed against the potential long-term benefits and harms, including consideration of the potential for neonatal survival without therapeutic options to sustain life beyond the neonatal period. Finally, *justice* in this setting must be considered on multiple levels: First, is the use of limited health care resources warranted when the beneficence of intervention is not well-established? Second, is the intervention available to all patients with the diagnosis of bilateral renal agenesis? And finally, is the potential benefit of intervention worth the long-term costs to the patient, the family, the health care system, and society?

33.4 Additional Ethical Considerations for Fetal Intervention in Cases of Bilateral Renal Agenesis

33.4.1 Uncertainty of Risks and Benefits of Intervention

There are only three reported cases of fetuses treated in utero with serial amnioinfusion that have survived to dialysis and kidney transplantation. The first case, reported in 2014, was initially diagnosed at 23 weeks with delivery at 28 weeks' gestation [3]. The second and third cases, reported from a single institution in 2019, underwent amnioinfusion from 24 to 28 weeks with delivery at 28 weeks, and from 26 to 32 weeks with delivery at 34 weeks, respectively [4]. All three cases survived to transplantation and suggest that bilateral renal agenesis may not be uniformly lethal. Data is lacking on the natural history of renal agenesis due to the inclusion of these cases with other underlying genetic anomalies in historical data and the lack of data on the prevalence of elective abortion in this setting [5]. Furthermore, there are no data on potential complications of amnioinfusion, limiting understanding of its risks to the fetus and mother prenatally. There are also no data on the risk of pulmonary, cardiovascular, dialysis complications, and those of prematurity in cases of amnioinfusion successfully leading to live birth [6]. Furthermore, data is lacking on developmental delay associated with early end stage renal disease, vascular implications of early hemodialysis, impact on family members, and long-term implications of early dialysis and transplantation on graft survival and overall prognosis in these patients. Current literature does not provide adequate data about the risks and benefits of fetal intervention to support offering serial amnioinfusion or other fetal intervention for bilateral renal agenesis as part of routine clinical practice.

33.4.2 Surgical Innovation Versus Medical Research

As surgical techniques continue to evolve in the field of fetal intervention, the line between surgical innovation and research has become less clear. Traditionally, the goal of surgical innovation is to offer a potential therapy to an individual patient whereas surgical research is intended to establish the effectiveness and generalizability of a new technique. (See Chaps. 49 and 50) For example, surgeons may tailor components of a well-established procedure such as surgical approach, instruments used, and incision size, for an individual patient without significantly deviating from the overall approach to surgical treatment [7]. However, in the setting of novel therapeutics, including fetal intervention, surgical innovation is often not based on previously accepted techniques and as a result, the efficacy of the treatment approach may not be well established [7]. Consequently, the treatment may be considered "experimental" even if the intent is to provide individual therapy.

This distinction between surgical innovation and research is an important one, as surgical research in a vulnerable population such as pregnant women has much stricter requirements for adequate informed consent than innovation [8]. Additionally, patients being offered novel techniques are at risk of therapeutic misconception or imputing clinical benefit to a therapy that is not yet proven [9]. Furthermore, the use of innovative procedures outside of the research setting may inhibit future formal research efforts [6]. Finally, surgeons should be transparent about their goals for treatment to ensure their obligation to the patient is fulfilled; in the setting of novel therapies, there is a greater risk for the surgeon to be motivated not only by the individual patient's wellbeing but also by the potential benefit to future patients offered by developing more effective techniques [7].

Due to these concerns about surgical innovation, we believe that the most ethical approach is to offer fetal interventions within a research setting, with clear delineation of the uncertainty of outcomes and clear standards to assess the effectiveness of a novel therapy. Chervenak and McCullough have offered an ethical framework to develop fetal interventions. In this framework, innovation is considered an initial step towards establishing the need for a controlled research study, with case reports or small case series identifying potential new therapies and providing the basis for hypothesis development. Prior to determining that the fetal intervention is ethically warranted in a research setting, Chervenak and McCullough outlined three questions to consider:

1. Based on prior animal studies or case series, is the proposed intervention expected to be lifesaving or prevent serious and irreversible harm to the fetus?
2. Compared to other potential study designs, is the intervention designed to involve the least risk for mortality and morbidity to the fetal patient?
3. Based on prior studies and theoretical risks for the current and future pregnancies, is the mortality risk and risk for injury or disability to the pregnant mother reliably expected to be low? [2, 9]

Clinical trials should also have clearly defined, predetermined endpoints to ensure adequate assessment of novel therapies prior to dissemination and implementation into clinical practice [7]. Use of this framework, which mirrors the IDEAL framework for the development and evaluation of surgical innovation [10, 11], offers an ethical approach to fetal intervention that respects the autonomy of the pregnant mother to make altruistic choices for her fetus. It also may identify gaps in current knowledge about the efficacy of these treatments.

33.4.3   Informed Consent

A comprehensive informed consent consists of four basic elements: (1) description of the clinical problem, the proposed treatment, and alternatives including no treatment; (2) discussion of risks and benefits of proposed treatment with comparisons to risks and benefits of alternatives and discussion of medical/clinical uncertainties regarding proposed treatment; (3) assessment of the patient's understanding of the information provided by the medical provider; and (4) solicitation of the patient's preference and consent for treatment [12]. (see Chap. 6) The extent of information provided is based on the physician's assessment of how it may impact diagnosis and treatment planning. Information should be provided in a way that is understandable to the average layperson and facilitates their meaningful participation in treatment planning.

To ensure adequate information for consent, patients must understand the "material risks" and expected benefits of treatment. However, there is no clear consensus on what constitutes a material risk. Patients often use short cuts to simplify the decision-making process, often leading to misunderstanding of the risks posed by a treatment [13]. Patients may also underestimate their own risks compared to other people [14]. These issues may be exacerbated in the setting of novel therapies, where patients may assume the treatment is more effective because it is new [9]. Additionally, knowledge about potential risks and benefits of the intervention are limited, with data about long term outcomes currently lacking [5]. As a result, counseling should be guided by "deliberative beneficence-based clinical judgment." [5].

An additional concern raised by the informed consent process in the setting of surgical intervention is that patients often idealize surgeons and accept surgical recommendations without meaningfully participating in the decision-making process [15]. As a result, the surgeon has a heightened responsibility to solicit patient feedback during the consent process. The physician must ensure that the patient understands the goals of intervention as research or innovation not as treatment. Germaine to the discussion is the general nature of the procedure to be performed and the expected outcomes; what to expect in the prenatal and neonatal periods; and the potential outcomes if the fetus survives to dialysis and transplant. Physicians should counsel families on current data about both the outcomes of observation (almost uniform neonatal mortality) and intervention (unknown despite rare case reports of successful survival to dialysis and transplant) [4, 5]. This discussion should include potential mortality risks in the prenatal and neonatal periods, as well as physical, developmental, psychosocial, and potential financial outcomes in cases of survival to neonatal dialysis and to transplantation, with acknowledgment of the uncertainty of outcomes given current data. Physicians should also provide counseling about maternal risks of fetal intervention, including preterm labor, infection, and potential risk to future pregnancies. Given the lack of generalizable data about the effectiveness of intervention, consent should be considered under the rubric of research with emphasis that the intervention is not yet proven to be clinically effective. As a result, words that infer efficacy ("treatment") or misattribute values to the treatment ("heroic" or "innovative") should be avoided [16]. Alternatives should also be discussed, including interruption of the pregnancy or comfort care if the mother declines enrollment in a research study. Finally, we recommend multidisciplinary counseling to aid in discussion with emphasis that intervention is an ongoing process and multiple decisions will need to be made after the initial decision for amnioinfusion or other fetal intervention.

33.5   Access to Care and Medical Justice: What Is Fair?

The principle of medical justice is founded on the idea that there is an element of fairness and equitable resource allocation with regard to medical decisions and treatments, including both resultant benefit and burden. Furthermore, in situations when services or resources are scarce, or treatments are novel and rare, a fair means of allocation should be determined. Decisions surrounding justice for fetuses with lethal anomalies undergoing intra-uterine interventions should be assessed beyond the fetal and immediate neonatal period. The ultimate goal resulting from this high risk innovative (often research-based) therapy is not just for immediate survival after delivery, but long-term well-being and quality of life. Given its complexity, fetal intervention may only be offered at a handful of large medical centers, each covering a vast geographic area. Offering fetal interventions within the confines of research allows those families without financial and medical reimbursement resources access to those pre-natal care options. This is one possibility for overcoming inequity of access to resources and safeguarding justice [16, 17]. Fetuses who have undergone intra-uterine intervention for lethal anomalies and survive as neonates will be closely enmeshed with a complicated, multidisciplinary medical team for weeks, months, years, and decades to follow. This is amplified, in particular, for families who live long distances from large fetal centers, often times requiring them to relocate to urban areas in order to best access care involved in fetal interventions, as well as potentially complicated long term ongoing care needs. Financial impact not only on families, but also on hospitals, healthcare systems and insurance providers must be taken into consideration, both short as well as long term. Surviving infants will chronically draw from medical systems that may already be strained.

In the case of children with adequate lung development born after amnioinfusion for renal agenesis, almost immediate initiation of neonatal dialysis is a necessary next step for a chance at survival. Infant and pediatric dialysis is known to represent a substantial burden for families and support systems and is even more pronounced in children of a very young age and those with comorbidities [18, 19]. Although limited to date, studies of the impact of pediatric dialysis on families show it is profound. They demonstrate that pediatric dialysis has the potential to disrupt family life and marriages [20, 21], results in more frequent academic setbacks in siblings and less time spent by parents with unaffected siblings. Parents may report experiencing a worse quality of life [22, 23] and that having a child with kidney disease requiring dialysis "is a pervasive and profoundly negative experience" [24]. Guidelines developed for decision making around initiation of renal replacement therapy in neonates and infants generally draw from multiple elements including presence of comorbidities; predictions for quality of life for the child and the family; availability of resources; and prognosis and potential for future organ transplantation [25]. Costs of neonatal and potential resultant lifetime renal replacement therapy are immense. Data from the International Pediatric Peritoneal Dialysis Network have demonstrated that the number of children under the age of three years taken on to renal replacement programs decreases significantly as the gross national income per capita falls [26]. The argument that cost should not be prohibitive in offering fetal therapy options to potential candidates is fair [17], however short-sighted. Downstream decisions, including short- and long-term decisions about renal replacement therapy interventions, are influenced by financial context.

Kidney transplantation is generally accepted as the best option for longer term renal replacement therapy, with dialysis to be used as a bridge to the ultimate goal. The decision to embark on amnioinfusion therapy prenatally to promote lung development in fetuses with renal agenesis, should be framed by the end-goal of renal transplantation and its impact on potentially amplifying the already unmatched supply and demand in potential donor organs versus recipients in need. Framed in the reality of scarce donor organ resources, the ethical considerations of proceeding with a fetal intervention that, in the *best*-case scenario, will result in drawing from a pool known to not have enough supply, is complex. A child listed on the deceased donor kidney transplant wait list, by nature of its age, is afforded a "pediatric advantage." This plays a part in donor allocation, resulting in shorter wait times for and younger organs allocated to children as compared to adults. Fairness in resource allocation pits a working middle-aged adult awaiting a deceased donor kidney against a fetus/neonate with a lethal anomaly who underwent a high-risk prenatal intervention and eventually listed as a pediatric recipient on the same deceased donor list. The role of justice is clearly complicated, and its equity is difficult to assess well.

33.6 Is There a Role for a Parent Advocate?

Decision making around surgical intervention for lethal fetal anomalies is complex. Based on existing models for solid organ living donor programs, we believe that an advocate for the expectant mother is necessary. An advocate could help identify possible stresses and disagreements related to benefits and risks to both the fetus and the mother as well as keep the focus on the best interests of the mother and fetus. The clinical/research team offering the potential innovative intervention to the expecting parent is committed to conveying accurate and detailed information in regards not only to the intervention, but also subsequent broader clinical, financial, psychological and social implications. It is impossible, however, for this team to be completely objective and thus conflict of interest is an obvious concern. Similarly, parents or families who have experienced surgical intervention for complex fetal diagnoses are also likely to be biased, given their potential direct, intense medical and psychosocial experiences. The concept of a designated "independent parent advocate" (IPA), is modeled after living donor liver programs (as need for surgical intervention here may mirror the urgency found in cases where prenatal intervention is being considered). In that setting, Organ Transplantation and Procurement Network policies have incorporated the requirement for "an independent donor advocate to ensure informed consent standards and ethical principles are applied to practice" should be developed [27, 28]. Similar to the case of living donor organ donation, pregnant mothers undergoing potential fetal intervention are a unique population—one that experiences no direct individual medical benefit. Thus, as successfully trialed in the solid organ living donor sphere, the role, job responsibilities and related boundaries of an IPA need to be carefully defined [29]. Ideally the IPA will provide an alliance to the pregnant mother, that is independent of needs of the fetus and provider team and understand enough of the fetal diagnosis and proposed intervention to be able to convey risks and benefits to both the pregnant mother and fetus. An individual who fits each of these criteria and possesses these crucial skill sets may be difficult to identify but is surely all the more important for this very unique circumstance.

33.7   Beyond Fetal Intervention: Recognizing and Addressing Conflict and Moral Distress of Providers and Parents

Moral distress is an emotional state of stress that arises when a healthcare provider feels a conflict between what he or she feels is ethically correct and what is possible to do within the constraints of the health care environment. It is increasingly recognized as an issue influencing the treatment of periviable neonates [30]. This may be especially true in cases where there is no standard of care and consequently uncertainty about the outcome of an intervention. In the setting of fetal intervention for bilateral renal agenesis, the outcome of early neonatal pulmonary support, dialysis, and other early interventions is unknown [16]. In our experience, providers may differ on what is appropriate to offer families or may disagree with decisions made by the family for ongoing care. Additionally, parental decisions may conflict with provider values and judgments, increasing moral distress for both the provider team and the family [31].

To address this uncertainty, some institutions have established guidelines for intervention to avoid futile care. However, how to define futile treatment is unclear [32, 33]. Is intervention futile if it has a 1% or 10% or 90% chance of survival? How do we gauge the risk of futility in the absence of data about outcomes? What if chances of success differ by institution [34]? One option to overcome the limitations of strict guidelines in this setting is to consider a prognosis-based gray zone, where the provider defers to parental judgment in cases where the outcome of intervention is not clear [33]. In our practice, we have utilized a hybrid approach. We start with general guidelines about when intervention, such as dialysis, has a reasonable chance of success as based on data from the neonatal dialysis experience in other conditions. We then make specific decisions about treatment with the parents on an individualized basis. We believe the use of general guidelines allows for transparency in our outcomes and helps to provide context to families making decisions in the setting of clinical uncertainty. We also maintain ongoing multidisciplinary team meetings with the family to reinforce the ongoing decision-making process surrounding any individual patient's care as well as the experimental nature of many of the interventions being considered. We believe that this approach allows for deference to parental values and judgment without creating an obligation on the medical team to provide treatment that we judge to be non-beneficial based on existing data. Finally, we recommend solicitation of second opinions from other centers with experience with fetal intervention and post-natal management in situations where the treatment team unanimously believe that further intervention will not be beneficial, recognizing that our ability to predict outcomes in these cases is limited by the lack of evidence to guide our decision-making and, as a result, our recommendations may be based on our own values and opinions rather than evidence-based judgment.

33.8 Case Resolution

The child underwent once-twice daily hemodialysis treatments for six months and was eventually transitioned to peritoneal dialysis. Access was obtained and rewired multiple times in both upper and lower extremities, as well as centrally. The patient was transferred to her home center at 9 months of age. She developed gradually worsening hydrocephalus due to superior vena cava syndrome. Venous drainage from the head occurred entirely via collateral vessels, requiring ballooning and stenting of vasculature every 2–3 months. She also had an absence of the inferior vena cava from the level of the liver to past the level of the bifurcation, with venous drainage occurring entirely via collaterals. Given these findings, the child was no longer a candidate for kidney transplantation. Second opinions were sought from multiple other pediatric transplant centers yielding similar responses. The child remains on peritoneal dialysis at 2 years of age.

33.9 Conclusion

The decision to proceed with surgical intervention for a lethal fetal anomaly is a very complex one and involves a thorough evaluation of the best interests of all parties involved, including the fetus, its family, the medical and psychosocial provider team, and society at large. A one-size-fits-all formula cannot be applied to any patient population. A nuanced, personalized approach to intervention and care needs to be a pillar for teams approaching these difficult clinical and ethical scenarios. Based on our experience and the literature, we advocate for a research-based approach to providing prenatal treatment in these cases to ensure adequate oversight of the intervention and its implications both in the prenatal period and in the longer term.

33.10   Selected References

- American Academy of Pediatrics Committee on Bioethics. Fetal therapy-ethical considerations. Pediatrics. 1999;103(5):1061–3. https://doi.org/10.1542/peds.103.5.1061.

  - Review by the American Academy of Pediatrics defining standards for discussions of fetal therapy with pregnant mothers.

- Bienstock JL, Birshner ML, Coleman F, Hueppchen NA. Successful in utero intervention for bilateral renal agenesis. Obstet Gynecol. 2014;124(2) (Part 2):413–5. https://doi.org/10.1097/aog.0000000000000339.

  - Case report of successful fetal intervention and transition to peritoneal dialysis for a patient with bilateral renal agenesis.

- Sugarman J, Anderson J, Baschat AA, et al. Ethical considerations concerning amnioinfusions for treating fetal bilateral renal agenesis. Obstet Gynecol. 2018;131(1):130–4. https://doi.org/10.1097/aog.0000000000002416.

  - Proposed ethical framework for fetal intervention in cases of bilateral renal agenesis.

- O'Hare EM, Jelin AC, Miller JL, et al. Amnioinfusions to treat early onset anhydramnios caused by renal anomalies: background and rationale for the renal anhydramnios fetal therapy trial. Fetal Diagn Ther. 2019;45:365–2. https://doi.org/10.1159/000497472.

  - Overview of the RAFT trial, a multi-center clinical trial to assess the efficacy of fetal intervention for bilateral renal agenesis or functional bilateral renal agenesis.

- Wilkinson D. Who should decide for critically ill neonates and how? The grey zone in neonatal treatment decisions. In: McDougall R, Delany C, Gillam L, editors. When doctors and parents disagree: ethics, paediatrics & the zone of parental discretion. The Federation Press; 2016.

  - Overview of the zone of parental discretion and the expansion of the grey zone of decision-making to cases of uncertain neonatal prognosis beyond gestational age alone.

References

1. American Academy of Pediatrics Committee on Bioethics. Fetal therapy-ethical considerations. Pediatrics. 1999;103(5):1061–3. https://doi.org/10.1542/peds.103.5.1061.
2. Chervenak FA, McCullough LB. Ethics of fetal surgery. Clin Perinatol. 2009;36:237–46. https://doi.org/10.1016/j.clp.2009.03.002.
3. Bienstock JL, Birshner ML, Coleman F, Hueppchen NA. Successful in utero intervention for bilateral renal agenesis. Obstet Gynecol. 2014;124(2, Part 2):413–5. https://doi.org/10.1097/aog.0000000000000339.
4. Sheldon CR, Kim ED, Chandra P, et al. Two infants with bilateral renal agenesis who were bridged by chronic peritoneal dialysis to kidney transplantation. Pediatr Transplant. 2019;23(6):e13532. https://doi.org/10.1111/petr.13532.
5. Thomas AN, McCullough LB, Chervenak FA, Placencia FX. Evidence-based, ethically justified counseling for fetal bilateral renal agenesis. J Perinat Med. 2017;45(5):585–94. https://doi.org/10.1515/jpm-2016-0367.
6. ACOG Committee on Ethics. ACOG Committee Opinion #352: innovative practice: ethical guidelines. Obstet Gynecol. 2006;108(6):1589–95.
7. Antiel RM, Flake AW. Responsible surgical innovation and research in maternal-fetal surgery. Semin Fetal Neonatal Med. 2017;22(6):423–7. https://doi.org/10.1016/j.siny.2017.05.002.
8. Mastroianni AC, Henry LM, Robinson D, et al. Research with pregnant women: new insights on legal decision-making. Hast Cent Rep. 2017;47(3):38–45. https://doi.org/10.1002/hast.706.
9. McCullough L, Jones JW, Brody BA. Informed consent: autonomous decision making of the surgical patient. In: LB MC, Jones JW, Brody BA, editors. Surgical ethics. Oxford University Press; 1986.
10. Barkun JS, Aronson JK, Feldman LS, Maddern GJ. Strasberg SM; for the Balliol Collaboration. Evaluation and stages of surgical innovation. Lancet. 2009;374(9695):1089–96. https://doi.org/10.1016/s0140-6736(09)61083-7.
11. Hirst A, Philippou Y, Blazeby J, et al. No surgical innovation without evaluation: evaluation and further development of the IDEAL framework and recommendations. Ann Surg. 2019;269(2):211–20. https://doi.org/10.1097/sla.0000000000002794.
12. Cordasco KM. Obtaining informed consent from patients: brief update review. In: Making health care safer II: an updated critical analysis of the evidence for patient safety practices. Agency for Healthcare Research and Quality; 2013.
13. Lloyd AJ. The extent of patients' understanding of the risk of treatments. Qual Health Care. 2001;(10, Suppl I):i14–8. https://doi.org/10.1136/qhc.0100014.
14. Weinstein ND. Optimism biases about personal risks. Science. 1989;246(4935):1232–3. https://doi.org/10.1126/science.2686031.
15. McNeally MF, Martin DK. An entrustment model of consent for surgical treatment of life-threatening illness: perspective of patients requiring esophagectomy. J Thorac Cardiovasc Surg. 2000;120(2):264–9. https://doi.org/10.1067/mtc.2000.106525.
16. Sugarman J, Anderson J, Baschat AA, et al. Ethical considerations concerning amnioinfusions for treating fetal bilateral renal agenesis. Obstet Gynecol. 2018;131(1):130–4. https://doi.org/10.1097/aog.0000000000002416.
17. O'Hare EM, Jelin AC, Miller JL, et al. Amnioinfusions to treat early onset anhydramnios caused by renal anomalies: background and rationale for the renal anhydramnios fetal therapy trial. Fetal Diagn Ther. 2019;45:365–72. https://doi.org/10.1159/000497472.
18. Bunchman TE. The ethics of infant dialysis. Perit Dial Int. 1996;16:S505–8. https://doi.org/10.1177/089686089601602s102.
19. Wightman AG, Freeman MA. Update on ethical issues in pediatric dialysis: has pediatric dialysis become morally obligatory? Clin J Am Soc Nephrol. 2016;11:1456–62. https://doi.org/10.2215/cjn.12741215.

20. Reynolds JM, Garralda ME, Jameson RA, Postlethwaite RJ. How parents and families cope with chronic renal failure. Arch Dis Child. 1988;63:821–6. https://doi.org/10.1136/adc.63.7.821.
21. Wiedebusch S, Konrad M, Foppe H, et al. Health-related quality of life psychosocial strains and coping in parents of children with chronic renal failure. Pediatr Nephrol. 2010;25:1477–85. https://doi.org/10.1007/s00467-010-1540-z.
22. Fielding D, Brownbridge G. Factors related to psychosocial adjustment in children with end-stage renal failure. Pediatr Nephrol. 1999;13:766–70. https://doi.org/10.1007/s004670050695.
23. Tsai TC, Liu SI, Tsai JD, Chou LH. Psychosocial effects on caregivers for children on chronic peritoneal dialysis. Kidney Int. 2006;70(11):1983–7. https://doi.org/10.1038/sj.ki.5001811.
24. Tong A, Lowe A, Sainsbury P, Craig JC. Parental perspectives on caring for a child with chronic kidney disease: an in-depth interview study. Child Care Health Dev. 2010;36:549–57. https://doi.org/10.1111/j.1365-2214.2010.01067.x.
25. Rees L. Renal replacement therapies in neonates: issues and ethics. Semin Fetal Neonatal Med. 2017;22:104–8. https://doi.org/10.1016/j.siny.2016.11.001.
26. Shaefer F, Borzych-Dulzulka D, Azocar M, et al. Impact of global economic disparities on practices and outcomes of chronic peritoneal dialysis in children: Insights from the International Pediatric Peritoneal Dialysis Registry. Perit Dial Int. 2012;32:399–409. https://doi.org/10.3747/pdi.2012.00126.
27. Advisory Committee on Organ Transplantation to HHS. US Department of Health and Human Services Recommendations 1-18. HRSA. 2002. https://www.organdonor.gov/about-dot/acot/acotrecs118.html. Accessed 8 Apr 2021.
28. Organ Transplantation and Procurement Network. Policy 14.3, living donation informed consent requirements. In: Notice of OPTN policy changes: align OPTN policy with U.S. Public Health Service Guideline, 2020. https://optn.transplant.hrsa.gov/media/4250/align_202phsguideline_202012_policynotice.pdf. Accessed 8 Apr 2021.
29. Hays R, Matas AJ. Ethical review of the responsibilities of living donor liver transplant. Clin Liver Dis. 2016;7(3):57–9. https://doi.org/10.1002/cld.533.
30. Janvier A, Prentice T, Lantos J. Blowing the whistle: moral distress and advocacy for preterm infants and their families. Acta Paediatr. 2017;106(6):853–4. https://doi.org/10.1111/apa.13852.
31. Prentice TM, Gillam L, Davis PG, Janvier A. The use and misuse of moral distress in neonatology. Semin Fetal Neonatal Med. 2018;23:39–43. https://doi.org/10.1016/j.siny.2017.09.007.
32. Wilkinson D, de Crespigny L, Xafis V. Ethical language and decision-making for prenatally diagnosed lethal malformations. Semin Fetal Neonatal Med. 2014;19:306–11. https://doi.org/10.1016/j.siny.2014.08.007.
33. Wilkinson D. Who should decide for critically ill neonates and how? The grey zone in neonatal treatment decisions. In: McDougall R, Delany C, Gillam L, editors. When doctors and parents disagree: ethics, paediatrics & the zone of parental discretion. The Federation Press; 2016.
34. Marmion PJ. Periviability and the 'god committee'. Acta Paediatr. 2017;106(6):857–9. https://doi.org/10.1111/apa.13806.

Part VIII
Critical Care

Chapter 34
Dealing with Families of Patients with Severe Brain Injury: How Long to Treat, When to Turn Off Support, Organ Donation

Maya A. Babu

Abstract Severe brain injured patients pose nuanced ethical dilemmas. The severity of the injury removes the patient's ability to consent, and results in family members having to take on the role of as decision maker. This chapter raises key issues around the injured patient, family discussions to guide treatment, and provides a framework to aid in the communication of difficult end-of-life topics.

Keywords Brain death · Informed consent · Empathy · Surrogate decision maker · Organ donation

> **Case**
>
> Patient GR is an 18-year-old man unbelted passenger involved in an 80-mph motor vehicle crash with two of his friends one Friday evening at 1:00 AM. The car hit a stationary object, GR was ejected and landed headfirst 60 ft away. He was unresponsive at the scene. Upon arrival, paramedics intubated him and rushed to the closest Level I trauma center where he was rapidly evaluated. With no clinical evidence of internal bleeding in the abdominal cavity, he was promptly taken for CT whole body imaging to assess his injuries. Findings included significant traumatic brain injury with diffuse cerebral edema and a subarachnoid hemorrhage. He remained unresponsive with an initial Glasgow Coma Score (GCS) of 3T [1]. The patient's mother and father arrived and spoke with the treating neurosurgeon who explained the severity of the head injury as well as the grave prognosis. Given the mechanism of the injury, the

M. A. Babu (✉)
Cleveland Clinic Martin Health, Port Saint Lucie, FL, USA
e-mail: Babum2@ccf.edu

© The Author(s), under exclusive license to Springer Nature Switzerland AG 2022
V. A. Lonchyna et al. (eds.), *Difficult Decisions in Surgical Ethics*, Difficult Decisions in Surgery: An Evidence-Based Approach, https://doi.org/10.1007/978-3-030-84625-1_34

477

findings on imaging, the neurologic exam, and the available data, the neuro-surgeon told the parents that the likelihood was 85–90% that the patient would persist in a minimally conscious state. The family was adamant that they wanted to pursue every possible medical treatment to keep their son alive, no matter the outcome.

34.1 Introduction

Surgical ethics is a field which strives to address the challenges faced by interventionalists when dealing with complex pathologies. Concepts such as informed consent are especially germane to surgeons as communicating the risks and expectations associated with a procedure guide much of what is ultimately performed. When a family is confronted by an unexpected event, such as trauma, the principles and foundation underlying communications with decision-makers become all the more sacred.

The scenario above is not uncommon for those who work in healthcare and care for trauma patients. Traumatic events are sudden and highly disruptive to families and communities. Families are often paralyzed by shock when informed that their loved one has suffered a devastating injury. Surgeons must be understanding and compassionate while remaining practical and honest in their descriptions of the patient's injury, severity and prognosis. Navigating this acute, devastating situation for families can pose several ethical challenges to the practitioner. In this chapter we will discuss in depth several of these challenges.

34.2 Search Strategy

A literature search was performed in the PubMed database using the search terms: brain injury AND informed consent; brain death; empathy AND trauma; organ donation AND brain death. Literature was limited to the English language and the years 2000–2020.

34.3 Discussion

34.3.1 Ethics of Head Trauma

There are multiple issues surrounding the ethics of treating a patient with head trauma. Head injury is divided into three categories: mild, moderate, and severe (see Table 34.1). A mild head injury is a Glasgow Coma Score (GCS) of 13–15. A score

Table 34.1 The Glascow Coma Score (GCS) [1]

Eye opening	Verbal response	Motor response
Spontaneously 4	Oriented 5	Obeys commands 6
To speech 3	Confused 4	Localizes to pain 5
To pain 2	Inappropriate 3	Withdraws from pain 4
None 1	Incomprehensible 2	Flexion to pain 3
	None 1	Extension to pain 2
		None 1

MILD head injury: 13–15
MODERATE head injury: 9–13
SEVERE head injury: < 8

between 9 and 13 is considered a moderate head injury while a score 8 or below is considered severe. Patients who have a moderate or severe brain injury are often unable to make decisions for themselves. These patients rely on a family member, guardian or surrogate to make decisions on their behalf. That decision maker becomes the primary conduit for communication with the healthcare providers.

Given their moribund state, several issues emerge in terms of how we care for and manage patients with severe brain injury. Firstly, we rely on the designated surrogate to make decisions on behalf of the patient. If the patient is young, this defaults to a parent or close relative. An older person may have a legally designated decision-maker. Communicating with this individual, who may or may not share the views held by the remaining family and friends, may pose a challenge, especially in situations in which withdrawal of care is considered. Legally and ethically, we strive to honor the patient's wishes for himself or herself. When there is strife among family members, it may take multiple conversations and even the assistance of the hospital's Ethics Committee to help identify and overcome the barriers towards consensus-building.

Secondly, the decision-maker is often overwhelmed with grief and shock at news of an unexpected traumatic event. Our recommendations for imaging studies or procedural intervention require consent, which may be delivered in a dire situation [2]. Ensuring that we as caregivers communicate the goals of an intervention, the risk and the alternatives helps maintain the value and intent of informed consent.

Thirdly, we rely heavily on the family's understanding of the patient's wishes (autonomy) and their comfort for making decisions on the patient's behalf. There may be unclear relationships or conflicts that the caregiving team may not be privy to. For instance, one patient I cared for had designated his ex-wife as his decision-maker. It was unclear to us if she had a financial conflict of interest (such as a life insurance policy) which might influence her decision-making regarding withdrawal of care. These are awkward, uncomfortable discussions but in withdrawal of support discussions, attempting to ascertain such information helps the care team work synergistically with the family towards what is best for the patient. Finally, there can be tension between the caregiver team and the family when the expectations for recovery are seemingly unrealistic. Families may want to continue with aggressive care while caregivers may feel that to be futile. Maintenance of a poor quality of life carries with it risks related to immobility, hygiene, and infection. The caregiving team can communicate this information with care, depth and precision, but the family may still choose a decision that does not align with the caregivers' recommendations. The duty of the caregiving team is to provide as much information as possible.

When clinical research is involved, clinician researchers are obligated to have the welfare of the research participant (beneficence) in their realm of awareness and concern. Especially in a moribund state, it is incumbent upon the clinical team to serve as advocates for the patient in dealing with researchers.

Considering interventions that are meant to sustain or lengthen life, we need to be mindful of nonmaleficience and inflicting as little harm as possible to reach a favorable outcome.

When patients in a moribund state are treated, the treating team must exercise concern for justice, equity and fairness. Keeping in mind the patient's injury, treatment should be approached with concern for the welfare of the patient.

34.3.2 Family Communication

We communicate often and with as much transparency as possible with the patient's family or decision-maker. We provide information in the plainest possible language. We ask our families what their understanding is of the patient's injury and whether the patient had communicated his or her wishes for long-term care prior to the injury. Families are usually overwhelmed by news of the traumatic injury. Repeated family communication helps answer evolving questions and also conveys to families the importance the caregiving team places in the care of their loved one.

34.3.3 Informed Consent

Informed consent poses its own challenges. We speak to a patient's family or guardian and provide as much information as we can as to prognosis and possible outcomes of procedures. There is debate in the literature as to how thorough an informed consent should be [3–5].

We convey to the family the procedures involved, the alternatives, the risks, the benefits, and the goals. We explain potential complications. No matter how long we communicate or the level of the language we use to convey this information, we don't necessarily have an assessment of the family's understanding prior to their acceptance of informed consent. We assume basic literacy and if the family appears confused, we ask for the assistance of additional family members or an interpreter when indicated. Despite these precautions, we cannot guarantee that the patient's family has complete understanding of the scope of the intervention described [6–9]. We utilize multiple caregivers to convey this information in the hopes that different word choice and different styles will convey the gravity of the situation to families.

Ultimately, we do have to make some assumptions as to literacy and basic competence when providing an informed consent. It is unrealistic, maybe impossible, for a surgeon, with an emergent situation to address, to have a detailed cognitive assessment or score by which to assess the understanding of a family prior to obtaining consent. We often have to act quickly and adeptly in order to have a favorable outcome. This is an area that has been debated in the ethics literature and is one that can be overcome with repeated family communication and use of plain-spoken language [6–8]. Legally, informed consent can have important ramifications. For instance, one study found that when informed consent is obtained in an office, malpractice risk can be decreased [10]. The area of research of obtaining informed consent in the context of devastating injuries can become murky. Researchers can blur the boundaries between clinical care and research in describing interventions for patients. It is vitally important that if research occurs in situations of trauma, that a third party obtain the research consent so that the family can delineate between the standard clinical care rendered and the care proposed by the research study.

34.3.4 Prognostication

It is difficult to provide accurate prognostication for a traumatized family. We do not have a crystal ball with which to predict how long a patient may survive or the level of devastation he or she may experience in the long term. What we can offer is a range of possible outcomes based upon our experience and the literature. We often paint for families the best-worst case scenarios [11]. When using this tool, the best-case scenario draws a picture of what the patient's life would be if recovery went as smoothly as possible and if the result did not offer the level of recovery that the patient would have desired, the family may allow support to be withdrawn. And, if the worst-case scenario would leave the patient and family in an unpalatable place, the family may be able to release their own wish for the patient's survival and make a decision in keeping with the patient's wishes to not remain on life support. The surrogate (family) must always act in a manner that abides by the wishes of the patient, or what one thinks the patient would have wanted.

Our goal is to provide the family with a realistic, probabilistic forecast. This consists of providing weights and percentages as to the likely outcome of certain scenarios. If a patient has a truly devastating head injury, then the likelihood of a miraculous recovery is vanishingly small. We do our best to use existing data such as the CRASH and IMPACT scores (see Table 34.2) to help families understand that it is not necessarily the initial injury which devastates the patient in the long term, but the related impairments which result from the initial injury which caused mortality [12]. These two frameworks input data from the field, such as presenting blood pressure or lab values, and help provide prognostic information in terms of chances of six month or beyond survival. Data from multiple patients was pooled to arrive at these diagnostic tools. Novel imaging modalities, such as functional MRI, may provide conflicting and inconclusive information for families as to whether

Table 34.2 Variables in the models predicting unfavorable outcome and mortality at six months

CRASH score	IMPACT score
Age	Age
Glasgow Coma Score	GCS motor score
Pupils reach to light	Pupil reactivity
Major extra-cranial injury	Hypoxia
CT scan available:	Hypotension
CT classification	CT classification
tSAH	tSAH on CT
	Epidural mass on CT
	Hb
	Glucose

CRASH: Corticosteroid Randomization After Significant Head injury
IMPACT: International Mission on Prognosis and Analysis of Clinical Trials in TBI
TBI: traumatic brain injury
tSAH: traumatic subarachnoid hemorrhage

their loved one is "awake." Helping to digest the meaning of such studies using simple language and without creating false hope is the aim of caregivers in communicating with families. It is important to acknowledge the family's hope for the best possible outcome and allow them to conclude that what they may hope for may not be the actual result [13].

34.3.5 Support

The duration we support a patient is impossible to predict a priori. Multiple factors are involved. The severity and circumstances of the injury, the characteristics of the patient such as age and co-existing morbidities, and the wishes of the family, are all important considerations when determining the duration for which support is provided. It takes time, sometime several weeks, until the patient's overall trajectory can be determined, and prognostication given. It also takes time for the family to adjust to the sudden change in their loved one and to be able to come to consensus for the next steps. There is no definitive timeline. Daily care, observations and reconsiderations of the patient's progress guides the decision-making.

34.3.6 Organ Donation

Organ donation may occur after declaration of brain death. It is challenging from the standpoint of the family. The subject of organ donation is delicate in the context of an acute traumatic injury. It is difficult for families to consider withdrawal of support and organ harvesting in a young person who has suddenly experienced devastating trauma.

With repeated communication and discussion with the family to convey an understanding of the gravity and severity of the injury, the subject of organ donation may be broached. We typically frame the discussion around that the person, or their soul is no longer with us. Their thinking, personality and aspirations are no longer present. Occasionally, families may challenge this notion, stating that only cardiac death represents "true death."

We focus on the knowledge of the wishes of the patient. The patient may have stated at some point that he or she would like to be an organ donor and provide an "opportunity for life" to another person. Is the family aware of any of these stated wishes? Families often appreciate the opportunity to have a portion of their loved one live on in another human being. It may be soothing to know that a family member did not die in vain and was able to help others live and that their soul may live on. We rely on multi-disciplinary teams, composed of spiritual services, social workers, practitioners who may be from their culture or tradition, to help explain the situation to the family in more familiar terms.

Experiencing a devastating loss triggers a flood of reactive emotions, and the anger, frustration or rage directed towards the care team should be approached with empathy and sympathy, although it can be difficult to do this at times. Allowing time for family to gather may help re-direct the conversation and allow them time to reflect. The participation of members of organ procurement agencies, apart from the critical care team, to discuss organ donation, will provide the family additional information with which to make a decision.

Another form of organ donation is donation after circulatory death (DCD). This is challenging to predict. Withdrawal of life-sustaining measures may occur without immediate "cardiac death". If the heart does not stop quickly enough and too much time passes without adequate perfusion of the organs, organ donation may no longer be possible. This can be an emotional rollercoaster for the family who has developed an expectation that their loved one will go on to help another. Expectation setting for families can be challenging but can occur. The act of pledging organ donation is an act of heroism for families. That the process is met with difficulty is not the ultimate end of their sacrifice or decision.

34.3.7 Framework for Communication with Families
(see Table 34.3)

There are many possible methods with which to communicate with families during the difficult time following a devastating brain injury. We recommend the following elements as a guide and a reminder of the principles that help facilitate an ethically supported discussion with families.

Table 34.3 Framework for communication

Honesty:	Sincerity, Transparency
Empathy:	Caring, Compassion
Repetition:	Multiple communications methods, Amplification
Time:	A period to absorb and reflect
Listen:	Understanding, Recognizing
Speak simply:	Easily accessible language, Avoidance of jargon

We recommend **honesty**. When families ask us about prognostication, whether an intervention will be successful, or whether their loved one suffers, honesty is truly the best policy. We often don't know. Conveying to a family that we do not know may seem incomplete but is often viewed as sincere. We do not want to give false information or false hope. Saying that we do not know is perfectly acceptable. Occasionally, a family may voice concern; "Well how could you not know?" In those situations, we should feel comfort in reassuring the family that we are here to provide honest information, and should we not have the answer, we will communicate as such.

We recommend **empathy**. It is impossible for us to live in the shoes of the family who is receiving devastating news. However, we all know what it is like to experience a set-back. Reminding ourselves of that vulnerability, the sadness, the hopelessness, and the devastation goes a long way in helping to empathize and connect with our families. It is important to convey that feeling as we are communicating devastating news with the family. There are no perfect words. Sincerity should come from the heart.

We recommend **repetition**. Repeating ourselves with clear simple language is acceptable. When we receive devastating news, we are not able to process every word. We are overwhelmed by emotion. Certain words or phrases dominate. Our own thoughts or questions cloud our thinking. "Did I say I love you to my son/my daughter today?" "Did I argue with him/her this morning?" "Could I have prevented this?" Family members are not necessarily listening to what you are communicating. We recognize this and recommend repeating key concepts to help the family understand the severity and consequences of the situation.

We recommend providing enough **time**. Oftentimes, a family needs an initial discussion of the severity of the situation followed with time to allow other family members to be communicated with and for reflection to occur. Another conversation in a day or two may be necessary to help solidify or reinforce the previous communication. Important discussions such as withdrawal of support should not be rushed into. It may take several days or even a week or two before a family has comfort with an important decision such as withdrawal of life-sustaining support.

We recommend **listening**. As physicians, we feel that we need to have all the answers. We feel that we need to lead and guide the discussion. We do not. Our most powerful communication can be sitting back and listening. I often ask the family before I speak to tell me about the patient. I ask what the patient likes to do in his or her spare time. I ask what his or her favorite color is. I ask what sports he or she likes to watch. These may seem like simple questions, but it helps us together to remember the patient. I want to know who we are talking about before we talk about that patient and what has happened to them. It is perfectly fine to listen.

We recommend that one **speak simply**. After years of schooling, understanding the complex language of medicine, being able to communicate this complex language in journal articles read by our colleagues, now is our opportunity to step back and to speak as simply as we know how. We communicate as if we are talking to a person who has no medical knowledge and is overwhelmed. We use simple words and try to explain ideas in several ways. Many a time, I have shared information with families thinking that I have conveyed the concept simply only to see a baffled look. I try again and I say to the family "I have not been clear, let me try again." I recognize that communication, despite our best efforts, may be incomplete. This helps put the family at ease as they understand that our goal is to help educate and inform them. Do not feel uncomfortable with your role as a listener and the need to revise your comments so that understanding can occur.

34.4 Case Conclusion

GR remained in a persistent vegetative state. The family opted to proceed to a long-term facility. After several months, he developed a pneumonia and sepsis secondary to a pressure ulcer. After several frank discussions with the patient's parents and sister, they opted to transition him to hospice, and he passed 10 days later. The patient's sister, who initially was vocal to have everything done, expressed a change of heart after she saw him suffer with illnesses and also saw her parents emotionally devastated by his clinical state. She expressed guilt for continuing to intervene which she now realized only prolonged his suffering.

34.5 Conclusion

We always wish that we have perfect information. Unfortunately, prognostication is a complicated dance. We rely on the best information we have available, not only related to the patient and his or her circumstance, but also to the latest data available [14]. Combining what we understand of the patient, his or her imaging and laboratory findings, the mechanism of injury, what the patient would want, as well as the available data of survival or outcome for the patient's injury, we make our best recommendation to the family. We have no crystal ball to predict the future. Being honest and upfront with our families when we have information to share is the best course of action. Ultimately, a family's decision relies on their comfort and understanding of their loved one's desired course of action. Where there is overall discomfort and anxiety there will be discomfort with decision-making. Our goal is to treat the family in addition to the patient with a severe brain injury because he/she is not in a position to make decisions for themselves. Our role is as a sherpa, guiding a family through the difficult decision-making process. We cannot and should not fault ourselves for not being able to provide precise estimates. Instead, providing a range of possibilities and a recognition that our data and our science in this area is imperfect is an appropriate, honest way to approach a family during this terrible time.

34.6 Selected References

- Weijer C, Peterson A, Webster F, et al. Ethics of neuroimaging after serious brain injury. BMC Med Ethics. 2014;15:41. https://doi.org/10.1186/1472-6939-15-41

  - This article offers insight as to the use of neuroimaging and how it can shape the ethics of discussing brain injury.

- Lloyd A, Hayes P, Bell PRF, Naylor AR. The role of risk and benefit perception in informed consent for surgery. Med Decis Making. 2001;21(2):141–9. https://doi.org/10.1177/0272989x0102100207

  - This article discusses how informed consent is framed for patients as the language used to discuss consent influences patient decision making.

- Chan Y, Irish JC, Wood SJ, et al. Patient education and informed consent in head and neck surgery. Arch Otolaryngol Head Neck Surg. 2002;128:1269–74. https://doi.org/10.1001/archotol.128.11.1269

  - This article discusses how informed consent can be utilized as an educational tool to inform patients as to scope and extent of surgery.

References

1. Teasdale G, Jennett B. Assessment of coma and impaired consciousness: a practical scale. Lancet. 1974;304(7872):81–4. https://doi.org/10.1016/s0140-6736(74)91639-0.
2. Weijer C, Peterson A, Webster F, et al. Ethics of neuroimaging after serious brain injury. BMC Med Ethics. 2014;15:41. https://doi.org/10.1186/1472-6939-15-41.
3. Del Carmen MG, Joffe S. Informed consent for medical treatment and research: a review. Oncologist. 2005;10:636–41. https://doi.org/10.1634/theoncologist.10-8-636.
4. Osuna E, Perez-Carceles MD, Perez-Moreno JA, Luna A. Informed consent. Evaluation of the information provided to patients before anaesthesia and surgery. Med Law. 1998;17:511–8.
5. Mishra PK, Ozalp F, Gardner RS, Arangannal A, Murday A. Informed consent in cardiac surgery: is it truly informed? J Cardiovasc Med. 2006;7:675–81. https://doi.org/10.2459/01.jcm.0000243001.59675.bf.

6. Lloyd A, Hayes P, Bell PRF, Naylor AR. The role of risk and benefit perception in informed consent for surgery. Med Decis Mak. 2001;21(2):141–9. https://doi.org/10.1177/0272989x0102100207.
7. Chan Y, Irish JC, Wood SJ, et al. Patient education and informed consent in head and neck surgery. Arch Otolaryngol Head Neck Surg. 2002;128:1269–74. https://doi.org/10.1001/archotol.128.11.1269.
8. Akkad A, Jackson C, Kenyon S, Dixon-Woods M, Taub N, Habiba M. Informed consent for elective and emergency surgery: questionnaire study. BJOG. 2004;111:1133–8. https://doi.org/10.1111/j.1471-0528.2004.00240.x.
9. Anderson OA, Wearne IMJ. Informed consent for elective surgery-what is best practice? J R Soc Med. 2007;100:97–100. https://doi.org/10.1177/014107680710000226.
10. Bhattacharyya T, Yeon H, Harris MB. The medical-legal aspects of informed consent in orthopedic surgery. J Bone Joint Surg. 2005;87:2395–400. https://doi.org/10.2106/jbjs.d.02877.
11. Kruser JM, Nabozny MJ, Steffens NM, et al. "Best case/worst case": qualitative evaluation of a novel communication tool for difficult in-the-moment surgical decisions. J Am Geriatr Soc. 2015;63:1805–11. https://doi.org/10.1111/jgs.13615.
12. Hicks R. Ethical and regulatory considerations in the design of traumatic brain injury clinical studies. Handb Clin Neurol. 2015;128:743–59. https://doi.org/10.1016/B978-0-444-63521-1.00046-7.
13. Hawley L, Hammond FM, Cogan A, et al. Ethical considerations in chronic brain injury. J Head Trauma Rehabil. 2019;34:433–6. https://doi.org/10.1097/HTR.0000000000000538.
14. Bernat JL. Ethical issues in the treatment of severe brain injury: the impact of new technologies. Ann N Y Acad Sci. 2009;1157:117–30. https://doi.org/10.1111/j.1749-6632.2008.04124.x.

Chapter 35
Burned Beyond Recognition: Ethics of Care

Chad M. Teven ⓘ

Abstract Several ethical issues arise in the care of acutely burned patients. These include medical decision-making, patient autonomy, informed consent, decisional capacity, and the patient-provider relationship. In the of case of severe or catastrophic burn injury, additional ethical concerns often develop that require consideration, such as surrogate decision-making, medical futility, withholding and withdrawing of treatment, and end of life care. Various approaches have been advocated as a strategy to manage the ethical challenges of burn care including moral principlism, which highlights the moral principles of beneficence, nonmaleficence, respect for patient autonomy, and distributive justice. An alternative strategy with clinical applicability is the "four-quadrant" approach, in which medical indications, patient preferences, quality-of-life, and contextual features are used to guide care. Regardless of the system employed, providers would benefit from a rational understanding of the ethical issues that frequently arise during the management of burn patients. Indeed, attentive application of clinical ethics in such cases often serves to facilitate the provision of optimal medical care while simultaneously ensuring the utmost respect for patient autonomy. This chapter will highlight ethical issues that arise in care of burn patients. Additionally, moral foundations, clinical considerations, and special cases will be discussed. Finally, an overview of various frameworks for addressing ethical challenges in burn care will be provided.

Keywords Burns · Capacity · Decision making · Informed consent · Medical ethics · Patient autonomy · Refusal of care · Withholding and withdrawing treatment · Medical futility · Catastrophic burn injury

C. M. Teven (✉)
Division of Plastic and Reconstructive Surgery, Department of Surgery, Mayo Clinic, Phoenix, AZ, USA

© The Author(s), under exclusive license to Springer Nature Switzerland AG 2022
V. A. Lonchyna et al. (eds.), *Difficult Decisions in Surgical Ethics*, Difficult Decisions in Surgery: An Evidence-Based Approach, https://doi.org/10.1007/978-3-030-84625-1_35

Case

John Smith (a fictionalized composite patient) is a 66-year-old male who was injured during an explosion while working in his shed. He was brought to the emergency room with extensive deep partial- and full-thickness burns to the face, trunk, arms, and legs totaling 80% total body surface area (TBSA). He initially presented alert and oriented, and was conversant with the medical team. He indicated a desire for palliation, repeatedly saying he did not want to be kept alive "by machines." Although no formal advance directive had been written, John indicated that his wife, Claudia, is who should be contacted to make medical decisions on his behalf if he became unable to. Soon after admission, the patient's pulmonary status worsened, and he lost consciousness. Without family present, the treating physician proceeded to intubate the patient. He was stabilized and transferred to burn intensive care unit (ICU) for ongoing management.

The patient's wife later arrived at the hospital and met with the clinical team. It was discovered by the fire department that the blast was intentional and was an attempt by John to injure himself. Claudia reported that he had a history of psychiatric illness (depression with rare psychotic features) but had not previously indicated a desire to harm himself. John had previously undergone pharmacologic treatment for his depression, but recently decided to stop taking his prescribed medications because he felt they were unhelpful. The medical team informed Claudia of the severity of John's condition, suggesting that his risk of mortality was at least 80% given the extent of his burn injuries, the presence of an inhalational component, and his comorbidities including coronary artery disease, chronic obstructive pulmonary disease, and smoking history. Recently, John had been experiencing significant functional disability due to is heart and lung disease. They further explained that should he survive the acute resuscitative period, John would require frequent trips to the operating room for debridement and grafting, long-term surgical reconstruction, and significant rehabilitation. As John's surrogate, Claudia was considered to be appropriate and rational in her thought process and demonstrated capacity. After two days of minimal clinical improvement, Claudia reported that John would "hate to live like this." She requested that no further life-sustaining interventions be provided, and that the patient receive only palliative care going forward. Surgical debridement was deferred per Claudia's request, which resulted in deterioration of the patient's condition due to burn sepsis. John remained unresponsive but occasionally groaned loudly, presumably from pain. A meeting between the care team, Claudia, and other members of the patient's family occurred, which featured discussion of medical futility as well as withdrawal of life-sustaining treatment including the ventilator. The patient's wife indicated her wish for cessation (i.e., withdrawal) of life-preserving care.

The clinical team considers whether it is ethically permissible to follow the patient's initial and the surrogate's ongoing wishes to withdrawal life support. In particular, some team members are concerned because of the mechanism of injury. In contrast, other team members worry that the care currently being provided is futile. As a result, the team would like to know whether the withdrawal of care is ethically forbidden or permissible. Further, the team questions whether there is in fact an ethical obligation to do so.

35.1 Introduction

Burn injuries constitute a significant public health crisis in the United States and across the world. In the United States in 2016, the American Burn Association reported nearly 500,000 burn injuries that received medical treatment, 40,000 of which required hospitalization [1]. The global incidence of injuries due to fire is approximately 1.1 per 100,000 population, disproportionately affecting low- and middle-income countries (LMIC) (incidence 1.3 per 100,000 population) compared to high-income countries (HIC) (incidence 0.14 per 100,000 population) [2]. In the United States and similar high-income countries, 40–50% of burn injuries occur in adults. Nevertheless, pediatric burns are a significant cause of morbidity in children, both in high-income and low-income regions. In the United States, burns constitute the fourth leading cause of accidental death [2].

The majority of global burn injuries are unintentional in nature. Less than 5% are the result of abuse, self-immolation, or other intentional cause. High-risk populations for burn injuries, both intentional and unintentional, consist of older adults, children, and women. In recent years, burn-related mortality in the United States has declined from 2.99 per 100,000 (1981) to 1.2 per 100,000 (2006). A similar trend has been observed around the world, with 5.3 deaths per 100,000 in 1990 and 4.9 deaths per 100,000 in 2010 [2]. Significant discrepancies exist between the number of deaths due to burns in high-income countries relative to the rest of the world. Of all burn deaths, nearly 90% occur in low- and middle-income countries, compared to 3% in high-income countries [2]. The exact reasons for this are uncertain, but factors that appear to increase the risk of burn injuries include nonwhite ethnicity, low household income and other socioeconomic factors, crowded living conditions, low education, and unemployment [2]. It is important to point out that while these socioeconomic factors play a role in individual risk and outcomes of burn, it is also imperative to recognize the associated system failure in many cases (i.e., none or inadequate burn units in LMIC).

In addition to an understanding of the incidence, prevalence, and risk factors associated with burn injuries, providers must be aware of the medical issues and complications that present in the setting of an acute burn injury. Severe burns are those in which >20% of the total body surface area (TBSA) is affected by non-superficial burns, or burns that are complicated by inhalation injury, chemical burns, high-voltage electrical burns, or major trauma [3]. Emergency management of severely burned patients is initially guided by Advanced Trauma Life Support (ATLS) and Advanced Burn Life Support (ABLS) protocols and includes assessment of airway, breathing, circulation, disability, exposure, and control of the environmental. Once the patient is stabilized, targeted therapy follows, which may include fluid resuscitation, prevention of hypothermia, escharotomy and/or fasciotomy, and potential transfer to the intensive care unit or a designated burn center. Severely burned patients that survive the acute period often experience long-term debilitating consequences of the injury, including functional deformity, significant pain, disability, and a protracted recovery. Numerous surgical procedures are generally required, acutely to excise nonviable skin and cover the resulting wounds, and in delayed fashion for reconstruction of scarring and contracture. Diminished quality-of-life (QOL) and psychological morbidity is also common after severe burn injury.

In addition to complicated and potentially fatal medical issues, severe burn injuries raise several ethical concerns (Table 35.1). To aid in assessment of and response to ethical issues, various frameworks have been developed that allow for a consistent approach to these problems [4]. The well-known framework of principlism described by Beauchamp and Childress analyzes issues in the context of four moral principles: respect for patient autonomy, beneficence, nonmaleficence, and justice (Table 35.2) [5]. Building upon this model, Jonsen et al. developed the "four-quadrant" approach to ethical analysis, in which medical indications, patient preferences, QOL, and contextual features (e.g., social, financial) are considered [6]. Regardless of the method employed, an important step toward appropriate application of ethically-sound principles in burn care management is an understanding of the common ethical issues that arise after severe burns. This chapter reviews the ethical considerations of burn care as reported in the literature. Additionally, an examination of the moral foundations, clinical considerations, and unique ethical cases that relate burn care management will be examined.

Table 35.1 Common ethical issues associated with severe burn injuries

• Patient autonomy
• Medical decision-making
• Capacity and competence
• Informed consent
• Patient-provider relationship
• Surrogate decision-making (i.e., substituted judgement, best interest standard)
• Refusal of treatment
• Medical futility
• Withholding and/or withdrawing of care/treatment
• End-of-life/palliative care
• Physician-assisted suicide and euthanasia
• Self-injury/immolation

Table 35.2 The ethical framework of moral principlism

Principle	Description
Respect for autonomy	Respect for the individual and his/her ability to make decisions with regard to one's own health and future; right to self-determination
Beneficence	To do and promote good; to prevent and remove evil or harm
Nonmaleficence	To do no harm; to avoid harming
Justice	Maximize benefit to patients and society while emphasizing equal worth, fairness, and impartiality

Adapted from Beauchamp and Childress [5]

35.2   Search Strategy

A literature review of all electronically available publications available as of November 22, 2020, was performed. An English-language search of three online databases (Medline, Scopus, and Web of Science) as well as manual inspection of citations in all identified articles from the online search was performed for publications from 2000 to 2020. The following keywords were used for the search: advanced directive, beneficence, burns, burn ethics, capacity, competence, consent, death and dying, decision making, end of life, euthanasia, futile care, informed consent, justice, medical ethics, nonmaleficence, patient autonomy, quality-of-life, palliative care, physician-assisted suicide, surrogacy, withholding and withdrawing of treatment.

All returned studies from the database queries utilizing the aforementioned key words and search strategy were reviewed for applicability. An initial title/abstract screen was performed to remove any results not pertaining to burn care and the ethics thereof. Studies without English or full text access were excluded. The most pertinent papers were ultimately selected.

35.3   Discussion

The care of acute burn injuries poses unique clinical challenges for the provider. In severe cases, such injuries may result in significant physiologic derangement that require intensive medical management as well as numerous invasive procedures in an effort to prevent death and severe disability. Further complexity is seen when burns are so severe that they leave the patient incommunicative, whether due to the injury or the required treatment (e.g., need for intubation in cases of severe inhalational injury). In such cases, patient autonomy is effectively lost, and decisions regarding a patient's care fall onto others. Such situations may prove morally distressing for providers and surrogates alike. While the medical management of severely burned patients has been described in detail, management of the ethical issues that arise in the care of such patients is less well defined [7].

35.4   Respect for Autonomy

Patient autonomy denotes respect for one's right to self-determination; that is, one's ability to make decisions with regard to their own health and future. While respect of autonomy has become a cornerstone of ensuring the ethical delivery of care, it is a relatively recent revelation in the context of biomedical ethics. Historically, medicine was practiced in a predominately paternalistic fashion, whereby providers were responsible for medical decision making. Although there remains a role for occasional paternalistic interactions between doctor and patient (e.g., incapacitated patients without a suitable surrogate), the value of patient preferences in managing severely burned patients should not be underestimated.

35.5   Shared Decision Making

A more recent model of medical decision making based in large part on the concept of patient autonomy is shared decision making (SDM). With SDM, provider and patient/surrogate enlist in an active interchange with the aim of facilitating a treatment plan that is understood and agreed to by all parties. Though SDM has limitations in certain situations, its use has been advocated as the pinnacle of patient-centered care [8]. Its application in the care of burn patients is especially appropriate. Burn management often results in a protracted course, involving acute and long-term surgical procedures, extensive therapy, and significant support. Achieving optimal results requires the input of patients, surrogates, and a multidisciplinary medical team comprised of physicians, surgeons, physiatrists, psychiatrists/psychologists, nurses, therapists, social workers, dieticians, counselors, clergy, and care managers.

35.6   Patient Capacity and Consent for Treatment

In the management of critically burned patients, the first step in safeguarding the value of patient autonomy—once acute medical issues have been addressed and the patient is stabilized—is an assessment of decisional capacity. In general, patients with normal cognition are deemed to have capacity. Capacity is a pre-requisite for the provision of informed consent. If a patient lacks capacity, a surrogate should be sought. A unique challenge to severe burns is whether patients are able to possess capacity acutely after the injury. Providers and burn survivors have previously cautioned that despite the patient's apparent ability to understand the situation, normal comprehension and decision making are negatively impacted after a traumatic event [9]. Similarly, surrogates may be unable to fully comprehend the clinical scenario and make appropriately informed decisions. Therefore, the medical team may find itself responsible for emergent decision-making in the acute setting. The medical team also has the responsibilities of educating patients/surrogates regarding the clinical situation and understanding their wishes and values [10]. This approach aims to increase autonomy and patient/surrogate decision-making once they feel comfortable. Finally, because capacity may be affected by several conditions that are difficult to detect acutely (e.g., burn shock, substance ingestion, pain, neurologic/psychiatric illness), providers must be deliberate in their assessment and treat each patient individually. In complicated cases, validated cognitive assessment tools and consultation to appropriate providers may be helpful.

35.7 Surrogate Decision Making

When patients lack capacity, a proxy or surrogate decision maker is identified. Ideally, this is documented in advance (e.g., advanced directive). In the absence of a predetermined proxy, state statutes dictate surrogate priority. Commonly, a surrogate will be a partner or other immediate relative. Several models of surrogate decision-making exist, including use of stated wishes (i.e., previous written/oral statements by the patient), substituted judgment, and best interest. No approach has been demonstrated to be superior; however, a shortcoming of surrogate decision making is that decisions made by surrogates are frequently inconsistent with decisions that would have been made by patients [11]. Efforts to mitigate such inconsistencies have been proposed. Brewster and colleagues developed a management model in which burn care teams simultaneously make acute medical decisions and comprehensively educate patients/surrogates on the clinical scenario until they are comfortable joining in the decision-making process [10]. It is important that the medical team and the surrogate have frequent and open communication.

35.8 Futility of Medical Treatment

The concept of medical futility is a relatively recent addition to the study of medical ethics, but it has become an important topic in the context of severely burned patients. It denotes treatment that will fail to provide any intended benefit, and its importance with respect to burn care stems from the established relationship between burn injury severity and mortality. Use of various clinical indicators (e.g., depth, TBSA, inhalational injury, patient age, comorbidities) allows for a reasonable prediction of survival estimate. Thus, authors have suggested that use of therapeutics in patients likely to die from their injury are futile and need not be provided. In contrast, authors including influential burn surgeon Bruce Zawacki believe that failure to initiate resuscitation due to medical futility is paternalistic and should be avoided [12].

Recently, it has becoming increasingly difficult to accurately predict burn survival—and therefore whether treatment is futile—due in large part to advancements in burn care management. Further, despite the development of myriad prediction scores (e.g., Baux, Smith, FLAMES), these models are all limited by superior predictive capacity for groups rather than individual patients [13]. Nevertheless, the withholding of treatment deemed to be futile is generally regarded as ethically permissible. Indeed, physicians should not provide treatment (or a therapy) that is ineffective or detrimental (negative effects > benefits). In contrast, treatment (or a therapy) that has a reasonable chance at providing benefit should not be withheld. For reference regarding what constitutes a reasonable chance of benefit, Schneiderman suggested that any intervention that produced no measurable benefit to the last 100 patients who are in the same situation as the patient in question does not have a reasonable chance for benefit [14]. Finally, when considering whether treatment would be futile, providers should consider its effect on autonomy and quality-of-life.

35.9 Withholding and Withdrawing Treatment

Closely tied to medical futility is the concept of withholding of treatment. Assuming patient autonomy, beneficence, and nonmaleficence have been considered, withholding treatment is usually ethically justified in the appropriate setting. For example, when patients formally express wishes to forego life-sustaining therapy (i.e., using an advanced directive) and also in cases in which the probability of benefit of an intervention (e.g., improve survival) is minimal. Withholding of treatment consists of not initiating an intervention; conversely, treatment withdrawal constitutes its discontinuation after it has already been started. Withholding treatment is often considered less emotionally taxing than withdrawing it, but the two are ethically equivalent. Just as one may refuse life-sustaining therapy preemptively (i.e., Do Not Resuscitate directive), one may request that life-sustaining therapy is halted.

Withholding and withdrawal of treatment are frequently encountered in burn management, often resulting in ethical challenges to patients, surrogates, and providers. While providing improved end-of-life care has become increasingly important of late, there is a paucity of research guiding appropriate implementation of effective palliation for end-of-life burn patients. Recently, Pham et al. used a stepwise withdrawal protocol in severely burned patients with the aim of standardizing symptoms palliation at the end of life [15]. The study found that use of their withdrawal protocol facilitated a more consistent provision of sedation and analgesia without accelerating death.

When a severe burn is likely to result in death, or a patient fails initial resuscitation efforts, or ongoing treatment efforts are ineffective, then it may be appropriate to suggest or agree to the withdrawal of life support [16]. When performed appropriately, treatment withdrawal facilitates earlier implementation of palliative measures and symptom relief. Moving forward, the burn community ought to evaluate developed palliative protocols effectively used in other settings (e.g., oncology) in order to identify novel strategies to improve end of life comfort in burn patients.

35.10   Special Consideration: Self-Immolation

Self-immolation is the act of committing suicide, generally by setting oneself on fire. It has frequently been used for political or religious purposes, often as an act of protest. In Western nations, the overall incidence of attempted suicide by burning is 2–6% of burn center admission. However, attempted suicide by self-immolation is associated with increased mortality, mean affected TBSA, complications (e.g., inhalation injury), and longer hospital stays [17]. Also, a high rate of psychiatric illness (43–90%)—depression, schizophrenia, personality disorders, substance abuse— has been associated with this patient population.

A clinical challenge in caring for burn patients that attempt suicide is determination of decisional capacity. Prior research regarding cognitive status in patients with psychiatric illness has been inclusive. Different psychiatric illnesses may affect decision-making differentially, with psychotic disorders (e.g., schizophrenia) likely to negatively impact cognition to a greater degree than mood disorders (e.g., depression) [18]. In the acute aftermath of severe burn injuries in attempted suicide, careful scrutiny of decisional capacity and formal psychiatric assessment is crucial.

It is not uncommon that requests for withdrawal/withholding of treatment are made by the patient and/or surrogate after a suicide attempt. The granting of such requests may be appropriate in specific (but not all cases), and should only be considered after careful deliberation among the treatment team, consulting services (e.g., psychiatric, ethics), and with the patient/surrogate. Brown and colleagues proposed an algorithm for withdrawal of life support after attempted suicide that recommends passage of time and gathering of evidence to permit greater probability of disability and improved clarity regarding a patient's values and desires before treatment is withdrawn [19]. Additionally, the algorithm holds that prior to granting the request, the treatment team should wait 72 hours (± depending on the clinical context) to allow adequate time to clarify the prognosis, ascertain and confirm patient/ surrogate wishes, and obtain formal assistance from psychiatry, ethics, and other providers as needed.

A notable aspect of this model is that the proximate cause of the critical illness is not relevant to the decision of treatment withdrawal. Though the scrutiny required in such cases should be higher than if not after a suicide attempt, any justification that is sufficient to permit withdrawal of care in patients without psychiatric illness (e.g., significant therapeutic burden without expected benefit) is sufficient to justify withdrawal of care in psychiatric patients. Applied to severely burned patients, significant injury that will result in permanent disability or death is often an appropriate justification for a withdrawal of treatment request. The actions that led to the patient's condition—whether accidental, intentional, or self-inflicted—are largely irrelevant to medical decision making. That is to say that although attempted suicide is often (though not always) an irrational decision, the decision to request comfort measures by a severely burned patient after attempted suicide may be rational, acceptable, and appropriate [20].

35.11 Special Consideration: Pediatric Burn Injuries

In addition to the numerous clinical and ethical issues that arise during the care of severely burned adults, management of severe pediatric burns may present with additional unique challenges. In general, pediatric patients are considered incompetent to make medical decisions. In contrast to capacity, which is a medical finding, competence is a legal state determined by statutory regulation or by a judge. Therefore, a guardian (usually a parent) is required to make decisions on the patient's behalf. Ethical challenges arise when intentional injury or factitious disorder imposed on another (FDIA), previously known as Munchausen syndrome by proxy[Diagnostic and Statistical Manual of Mental Disorders (DSM 5) ICD-10 20201 F68.A], is suspected. Engagement of other family, the ethics committee, and/or child protective services may be helpful in such cases.

Discussion of medical futility and the withholding/withdrawal of treatment in children is also complicated. While rare instances exist in which withholding of treatment from children may be appropriate (i.e., treatment that would delay imminent death without alleviating suffering), most authors contend that measures that optimize survival ought to be attempted initially [21]. Severe burn injuries may result disfigurement, deformity, disability, and reduced QOL. Because a child's cognition is not be fully developed, providers, therapists, developmental psychologists, and counselors with pediatric expertise should be enlisted to aid in the child's rehabilitation.

Finally, ethical concerns may arise when parents and providers disagree on medical management. In such cases, open communication between care team and parents is paramount. Ultimately, parents' wishes should be considered, but the best interests of the child take priority [9]. In times of disagreement, it may be beneficial to elicit support from consulting providers, the ethics committee, hospital administration and/or federal and state governmental agencies as needed.

35.12 Case Analysis

The case presented at the start of the chapter raises several ethical issues that have been discussed herein. After presentation to the hospital, patient John Smith indicated his desire for comfort measures, stating that he did not want to be kept alive "by machines." Soon thereafter, he becomes unconsciousness, ostensibly losing decisional capacity. Initially, one must determine whether John has capacity when first presenting to the hospital. Normally, appropriate adults are determined to have capacity in the absence of contradictory evidence. In the current case, the severe burn injury was the result of attempted suicide. Therefore, a standard capacity assessment would be insufficient. A more deliberate approach utilizing validated assessment tools and formal psychiatric evaluation is necessary to conclusively determine capacity. Thus, one cannot presume John demonstrates capacity on arrival despite his initial coherence.

Soon thereafter, John decompensates, erasing any remaining question of capacity. In such cases, providers must identify a surrogate, ideally who has been designated prior to the injury and is knowledgeable of the patient's values and desires. It is also important to substantiate the adequacy of a surrogate. Although an advanced directive was absent from the current case, John indicated that his wife Claudia would serve as his surrogate, a decision that was consistent with state guidelines regarding surrogacy order. Upon her arrival to the hospital to meet with the medical team, Claudia was found to demonstrate capacity, to possess a rational thought process, and therefore to be an adequate surrogate. Moving forward, the medical team is responsible for fully educating Claudia regarding John's condition, treatment strategy, and prognosis. Further, the team will turn to Claudia to make medical decisions for John.

An additional complicated factor unique to the current case is the mechanism of injury (i.e., attempted suicide by self-immolation). Due to John's suicide attempt, this information is important in determining how to provide the best care to John at the present time. Formal psychiatric assessment is helpful, especially if John were lucid, even while unconscious. Further, the mechanism of injury is relevant insofar as it may alter the course and strategy of management. Attempted suicide in of itself does not prevent withdrawal of treatment in this case once it is clear that John's condition is worsening and will likely result in death. However, additional steps and added scrutiny are necessary to ensure that such a decision is rational and appropriate. Indeed, a request to withdraw treatment is reasonable in the setting of a severe burn injury with a high probability of mortality. Therefore, treatment withdrawal is reasonable and ethically permissible. In fact, it facilitates patient autonomy by respecting his surrogate's—and therefore his—wishes.

In contrast, it would be ethically dubious to withhold care on the grounds of medical futility. The provided information is inadequate to conclude that continued treatment is futile. While John's clinical status is noted to be deteriorating, it is plausible that initiation or aggressive treatment may offer a survival benefit.

Finally, it would be ethically acceptable to honor Claudia's wishes to provide palliative care in place of life-sustaining treatment to John.

As a final point, it is important to recognize that the case in question and whether various decisions are ethically sound are context dependent. For example, if John's burns were <20% TBSA and he suffered from minimal inhalation injury, the prognosis would be vastly different. Acute and long-term care would likely be different as well. The decision-making calculus thus must take into account this new information. It would be reasonable, given a decreased need for urgent decision-making, to obtain formal assessment of John's cognitive status (e.g., psychiatric consult for use of validated instrument). The goal in any case is respect for one's autonomy.

Thus, if John was deemed to have capacity, his active input would be crucial to properly guiding medical decision-making in an ethical fashion.

35.13   Concluding Remarks

The care of patients with significant burns is associated with numerous clinical and ethical challenges. Patients are best served when care is provided in a multi-faceted fashion by a multidisciplinary team at a center that specializes severe burn management. Upon initial assessment, providers are to provide care consistent with ATLS and ABLS protocols. Once the patient has been initially stabilized, a thorough history and physical examination should be performed to identify further injury as well as factors within the patient's history that are relevant to current management (e.g., mechanism of injury, past medical history, current medications, substance use, etc.). The provider must determine whether the patient is cognitively appropriate and has decisional capacity. In pediatric patients or if there is any question regarding the patient's ability to make appropriate decisions and provide informed consent, a guardian and/or surrogate decision maker should be sought. Ideally, the care team will have been in contact with the patient's family. After initial resuscitation and management of acutely life-threatening injuries, a more detailed assessment is performed, studies are obtained, and management plans are crafted. Patients and/or surrogates should be included in decision making to the level with which they are comfortable. Ongoing education regarding the clinical scenario provided by the provider and care team are important. The provider should approach both the medical and ethical issues that may arise in systematic fashion. Finally, an ethical framework (e.g., four-quadrant approach) may be applied to facilitate the provision of ethical treatment. Management of severe burn injuries presents with unique clinical and ethical challenges; however, application of sound ethical principles will serve to optimize treatment for this patient population.

35.14   Selected References

- Beauchamp T, Childress J. Principles of biomedical ethics. 8th ed. Oxford University Press; 2019.
  - Beauchamp and Childress's groundbreaking work on moral principlism with elucidation of the principles of beneficence, nonmaleficence, respect for autonomy and justice.
- Jonsen AR, Siegler M, Winslade WJ. Clinical ethics: a practical approach to ethical decisions in clinical medicine. 8th ed. McGraw-Hill; 2015.

- – The authors utilize their four box method as a clinically relevant approach to ethical case analysis. They are: medical indications, patient preferences, respect for autonomy and contextual (social, financial, etc.) features.

- Barry MJ, Edgman-Levitan S. Shared decision making—the pinnacle of patient-centered care. N Engl J Med. 2012;366:780–1

  - – Perspective on shared decision making from president of the Informed Medical Decisions Foundation, a foundation that aims to advance evidence-based shared decision making.

- Zawacki BE. Ethically valid decision making. In: Herndon DN, editor. Total burn care. New York: Elsevier; 1996.

  - – A recognized authority on surgical burn treatment discusses valid and ethical decision-making in the care of burn patients.

References

1. American Burn Association. Burn incidence fact sheet. https://ameriburn.org/who-we-are/media/burn-incidence-fact-sheet/. Accessed 16 Dec 2020.
2. Peck MD. Epidemiology of burn injuries globally. In: Jeschke MG, Collins KA, editors. UpToDate. 2019. https://www.uptodate.com/contents/epidemiology-of-burn-injuries-globally. Accessed 16 Dec 2020.
3. Gauglitz GG, Williams FN. Overview of the management of the severely burned patient. In: Jeschke MG, Collins KA, editors. UpToDate. 2020. https://www.uptodate.com/contents/overview-of-the-management-of-the-severely-burned-patient. Accessed 16 Dec 2020.
4. Teven CM, Gottlieb LJ. The four-quadrant approach to ethical issues in burn care. AMA J Ethics. 2018;20:595–601.
5. Beauchamp T, Childress J. Principles of biomedical ethics. 8th ed. Oxford University Press; 2019.
6. Jonsen AR, Siegler M, Winslade WJ. Clinical ethics: a practical approach to ethical decisions in clinical medicine. 8th ed. McGraw-Hill; 2015.
7. Lee RC, Teven CM. Acute management of burn/electrical injuries. In: Song DH, editor. Lower extremity, trunk and burns. Elsevier; 2017. Neligan P, ed. Plastic surgery. 4th ed. vol 4. p. 392–423.
8. Barry MJ, Edgman-Levitan S. Shared decision making—the pinnacle of patient-centered care. N Engl J Med. 2012;366:780–1.
9. Cole P, Stal D, Hollier L. Ethical considerations in burn management. J Craniofac Surg. 2008;19:895–8.
10. Brewster LP, Bennet BK, Gamelli RL. Application of rehabilitation ethics to a selected burn patient population's perspective. J Am Coll Surg. 2006;203:766–71. https://doi.org/10.1916/j.jamcollsurg.2006.06.024.
11. Taye H, Magnus D. Suicide and the sufficiency of surrogate decision makers. Am J Bioeth. 2013;13:1–2. https://doi.org/10.1080/15265161.2013.769827.
12. Zawacki BE. Ethically valid decision making. In: Herndon DN, editor. Total burn care. New York: Elsevier; 1996.
13. Halgas B, Bay C, Foster K. A comparison of injury scoring systems in prediction burn mortality. Ann Burns Fire Disasters. 2018;31:89–93. PMID: 30374258

14. Schneiderman LJ. Defining medical futility and improving medical care. Bioeth Inq. 2011;8:123–31. https://doi.org/10.1007/s11673-011-9293-3.
15. Pham TN, Otto A, Young SR, et al. Early withdrawal of life support in severe burn injury. J Burn Care Res. 2012;33:130–5. https://doi.org/10.1097/bcr.0b013e31823e598d.
16. Atiyeh B. End-of-life (EOL) comfort care and withdrawal of life support (WLS) of severely burned patients: a review of the literature. Ann Burns Fire Disasters. 2020;33:154–61.
17. Castana O, Kourakos P, Moutafidis M, et al. Outcomes of patients who commit suicide by burning. Ann Burn Fire Disasters. 2013;26:36–9.
18. Karlawish J. Assessment of decision-making capacity in adults. In: DeKosky ST, Mendez MF, editors. UpToDate. 2020. https://www.uptodate.com/contents/assessment-of-decision-making-capacity-in-adults. Accessed 17 Dec 2020.
19. Brown SM, Elliott CG, Paine R. Withdrawal of nonfutile life support after attempted suicide. Am J Bioeth. 2013;13:3–12. https://doi.org/10.1080/15265161.2012.760673.
20. Teven CM, Angelos P. Comfort care after self-immolation: is the physician complicit? Am J Bioeth. 2020;20:123–5. https://doi.org/10.1080/15265161.2020.1782514.
21. Rode H, Millar AJW, Castle B, Lyle J. Ethical decision making in severe pediatric burn victims. S Afr Med J. 2001;101:17–9.

Chapter 36
Rationing Ventilators

Samuel Reis-Dennis ⓘ and Megan K. Applewhite ⓘ

Abstract In times of overwhelming crisis, most recently experienced in the context of the novel coronavirus disease 2019 (COVID-19), hospitals and medical facilities are likely to experience a shortage of valuable resources. When the number of ill patients exceeds the number of resources available, bioethicists may be asked to create structural frameworks to help institutions allocate resources fairly. When writing these guidelines, ethicists must attend to a range of considerations in order to create a functional document that will work to promote public health. Here, we highlight and discuss some of the most challenging questions that are likely to arise when crafting guidelines and implementing ventilator allocation frameworks. First, we discuss some foundational principles of ventilator distribution. Next, we examine the ethics of some specific ventilator allocation criteria. Finally, we consider the difficulties of operationalizing allocation guidelines.

Keywords Ventilators · Ventilator allocation · Ethics · COVID-19 · Resource allocation · Pandemic · triage · Limited resources

S. Reis-Dennis
Alden March Bioethics Institute, Albany Medical College, Albany, NY, USA
e-mail: resides@amc.edu

M. K. Applewhite (✉)
Department of Surgery, Alden March Bioethics Institute, Albany Medical College,
Albany, NY, USA
e-mail: applewm@amc.edu

© The Author(s), under exclusive license to Springer Nature
Switzerland AG 2022
V. A. Lonchyna et al. (eds.), *Difficult Decisions in Surgical Ethics*, Difficult
Decisions in Surgery: An Evidence-Based Approach,
https://doi.org/10.1007/978-3-030-84625-1_36

503

Case

In the midst of a pandemic, the intensive care units are full. The operating room ventilators are being used in the emergency department to provide respiratory support to those in failure in order to optimize their likelihood of recovery. There is one more ventilator available. Three patients were just seen in the ED, each hypoxic, each having been determined to require mechanical ventilation.

- *Patient 1*: 25 years old, known intravenous drug abuser, HIV-positive with high viral load, nonadherent with medications, multiple prior visits to the trauma bay for penetrating wounds associated with gang violence
- *Patient 2*: 55 years old, obese, hypertension, poorly controlled type 2 diabetes, pastor, volunteer at the local food bank, single father of three adopted children
- *Patient 3*: 75 years old, retired cardiologist, runs half-marathons, plays golf on weekends, still attends medical grand rounds every week at the hospital, very active with medical student and resident education.

All three patients are being maintained on high-flow oxygen but are worsening. How should the ventilator be allocated? Should only one of these candidates get a ventilator, or should all currently ventilated patients be reassessed for their likelihood of successful extubation and evaluated alongside the three new patients?

36.1   Introduction

In times of overwhelming crisis, the supply of certain resources may become inadequate for the number of individuals who medically require them. The Coronavirus disease 2019 (COVID-19) pandemic, has given rise to worries about such scarcity with respect to ventilators. Here, we review some of the pivotal questions those writing guidelines for allocating ventilators during times of scarcity must face. First, we discuss some foundational principles of ventilator distribution that will inform the selection of specific allocation criteria. Next, we survey various allocation criteria for ventilator distribution. Finally, we discuss the difficulties of operationalizing allocation guidelines. In the process, we consider beneficence-based ambitions such as maximizing the number of lives, life-years, and quality-adjusted life-years saved, as well as autonomy-based ideals such as respect, dignity, and deference to democratic institutions (see Table 36.1).

Table 36.1 Ethical principles of ventilator rationing

Principle	Application to allocation of ventilators
Autonomy	Allocation criteria should reflect a basic respect for all persons as autonomous reasoners with dignity. Such respect requires transparency and may, in some cases, require endorsing allocation frameworks developed by democratic institutions. Democratically developed guidelines can indirectly reflect the will of the people and promote accountability.
Beneficence	Allocation criteria should endeavor to save lives, although this goal must be conditioned by other values, such as respect for persons
Non-maleficence	Removing patients with poor clinical outlooks from ventilators could be harmful to those patients. In conditions of scarcity, such measures may be justified by other values, such as justice and beneficence.
Justice	Allocation criteria should be fair and transparent. They should not be based on morally irrelevant factors such as the ability to pay or personal relationships.

36.2 Search Strategy

The central points addressed in this chapter are ones that the authors personally encountered when writing ventilator allocation guidelines for their institution that were ultimately adopted by many regional hospitals for use during the COVID-19 pandemic. In their research, the authors searched the keyword terms above in PubMed and JStor and queried North American hospital bioethics leadership via the Association of Bioethics Program Directors. No strict limits were placed on the searches, but rather, recent articles that had been widely read and cited were considered. The authors also consulted publicly available state allocation guidelines, focusing especially on New York's guidelines, which were initially developed for H1N1 influenza. New York's framework was widely discussed and used with varied modifications depending on institutional need.

36.3 Discussion

36.3.1 The Goals of Resource Allocation

Resource allocation schemes will differ insofar as they aim to realize varying ethical and practical goals. We survey some possible ambitions here:

36.3.2 Saving Lives

To some, it will seem obvious that ventilator allocation policies ought to aim to maximize the number of total lives saved. It is clear that saving lives is a central goal of allocation, and that guidelines that failed to promote this goal to some degree would be failures. But saving lives cannot be the sole ambition of allocation policy. It would be obviously impermissible, for instance, to use slave labor to produce more ventilators, even if doing so would save the most lives. The example is extreme, of course, but it serves to starkly illustrate the point that there are some values we may not sacrifice even in the name of reducing mortality.

Potential re-allocation of ventilators away from patients living in long-term ventilation facilities also forces us to confront the limits of our ambition to save lives. Every ventilator allocated to a long-term-use patient could, in theory, be redistributed to save multiple lives during a crisis. States such as New York have explicitly rejected the redistribution of ventilators from long-term-use facilities on the grounds that seizing ventilators from long-term-use patients would violate our duty to care for the vulnerable by unduly victimizing disabled people [1]. At the very least, it seems that such redistribution is not *obviously required*, and this, again, suggests that ventilator allocation must do more than merely maximize the number of lives saved.

36.3.3 Saving Life-years

The ambition of saving the most life-years suffers from the same over-simplicity as the goal of saving the most lives. Still, it does have specific virtues and pitfalls that are worth noting. For one, it reflects the widely held intuition that, all other things equal, the youngest patients, who have yet to live full lives, should be prioritized over the oldest patients, who already have [2]. On the other hand, the use of life-years involves calculating patients' future long-term life expectancies, a task that introduces practical and ethical complications. Such calculation is difficult and potentially impossible given crisis conditions and time constraints. Moreover, our best estimates of long-term life expectancy may be based on factors such a patient's race, neighborhood, or income. And they would almost certainly involve considering comorbid conditions strongly linked with poverty, poor access to health care and healthy food, and other morally irrelevant social factors. As a result, the use of life-years raises the threat of discrimination and would serve to entrench racial and economic disparities in health [3].

36.3.4 Saving Quality-adjusted Life-years

The use of "quality-adjusted life-years" inherits the problems of schemes that aim to save the most lives or the most life-years. It also introduces the fraught task of judging quality of future life. This ambition, though perhaps philosophically interesting, is both famously difficult and outside the traditional purview of state and hospital officials [4].

36.3.5   Realizing or Upholding Shared Values

If lifesaving cannot be the only goal of resource allocation policy, what other values should allocation schemes strive to realize or uphold? One might attempt to answer this question generally, by appealing to "the values of the community," "the values of the hospital," or, even more abstractly, some conception of absolute moral truth. Each of these approaches raises difficulties. The values of the community may not be monolithic or conducive to a uniform framework. Indeed, it may be challenging to articulate them at all. Even if such articulation were successful, community values may not be ultimately defensible. Appeals to the values of the hospital face this latter problem as well. The aspiration to ground allocation policy in absolute moral truths quickly runs into familiar questions about what these truths are and how we come to know them.

Another alternative is to ground the guiding values of allocation policy in a public and democratic *process*. This approach might involve reliance on local, state, or federal guidelines formulated by task forces convened by public officials whom voters can hold accountable in elections.

36.3.6   To What Extent Should Allocation Policy Adhere to Government Guidelines?

The extent to which ventilator allocation frameworks ought to deviate from available government guidelines will depend in part on the overarching goals of the allocation scheme, as discussed above. Insofar as allocation frameworks adhere to state guidelines, they maintain a connection to a democratic process. State frameworks are publicly available, and, because they are the product of government, their use enables at least some level of accountability. Moreover, such guidelines can be consistently applied across a region, promoting fairness and reducing the chances that those with the means to do so will "shop" for the hospital whose idiosyncratic guidelines give them the best odds of receiving a ventilator at the expense of less fortunate patients who may be more clinically-appropriate candidates.

On the other hand, state guidelines may be insufficiently responsive to the particular needs of the communities and hospitals that require them. Physicians and patients face challenges specific to particular places—not all hospitals in an area may be struggling in exactly the same ways—and times—guidelines that made sense for influenza may not make sense for Covid-19, for example. State and federal guidelines may not have the flexibility to meet these needs.

36.3.7 Who Should Make Allocation Decisions?

One might think that attending physicians are better positioned than independent committees to make allocation decisions, as critical care and emergency physicians have a wealth of experience with triage. They also have the best sense of their patients' clinical outlooks, and deep understanding of their needs. These relationships, however, although essential to good patient care, can bias allocation decisions. Triage committee members who do not have access to identifying patient information must base their decisions solely on criteria that can be applied uniformly to all candidates.

Additionally, the use of triage committees (which could include critical care physicians, nurses, ethicists, social workers, chaplains, lawyers, hospital leadership, and community members) introduces a valuable oversight and accountability mechanism, ensuring that allocation decisions are always discussed by a group. Relatedly, the use of triage committees relieves attending physicians of the burden of allocation. Expecting doctors, who are already providing medical care during the crisis, to make all allocation decisions on their own would be both practically unrealistic and ethically unreasonable. Bedside providers should be allowed to focus on healing their patients; they should not have to assume ultimate responsibility for deciding to prioritize the needs of other patients at the expense of their own.

For these reasons, many state and hospital policies recommend that triage committees or triage officers (if the hospital has inadequate personnel for a full triage committee) should make allocation decisions [5, 6]. Still, communication between triage committees and medical teams is essential, and attending physicians have important roles to play in the implementation of any successful allocation framework.

36.4 Evaluation of Possible Allocation Criteria

36.4.1 First-come, First-serve

When used as a primary criterion, first-come, first-serve undermines the goal of saving lives. Such a policy would lead to preventable deaths when early-arriving patients, unlikely to survive even with ventilation, receive priority treatment over later-arriving patients more likely to survive with ventilation.

As a secondary (tie-breaking) criterion, first-come, first-serve advantages those with the means to travel to hospitals with the space to accommodate them. There is nothing morally wrong with traveling to a hospital with empty beds, but the people who arrive first should not necessarily maintain "highest priority" status if resources do become scarce.

36.4.2 Lottery

As a primary criterion, a pure lottery system would give everyone an equal chance to receive access to scarce therapy. In this way, it facilitates a certain form of fairness. It is worth noting, however, that this does not imply that non-lottery systems are unfair. Here, it is worth distinguishing between the "total" or even "metaphysical" fairness of a lottery system, and a more practical, everyday sense of fairness. This latter sense is expressed in our best examples of equitable hiring practices, for example, or in genuine meritocracies. For example, there may be some sense in which it is "unfair" that not everyone is tall and skillful enough play professional basketball, but this is not grounds for a genuine ethical complaint that the NBA's draft process is unfair in the everyday sense of the concept.

A lottery process removes bias, but does so at the expense of precision. If used as a primary criterion, it would lead to unnecessary deaths when patients likely to survive with ventilator support lose lotteries to patients unlikely to survive even with therapy. As a final tiebreaker, however, lotteries retain the virtue of removing bias, and offer a sense of closure.

36.4.3 Age

Using age as an allocation criterion reflects the widely shared intuition that younger people who have not had the chance to experience life's major stages should be given the chance to do so [2]. On the other hand, using age as a criterion discriminates against older patients.

Some might argue that using age as a primary criterion increases the chances that patients who are more likely to benefit from treatment actually receive it. But if this is one's goal, then mortality risk would make more sense than age as a primary criterion. The reason is straightforward: some younger people are less healthy than some older people, and so age is at best a rough proxy for mortality risk. For example, the prognosis of a healthy 60-year-old may be much better than that of an unhealthy 45-year-old.

36.4.4 Mortality Risk

The use of purely clinical factors, objective measures of a patient's risk of death with and without treatment, as primary allocation criteria can provide a sense of fairness by eliminating explicit consideration of non-medical factors including age and occupation. The use of defined clinical factors also reflects the understandable concern to save as many lives as possible, although, as we have seen, this goal requires ethical limits. The primary reason to use mortality risk to make allocation decisions is simple: inefficient use of scarce resources will result in needless death. It would be wasteful to use scarce ventilators on patients who would be likely to survive even without ventilation, or on patients who would not survive even with ventilator support. The use of mortality risk as a primary criterion guides triage officers to make decisions based on clinical data, helping them to make the most efficient use of scarce resources. It prevents doctors from having to pursue treatments likely to be ineffective, or from letting patients die when a more effectual distribution of resources would have allowed them to live.

Those who opt to use mortality risk as a criterion must decide how to measure it. Here, we survey two options: short-term morality risk—the likelihood that a patient will survive his or her current hospitalization, and long-term mortality risk—the likelihood that a patient will survive for a year after receiving treatment.

36.4.5 Long-term Mortality Risk

A scheme that uses long-term mortality risk as a primary criterion would privilege those patients who would be likely to survive for at least one year *if and only if* they received access to a ventilator. The use of long-term mortality risk as a primary criterion helps to ease the intuitive pressure against allocating resources to those likely to die within a year of receiving treatment at the expense of those likely to survive beyond a year. However, the use of long-term mortality risk as a criterion raises various ethical issues. Perhaps most glaring is the fact that such a scheme could entrench unjustifiable disparities in health. Using such a framework, patients with comorbid conditions would be less likely than patients without comorbid conditions to receive access to ventilators. The development of comorbid conditions is strongly linked with poverty, poor access to healthy food, poor access to health care, and other social factors [3]. An allocation policy that favored patients with low long-term mortality risk would widen the gulf between the well-served and the under-served.

This is a serious concern, and one that cannot be adequately addressed in ventilator allocation policy alone. While we must be willing to admit that the use of long-term mortality risk will entrench health disparities, we need not conclude that this settles the question of whether long-term mortality risk is an ethically acceptable allocation criterion. Perhaps the wrong of allowing healthier patients to die in order to save the lives of patients likely to die within a year outweighs the wrong of deepening disparities in health. On the other hand, we have seen that simply maximizing the number of life-years saved cannot be the only goal of allocation policy, and so appealing to longevity alone would also be insufficient to justify the use of mortality risk as a primary allocation criterion.

36.4.6   Short-term Mortality Risk

The use of short-term mortality risk significantly mitigates the risk of deepening unjustifiable health disparities. The aspiration of a scheme that relied on short-term clinical outlook as a primary criterion would be to allocate resources to those patients who would be likely to survive their current hospitalizations *if and only if* they received therapy. A framework that accomplished this goal would not serve to entrench health disparities by disadvantaging a patient with comorbid conditions *unless* those conditions made it the case that the patient would be unlikely to survive his current hospitalization *even if* he received ventilator access. Indeed, if members of marginalized groups are more likely to become infected and seriously ill, they may be more likely to be members of the patient cohort that a such a framework would favor (patients who would survive their current hospitalization if and only if they received treatment).

On the other hand, a policy that only considered short-term mortality risk would allow for a form of inefficiency because it would fail to maximize the number of life-years saved. One might argue that a young person very likely to live a full life after a short time on a ventilator should receive a higher priority than an older, sicker person likely to die within a year of receiving ventilatory support.

36.4.7   Health Care Worker Status

Use of health care worker status as a primary allocation criterion would lead to unnecessary death if a health care worker received priority despite being likely to die even after receiving access to a ventilator. In such cases, both the health care worker and the patient the health care worker supplanted would be unlikely to survive their hospitalizations. This problem would not arise, however, if health care worker status served as a secondary criterion, used only to break ties between ventilator candidates whose clinical pictures were on a par.

One argument in favor of using health care worker status as an allocation criterion is that health care workers *earn* priority as a reward for, or as insurance against, the risk they undertake in the name of the public good during a crisis. Another is that health care workers have tremendous instrumental value to life-saving efforts. The first argument is backward-looking: it focuses on what we owe to health care workers given contributions and sacrifices they have already made. The second argument is forward-looking. Because it is based on the instrumental value of health care workers in the future, it depends on the two assumptions: first, that health care workers are genuinely scarce, and, second, that health care workers who receive ventilation will regain the strength to return to work during the crisis.

Both arguments raise questions about the definition of "health care worker." Should this category be understood to cover EMTs and physicians' assistants, for example? What about medical students? What about custodians who sanitize hospital rooms? The answer may depend on one's justification for using health care worker status as a criterion in the first place. Students just beginning medical school, for example, may have high future instrumental value but not yet have "earned" priority by placing themselves in harm's way. Hospital custodians have placed themselves in harm's way but may be relatively easier to replace and therefore not as instrumentally valuable to future life-saving efforts.

The question of who counts as a health care worker leads naturally to a more general question: if priority is based on having placed oneself in harm's way, or on future instrumental value, why limit it to health care workers? Firefighters, for example, endanger themselves and make sacrifices in the name of the public good every day; educators, scientists, and a wide range of essential employees may have high future instrumental value.

36.4.8   Other Patients Requiring Ventilation

Thousands of people require chronic ventilation either in private homes or nursing facilities. Earlier, we briefly discussed arguments for and against seizing chronic-use ventilators in the name of maximizing total lives saved, but the ethics of long-term ventilation during a crisis go beyond this vision of extreme utilitarianism. Indeed, one might argue that patients who rely on chronic ventilation should receive priority treatment when they leave their permanent residences and present to hospitals during ventilator shortages. Such patients have come to rely on ventilation to such an extent that their ventilators may take on the status of body parts [7]. To deprive them of ventilation, according to such a view, could amount to a serious violation.

Opponents of affording priority to patients who require chronic ventilation might reject the thesis that a ventilator can take on the status of a body part, or might appeal to the fact that the hospital's ventilator is a different ventilator from the long-term machine that may have acquired body-part status. Such opponents might argue that hospitals ought to treat all patients equally regardless of whether they require chronic ventilation or not. Moreover, they might note that giving patients who require chronic ventilation priority would lead to unnecessary death if chronic-ventilator status served as a primary criterion. If a ventilator were allotted to such a patient who was not likely to live even with treatment, a person likely to survive with ventilation would be at risk of preventable death. These arguments would also apply to the question of whether hospital patients who require ventilation acutely, but for reasons unrelated to the crisis, ought to be subject to triage guidelines along with newly-arriving patients.

36.4.9   Operationalizing Allocation Guidelines

Addressing the above points and determining what ethical principles are priorities as well as what criteria to use for allocation are critical in the structure of ventilator allocation guidelines. However, even after these considerations have been addressed, health care institutions must face the equally significant challenge of operationalizing the guidelines. Issues related to avoiding bias, assessing and communicating mortality risk, determining when, how, and where triage teams should meet, and minimizing triage team burnout must be addressed even after the creation of a defensible framework.

36.4.10 How/Where/When do Triage Teams Meet?

During a pandemic, working remotely can minimize disease propagation in the community. Meeting on a video-based internet platform is likely the safest way to meet, but the security of the platform must be considered.

Institutions must also decide how frequently the teams will meet. If there is only one clinical score collected daily on each patient, should the triage teams meet once a day at a structured time? Or does it make more sense to meet when needed, when a new patient is determined to require ventilation? We recommend the former (a structured once-daily meeting) in order to minimize the risk of burnout of the triage teams. Such difficult decisions will likely lead to moral injury of the triage team members even in the best scenario and minimizing repeated meetings and disruptions to home life and sleep is ideal.

Additionally, in order to mitigate the possibility of burnout and depression from the anxiety of participating in such life-and-death decision-making, having a structured and regular debriefing for triage team members is advisable. Hospital therapists, chaplains, and others should develop a plan to optimize wellness in this group as early as possible.

36.4.11 Calculating the Objective Mortality Risk Score

It is of critical importance that all demographic and other identifying information be separated from objective scoring for triage in order to eliminate bias. To this end, triage team members should not be the individuals collecting data for the scoring system, either at the bedside or in the electronic medical record. One such mortality risk score used is the Modified Sequential Organ Failure Assessment (MSOFA) (see Table 36.2) [8]. The MSOFA includes evaluating severity of end organ disease by measuring respiratory function (SpOx/FiO2), liver function (presence or absence of scleral icterus/jaundice), cardiovascular function (hypotension, requirement of vasoactive medications), central nervous system function (Glasgow Coma Score), and renal function (creatinine). There are also other such scales, and regardless of which assessment tool is utilized, it would stand to reason that the clinical bedside team would collect those data to calculate the MSOFA (or other tool) score of each patient and deliver them to the triage team, but with large volumes of patients being considered and a resulting large number of doctors and midlevel running teams to

Table 36.2 Modified sequential organ failure assessment score [8]

Organ system	0	1	2	3	4
Respiratory SpO$_2$/FiO$_2$	>400	≤400	≤315	≤235	≤150
Liver	No scleral icterus or jaundice			Scleral icterus or jaundice	
Cardiovascular, hypotension	No hypotension	MAP < 70 mm Hg	Dopamine ≤ 5 or dobutamine, any dose	Dopamine > 5, epinephrine ≤ 0.1, norepinephrine ≤0.1	Dopamine > 15, epinephrine > 0.1, norepinephrine > 0.1
CNS, Glasgow Coma Scale	15	13–14	10–12	6–9	<6
Renal, creatinine, mg/dL	<1.2	1.2–1.9	2.0–3.4	3.5–4.9	>5.0

Dopamine, dobutamine, epinephrine, and norepinephrine doses in micrograms per kilogram per minute. CNS, central nervous system: MAP, mean arterial pressure

Reprinted with permission from Cambridge University Press

take care of them, a very simple and straightforward mechanism must be in place to facilitate 100% compliance with routine score collection.

What is "routine score calculation"? Should each patient have one score calculated every day at the time of rounds, or should every ventilated patient's score be calculated only when a new patient requires a ventilator? It is impractical to think that the medical teams can retrieve the data to calculate scores on demand. Although the MSOFA scores may be dynamic based on changes in clinical status, it is much more reasonable to have a once-daily calculation resulting in a once-daily triage team meeting. If new patients require ventilation after that meeting, then their scores should be calculated and compared to the scores that were calculated earlier that day in order to allocate as appropriate (see Fig. 36.1).

One challenge of having the medical rounding teams collect the scores is facilitating good communication between the medical and triage teams. Ideally, an app (none currently available) would allow the medical team to enter data on a specific patient, which is then anonymized and made available to the triage team. The goal would be for the triage team to have sequential scores on the same patients in order

Step 2 – Mortality Risk Assessment Using SOFA[1]	
Color Code and Level of Access	**Assessment of Mortality Risk/ Organ Failure**
Blue No ventilator provided. Use alternative forms of medical intervention and/or palliative care or discharge. Reassess if ventilators become available.	Exclusion criterion OR SOFA > 11
Red Highest Use ventilators as available	SOFA < 7 OR Single organ failure[2]
Yellow Intermediate Use ventilators as available	SOFA 8 – 11
Green Use alternative forms of medical intervention or defer or discharge. Reassess as needed.	No significant organ failure AND/OR No requirement for lifesaving resources

[1]If a patient develops a condition on the exclusion criteria list at any time from the initial assessment to the 48 hour assessment, change color code to blue. Remove the patient from the ventilator and provide alternative forms of medical intervention and/or palliative care.
[2]Intubation for control of the airway (without lung disease) is not considered lung failure.

Fig. 36.1 Triage chart for Step 2 [1]. A triage officer/committee allocates ventilators according to the color code assigned. (Source: New York State Department of Health Task Force on Life and the Law. November 2015. {Public domain})

to track their progress, and so the app would need to have patient identifiers on the rounding team's side to allow them to enter data on the right patients that would then correspond only to a "subject number" that is anonymized on the triage team side.

36.4.12 Comorbid and Frailty Indexes

In the case of the New York State Ventilator Allocation Guidelines as well as other structured allocation policies, the SOFA (sequential organ failure assessment) score is utilized to initially evaluate all patients. Above we described a similar, but more readily calculable score, the MSOFA. With COVID-19, there are several other comorbidities not accounted for in the SOFA/MSOFA score that have been found to coincide with worse outcomes. Based on these findings, an institution may decide to employ a comorbidity index or a frailty index that incorporates poor prognostic comorbidities into short or long-term mortality assessments. One such example of a frailty index is the modified frailty index 5 (mFI-5) [9]. The comorbitidies included on mFI-5 are diabetes mellitus requiring medication, hypertension requiring medication, functional status (dependency), history of COPD or pneumonia, and history of congestive heart failure within 30 days. If a comorbidity index is used, it would need to be carefully selected to reflect comorbidities that are known to minimize the success of mechanical ventilation in a given patient population. Additionally, institutions would need to decide whether to use such an index as the primary triage criterion or as a tiebreaker. And, as we noted above, institutions should keep in mind that while the use of these indices can maximize preservation of life-years, it can also exacerbate pre-existing health disparities insofar as patients with comorbid conditions necessarily receive lower scores.

Cases

To review and revisit the case that started our discussion:

- *Patient 1*: 25 years old, known intravenous drug abuser, HIV-positive with high viral load, nonadherent with medications, multiple prior visits to the trauma bay for penetrating wounds associated with gang violence
- *Patient 2*: 55 years old, obese, hypertension, poorly controlled type 2 diabetes, pastor, volunteer at the local food bank, single father of three adopted children
- *Patient 3*: 75 years old, retired cardiologist, runs half-marathons, plays golf on weekends, still attends medical grand rounds every week at the hospital, very active with medical student and resident education.

All three patients are being maintained on high-flow oxygen but are worsening. How should the ventilator be allocated? Should only one of these candidates get a ventilator, or should all currently ventilated patients be reassessed for their likelihood of successful extubation and evaluated alongside the three new patients?

A MSOFA or SOFA score should be calculated on each patient based on their end organ function, and a blinded triage team should triage the patients accordingly into the appropriate color-coded risk category. Following this, if there are any ties, we would advocate either going to a lottery system or to calculate a 5-item mFI and determine the patient most likely to benefit from the ventilator based on these criteria. As mentioned previously, utilizing a direct lottery following a tied MSOFA/SOFA is one way of minimizing the known disparities in healthcare leading up to the hospitalization that are known to disproportionately affect minority patients.

36.5 Conclusion

In developing a justifiable plan for distributing scarce ventilators during overwhelming crisis, institutions must determine the goals of their resource allocation frameworks, select specific allocation criteria, establish triage teams, and determine how to effectively implement their guidelines. The needs and capabilities of institutions will vary widely, but understanding the ethical principles, arguments, and ideals at issue is critical to responsible decision-making at the hospital, community, and state levels.

36.6 Selected References

- Persad G, Wertheimer A, Emanuel EJ. Principles for allocation of scarce medical interventions. Lancet. 2009;373(9661):423–431. https://doi.org/10.1016/s0140-6736(09)60137-9

  – Helpfully outlines various possible allocation criteria and defends the influential "whole lives" model of allocation.

- Antommaria AHM, Gibb TS, McGuire AL, et al; for a Task Force of the Association of Bioethics Program Directors. Ventilator triage policies during the COVID-19 pandemic at U.S. Hospitals associated with members of the Association of Bioethics Program Directors. Ann Intern Med. 2020;173:188–194. https://doi.org/10.7326/m20-1738

  – Summary and analysis of ventilator triage policies developed by bioethicists at major US hospitals during the Covid-19 pandemic.

- Emanuel EJ, Persad G, Upshur R, et al. Fair allocation of scarce medical resources in the time of Covid-19. N Engl J Med. 2020;382:2049–2055. https://doi.org/10.1056/nejmsb2005114

  - Overview of values that might guide an ethical allocation policy that offers recommendations specific to the context of the Covid-19 pandemic.

References

1. New York State Task Force on Life and the Law. Ventilator allocation guidelines. New York State Dept of Health; 2015.
2. Persad G, Wertheimer A, Emanuel EJ. Principles for allocation of scarce medical interventions. Lancet. 2009;373(9661):423–31. https://doi.org/10.1016/s0140-6736(09)60137-9.
3. Graham H. Social determinants and their unequal distribution: clarifying policy understandings. Milbank Q. 2004;82(1):101–24. https://doi.org/10.1111/j.0887-378x.2004.00303.x.
4. Hausman DM. Valuing health: a new proposal. Health Econ. 2010;19(3):280–96. https://doi.org/10.1002/hec.1474.
5. Antommaria AHM, Gibb TS, McGuire AL, et al; for a Task Force of the Association of Bioethics Program Directors. Ventilator triage policies during the COVID-19 Pandemic at U.S. Hospitals associated with members of the Association of Bioethics Program Directors. Ann Intern Med. 2020;173:188–194. https://doi.org/10.7326/m20-1738
6. Emanuel EJ, Persad G, Upshur R, et al. Fair allocation of scarce medical resources in the time of Covid-19. N Engl J Med. 2020;382:2049–55. https://doi.org/10.1056/nejmsb2005114.
7. Preester HD, Tsakiris M. Body-extension versus body-incorporation: is there a need for a body-model? Phenomenol Cogn Sci. 2009;8:307–19. https://doi.org/10.1007/s11097-009-9121-y.
8. Grissom CK, Brown SM, Kuttler KG, et al. A modified sequential organ failure assessment score for critical care triage. Disaster Med Public Health Prep. 2010;4:277–84. https://doi.org/10.1001/dmp.2010.40.
9. Subramaniam S, Aalberg JJ, Soriano RP, Divino CM. New 5-factor modified frailty index using American College of Surgeons NSQIP data. J Am Coll Surg. 2018;226(2):173–181.e8. https://doi.org/10.1016/j.jamcollsurg.2017.11.005

Part IX
Do Not Resuscitate/Palliative Care/End of Life

Chapter 37
Peri-Operative DNR: An Ethical Dilemma

Michael Shapiro ⓘ, Eric A. Singer ⓘ, and Pringl Miller ⓘ

Abstract Patients with pre-existing "Do Not Resuscitate (DNR)" orders are increasingly candidates for palliative surgical procedures. Many surgeons and anesthesiologists are uncomfortable operating on a patient with a DNR order in effect. Thus, there has been a long tradition of suspending DNR orders when patients undergo anesthesia for surgery, but this may not align with the patient's goals of care. Respect for the patient's autonomy requires a multidisciplinary exploration of the patient's goals and values, and a discussion of how the circumstances of a cardiac arrest in the operating room may differ. Following such a reconsideration of the DNR order, now required by all of the involved societies, the patient may choose to maintain, suspend, or modify their DNR order.

Keywords DNR · Suspension of DNR · Required reconsideration · Resuscitation
Anesthesia · Perioperative care · Goals of care · Autonomy · Palliative surgery
Surgical palliative care

M. Shapiro (✉)
Department of Surgery, Rutgers New Jersey Medical School, University Hospital,
Newark, NJ, USA
e-mail: Michael.shapiro@rutgers.edu

E. A. Singer
Section of Urologic Oncology, Rutgers Cancer Institute of New Jersey and Rutgers Robert
Wood Johnson Medical School, New Brunswick, NJ, USA

P. Miller
Department of Medical Education, Physician Just Equity, San Francisco, CA, USA

© The Author(s), under exclusive license to Springer Nature   521
Switzerland AG 2022
V. A. Lonchyna et al. (eds.), *Difficult Decisions in Surgical Ethics*, Difficult
Decisions in Surgery: An Evidence-Based Approach,
https://doi.org/10.1007/978-3-030-84625-1_37

Case

Mr. P was a 72-year-old man four years status post a colectomy for colorectal cancer who was recently diagnosed with recurrent nonresectable colorectal cancer metastasis. He suffered a new sub-trochanteric hip fracture after tripping over his grandchild's toy in the yard. There was no evidence that the hip fracture was pathological. Mr. P's metastatic disease was otherwise stable on chemo and biologic therapy. The orthopedic surgeon recommended operative stabilization of the fracture to enable continued mobility and quality of life. Mr. P had an advance directive (AD) that included a "Do Not Resuscitate (DNR)" order, and a DNR order was entered into his electronic medical record (EMR) upon admission. Mr. P favored surgery to confer the best possible functional status for the future, recognizing that the recovery process would be difficult and that his postoperative function may not return to baseline. However, he wished to maintain his DNR order should he have a cardio-pulmonary arrest that was not considered to be rapidly reversible perioperatively. The patient's family is concerned that adhering to his AD might deprive them of quality time with him.

37.1   Introduction

The case presented above has become a common clinical scenario on surgical services posing recurrent ethical dilemmas as our population ages with increasing frailty, and may lead to confusion, frustration, moral distress, and conflict between surgeons, anesthesiologists, nurses, patients, and their families. In the United States, an estimated 15% of end-of-life patients with a DNR order may be scheduled for surgery or interventional procedures [1–4]. This occurrence may introduce tensions around honoring patient autonomy, providing beneficent care, avoiding non-maleficent care, and acting justly. Within the goals of palliative surgery these ethical principles should align with gaining time, improving quality of life, decreasing pain, or treating isolated problems such as fractures [5]. Patients presenting for surgical care with a DNR order often create confusion for the surgical team [6] and anesthesiologists frequently face moral distress when they provide anesthesia care to patients with DNR orders [7]. The optimal start to this case is a multidisciplinary approach to the question, an understanding of the development and proper role of attempted resuscitation in the delivery of care, and an exploration of how such interventions may, or may not, comport with the patient's goals of care. Ultimately, it is the surgeon's responsibility to help patients work through a decision that will provide them with "their" best outcome.

37.2 Search Strategy

PubMed was searched for English language publications using the key words: DNR, Suspension of DNR, Required Reconsideration, Resuscitation, Anesthesia, Perioperative Care, Goals of Care, Autonomy, Palliative Surgery, and Surgical Palliative Care. Manuscripts published in high impact journals representing surgery, anesthesiology, and nursing perspectives were sought out.

37.3 Discussion

While there are many ways to evaluate ethical issues, the four principles of autonomy, beneficence, nonmaleficence, and justice are a common lens through which to view an ethical dilemma (see Table 37.1). Most ethical dilemmas are not simply a matter of choosing "right" over "wrong" but have to do with recognizing and resolving conflicting principles or obligations. In the case above, how does the care team simultaneously respect a patient's wishes (autonomy) while ensuring the best outcome (beneficence) and avoiding harm (nonmaleficence) and the equitable

Table 37.1 Ethical principles as applied to a DNR case

Ethical principle	Peri-operative DNR case application
Autonomy	As proposed by Cohen and Cohen[*], the standard of care for shared-decision making for surgical patients with pre-existing DNR orders is a discussion called "required reconsideration". A required reconsideration discussion is explicitly designed to honor a patient's autonomy and right to maintain a DNR order perioperatively. By exploring a patient's rationale for having their DNR order to begin with as well as their current treatment preferences, goals, and values, surgeons can gain critical information that informs whether to council a patient to maintain or suspend their DNR order perioperatively. [*]Cohen CB, Cohen PJ. "Required Reconsideration of 'Do-not-resuscitate" Orders in the Operating Room and Certain Other Treatments." *Law, Medicine, and Heath Care*. 1992;20(4):354–363.
Beneficence	Required reconsideration discussions provide a framework that seeks to align each patient's preferences, goals, and values with the care delivered. Without dedicated discussions about the benefits and burdens of a perioperative DNR order, surgical care can deviate from the principle of beneficence and patient-centered care.
Non-maleficence	In order to avoid inflicting unnecessary harm on patients during the perioperative period, required reconsideration discussions should provide surgeons the necessary information that supports a patient's preferences, goals, and values aligning perioperative care accordingly.
Justice	All patients deserve receiving the standard of care and evidence based-practice options. Required reconsideration has become the professional ethical standard of care for establishing what is in the patient's best interests regarding their pre-existing DNR order during the perioperative period.

treatment of similar patients in need (justice)? We will explore options to resolve these conflicting obligations below.

37.3.1   History of Cardiopulmonary Resuscitation (CPR)

The ability to treat cardiac arrest caused by arrythmia became possible with the advent of external cardiac pacing and defibrillation in the 1950s [8–10]. While defibrillation could temporarily cause the return of spontaneous circulation (ROSC), survival to hospital discharge was rare [8]. Most importantly, defibrillation was only successful when initiated soon after the onset of the arrhythmia, making the operating room, with its constant monitoring of heart rhythm and vital signs, the environment where defibrillation could have the greatest efficacy.

37.3.2   Contemporary Experience
with Cardiopulmonary Resuscitation

While ROSC is obtained in approximately 40% of patients, only one patient in 10 will live long enough to be discharged from the hospital [9–12]. Sepsis within 24 hours, cancer, metastatic cancer, dementia, African American race, serum creatinine ≥ 1.5 mg/dL, and coronary artery disease were factors associated with a failure to survive to hospital discharge [11]. American College of Surgeons (ACS)-National Surgical Quality Improvement Program data between 2005–2010 demonstrated that 85.9% of cardiopulmonary events in surgical patients occurred postoperatively, varying by specialty (1 in 33 for cardiac surgery vs 1 in 258 for general surgery). 70% of patients died within 30 days postoperatively [13]. Kalkman et al. similarly published that in the perioperative setting the survival rate after cardiopulmonary resuscitation is approximately 25% [14] with 45–66% of survivors experiencing a favorable neurologic outcome, defined as being able to live independent lives with or without mild neurologic impairments (quality survival) [15–17]. However, other reports have indicated that few of those survivors live longer than five years, many suffering from significant neurological disability, requiring chronic institutional care that fails to restore independent living. As expected, younger patients with fewer comorbidities who experience a witnessed ventricular fibrillation arrest that is promptly treated with defibrillation have higher survival rates [18].

37.3.3   An Unintended Consequence of Cardiopulmonary Resuscitation

Through the 1960s and 70s, with the development of standardized techniques, CPR became routine *therapy* for any patient who died in the hospital, including those for whom cardiac arrest was the predicted terminal event of a dying process. In 1974, the American Medical Association recommended that decisions not to resuscitate be entered into the medical record, and communicated to all attending staff, to avoid confusion and moral distress on the part of hospital staff [19]. Then, in 1976, the first hospital policy concerning "orders not to resuscitate" was published by Rabkin et al. [20] Although the policy recognized the "growing concern that it may be inappropriate to apply technologic capabilities to the fullest extent in all cases and without limitation," it nonetheless erred on the side of intervention, stating, "it is the general policy of hospitals to act affirmatively to preserve the life of all patients, including patients who suffer from irreversible terminal illness." The policy thus mandated attempts at resuscitation in all patients without a DNR order, creating the perverse outcome in which resuscitation became the only medical intervention requiring a medical order *not* to be performed. Increasingly, however, this default position is being questioned, even in the lay literature [21].

37.3.4   Popular Perception and the Medical Reality of CPR Outcomes

Unfortunately, the majority of the lay public obtain their understanding about CPR from popular media, e.g., television, where the outcome of attempted resuscitation is far better than in real life. For example, one study found that 75 percent of TV patients who receive CPR are alive immediately after, and 67 percent of patients survive in the long term [22]. Patients and families tend to have unrealistic expectations about the utility of CPR relative to their loved one's goals and functional expectations, over-estimating its benefit, and under-estimating its associative morbidity. A recent study of patients and their companions in the emergency department waiting area of a tertiary care hospital found the majority of those surveyed estimated that the success rate of CPR was over 75% in all situations [23]. Patients may make decisions about their preference for CPR based on incorrect data, and not in accord with their goals and preferences [23].

37.3.5 DNR Orders Should Be Discussed in the Context of Goals of Care

Much of the confusion concerning executing DNR orders results from considering this decision in isolation (i.e., "I don't want to die"), rather than as a part of a holistic discussion of a patient's overall goals of care in their particular health circumstances (i.e., "I have terminal disease and want to minimize my suffering"). The right that a patient has to direct their healthcare decisions stems from the ethical principle and legal precedents that honor patient autonomy and the right of persons for self-determination respectively.

37.3.6 Self Determination and the Right to Refuse Life-Prolonging Treatment

The legal basis for the patient's right to refuse unwanted medical treatment, and the duty for clinicians to provide informed consent, derives, in the US, from an opinion by Benjamin Cardozo in 1914, *Schloendorff v. Society of New York Hospital*: "Every human being of adult years and sound mind has a right to determine what shall be done with *his* own body; and a surgeon who performs an operation without *his* patient's consent commits an assault for which *he* is liable for damages. This is true except in cases of emergency where the patient is unconscious and where it is necessary to operate before consent can be obtained" [24].

The right of patient self-determination in deciding to refuse medical treatment was extended in 1976 (the same year as the first hospital policy regarding DNR was published [21]) by the New Jersey Supreme Court in the case of Karen Ann Quinlan, a 21-year-old woman in a persistent vegetative state. Her father petitioned the court to be appointed her guardian so that he could remove her from the ventilator and withdraw unwanted life-sustaining medical treatment. *In the Matter of Karen Ann Quinlan*, the court recognized a legal right of privacy permitting a patient (or their legal agent) to refuse medical treatment, even if the patient should die as a result [25].

The ethical concept of patient autonomy became further elucidated in 1977 by the publication of *Principles of Biomedical Ethics* by Beauchamp and Childress and and *The Belmont Report* in 1979. *The Belmont Report*, written by the National Commission for the Protection of Human Subjects of Biomedical and Behavioral Research, established guidelines for basic ethical principles to protect human subjects in biomedical and behavioral research conducted in the US. The report described the ethical principles of "respect for persons (beneficence, and justice)" [26]. They defined "an autonomous person as an individual capable of deliberation about personal goals, and of acting under the direction of such deliberation." They further noted that "to repudiate a person's considered judgments, to deny an individual the freedom to act on those considered judgments, or to withhold information necessary to make a considered judgment" showed a lack of respect for a person's autonomy [26].

Beachamp and Childress proposed four principles that guide ethical decision-making: autonomy, beneficence, non-maleficence and justice [27]. Although these principles are considered to be of equal value, patient autonomy has clearly become the predominant consideration. In fact, it has been suggested that the tyranny of physician beneficence has been replaced by the tyranny of patient autonomy [28]. It is clear that patient goals are critically important in making patient-concordant medical decisions. The role of the patient in providing direction to their healthcare provider in the form of an advance directive was enshrined in law in the 1990 Patient Self-Determination Act [29].

Respect for patient autonomy requires more than solely providing patients (and families) with factual information and then leaving decision-making to them without the benefit of expert guidance. As noted by Emanuel and Emanuel [30], this approach (which they call the "informative model") "assumes the patient's values are well-defined and known, and that the clinician's values, or the clinician's interpretation of the patient's values, have no place in medical decision-making". Recognizing that many patients have not thought deeply about their values, or how those values might direct their medical decision-making, the Emanuel's instead advocate for a "deliberative model," where the physician's role is to assist the patient in recognizing and defining goals and values appropriate to their clinical situation, and then using those goals and values to help patients reach an appropriate medical decision. The surgeon is thus guiding, not coercing, the patient in their development of goals and values relative to the information available facilitating healthcare decisions that uphold their values.

37.3.7   When Is Maintaining a Perioperative DNR Appropriate?

Before exploring the question of DNR in the OR, it is necessary to understand why a patient might choose, or a physician recommend, a DNR order in general. This, of course, requires an understanding of the patient's values and goals of care. It also requires acknowledgement that a DNR order does not mean "do not treat" or "do not care." It does mean that, in the event of a cardiac or respiratory arrest, within the context of low likelihood of preserved acceptable quality of life there will be no attempt at resuscitation, thereby allowing a natural death to proceed. Respect for patient autonomy recognizes the patient's right to refuse unwanted interventions that might interfere with a natural death and one that has the potential to be less painful, harmful, and more peaceful. Survey data informs us that most patients prefer to die painless peaceful deaths, when possible, at home surrounded by loved ones. It is incumbent upon us as surgeons who care for seriously ill patients to provide guidance in clinical decision making that is best aligned with a patient's preferences, goals, and values. Cardiac arrest is the final common pathway of any dying process. A DNR order should not be interpreted as a patient desiring death or that the patient "is giving up". A DNR order often represents a rational and well-reasoned decision based on the acceptance of death and the wish not to prolong the dying process. A DNR order is merely the manifestation of this understanding in the best of circumstances with a patient who has decision making capacity or their designated surrogate. It is imperative that when practicing within the ethical principles of care that autonomy, beneficence, non-maleficence, and justice be applied at the end of life. [31] Unfortunately, in our highly medicalized culture clinicians have not done the best job normalizing death as a natural occurrence of life. Our death defying and denying society makes it difficult for surgeons to engage in preparedness planning in a way that is transparent and supportive. With the knowledge that surgeons have—namely that an attempt at resuscitation merely prolongs the dying process and increases suffering, rather than prolonging a meaningful life (from the patient's perspective), surgeons have an ethical obligation to share their knowledge with patients in order to adjust their expectations and find a care plan that honors their dignity at the end of life. To avoid transparent discussions that often counter what is understood by popular media is inconsistent with the ethical principle of beneficence and might be viewed as maleficent. The vast majority of patients who die in the hospital do so with an existing DNR order, and review of these cases failed to find any ethical objections in those patients [32, 33]. Briefly, there are three situations in which a DNR decision is appropriate [34]:

- When a patient makes an informed decision to decline CPR
- In those situations where CPR is known to be nonbeneficial
- When the physician and patient (or designated surrogate decision maker) recognize the burdens of CPR would outweigh the benefits.

In order for patients and surrogate decision makers to make patient-centered decisions, it is imperative to provide realistic information and paint a picture of the best and worst-case scenario so that they can picture themselves on the other end of an unsuccessful resuscitation. Breaking bad news is a skill to be developed because no one likes to deliver unfavorable information due to the risk of upsetting patients. Research tells us that patients prefer honesty and transparency and that honesty and transparency promote trust in the patient-physician relationship. Given that most patients prefer to be told directly what their prognosis is, surgeons need to learn how to articulate specifics about the natural history of a disease, the anticipated outcome of CPR, the probability of a successful resuscitative effort, survival to hospital discharge, the morbidity associated with CPR (including anoxic brain injury and blunt physical trauma), and the reality of how attempted CPR will impact future quality of life. When patients are properly informed about the process of CPR and the expected outcomes, many opt out of receiving CPR [35].

A not so infrequent ethical dilemma that arises in surgical practice is the tension when surgeons articulate that CPR is likely to be nonbeneficial but the patient or their designated surrogate decision maker disagrees and insists on being resuscitated. In this scenario it has been suggested that a sham attempt at resuscitation may actually be beneficial for the patient and family by providing "symbolic comfort", even when likely to fail, or even cause harm to the patient [36]. One author has suggested that it is appropriate to perform CPR on a patient who "might already be dead" for the psychological benefit of the grieving family [37], though this has been widely criticized [38].

37.4 Perioperative DNR Orders Still Elicit Tension Despite Clear Professional Guidelines

37.4.1 Society Guidelines and Position Statements

The issue of DNR orders during anesthesia for surgery was first raised by Truog in 1991 [39]. He noted at that time that few, if any, hospitals had specific policies regarding DNR orders in the OR; those few that did required automatic suspension of the patient's DNR order. There are several reasons why suspension of a DNR order might be appropriate during anesthesia; these include the inherent risk of induction of anesthesia, which often necessitates interventions associated with resuscitation (intubation, paralytics, inotropic medications). It then becomes important to define the meaning of DNR—does it mean only no chest compressions or defibrillation? Herein lies the confusion implicit in where "maintaining homeostasis" in a critically ill patient ends and "resuscitation" begins. Secondly, witnessed cardiac arrests occurring during an intervention are more easily reversed, with better survival than those occurring on the ward [40]. Finally, Truog noted that the presence of a DNR order might alter the anesthetic approach used, providing less than optimal anesthesia in an attempt to maintain stability. For all these reasons, Truog concluded that it may be appropriate to suspend a DNR order in the peri-operative period, but that rigid policies regarding the management of DNR orders would be contrary to the concept of patient autonomy.

From an ethical perspective, then, to honor patient autonomy would call into question automatic suspension of a pre-existing DNR order unless that decision was shared by the patient. For the patient who desires to proceed with surgery in which an alternative form of anesthesia is not possible, unilateral clinician suspension of a pre-existing DNR would be paternalistic, potentially coercive, and not necessarily aligned with patient centered care.

The first official professional society statement focused on the issue of perioperative DNR followed Truog's sentinel paper. The American Society of Anesthesiologists (ASA) first issued in 1993 ethical guidelines for perioperative DNR orders. This statement was updated and revised in 2018 [41]. Similarly, professional society statements on perioperative DNR were published by the American College of Surgeons (ACS) [42] and the Association of periOperative

Registered Nurses (AORN) [43]. These professional society statements collectively represent a consensual guideline that mandatory suspension of a DNR order perioperatively is unethical. Furthermore, each statement reinforces the ethical requirement proposed by Cohen and Cohen for principal clinicians to have a required reconsideration discussion with the patient or their surrogate decision maker [44]. This ethical responsibility usually lies with the attending surgeon and anesthesiologist, preferably as a team at the same time to explain issues related to the administration of anesthesia and the proposed procedure, and to clarify the patient's wishes regarding the DNR order perioperatively. The patient or their surrogate decision maker would then have the opportunity to suspend the DNR order, maintain the DNR order, or provide details of their preferences regarding specific aspects of and reasons for resuscitation (e.g., if extubation is not possible withdraw life-sustaining medical treatment, or if cardiac arrest caused by an easily remediable problem, please attempt resuscitation; otherwise, please do not attempt resuscitation). Integral to the preoperative DNR decision for suspension is the duration for which the suspension will last. The required reconsideration discussion must include the patient's preferences for how long they would want to be subjected to resuscitative efforts and life-sustaining medical therapy during the postoperative period. In most cases, the suspension would extend through the post-anesthesia care unit (PACU). However, for some patients who recover in the intensive care unit due to prolonged mechanical ventilation the duration of life support might last longer whether intended or unintended [45] which is why a discussion about expectations, goals, values and preferences is critical preoperatively. Understanding that said expectations, goals, values and preferences may change over time, this discussion or series of discussions must then be clearly documented in the patient's electronic medical record, so that all members of the treatment team are informed of the parameters of patient centered care. Not all treatment team members will necessarily feel comfortable with a perioperative DNR order, it is therefore important to recognize and plan for the potential that members of the treatment team might need to be replaced due to a moral, ethical, or conscientious objection. Such individuals must be permitted to withdraw from their involvement in the case without penalty and be replaced with an alternate equally qualified team member [41, 42, 43].

Despite uniform agreement among the key operative professional societies since the early 1990s, almost 30 years ago, adopting these professional society position statements encouraging a "required reconsideration" discussion has been slow to permeate clinical practice. Anesthesia residency programs surveyed between 1991 and 1997, with subsequent follow-up, noted the percentage that had DNR policies, and mandated suspension, dropped from 81% to 26% [46]. A significant number of those still with mandated suspension had not revised their policies following the ASA 1993 Ethical Guidelines [41].

Unfortunately, even today it is not uncommon for surgeons to be approached by OR nursing or anesthesia staff about a DNR order with the expectation that it would be automatically suspended before the patient goes to the OR, even in hospitals that have perioperative DNR policies to the contrary. Further, many surgical trainees and surgeons believe the required pre-operative conversation exists merely to inform the patient they need to suspend their DNR.

In a 2013 study of patient and doctor attitudes, the patient response rate was 84% and 92% of the patients believed a discussion about perioperative resuscitation plans should occur between the doctor and the patient [47]. Over half of the patients (57%) agreed that pre-existing DNR requests should be suspended while undergoing a surgical procedure with anesthesia. The response rate for anesthesiologists and surgeons was 53% and 22% respectively. Thirty percent of respondents believed that DNR orders should be automatically suspended intraoperatively. Fifty-two percent disagreed with that practice while 17% were unsure. Anesthesiologists (18%) were significantly less likely to unilaterally suspend DNR orders than surgeons (38%). In a scenario-based assessment, 54% of doctors were unlikely to follow the patient's DNR request, while 28% were likely to comply and 18% were unsure. After completing a general question assessment regarding perioperative DNR, over half (55%) agreed that DNR requests were illogical during surgical procedures (anesthesiologists 54% surgeons 75%). Half of all doctor respondents agreed with the statement that intraoperative DNR orders should be respected because resuscitative issues are based on a patient's value system rather than doctor preferences. What survey data has revealed over time beginning before perioperative DNR guidelines until the present is that anesthesiologists have changed their attitudes and beliefs more dramatically in favor of patient autonomy than have surgeons despite very similar professional society guidelines [48].

As the frequency of perioperative DNR scenarios increases, we must integrate an ethical and palliative care approach to cases like Mr. P's. An intentional exploration of how attempted resuscitation during perioperative care may, or may not, comport with the patient's values and goals of care is essential [49]. By collaborating with all treatment team members, confusion, frustration and moral distress can be prevented. Similarly, from a clinical medical ethics perspective, surgeons should respect the dignity and autonomy of patients and honor the right of the patient with decision making capacity to choose among treatments, including those that may or may not prolong life [49].

37.4.2 Integrating Required Reconsideration into Ethical Surgical Practice

How then, does one ascertain the patient's goals of care, and apply them to the question of DNR in the operating room? Although patient autonomy may be the principal driver of this process, goals must be medically realistic, balancing beneficence, non-maleficence and justice. Further, while patients may refuse unwanted interventions, they do not have the right to insist on medically unindicated procedures. Surgeons are not obligated to offer patients unindicated and nonbeneficial treatment and should refuse inappropriate requests [49].

There is an extensive literature describing how to conduct a structured goals of care discussion [50–52], which is beyond the scope of this discussion.

As noted previously, helping patients define their values and express their goals of care requires an exploration [53], and often assistance in their recognition of their values and care preferences [30]. For some patients, this may be a preference to extend life, regardless of perceived quality or prolonged suffering. Other patients may value cognitive ability, or avoidance of suffering. For some patients, these are issues they may not have previously considered in depth, or even actively avoided. A nuanced understanding of the patient's values will allow the surgeon and anesthesiologist to have a meaningful discussion of appropriate perioperative interventions and ultimately identify the primary goals of care from the patient's perspective so that the surgeon's care can achieve the patient's objectives [49]. Ideally, these discussions should be held with the patient's support system present, so they can also listen to the patient and understand the issues of importance, always taking into account cultural norms and preferences.

All too often, the approach to interventions in the ICU and operating room have been "procedure-directed," using a checklist approach to which procedures (e.g., intubation, chest-compression, defibrillation) may be used [46]. Such an approach is simple, particularly with frequent hand-offs between clinicians, and does not require a real understanding of the patient's values and goals. A "goal-directed" approach, on the other hand, while requiring a more detailed and thoughtful discussion with the patient, permits the care team to tailor their response to the preferences of the patient in any particular situation [46, 54]. Thus, for a patient who values cognitive ability over all else, the OR team might treat a quickly reversible cause of cardiac arrest, while recognizing that extended resuscitation efforts are not compatible with the patient's wishes. Those treatment decisions would be different if the team understood the patient valued life over all other considerations, or, at the other extreme, considered their current life conditions intolerable.

37.5   Case Conclusion

How, then, might one structure an appropriate goals of care discussion for Mr. P? The discussion needs to occur with enough time to allow for reflection—in the OR holding area there is not enough time nor is the location appropriate. Ideally, one would like the principal members of the operative team, the attending surgeon and anesthesiologist responsible for the care of the patient, to be present together during this required reconsideration discussion. Other important contributors may include the patient's primary nurse, and members of the palliative care team including pastoral care, if the patient desires that. Mr. P's family, or at least his healthcare surrogate decision maker, should also be present. If all relevant members of the team cannot meet together, there must be a mechanism to communicate the discussion to those not present, but it is preferable for all team members to provide information, and to hear the same thing from the patient together. The goal is to come to an understanding of the patient's values, not to impose values on them.

When the meeting was held with Mr. P, he noted that his quality of life was currently acceptable, but he also came to recognize that he was going to die from his cancer and accepted that. He was concerned that later in his disease process he may have a great deal of discomfort, which he would like to avoid. Thus, should he suffer an intra-operative arrest, he does not want attempts at resuscitation to bring him back only to confront more suffering in the future. It was explained to him that cardiopulmonary arrests in the OR are often more easily reversed than elsewhere, and the palliative care team explained options for pain control, should pain become a burdensome symptom in the future. After carefully considering all the information provided, Mr. P elected to maintain his DNR status throughout the perioperative period. His fracture was repaired without incident, and he was discharged to a rehabilitation facility in a timely manner.

37.6   Concluding Remarks

CPR is merely one intervention of many designed to help patients to achieve their goals of care. It is not appropriately viewed as a stand-alone, yes or no decision, but is more usefully discussed in the context of the patient's overall values and goals of care. A DNR order in the perioperative period is a unique circumstance, given the effects of anesthetic agents, surgical interventions and continuous monitoring, and thus requires a separate discussion called *Required Reconsideration* [44, 55]. Important concepts include advocating for patient autonomy in making a well-informed shared decision with the treatment team, maximizing beneficence, as viewed by both the patient and their caregivers, and minimizing the opportunity for confusion, misunderstanding and maleficent care improving patient satisfaction and reducing adverse outcomes. It is also important to recognize disabilities, language barriers, cultural preferences, and health equity in goals of care discussions again honoring the ethical principles of autonomy, beneficence, non-maleficence and justice.

37.7   Selected References

- Cohen CB, Cohen PJ. Required Reconsideration of 'Do-not-resuscitate' Orders in the Operating Room and Certain Other Treatments. Law Med Health Care. 1992;20 [4]:354–363. doi:https://doi.org/10.1111/j.1748-720x.1992.tb01216.x

  - The authors established "required reconsideration" as the optimal mechanism for respecting patient autonomy while enabling the provision of invasive or high-risk procedures.

- American Society of Anesthesiologists. Committee on Ethics. Ethical Guidelines for the anesthesia care of patients with do-not-resuscitate (DNR) orders or other directives that limit treatment. Approved by the ASA House of Delegates, reaffirmed October 17, 2018. Accessed January 21, 2021. https://www.asahq.org/standards-and-guidelines/ethical-guidelines-for-the-anesthesia-care-of-patients-with-do-not-resuscitate-orders-or-other-directives-that-limit-treatment
- American College of Surgeons. Committee on Ethics. Statement of the American College of Surgeons on advance directives by patients: 'do not resuscitate' in the operating room. 2014. Accessed January 21, 2021. https://www.facs.org/about-acs/statements/19-advance-directives
- Association of periOperative Registered Nurses. Perioperative care of patients with do-not-resuscitate (DNR) orders. 1994. Accessed April 26, 2021. https://www.aorn.org/guidelines/clinical-resources/position-statements

  - These three references demonstrate important alignment between the professional societies representing surgeons, anesthesiologists, and perioperative nurses and their unanimity that the automatic suspension of DNR orders is unethical. Required reconsideration of advance directives should be considered the standard of care.

References

1. Association of periOperative Registered Nurses. AORN Position Statement on Perioperative Care of Patients with Do-Not-Resuscitate Orders. 2020. Accessed January 24, 2021. https://www.aorn.org/guidelines/clinical-resources/position-statements.
2. ECRI. Do-Not-Resuscitate Orders. Health System Risk Management. February 2, 2018. Accessed January 24, 2021. https://www.ecri.org/search-results/member-preview/hrc/pages/eth3.
3. La Puma J, Silverstein MD, Stocking CB, Roland D, Siegler M. Life-sustaining treatment. A prospective study of patients with DNR orders in a teaching hospital. Arch Intern Med. 1988;148(10):2193–8. https://doi.org/10.1001/archinte.1988.00380100067015.
4. Scott TH, Gavrin JR. Palliative surgery in the do-not-resuscitate patient: ethics and practical suggestions for management. Anesthesiol Clin. 2012;30(1):1–12. https://doi.org/10.1016/j.anclin.2012.02.001.
5. Guarisco KK. Managing do-not-resuscitate orders in the perianesthesia period. J Perianesth Nurs. 2004;19(5):300–7. https://doi.org/10.1016/j.jopan.2004.08.002.
6. Ball KA. Do-not-resuscitate orders in surgery: decreasing the confusion. AORN J. 2009;89(1):140–50. https://doi.org/10.1016/j.aorn.2008.10.001.
7. Truog RD, Waisel DB. Do-not-resuscitate orders: from the ward to the operating room; from procedures to goals. Int Anesthesiol Clin. 2001;39(3):53–65.
8. Zoll PM. Resuscitation of the heart in ventricular standstill by external electric stimulation. N Engl J Med. 1952;247(20):768–71. https://doi.org/10.1056/nejm195211132472005.
9. Zoll PM, Linenthal AJ, Gibson W, Paul MH, Norman LR. Termination of ventricular fibrillation in man by externally applied electric countershock. N Engl J Med. 1956;254(16):727–32. https://doi.org/10.1056/nejm195604192541601.

10. Lown B, Neuman J, Amarasingham R, Berkovits B. Comparison of alternating current with direct current electroshock across the closed chest. Am J Cardiology. 1962;10:223–33. https://doi.org/10.1016/0002-9149(62)90299-0.
11. Ebell MH, Becker LA, Barry HC, Hagen M. Survival after in-hospital cardiopulmonary resuscitation. A meta-analysis J Gen Intern Med. 1998;13:805–16. https://doi.org/10.1046/j.1525-1487.1998.00244.x.
12. Peberdy MA, Ornato JP, Larkin GLL, et al. For National Registry of cardiopulmonary resuscitation investigators. Survival from in-hospital cardiac arrest during nights and weekends. JAMA. 2008;299(7):785–92. https://doi.org/10.1001/jama.299.7.785.
13. Kazaure HS, Roman SA, Rosenthal RA, Sosa JA. Cardiac arrest among surgical patients: an analysis of incidence, patient characteristics, and outcomes in ACS-NSQIP. JAMA Surg. 2013;148(1):14–21. https://doi.org/10.1001/jamasurg.2013.671.
14. Kalkman S, Hooft L, Meijerman JM, Knape JTA, van Delden JJM. Survival after perioperative cardiopulmonary resuscitation: providing an evidence base for ethical management of do-not-resuscitate orders. Anesthesiol. 2016;124(3):723–9. https://doi.org/10.1097/aln.0000000000000873.
15. Constant A, Montlahuc C, Grimaldi D, et al. Predictors of functional outcome after intraoperative cardiac arrest. Anesthesiol. 2014;121(3):482–91. https://doi.org/10.1097/aln.0000000000000313.
16. Ramachandrans K, Mhyre J, Kheterpal S, et al. For the American Heart Association's get with the guidelines-resuscitation investigators. Predictors of survival from perioperative cardiopulmonary arrests: a retrospective analysis of 2,524 events from the get with the guidelines – resuscitation registry. Anesthesiol. 2013;119(6):1322–39. https://doi.org/10.1097/aln.0b013e318289bafe.
17. Braz LG, Braz JRC, Módolo NSP, Nascimento PD Jr, Shuhama AP, Navarro LHC. Cardiac arrest during anesthesia at a tertiary teaching hospital: prospective survey from 1996 to 2002 [in Portugese]. Rev Bras Anestesiol. 2004;54(6):755–68. https://doi.org/10.1590/s0034-70943004000600002.
18. Andersen LW, Holmberg MJ, Berg KM, Donnino MW, Granfeldt A. In hospital cardiac arrest: a review. JAMA. 2019;321(12):1200–10. https://doi.org/10.1001/jama.2019.1696.
19. Standards for cardiopulmonary resuscitation (CPR) and emergency cardiac care (ECC). V. Medicolegal considerations and recommendations. JAMA. 1974;227(7 Suppl):864–6. https://doi.org/10.1001/jama.227.7.833.
20. Rabkin MT, Gillerman G, Rice NR. Orders not to resuscitate. N Engl J Med. 1976;295(7):364–6. https://doi.org/10.1056/nejm197608122950705.
21. Span P. CPR, by default. *New York Times*. January 31, 2020. Accessed April 25, 2021. https://www.nytimes.com/2020/01/31/health/cpr-elderly.html.
22. Diem SJ, Lantos JD, Tulsky JA. Cardiopulmonary resuscitation on television – miracles and misinformation. N Engl J Med. 1996;334(24):1578–82. https://doi.org/10.1056/nejm199606133342406.
23. Bandolin NS, Huang W, Beckett L, Wintemute G. Perspectives of emergency department attendees on outcomes of resuscitation efforts: origins and impact on cardiopulmonary resuscitation preference. Emerg Med J. 2020;37(10):611–6. https://doi.org/10.1136/emermed-2018-208084.
24. *Schloendorff v. Society of New York Hospital*. 211 N.Y. 125, 105 N.E. 92 (1914).
25. *In Re Quinlan*. 70 N.J. 10 (1976). 355 A.2d 647.
26. National Commission for the Protection of Human Subjects of Biomedical and Behavioral Research. *The Belmont Report: Ethical Principles and Guidelines for the Protection of Human Subjects of Research*. US Government Printing Office; 1979.
27. Beachamp TL, Childress JF. Principles of biomedical ethics. 8th ed. Oxford University Press; 2019.
28. Schneider CE. The practice of autonomy: patients, doctors and medical decisions. Oxford University Press; 1998.

29. The Patient Self-Determination Act. Omnibus Budget Reconciliation Act of 1990. Public Law No. 101–508. §§ 4206 & 4751, 104 Stat. 1388–115 & 1388–204.
30. Emanuel EJ, Emanuel LL. Four models of the physician-patient relationship. JAMA. 1992;267(16):2221–6. https://doi.org/10.1001/jama.1992.03480160079038.
31. Burns JP, Truog RD. The DNR order after 40 years. N Engl J Med. 2016;375(6):504–6. https://doi.org/10.1056/nejmp1605597.
32. Aune S, Herlitz J, Bang A. Characteristics of patients who die in hospital with no attempt at resuscitation. Resuscitation. 2005;65(3):291–9. https://doi.org/10.1016/j.resuscitation.2004.11.028.
33. Fritz Z, Heywood R, Moffat S, Bradshaw L, Fuld J. Characteristics and outcome of patients with DNACPR orders in an acute hospital: an observational study. Resuscitation. 2014;85(1):104–8. https://doi.org/10.1016/j.resuscitation.2013.08.012.
34. Mockford C, Fritz Z, George R, et al. Do not attempt cardiopulmonary resuscitation (DNACPR) orders: a systematic review of the barriers and facilitators of decision-making and implementation. Resuscitation. 2015;88(3):99–113. https://doi.org/10.1016/j.resuscitation.2014.11.016.
35. Schonwetter RS, Walker RM, Kramer DR, Robinson BE. Resuscitation decision making in the elderly: the value of outcome data. J Gen Intern Med. 1993;8(6):295–300. https://doi.org/10.1007/bf02600139.
36. Bremer A, Sandman L. Futile cardiopulmonary resuscitation for the benefit of others: an ethical analysis. Nurs Ethics. 2011;18(4):495–504. https://doi.org/10.1177/0969733011404339.
37. Truog RD. Is it always wrong to perform futile CPR? N Engl J Med. 2010;362(6):477–9. https://doi.org/10.1056/nejmp0908464.
38. Paris JJ, Angelos P, Schreiber MD. Does compassion for a family justify providing futile CPR? J Perinatol. 2010;30:770–2. https://doi.org/10.1038/jp.2010.105.
39. Truog RD. Do-not-resuscitate orders during anesthesia and surgery. Anesthesiol. 1991;74(3):606–8. 2001038.
40. Peatfield RC, Sillett RW, Taylor D, McNichol MW. Survival after cardiac arrest in hospital. Lancet. 1977;309(8024):1223–5. https://doi.org/10.1016/s0140-6736(77)92435-7.
41. American Society of Anesthesiologists. Committee on Ethics. Ethical Guidelines for the anesthesia care of patients with do-not-resuscitate (DNR) orders or other directives that limit treatment. Approved by the ASA House of Delegates, reaffirmed October 17, 2018. Accessed January 21, 2021. https://www.asahq.org/standards-and-guidelines/ethical-guidelines-for-the-anesthesia-care-of-patients-with-do-not-resuscitate-orders-or-other-directives-that-limit-treatment.
42. American College of Surgeons. Committee on Ethics. Statement of the American College of Surgeons on advance directives by patients: 'do not resuscitate' in the operating room. 2014. Accessed January 21, 2021. https://www.facs.org/about-acs/statements/19-advance-directives.
43. Association of periOperative Registered Nurses. Perioperative care of patients with do-not-resuscitate (DNR) orders. 1994. Accessed April 26, 2021. https://www.aorn.org/guidelines/clinical-resources/position-statements.
44. Cohen CB, Cohen PJ. Required reconsideration of 'do-not-resuscitate' orders in the operating room and certain other treatments. Law Med Health Care. 1992;20(4):354–63. https://doi.org/10.1111/j.1748-720x.1992.tb01216.x.
45. Clemency MV, Thompson NJ. Do not resuscitate orders in the perioperative period: patient perspectives. Anesth Analg. 1997;84(4):859–64.
46. Truog RD, Waisel DB, Burns JP. DNR in the OR: a goal-directed approach. Anesthesiol. 1999;90(1):289–95. https://doi.org/10.1097/00000542-199901000-00034.
47. Burkle CM, Swetz KM, Armstrong MH, Keegan MT. Patient and doctor attitudes and beliefs concerning perioperative do not resuscitate orders: anesthesiologists' growing compliance with patient autonomy and self-determination guidelines. BMC Anesthesiol. 2013;13(2) https://doi.org/10.1186/1471-2253-13-2.
48. Kopecky K, Pelletier P, Miller P. Strategies for collaborative consideration of Patient's resuscitation preferences. AMA J Ethics. 2020;22(4):E325–32. https://doi.org/10.1001/amajethics.2020.325.

49. American College of Surgeons. Statement on Principles of Palliative Care. 2005. Accessed on January 24, 2021. https://www.facs.org/about-acs/statements/50-palliative-care.
50. McGreevy C, Kunac A, Chokshi R, Smith JH, Mazza D, Mosenthal AC. Discussing goals of care preoperatively in high-risk oncologic surgery [ASCO Abstract 38]. J Clin Oncol. 2015;33(29, suppl):38. https://doi.org/10.1200/jco.2015.33.29_suppl.38.
51. Kunac A. Shared decision-making and goals-of-care discussion in the preoperative visit. In: Mosenthal AC, Dunn GP, editors. Surgical Palliative Care. Oxford University Press; 2019.
52. Taylor LJ, Nabozny MJ, Steffens NM, et al. A framework to improve surgeon communication in high-stakes surgical decisions: best case/worst case. JAMA Surg. 2017;152(6):531–8. https://doi.org/10.1001/jamasurg.2016.5674.
53. Pellegrino ED. Toward a reconstruction of medical morality. Am J Bioeth. 2006;6(2):65–71. https://doi.org/10.1080/15265160500508601.
54. Jackson SH, Van Norman GA. Goals and values-directed approach to informed consent in the "DNR" patient presenting for surgery: more demanding of the Anesthesiologist? Anesthesiol. 1999;90(1):3–6. https://doi.org/10.1097/00000542-199901000-00003.
55. Shapiro ME, Singer EA. Perioperative advance directives: do not resuscitate in the operating room. Surg Clin N Am. 2019;99(5):859–65. https://doi.org/10.1016/j.suc.2019.06.006.

Chapter 38
Goals of Care with Palliative Surgery

Shuddhadeb Ray (iD), **Douglas Brown, and Piroska Kopar** (iD)

Abstract Almost all surgical procedures have a palliative component to them in that they aim to relieve symptoms of some disease process or injury. Some patients who have life-threatening illnesses or are at the end of their lives may still benefit from surgical procedures, even if the goal of the therapy is not curative. In this chapter, we explore the reasoning prerequisite to offering palliative surgical procedures. The surgeon, the patient, and/or the patient's surrogate may be confused about the goals of care for palliative surgical therapy. The patient's goals of care may change as the disease progresses and curative management may transition into palliative management. It is important to explore goals of care at pivotal decision points with the patient, family members, and friends in a multidisciplinary care setting that ideally includes the patient's primary care physician, relevant specialists, critical care team, and surgeon in order to fully explore all palliative options and set realistic goals and expectations in line with the patient's wishes and values prior to offering palliative surgical therapy.

Keywords Palliative surgery · Surgical ethics · Goals of care · Outcome measures Complications · Surrogate decision-maker

S. Ray (✉)
Department of Surgery, Washington University School of Medicine, St. Louis, MO, USA
e-mail: sray@wustl.edu

D. Brown · P. Kopar
Department of Surgery, Center for Humanism and Ethics in Surgical Specialties, Washington University School of Medicine, St. Louis, MO, USA
e-mail: debrown@wustl.edu; pkopar@wustl.edu

© The Author(s), under exclusive license to Springer Nature Switzerland AG 2022

V. A. Lonchyna et al. (eds.), *Difficult Decisions in Surgical Ethics*, Difficult Decisions in Surgery: An Evidence-Based Approach,
https://doi.org/10.1007/978-3-030-84625-1_38

Search Strategy

Medline, EMBASE, and Google Scholar were searched without filters or language restrictions from inception to July 10th, 2020, using a combination of the terms: palliative care, palliative surgery, palliative goals of care, palliative surgery ethics. 10,369 articles were found in this manner and 40 were screened manually based on relevance to ethics and palliative surgery, and fourteen were chosen as references for this chapter due to relevance.

Case

A 74-year-old male presents to his primary care doctor with abdominal discomfort and unintentional weight loss. Further work-up reveals intermittent blood in his stools. He is referred to gastroenterology. Upper and lower endoscopy is performed and reveals a 3-centimeter mass in his transverse colon that is biopsied and found to be adenocarcinoma. Imaging shows that the tumor has grown through the wall of the colon but staging shows that the patient does not have any evidence of metastatic disease or involved lymph nodes. The patient is referred to a colorectal surgeon who discusses surgical options with the patient. The patient undergoes a partial colectomy with accompanying lymph node dissection and does well post-operatively without the need for adjuvant therapy.

Case continued

The now 76-year-old patient, after his successful prior colon cancer resection, on surveillance imaging, is noted to have a recurrence of a mass at his prior colon resection site. Repeat colonoscopy and biopsy confirms recurrence of colon cancer. Further work-up and cancer staging show no signs of metastatic disease and he is prepared for another operation for possible resection of this local recurrence. At operation, however, small nodules are found throughout the peritoneal cavity without the presence of ascites. Biopsy confirms metastatic disease. The operation is stopped, and the patient is referred for palliative chemotherapy.

38.1 Introduction

Medical and surgical care should strive to address issues beyond the physiologic state of the disease process being treated. Patients who have advanced illness, particularly cancer diagnoses, often suffer from poor symptom control and struggle with medical decision-making. Patients' families may also suffer physically, mentally, and even economically [1]. Attention to palliative care in the United States has increased following the publishing of an Institute of Medicine Report in 1997 that evaluated challenges associated with end of life care [2]. Palliative care is described by the World Health Organization as "an approach that improves the quality of life of patients and their families facing the problems associated with life-threatening illness, through the prevention and relief of suffering by means of early identification and impeccable assessment and treatment of pain and other problems, physical, psychosocial, and spiritual" [3]. By extension, palliative surgery focuses on using surgical procedures as a part of the management plan to reach palliative goals. The goal of palliative surgery is not to cure an ailment, but to ease suffering, including but not limited to when patients are at life's end or are facing a life-threatening illness.

Recently, the role of the surgeon has become more prominent in the palliative care process. The American College of Surgeons (ACS) has defined palliative surgery as "surgical procedures used with the primary intention of improving quality of life or relieving symptoms caused by an advanced disease" [4] and the ACS published a statement of principles of palliative care for its membership (see Table 38.1) [5].

Table 38.1 Statement of principle of palliative care, American College of Surgeons [5]

Statement of principles of palliative care
1. Respect the dignity and autonomy of patients, patients' surrogates, and caregivers.
2. Honor the right of the competent patient or surrogate to choose among treatments, including those that may or may not prolong life.
3. Communicate effectively and empathically with patients, their families, and caregivers.
4. Identify the primary goals of care from the patient's perspective, and address how the surgeon's care can achieve the patient's objectives.
5. Strive to alleviate pain and other burdensome physical and nonphysical symptoms.
6. Recognize, assess, discuss, and offer access to services for psychological, social, and spiritual issues.
7. Provide access to therapeutic support, encompassing the spectrum from life-prolonging treatments through hospice care, when they can realistically be expected to improve the quality of life as perceived by the patient.
8. Recognize the physician's responsibility to discourage treatments that are unlikely to achieve the patient's goals, and encourage patients and families to consider hospice care when the prognosis for survival is likely to be less than a half-year.
9. Arrange for continuity of care by the patient's primary and/or specialist physician, alleviating the sense of abandonment patients may feel when "curative" therapies are no longer useful.
10. Maintain a collegial and supportive attitude toward others entrusted with care of the patient.

The case scenario presented above represents initially treating the patient surgically with a curative intent. It is important to remember that all surgical care has a palliative intent embedded within its care goals. Some part of all surgical care focuses on minimizing symptomatology and suffering. The patient in the scenario above may find relief from his abdominal discomfort, so his symptoms are palliated, and while he does face a possible life-threatening illness, the goal of his initial surgical care is to cure him of his disease and restore him to his prior quality of life. For the purposes of this chapter, we will focus more on how to approach goals of care when the outcome of surgical interventions aim to palliate patient symptoms when there are no surgical options for curing them of a disease.

38.2   What Palliative Surgery Is and Is Not

The second surgery in the case scenario above illustrates a common misconception among surgeons regarding palliative surgery. Surgery with a curative intent in which a tumor is not fully resected, leaving behind residual tumor, is not palliative surgery. A majority of surgical oncologists responding to a 2002 Society of Surgical Oncology survey reflected this mistaken view of 'palliative surgery'. The survey responses revealed that many surgeons equate palliative surgery with non-curative surgery [6].

The patient in the case scenario above had a surgical procedure that may be described as non-curative surgery in that his disease process, colon cancer, could not be cured with his planned surgery. However, he was not palliated of any specific symptoms. It is also important to distinguish palliative surgery from palliative care for surgical patients, which describes attaining the goals of palliative care for patients after they have had surgery but do not need another operation.

Many surgical procedures are considered palliative in that they aid in treating the symptoms of patients at the end of their lives or with life-threatening illnesses. The most common surgical palliation occurs in the care of patients with cancer. Palliative surgical procedures are now routinely included among the therapies offered at comprehensive cancer centers. At one tertiary cancer center, 12.5% of surgical cases could be classified as palliative procedures [7]. In cancer care, surgical procedures may be helpful for cancer-associated pain, bleeding from tumors, obstructions such as intestinal obstructions, and malignant fluid re-accumulations. Specific examples of palliative procedures for cancer patients include:

palliative tumor resection to address bleeding or obstruction such as an obstructing or bleeding gastric cancer

drainage of fluid accumulation as can be seen in metastatic disease to the pleural spaces from a number of cancers, which can also be treated with pleurodesis or placement of an indwelling pleural catheter that can be intermittently drained to aid respiration

intestinal bypass operations to aid obstructions from gastrointestinal malignancies including colon caner cancers amenable to debulking procedures where tumor burden is relieved, which may help symptomatology but does not cure the cancer itself (e.g., therapy for unresectable malignant mesothelioma, multiorgan colorectal cancer metastases, and certain cases of peritoneal carcinomatosis)

Case continued

Our 76-year-old patient with metastatic colon cancer, while undergoing palliative chemotherapy, presents to the emergency room with nausea, vomiting, and increasing abdominal pain and distension. He notes he has not had a bowel movement in 3 days. Cross-sectional imaging shows distended loops of small bowel and mesenteric nodularity likely to be metastatic disease throughout the peritoneal cavity. There is no ascites, and a single transition point is identified with distal small bowel decompression. He is diagnosed with a malignant bowel obstruction and admitted to the hospital. A nasogastric tube is placed for gastrointestinal decompression and combined with anti-emetics to relieve the patient's nausea. The surgeon is consulted to evaluate the patient for possible surgery to relieve his small bowel obstruction. The patient wants to know what his quality of life will be after surgery.

The patient has now presented with a life-threatening complication, quite possibly near the end of his life, with a surgical problem that is difficult to manage. Malignant bowel obstruction represents a particularly problematic decision in that surgery may be able to relieve the patient's obstruction, but then the patient may be confined to care in the hospital for his post-operative care and exhaust many of the few remaining weeks he has to survive. These patients are also often poor candidates for surgery due to malnutrition and deconditioning associated with their gastrointestinal malignancy [8]. This scenario illustrates a common ethical dilemma that must be addressed in a timely fashion by the care team. In current medicine, these patients may be admitted to an oncology service. Additionally, if they are particularly ill, they may be admitted to the intensive care unit with a team of critical care specialists managing their care. Due to advanced illness, a palliative care physician may be consulted to help manage the patient's symptoms and goals of care. The surgeon is added to this multidisciplinary care team, a hallmark of modern medicine, in which physicians and healthcare professionals from multiple fields must coordinate and effectively communicate their care plans to provide the best possible care for the patient.

38.3   Ethical Framework

Multiple care teams are seeing the patient in the above scenario who has a malignant bowel obstruction and is now admitted to the hospital for further management. How is the patient encouraged to trust the care team? The answer lies with each of the

Table 38.2 Core ethical principles and the goals of surgery

Ethical responsibility	Curative/Restorative surgery	Palliative surgery
To avoid additional harm to the patient (i.e., non-maleficence)	Prevent post-operative complications, pain, or functional debility and allow restoration of quality of life acceptable to the patient	Prevent post-operative complications, and prevent further pain or debility brought on by the patient's advanced or terminal disease process
To deliver benefit to the patient (i.e., beneficence)	A recovery of quality of life acceptable to the patient results from a successful surgical intervention.	Pain/suffering no longer undermine the patient's quality of life (or dying) after a successful surgical intervention.
To respect the patient's goals (i.e., patient self-determination)	The patient is discharged with a feasible return to pre-operative quality of life after a successful surgical intervention.	Pain/suffering no longer keep the patient from experiencing a desired quality of life (or dying) after a successful surgical intervention.
To protect the patient from bias (i.e., fairness or justice)	The patient's demographics do not alter the outcome after a successful surgical intervention.	The patient's demographics do not alter the outcome after a successful surgical intervention.

pillars of clinical ethics (see Table 38.2), i.e., beneficence, non-maleficence, self-determination or autonomy, and fairness or justice. The medical team aims to make a positive valued difference in the patient's wellbeing (beneficence) while being careful to avoid harming the patient (non-maleficence), honor the patient's wishes in accordance with their values (autonomy), be free of bias, and good stewards of medical resources (justice or fairness). In addition, the medical and surgical teams must effectively and professionally communicate amongst themselves, and with the patient. The patient must have sufficient time to clarify his preferences, ask questions, and reconsider the focus of care as new information arises or management plans change.

This trust is difficult to establish and fragile. Most patients requiring evaluation for a palliative surgical procedure have a life-threatening condition or are at the end of their lives. They represent a vulnerable patient population, and their families are also vulnerable due to significant stresses on both the patient and family that may be physical, psychological, social, or even economic in nature. These stresses may significantly strain effective communication between the patient and his family, and also with the care team.

The surgeon must weigh a duty to benefit the patient without causing avoidable harm. Surgeons have historically been stereotyped as authoritative and paternalistic, thereby prone to undermine the patient's and the patient's families' autonomy [4]. From a more pragmatic standpoint, the array of surgeries available to the surgeon to help aid the patient can be the source of distrust. Palliative surgical procedures are some of the least studied in the surgical profession. There is scant medical evidence that demonstrates support for many such procedures even though they may theoretically be expected to help alleviate patient symptoms. Thus, palliative procedures are often offered to patients based on the discretion of the surgeon or the palliative care team, creating significant variance in what is offered to patients. This complexity may be further compounded by the care providers' lack of familiarity with existing procedures that may help palliate the patient. Palliative surgeries aid the patient's quality of life and relieve suffering. In some cases, the palliative goal is not achieved, in which case further harm may have been done to that patient. This uncertainty may account for some of the variability in what may or may not be offered to patients in terms of palliative surgical procedures. The potential for miscommunication when multiple medical teams and family members are involved in decision-making for a patient's clinical care is obvious. Palliative care discussions are additionally challenging when the patient, family, or even care givers insist that they want to "do everything". This appeal has different connotations that can lead to significant confusion about the patient's goals of care.

Goals of care may be curative, rehabilitative, life-prolonging, or comfort focused [9]. In this regard, there should be ongoing goals-of-care discussions for all medical and surgical therapies. The point of these patient-centered discussions is to establish the patient's healthcare preferences so that their management remains consistent with their values, with help from family or surrogate decision makers. All surgical procedures that are not emergent are preceded by a discussion with the patient or family/surrogate decision-maker about the risks and benefits of the procedure in an informed consent process. This discussion presents an opportunity for clarification of the patient's goals of care and has the additional benefit of involving all of the same stakeholders in the overall care of the patient including the patient, their family or surrogate decision-maker, the primary care team, the palliative care team, and the surgical team. Medicine necessitates collaboration among these complex, multi-disciplinary care teams. For a patient being evaluated for palliative surgery, management often involves a service such as hospital medicine taking primary care of the patient, with a palliative care service assisting to make recommendations, and with the possible addition of a surgical service to address surgical palliation. It is particularly important that the surgeon approach the patient with a plan in coordination with these other care services to offer therapy that is clear and in line with the patient's values.

38.4   Discussion: Ethical Analysis

The priority of palliative surgery is to reduce pain and suffering. When a consult is sought for a palliative surgical procedure, the most important factor patients consider is the physical impact of uncontrolled symptoms [7]. Secondary decision-altering factors include the social impact of symptoms and maintaining hope. Treatments that in the care team's best professional judgment will not have a reasonable chance of benefiting the patient and will serve only to prolong the dying process or place undue burden on the patient should not be offered, initiated, or continued. Pain and suffering are of course not isolated to the patient. The patient's family and friends often report significant distress linked to the uncertainty of the patient's clinical situation and prognosis.

It is difficult to establish outcome measures by which to define success in palliative surgery. Unlike outcomes measured for curative surgery (e.g., survival or event-free or cancer-free survival), only the patient or patient's family can finally determine the benefit of palliative surgery. Complications after palliative surgeries are common though not numerically defined for all palliative procedures. These complications can significantly limit the palliative effect of the surgery. For cancer patients, a significant postoperative complication following a palliative procedure diminished the chances of symptom resolution to just 17% in a study of 59 patients who underwent palliative surgery for advanced malignancies [10]. While there is no standardized or validated tool to measure outcomes in palliative surgery, there are a few measures currently being used to predict procedural success e.g., the absence of post-operative complications, and the need for prolonged hospitalization. One tool that is favorably reviewed is the Palliative Surgery Outcome Score (PSOS). The PSOS calculates the number of symptom-free, non-hospitalized days as a fraction of the number of post-operative life days (up to 180 days). Both patients and their families have identified a PSOS value of 0.7 as an acceptable positive outcome [11]. This score can be applied to any palliative surgery situation, but the validating study was completed for patients with advanced malignancies. As focus and research on palliative surgery grows, additional tools for reliably and meaningfully measuring outcomes of palliative surgery should emerge.

Prior to any surgical procedure, the surgeon and patient exchange information and preferences in an informed consent process. This process can be particularly complicated prior to palliative procedures. While the details of the informed consent process may vary based on the medical society or group defining the critical steps, most standards include the core elements of: competence and voluntariness of the patient, disclosure of procedural risks and assessment of patient understanding, and a decision or authorization for the procedure to continue [12]. Since the outcomes of palliative procedures remain poorly measured, discussions with patients and families about procedural outcomes often lack medical evidence. Patients requiring palliative surgery are more likely to lack decisional capacity due to their advanced illness. If a patient lacks decisional capacity, an appropriate surrogate (usually but not necessarily a close family member) should assist in the decision making (1) ideally/preferably by representing the patient's known values and goals or (2) if such are not known, then by promoting the patient's best interests. However, the care team is not obligated to adhere to a surrogate's input if the surrogate seems to lack decisional capacity or their decision seems to be contradictory to the patient's expressed values or goals (see Chap. 39). In such circumstances, utilizing Social Services, Spiritual Care (see Chap. 19), the Ethics Committee, and/or Risk Management is strongly encouraged. If no other options exist, the hospital may pursue action through the courts to establish a guardian for the patient. In the case of suspected patient abuse or neglect, the appropriate administrative agency should be notified. The informed consent process provides an opportunity to review and further discuss goals of care for the patient's disease process as a whole and advance directives, beyond just the surgical procedure.

In reviewing goals of care for a patient being assessed for palliative surgery, clarifying what is medically and surgically feasible becomes particularly important.

Patients and their families may see the involvement of a surgeon as new hope for cure or improved chances of survival. Surgeons may be concerned that being frank will risk taking hope away from the patient and family. A survey of physicians about palliative surgery in patients with advanced cancer found that the greatest ethical dilemma for surgeons was providing patients and their families with honest information without destroying hope [13]. Ethically skilled care team members are prepared to move discussions with patients or surrogates toward consensus regarding the patient's outcome/discharge expectations. A patient's expectations may be restoration to preadmission functional status, relief from pain and suffering, survival regardless of quality of life, or survival long enough for desired closure. Quality of life outcomes that may be unacceptable to a patient include being permanently unconscious, being permanently unable to remember or make decisions or recognize loved ones, being permanently bedridden and dependent on others for activities of daily living, being permanently dependent on hemodialysis, or being permanently dependent on artificial nutrition and/or hydration. A 'Goals of Care— Communication Template' (see Table 38.3) can help frame/guide this discussion [14].

The focus of care for most patients is to restore the patient to a level of function compatible with the patient's expectations, with all appropriate therapies being initiated and continued. Not all patients who are assessed for palliative surgery will benefit from a procedure. If the care team concludes that the desired restoration cannot be achieved with surgical palliation, further discussion with the patient and family members is needed in order to reconsider the expectations for the hospitalization. Based on this discussion, current management may not be escalated, additional interventions may not be introduced, and current life-sustaining treatments may be discontinued so as not to place undue burden on the patient. Regardless of the patient's suitability as a surgical candidate, the duty of the care team is to further discuss goals of care (see Chap. 7) and expectations as the situation changes with gradations of palliation. It is important to remember that the surgeon is not merely a technician, but a member of the multidisciplinary care team that must address the patient's needs whether a surgical procedure is planned or not. In some cases, the focus of care should shift to concentration on the patient's comfort during the dying process.

Case Closure

Our 76-year-old patient with metastases and malignant bowel obstruction is seen by the surgeon and discusses the case with the multidisciplinary health care team. The surgeon offers exploratory laparotomy and possible small bowel resection, bypass, or diversion for relief of his obstruction as cross-sectional imaging shows a single transition point. He emphasizes that while the patient's symptoms may be relieved if the surgery is successful, there is an approximate 50% chance of recurrence of his obstruction in the coming month, and the surgeon quotes him a 25–30% risk of mortality in the same time frame. After deliberation with his family, and due to his advanced symptoms, the patient decides to undergo surgery. During surgery, the patient's small bowel obstruction is treated with short-segment small bowel resection and primary anastomosis. The patient recovers in the following week, has minor drainage from his surgical wound, is able to restart per oral intake, and is discharged home with opioids for pain control.

Approximately five weeks later, he presents once again to the hospital with another small bowel obstruction. His symptoms are partially relieved with insertion of a nasogastric tube. The palliative care team sees him once again along with the surgeon. The surgeon this time does not recommend redo surgery because it is unlikely to help him symptomatically and is even a higher risk than the first time around. The patient and his family are thankful for the past month he was able to spend with them, but now they decide to forego any further invasive interventions. The medical care team controls his symptoms with a combination of nasogastric drainage, anti-emetics, pain medications, and anti-secretory agents. He goes home with hospice care where he passes away approximately one week later.

Table 38.3 Goals of Care—Communication Template [14]

<u>**PART A: Document Goals of Care**</u>

Based upon comprehensive discussion between the patient _____ (or surrogate) and the treating physician, the following explanation best describes the patient's current goals of care:

_____

EXAMPLES include but are not limited to: "return to prior living situation at previous functional status" or "return to prior living situation after physical therapy" or "remain in my home" or "be free of pain or breathlessness" or "maintain my privacy and dignity" or "be able to interact with my loved ones" or "attend my granddaughter's graduation".

NOTE: "Do everything" is NOT a goal of care. Ask the patient (or surrogate) what 'everything' is intended to achieve.

NOTE: To set realistic goals, the patient (or surrogate) needs a clear description of what to expect.

Discuss and document if the patient wants aggressive **life-support measures** stopped and wants treatment instead to focus on comfort and dignity if any one or combination of the following is the most likely outcome:

_____ being permanently unconscious (i.e., completely unaware of surroundings with no chance of regaining consciousness)

_____ being permanently unable to remember, understand, make decisions, recognize loved ones, have conversations

_____ being permanently bedridden and completely dependent on the assistance of others to accomplish daily activities (e.g., eating, bathing, dressing, moving)

_____ being permanently dependent on mechanical ventilation

_____ being permanently dependent on hemodialysis

_____ being permanently dependent on artificial nutrition (tube feedings) and/or intravenous hydration for survival

_____ death likely to occur within days to weeks and treatments are only prolonging the dying process

_____ other(specify): _____

_____

Table 38.3 (continued)

PART B: Document Focus of Care
Based upon the above understanding of the patient's goals of care: □ The focus of care will be to restore the patient to a level of function compatible with the goals outlined above. Specific testing and treatments will be ordered by the patient's physicians with the intent to achieve these goals. □ The focus of care will concentrate on the patient's comfort. Treatments that serve only to prolong the process of dying or place undue burden on the patient will not be initiated or continued.
PART C: Recommend Resuscitation Status

1. Based on the current condition, prognosis and comorbidities, and on weighing likely benefits, harms and goals outlined above --
   A. The treating physician **does / does not (circle one)** recommend <u>CPR</u> in the event of cardiac arrest.
   B. The treating physician **does / does not (circle one)** recommend <u>intubation</u> in the event of impending respiratory arrest.
   C. The treating physician at this time **cannot make a definitive recommendation(circle)** regarding CPR or intubation.
2. These recommendations have been discussed with the patient (or surrogate) with reassurance that if resuscitation is not performed, treatment will be provided with the goal of comfort and dignity: **Yes / No**
3. For the patient (or surrogate) who decides to be resuscitated (i.e., Code 1) despite the treating physician's recommendation against such, the treating physician has discussed the likely immediate consequences of CPR if successful: **Yes / No**
4. **Person with whom to speak if the patient lacks decisional capacity:**
Name: _____ Relation: _____
Phone Number: _____

38.5   Conclusion

Palliative surgery continues to grow as an essential component of comprehensive palliative care services. The success of a palliative surgical procedure is difficult to measure in quantitative terms, leaving the final assessment to the patient or their family members. The ethically sound delivery of palliative care including palliative surgical procedures requires a multidisciplinary care team that effectively communicates and delivers procedural options and outcomes aligned with the patient's preferences and values.

Acknowledgement   We thank Drs. Laureen Hill and Johnathan Green for their participation in the development of Table 38.3: 'Goals of Care—Communication Template'.

38.6   Selected References

- Dunn GP. Palliating patients who have unresectable colorectal cancer: creating the right framework and salient symptom management. Surg Clin. 2006;86(4):1065–92. https://doi.org/10.1016/j.suc.2006.05.008.

  – The author, a colorectal surgeon and palliative care specialist, describes the work-up and palliation of patients with unresectable colorectal cancer. Barriers to proper palliation, a comprehensive multidisciplinary approach to palliative needs assessment, and different models to deliver palliation are discussed. How specific symptoms may be addressed, including appropriate surgical therapies and how to assess the needs of the patient's family are detailed.

- Krouse RS, Nelson RA, Farrell BR, et al. Surgical palliation at a cancer center: incidence and outcomes. Arch Surg. 2001;136(7):773–8. https://doi.org/10.1001/archsurg.136.7.773.

  – This is a retrospective review of surgeries at a NCI-designated comprehensive cancer center over a one year period with a one year follow-up. They enumerate the indications, risks, and outcomes of surgical interventions on cancer patients. A significant portion of these procedures, 12.5% (240 of 1915), are completed with palliative rather than curative intent.

- Hofmann B, Håheim LL, Søreide JA. Ethics of palliative surgery in patients with cancer. Br J Surg. 2005;92(7):802–9. https://doi.org/10.1002/bjs.5104.

  – The authors go beyond the clinical decision-making process for patients with advanced malignancies that may benefit from palliative surgery and explore the moral and ethical challenges these situations present. These challenges are analyzed in terms of the core ethical principles describing respect for patient autonomy, 'duty to help', benevolence, and delivering proper information to patients. The lack of a standardized vocabulary and limited clinical evidence to guide the discussion about palliative procedures provides additional methodological and moral challenges.

- McCahill LE, Krouse RS, Chu DZJ, et al. Decision making in palliative surgery. J Am Coll Surg. 2002;195(3):411–22; discussion 422–3. https://doi.org/10.1016/s1072-7515(02)01306-6.

  – A survey of 110 questions consisting of case vignettes evaluated how surgeons selected treatment for symptomatic patients with advanced malignancies and what ethical dilemmas they encounter in the act. The most common ethical dilemmas were providing patients with honest information without destroying hope and preserving patient choice. The most common barriers were referral to surgery by other specialists and limitations imposed by managed care.

References

1. Dunn GP. Palliating patients who have unresectable colorectal cancer: creating the right framework and salient symptom management. Surg Clin. 2006;86(4):1065–92. https://doi.org/10.1016/j.suc.2006.05.008.
2. Institute of Medicine (US) Committee on Care at the End of Life. Approaching death: improving care at the end of life (Field MJ, Cassel CK, editors). National Academies Press (US); 1997. http://www.ncbi.nlm.nih.gov/books/NBK233605/. Accessed 16 Oct 2020.
3. World Health Organization. Palliative care. WHO; August 5, 2020. https://www.who.int/cancer/palliative/definition/en/. Accessed 16 Oct 2020.
4. Dunn GP, Martensen R, Weissman D. Surgical palliative care: a resident's guide. American College of Surgeons; 2009. https://www.facs.org/~/media/files/education/palliativecare/surgicalpalliativecareresidents.ashx. Accessed 25 Oct 2020
5. American College of Surgeons. Statement of principles of palliative care. American College of Surgeons; August 10, 2005. https://www.facs.org/about-acs/statements/50-palliative-care. Accessed 25 Oct 2020.
6. McCahill LE, Krouse R, Chu D, et al. Indications and use of palliative surgery-results of Society of Surgical Oncology survey. Ann Surg Oncol. 2002;9(1):104–12. https://doi.org/10.1245/aso.2002.9.1.104.
7. Krouse RS, Nelson RA, Farrell BR, et al. Surgical palliation at a cancer center: incidence and outcomes. Arch Surg. 2001;136(7):773–8. https://doi.org/10.1001/archsurg.136.7.773.
8. Paul Olson TJ, Pinkerton C, Brasel KJ, Schwarze ML. Palliative surgery for malignant bowel obstruction from carcinomatosis: a systematic review. JAMA Surg. 2014;149(4):383–92. https://doi.org/10.1001/jamasurg.2013.4059.
9. The Joint Commission. Goals of Care. In: Specifications Manual for Joint Commission National Quality Measures (v2018A). The Joint Commission; 2018. https://manual.jointcommission.org/releases/TJC2018A/DataElem0708.html. Accessed 25 Oct 2020.
10. Hofmann B, Håheim LL, Søreide JA. Ethics of palliative surgery in patients with cancer. Br J Surg. 2005;92(7):802–9. https://doi.org/10.1002/bjs.5104.
11. McCahill LE, Smith DD, Borneman T, et al. A prospective evaluation of palliative outcomes for surgery of advanced malignancies. Ann Surg Oncol. 2003;10(6):654–63. https://doi.org/10.1245/aso.2003.06.011.
12. Beauchamp TL, Childress JF. Principles of biomedical ethics. 8th ed. Oxford University Press; 2019.
13. McCahill LE, Krouse RS, Chu DZJ, et al. Decision making in palliative surgery. J Am Coll Surg. 2002;195(3):411–22; discussion 422–3. https://doi.org/10.1016/s1072-7515(02)01306-6.
14. Brown D. Surgical ethics: theory and practice background. In: Ferreres AR, editor. Surgical ethics: principles and practice. Switzerland: Springer Nature; 2019. p. 27–43. https://doi.org/10.1007/978-3-030-05964-4_3.

Chapter 39
Ethical Conflicts in Surrogate Decision Making

Leah Conant ⓘ and Piroska Kopar ⓘ

Abstract Once patients are too sick to make healthcare decisions for themselves, this task is relegated to their surrogate decision makers. Because of the complexity and ever-changing nature of these decisions, it is not surprising that conflicts arise between various stakeholders in this process. Furthermore, the variability of state law on surrogate decision making may further cloud decision-making, ultimately delaying, and sometimes undermining, patient care. This chapter examines the nature and causes of conflicts in surrogate decision making, outlines the ethical dilemmas embedded therein, and offers an overview of practically useful approaches to the resolution of ethically challenging surrogate decision making.

Keywords Surrogate decision-making · Conflict in medical decisions
End-of-life care · Palliative care · Goals of care

> **Case**
> Mrs. S, a 69-year-old woman, was admitted to the intensive care unit with COPD exacerbation after undergoing an exploratory laparotomy with lysis of adhesions for a small bowel obstruction. Her medical history included coronary artery disease with multiple cardiac stent placements. The most recent echocardiogram showed severe mitral regurgitation. Her COPD exacerbation

L. Conant
Washington University in Saint Louis School of Medicine, Saint Louis, MO, USA
e-mail: lconant@wustl.edu

P. Kopar (✉)
Department of Surgery, Center for Humanism and Ethics in Surgical Specialties, Washington University in St. Louis School of Medicine, St. Louis, MO, USA
e-mail: pkopar@wustl.edu

© The Author(s), under exclusive license to Springer Nature Switzerland AG 2022
V. A. Lonchyna et al. (eds.), *Difficult Decisions in Surgical Ethics*, Difficult Decisions in Surgery: An Evidence-Based Approach,
https://doi.org/10.1007/978-3-030-84625-1_39

became complicated by a ventilator associated pneumonia and she went into acute cardiac failure resulting in multiorgan system dysfunction. Her renal function worsened acutely, and she developed liver failure. A family meeting was held in which the attending surgeon relayed her own personal conversation with the patient prior to her intubation, according to which the patient did not want to pursue aggressive life prolonging measures. The family present included the patient's elderly mother and daughter-in-law. The patient's son was available by telephone only. Applicable state laws did not specify a hierarchy for surrogates, but all three involved family members wanted to press on with life-prolonging measures despite the physician's hesitation in offering them.

39.1   Introduction

While the doctor–patient relationship is well established historically, professionally, and legally, the relationship of the physician to the patient's family is less well delineated. Surrogate decision makers are asked to exercise substituted judgment when making medical decisions for their loved ones based on their intimate knowledge of the sick person's values. Paradoxically, it is precisely this closeness that sometimes creates a conflict of interest and confuses the decision-making process (see Table 39.1). It can be psychologically taxing to separate one's own wishes for a loved one from the wishes of the patient (1).

Although under most circumstances the goals of the patient and her family align seamlessly, when the patient is no longer able to make decisions for herself, the question arises—"What do we, as physicians, owe our patients' families?" Palliative care, as defined by the World Health Organization, aims to provide care for both the

Table 39.1 Elements of ethics and their application to patients without decision making capacity

Elements of Ethics	Autonomy	Beneficience	Nonmaleficence	Justice
	When approached with difficult decisions, surgeons must focus on the patient's wishes, even when family may try to convince the medical team others.	In critically ill patients, the medical team must abstain from futile care that will not aid in improving the patient's overall status and/or achieves the patient's goals.	If a surgeon provides futile care or care that does not align with the patient's values, they are in fact inflicting harm on the patient. Such care should be ceased immediately upon detection.	Providing all patients with the highest level of care, regardless of their background, especially when making difficult decisions.

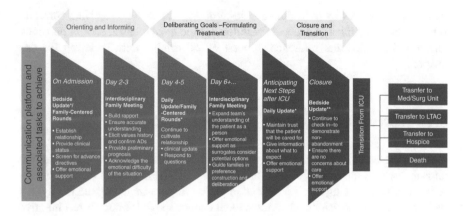

Fig. 39.1 Communication platform for critically ill patients

patient and the family (2). Prioritizing both the patient's and her family's goals for the patient's care almost inevitably leads to some conflicts. Difficult medical decisions are fraught with stress, guilt, and unease, especially at the end of life and in critical conditions (3). Without clear and accessible advanced directives, the concordance between the wishes of patients and the predictions of surrogate decision makers is estimated at 68% (4). And, even when a patient's advanced directive is available for guidance, literature shows that as their illness evolves, patients tend to change their minds about their goals of care. (1, 4)

Amidst such uncertainty and under emotional duress, it is indeed challenging to navigate surrogate decision making for both the patient's family and the medical team. An ethical dilemma arises when the wishes of the surrogate decision maker do not appear to represent those of the patient. This challenge, in turn, can lead not only to a counterproductive tension between the medical team and the surrogate decision maker, but may ultimately commit the patient to a fate in direct opposition to her goals and values. Management strategies to navigate such conflicts include early recognition, frequent and open lines of communication, a multidisciplinary approach, and, most importantly, tactful refocusing on the patient's personal goals (see Fig. 39.1) (5).

39.2 Search Strategy

We conducted a search of PubMed and Scopus using the following terms: physician patient relations, patient communication, patient conflict, end of life care, major medical decision, terminal care, family conflict. Given the significant differences in how individual cultures handle end of life care and surrogate decision making, we included only articles from the United States and Canada for review. We further narrowed our search by excluding articles written prior to 2000 to obtain currently relevant data on clinical practice. In addition, we included relevant articles and book chapters for contextual reference. A total of 24 articles were reviewed for this chapter.

39.3   Discussion

The World Health Organization defines the palliative care specialty as a "field that aims to improve the care of patients and families." (2) Although the practice of surrogate decision making is not restricted to palliative care, including the family in a patient's medical decisions when the patient cannot speak for herself has intuitive appeal. When we, as physicians, commit to caring for two or more closely linked, but still separate individuals, the question necessarily arises: in what measure or ratio do we prioritize these professed obligations should they ever conflict? To address this question, we must have an understanding of the process, accuracy, and the dynamics of surrogate decision making before we attempt to evaluate potential remedies to resolving such conflicts as described in the literature.

39.3.1   Decisional Capacity

Patients with decisional capacity have an absolute right to refuse any and all medical treatments. Patients may also request certain treatments whose likely outcomes align with their personal values and goals. Although no physician may be coerced into providing non-beneficial or futile care, the quality-of-life measures and the amount of risk a patient is willing to assume for a projected benefit are highly variable and exceedingly personal. A particular patient, for example, may accept that the outcome of a course of treatment may lead to life in a nursing home, whereas for another patient such a result might be unacceptable (6).

Decision-making capacity may be assessed by any physician and does not need the expertise of a psychiatrist. Such an assessment ascertains the patient's ability to explain any proposed intervention (including risks and benefits) and to demonstrate a logical connection between causes and effects. Although medical professionals may, at times, disagree with the weight a patient assigns to a treatment option, as long as the patient is able to express her own decision in this manner, the patient is determined to have decisional capacity for this particular decision. Of note, decisional capacity may vary by the complexity of the decision and a patient's decisional capacity may also fluctuate depending on her clinical condition (7).

39.3.2 Surrogate Decision Making

When a patient lacks decisional capacity, the clinical team turns to a surrogate decision maker for answers. If the patient has a legally executed durable power of attorney for healthcare (DPOAH), then this person should assume the role of decision making for the patient for as long as the patient lacks decisional capacity. Alternatively, the identity of surrogate decision makers varies legally by state and ethically by patient scenario. Several databases exist that list state specific laws on the matter, making it imperative that a clinician is familiar with the relevant state laws of her practice. In states with no strict surrogate hierarchy, any one person may be named the surrogate decision maker who the clinical team judges to be best positioned to represent the patient's own wishes. Careful and thorough documentation of the reasons for relying on one potential surrogate over another is necessary. The surrogate decision maker is asked to exercise substituted judgment, which means that he or she should, to the very best of his or her ability and knowledge of the patient's values and goals, make decisions the same way the patient would were she able to participate. When substituted judgment is exercised properly, the surrogate becomes an extension of the patient's autonomy. (1, 8)

39.3.3 Complicating Factors in Surrogate Decision Making

Several factors may complicate the surrogate's decision-making process. First, understanding of the patient's goals and values can be incomplete. While an advance directive may exist stating the patient's preferences and/or the patient may have discussed her wishes with her family in great detail, it is unlikely that such a document or discussion had addressed all possible situations (9). In addition, data show that as patients' conditions decline, they tend to accept a quality of life previously rejected (10). For example, a patient who may have signed a living will that does not allow for prolonged mechanical ventilation may be more amenable after several weeks in the hospital on a ventilator. Studies show that amidst these uncertainties, adult children serve as the least accurate and spouses as the most accurate proxies. One reason for this anomaly is the likelihood that adult children are more vulnerable to the influences of other family members than are spouses (8). Additional influences that threaten substituted judgment are psychological factors such as grief, guilt, and a sense of helplessness (11).

39.3.4   Conflict in Surrogate Decision Making

Conflict around surrogate decision making is common. One study found that in 63% of cases either the physician or the surrogate perceived conflict (12). There are many potential sources of conflict that may arise both among family members and between the physician and the surrogate decision maker(s). Different religious and cultural beliefs, language barriers, and perceived abandonment are examples of possible instigators of conflict (13). The greatest source of conflict, however, is stress experienced by the surrogate(s) and the physician. Family members are usually not accustomed to dealing with death. This finality can cause great distress, leading proxies to make decisions that may not align with the patient's wishes. When feeling anxious, surrogates will often choose the path of least resistance or the easiest decision, which in most cases is continuing life-prolonging interventions (3).

The decision to remove life-sustaining interventions is a weighty one and not infrequently surrogates avoid even discussing this possibility. A surrogate who feels forced to make a difficult choice in the midst of conflict is likely to act in a way to sooth his own distress, even when this is clearly counter to the patient's wishes. One study found that in a contentious situation, families tend to opt for continuing aggressive measures, whereas physicians lean towards withdrawing treatment (9, 14). When the conflict exists between various members of the family, surrogates may inappropriately choose life-prolonging care so as to appease other family members, a convenance particularly evident among siblings. The greater the conflict the less accurate the surrogate's decision making becomes (14). Addressing conflict between physicians and surrogates is important to maintain optimal care for the patient, to aid the family in the grieving process, and to reduce physician burnout. (11)

It is difficult for physicians to respect the surrogate decision maker's representation of the patient's wish when clear evidence exists to the contrary. For example, a surrogate may want to proceed with placement of a tracheostomy when the patient's living will specifically forbid it. As previously mentioned, however, patients may change their minds about accepting life-prolonging and life-sustaining measures more readily the sicker they are. Because of this shift in patients' goals of care that evolves along with the state of their illness, surrogate decision making is relied on more heavily than written living wills. Still, there are frequent instances in which a patient has independent and in-depth conversations with her physician shortly before having to face a difficult medical decision that strongly suggest that the patient's goals of care are more in line with comfort measures than with aggressive interventions. Similarly, family accounts of a patient's values may direct the physician toward life-prolonging and invasive procedures that would directly counter the patient's autonomous choice (14).

39.3.5   *Ethical Principles in Surrogate Decision Making*

When examining conflicts surrounding surrogate decision making, it is important to employ the landmark principles of bioethics—i.e., autonomy, nonmaleficence, beneficence, and justice. (see Table 39.1). Applying these principles in surrogate decision making is both a function of how much weight we give to each principle and also of the exact understanding of each principle. The way we understand autonomy, in particular, has evolved significantly over time and cultural context. The most conservative view on patient autonomy is also the oldest one in Western Civilizations. Built on the idea of individual autonomy as defined by Immanuel Kant, each person (or patient) must be viewed as an end in herself and never as a means to someone else's end (15). In practical terms, this view means that a patient's choice about her own personal body or self should always remain the primary objective and should never be sacrificed for the good of anything or anyone else. The process of informed consent embodies this interpretation of autonomy in that informed consent is only valid when given free of any coercion or undue influence and following a rational process. It is this individualistic interpretation of autonomy that is embraced by Beauchamp and Childress and taught in US medical schools (16).

Relational bioethics, in contrast to principlism, views each individual as primarily a social being, defined by her personal relationships and embedded in her own cultural microcosm. Relational bioethics builds on feminist bioethics, according to which no patient exists in a vacuum prior to entering the hospital (17). True autonomy, therefore, is achieved only when one is united with and active in one's own social sphere. Family members, as active representatives of the patient's normal social surroundings, enhance a patient's autonomy and therefore should be viewed as an extension of the patient even when the patient has decision making capacity (18). The relational understanding of autonomy is supported by empiric data from outpatient cancer patients that showed a sense of increased empowerment and freedom in medical decision making in cancer patients whose families were actively engaged in the process (19).

Indeed, when patients and family agree with the medical recommendation of the physician, communication tends to be straightforward. In these instances, the presence of family by the bedside seems to augment the recovery of the patient or else the transition of the patient's care to palliation. Tensions arise, however, when patients and members of her close support system disagree. If we accept the relational view of autonomy above, we are obliged to consider our commitments as physicians to the family and/or surrogate decision maker(s) in addition to the patient.

The degree to which family members ought to be considered in their own right in surrogate decision making has been debated in the literature. Expert opinion on the matter varies from viewing the family as simply a support system for the patient to identifying surrogate decision makers as independent stakeholders with possibly equal or even higher stakes than the patient. Pointing to the principle of justice, some scholars have argued that because it is the family who must shoulder the burden of caring for the ill patient were she to leave the hospital, it is only fair that we extend our clinical obligation to include them in equal parts (20). Others have proposed that although the family is an essential component of the patient's identity, and hence autonomy, we must as clinicians reorient the family to center decisions on the patient to at least a greater degree than on those who are not sick. Being sick, these writers argue, changes the balance between individual autonomy and justice because of the greater vulnerability associated with being ill. Consequently, although the family are true stakeholders in end-of-life decision making, their personal wishes should be factored into a lesser degree than those of the patient (18, 21). A common theme among proponents of honoring relational autonomy in surrogate decision making is that they identify the physician as the mediator between patient and family interests.

39.3.6   The Physician's Role in Surrogate Decision Making

Due to the many challenges surrounding surrogate decision making for patients, physicians must play an active and steering role. It is often easier to avoid conflict, take the path of least resistance, simply present a menu of medical choices to the family, and proceed with whichever they select. Such an approach, however, is not only unprofessional and unethical, but may also lead to preventable suffering for the patient. As physicians we have an ethical responsibility to do no harm. The concept of harm is both objective and subjective. We encounter subjective harm when dealing with patients for whom surrogates are deciding. Placing a tracheostomy, for example, in itself may not be harmful. But being maintained on a ventilator for a prolonged time contrary to a patient wish is subjectively harmful, or qualitatively non-beneficial. It is incumbent upon the physician to frame the conversation with the family using the principles of substituted judgment.

Providing care that is beneficial and respects patient autonomy requires that all conversations with surrogate decision makers focus, from the very beginning, on the patient's goals and values. It is helpful to review with the family what the patient's quality of life was like prior to admission to the hospital and what values she held. Creating a narrative around the patient's life early in the physician-family communication helps center the focus on the patient's personhood (9). Open-ended questions that inquire about the patient's source of joy and satisfaction in life are particularly helpful in this process. Asking yes or no questions may feel accusatory to family members and prove counterproductive to the physician-family relationship. Family conferences need not be long to be effective. Showing empathy and an interest in the patient as a person develops trust between the physician and the family, leading to less conflict in surrogate decision making and greater family satisfaction (5).

39.3.7 *Managing Conflict in Surrogate Decision Making*

The single most effective way to manage conflict in surrogate decision making is to be proactive. Avoiding conflict does not amount to managing it. If there is reasonable evidence that the surrogate decision maker is not acting in accordance with the patient's own wishes, a conflict exists. Simply following the wishes of the surrogate decision maker does not constitute resolution of this conflict and the physician is ethically bound to address it. The physician should feel empowered to advocate for the patient in the spirit of both beneficence and non-maleficence (6).

Several successful strategies of conflict prevention have been described in the literature. The first is early and open communication with the patient herself about her values and goals when possible. In one national survey, the five most important considerations for patients at the end of life were identified as freedom from pain, freedom from anxiety, freedom from shortness of breath, being kept clean, and being physically touched. Additionally, patients valued a physician who would discuss death and dying openly and with whom they could share their own fears (13). Physicians should encourage patients to discuss their goals and wishes with their family members in advance along with their physician. Managing expectations and understanding the patient's values and goals made under calm circumstances can significantly reduce the stress of surrogate decision making. For example, if a patient has a new cancer diagnosis, even if she is likely to survive, the physician should encourage the patient to begin discussing what she values most with her family members and potential surrogate decision makers. Creating and maintaining trust through open communication with both the patient and her family leads to the development of lasting trust and the reduction of conflict.

Once a patient is decisionally incapacitated, it is important to create an environment where communication between the surrogate and the medical team is readily available in order to ensure that conflicts are being addressed as they arise. When there is a shift in the focus of care from aggressive to comfort care, anticipatory guidance from the attending physician can aid in reducing conflict with surrogates (5). One systematic review found prognostication, conflict mediation, empathic communication, and family-centered aspects of care as the most important competencies for providing palliative care that is helpful for both patient and family in critical care settings. It is critically important for the physician to stress explicitly that neither the patient nor the family will be abandoned by the medical team should the patient's goals of care transition to withdrawing or withholding life-sustaining interventions. (22)

One opportunity to foster trust and open communication between the medical team and the family is during bedside rounds with the family present. Although rounds are focused on the details of system-specific medical management plans and are often time-limited, for select patients and families they may serve as a convenient time to address the patient's goals and values along with her medical plan. Doing so at the bedside incorporates valuable input from the patient's nurse, who is the person most intimately familiar with the patient's minute to minute condition at

Table 39.2 Steps for managing cases of suspected undue influence

Step	Goal	Method
1: Consult the medical team	To determine whether the patient has expressed specific treatment preferences to one of them	Team meeting with staff involved in care of patient or separate conversations ("Has Mrs. B said anything to you about how she feels about the current treatment plan? Has she exhibited any behaviors that would make you suspect she may not be on board?")
2: Engage the patient	To ascertain patient's authentic treatment preferences	In person discussion with patient, without family present if possible ("I just wanted to check with you to see how involved you'd like to be with your care and to make sure you're comfortable with our current treatment plan. Have you spoken with your [spouse, child, sibling, and so on] about how you're feeling? May I ask why not?")
3: Organize a family meeting	To provide a forum for open communication between patient and family members who may be exerting undue influence	Physical meeting with patient and family, as well as other team members (social work, ethics, chaplaincy, palliative care, and so on)
4: Reevaluate the treatment plan	To ensure the current treatment plan is a valid expression of relational autonomy (Goal is not to change patient's mind)	Ask the patient whether, given everything that has been discussed, she would like to proceed under the current goals of care
5: Continue to empower the patient	To respect the autonomy of the patient by reminding the patient that she is free to change the treatment plan at any time	Periodic communications with the patient ("Are you still comfortable with the direction we are headed in? Let me know if you want to talk again about the goals of care.")

this point. Such bedside rounds and family discussions also allow the physician to assess the family's receptiveness to further conversations and to gauge family dynamics. Family centered electronic communication portals and telephone updates in the absence of physically present family members may also serve the same role and may be done with greater time flexibility. Both bedside rounds and telephone updates aid in building rapport and trust with the family and ultimately in providing better care for the patient. Including the family in the patient's care with frequent updates and opportunities for contribution is not overriding the patient's autonomy, but rather is supporting relational autonomy (see Table 39.2) (23).

Patients in critical care settings are often managed by more than one medical team. Multidisciplinary family meetings with all relevant specialties in attendance can be a powerful tool in demonstrating to the family the medical team's commitment to the patient. Such meetings are also helpful in addressing medical uncertainties by coordinating the collective expertise of physicians from multiple specialties. When prognostic uncertainties still remain, a trial of therapy is warranted. A trial of therapy refers to introducing or continuing an intervention with a reasonably set time limit to allow for improvement. If the patient does not improve, then she may be said to have failed the trial of therapy, indicating that we must reassess the goals of our care. For example, if a patient with refractory septic shock already on maximal doses of vasopressors and broad-spectrum antibiotics from an infection without a clear source is not improving, we might suggest a trial of therapy in the form of repeating a full infectious workup and giving stress dose steroids empirically. We might say that some improvement within 72 hours would be reasonably expected and communicate these parameters to the family. If a trial of therapy determines that a patient is no longer responsive to therapy thus signaling the progression of her illness to its end stages, the physician now has objective evidence upon which to recommend the refocusing of goals toward palliation and comfort care. (3, 24)

On occasion, despite all of our efforts to prevent conflict in surrogate decision making, a conflict nevertheless persists. It may happen, for example, that the surrogate decision maker derives financial benefit from prolonging the patient's life, or vice versa, leading him or her to make decisions more in line with his or her own personal gain than exercising substituted judgment. Such undue influence undermines the physician's duty to preserve the patient's autonomy. In states with no legal hierarchy of surrogate decision makers, the solution to such an overt conflict of interest is for the clinical team to turn to another family member or friend who appears to be representing the patient's wishes more accurately. Any such change in surrogate decision making must be clearly documented along with the reasons that prompted the change. In states that do have strict surrogate hierarchies, consulting the hospital ethics committee would be warranted to engage an objective third party to assess the appropriateness of the surrogate decision maker and offer recommendations for an ethically feasible way forward.

Frequently, the conflict of interest that clouds the surrogate's judgment in respecting the patient's wishes is not financial, but emotional. The first step in addressing this problem is to recognize it. Family members may act out of profound anger, sadness, or stress, without even recognizing their own motivations. In such cases, the physician must guide the surrogate(s) back to the appropriate focus of the medical care: the patient. The medical team can honor the family by trying to minimize their stress while also pursuing a course of action that is in the best interest of the patient and in line with her previously stated wishes. This navigation can be achieved through the open communication methods described above and anticipatory guidance when there is going to be a shift in care. At times the physician will have to rely on her moral courage to oppose family requests that are clearly against the patient's wishes. In these instances, the physician should calmly and with empathy discuss with the family that her primary duty to the patient lies in doing no harm. The backup of an ethics consult may prove helpful but is not necessary in these clinical situations. Emphasizing that the medical team will not abandon the family or the patient in such instances is paramount and offering third party services to help the family process the loss can mitigate any conflict. A visit with a chaplain or a social worker should be offered to the family under these difficult circumstances.

Conversely, situations may arise in which the physician recommends a therapeutic intervention for the patient for which the surrogate does not give consent. This results in a pause in treatment as the physician cannot proceed without signed consent from the surrogate. The impasse in treatment can lead to the inappropriate and preventable deterioration of patient or to missing a window of therapeutic opportunity that, in the professional opinion of the physician, is indicated for the patient's condition. Currently, there are only four states that sanction a physician's ability to override the surrogate's refusal for a therapeutic intervention. These states are Arizona, South Dakota, Pennsylvania, and Ohio (8).

39.4   Case Revisited

Conversations over multiple days with the family continued as Mrs. S' condition continued to deteriorate. The attending physician from the intensive care unit invited the patient's surgeon, cardiologist, and pulmonologist to join the family conference. The values and goals of the patient were reiterated and actually agreed upon by all participants, including the son who was only available via telephone. On several occasions, family members voiced their agreement that the patient would not want to continue with aggressive measures. Yet, they continued to object to transitioning to comfort care, citing both religious expectations and their own inability to deal with losing the patient. After the third meeting with everyone present, the attending physician in the ICU informed the family that she would remove Mrs. S from the ventilator that day and allow her to pass in accordance with her wishes. She did so calmly and with empathy, explaining that she had to uphold her dedication to the principle of non-maleficence in order to preserve her professional integrity. The intensivist stressed that the disease process facing Mrs. S thwarted all attempts at her recovery. Now, it is the medical team's responsibility to aggressively care for her comfort in her final hours. She further promised that she would not abandon the patient while dying and asked for the aid of the chaplain and the social worker in processing the family's grief, anger, and loss of their loved one.

39.5   Conclusion

Surrogate decision making is fraught with uncertainties and such situations easily lend themselves to creating conflict around how to proceed in a patient's medical care. Uncertainties arise both from the lack of a complete understanding of the patient's own wishes and also from the unpredictability of how patients may change their minds with what goals and values they find acceptable as their disease progresses. Conflicts may arise among family members and between surrogate decision makers and the clinical team. The best approach to avoiding such conflicts is through prevention by early and frequent communication with the family. Not one form of communication is best, and each patient and encounter is different. There is no universal way to satisfy all patients and surrogates, but the earlier the medical possibilities are discussed the more fruitful future cooperation is likely between family and physician. A useful graphic for how to utilize the various forms of communication with families and patient in Fig. 39.1.

Central tenets of managing potential conflicts in surrogate decision making include inquiring about the patient as a person with her goals and values identified early and clearly; encouraging the surrogate(s) to exercise substituted judgment, and invoking the physician's duty to the patient to, above all, do no harm. Addressing these conflicts takes both practice and moral courage. In the spirit of palliative care and relational autonomy, attending to the family's distress is also incumbent on the clinical team. Social work or chaplaincy consults may help alleviate some of the moral distress of the family, which ultimately is an extension of the patient and whose care, therefore falls within the scope of our obligations as physicians.

39.6   Selected References

- Bernat JL. *Ethical issues in neurology.* 2nd ed. Butterworth-Heinemann; 2002; 87–91.

  - Family members serving as surrogate decision makers must abide by three standards defined by ethics and the law: The standard of expressed wishes, substituted judgement, and best interests. With expressed wishes, the surrogate decision makers must act on the goals and values expressed by the patient prior to their current illness rendering them incapacitated. If the patient's wishes were not previously expressed, the surrogate must use substituted judgement, applying the patient's values to the situation. If there is no evidence as to the patient's wishes, the surrogate must rely on best interest in the situation, for example, considering the patient's suffering and the potential burdens as a result of any treatment.

- Seaman JB, Arnold RM, Scheunemann LP, White DB. An Integrated Framework for Effective and Efficient Communication with Families in the Adult Intensive Care Unit. Ann Am Thorac Soc. 2017;14(7):1015–10. https://doi.org/10.1513/annalsats.201612-9655OI

  - Time and care are required for a surrogate to make accurate decisions regarding a patient's care. Anxiety, stress, and guilt can lead to inaccurate choices that do not align with the patient's goals and values. Providing family members with safe spaces to discuss, understand, and ask questions regarding the care of a patient are paramount in making difficult decisions regarding a patient's care.

- Schuster RA, Hong SY, Arnold RM, White DB. Investigating Conflict in ICUs-Is the Clinicians' Perspective Enough? Crit Care Med. 2014;42(2):328–335. https://doi.org/10.1097/ccm.0b013e3182a27598

  - Conflict is perceived by either the physician or surrogate decision maker in approximately 63% of cases in the intensive care unit. Satisfaction with the physician's bedside manner was associated with lower perception of conflict.

References

1. Bernat JL. Ethical issues in neurology. 2nd ed. Butterworth-Heinemann; 2002. p. 87–91.
2. World Health Organization. PAHO. Covid-19 has infected some 570,000 health workers and killed 2500 in the Americas, PAHO Director says. September 2, 2020. Accessed January 11, 2021. https://www.paho.org/en/news/2-9-2020-covid-19-has-infected-some-570000-health-workers-and-killed-2500-americas-paho.
3. Shalowitz DI, Garrett-Mayer E, Wendler D. The accuracy of surrogate decision makers: a systematic review. Arch Intern Med. 2006;166(5):493–7. https://doi.org/10.1001/archinte.166.5.493.
4. Hinkle LJ, Bosslet GT, Torke AM. Factors associated with family satisfaction with end-of-life care in the ICU: a systematic review. Chest. 2015;147(1):82–93. https://doi.org/10.1378/chest.14-1098.
5. Kopar PK, Brown DE, Turnbull IR. Ethics of codes and codes of ethics: when is it ethical to provide cardiopulmonary resuscitation during the COVID-19 pandemic? Ann Surg. 2020;272(6):930–4. https://doi.org/10.1097/sla.0000000000004318.
6. Moore RF. A guide to the assessment and Care of the Patient Whose Medical Decision-Making Capacity is in question. Med Gen Med 1999:E7. PMID: 11104409.
7. Venkat A, Becker J. The effect of statutory limitations on the authority of substitute decision makers on the care of patients in the intensive care unit: case examples and review of state laws affecting withdrawing or withholding life-sustaining treatment. J Intensive Care Med. 2014;29(2):71–80. https://doi.org/10.1177/0885066611433551.
8. Mehter HM, McCannon JB, Clark JA, Wiener RS. Physician approaches to conflict with families surrounding end-of-life decision-making in the intensive care unit. A qualitative study. Ann Am Thorac Soc. 2018;15(2):241–9. https://doi.org/10.1513/annalsats.201702-105OC.
9. Lee MA, Smith DM, Fenn DS, Ganzini L. Do patients' treatment decisions match advance statements of their preferences? J Clin Ethics 1998;9(3):258–262. PMID: 10029826.
10. Kramer BJ, Boelk AZ. Correlates and predictors of conflict at the end of life among families enrolled in hospice. J Pain Symptom Manag. 2015;50(2):155–62. https://doi.org/10.1016/j.jpainsymman.2015.02.026.
11. Schuster RA, Hong SY, Arnold RM, White DB. Investigating conflict in ICUs-is the clinicians' perspective enough? Crit Care Med. 2014;42(2):328–35. https://doi.org/10.1097/ccm.0b013e3182a27598.
12. Steinhauser AE, Christakis NA, Clipp EC, McNeilly M, McIntyre L, Tulsky JA. Factors considered important at the end of life by patients, family, physicians, and other care providers. JAMA. 2000;284(19):2476–82. https://doi.org/10.1001/jama.284.19.2476.
13. Parks SM, Winter L, Santana AJ, et al. Family factors in end-of-life decision-making: family conflict and proxy relationship. J Palliat Med. 2011;14(2):179–84. https://doi.org/10.1089/jpm.2010.0353.
14. Kant: Groundwork of the Metaphysics of Morals: Edition 2 (revised). In: Gregor M, Timmermann J, Korsgaard CM, editors. Cambridge University Press; 2012; p. 37–108.

15. Beauchamp TL, Childress JF. Principles of biomedical ethics. 8th ed. Oxford University Press; 2019. Chapter 4
16. Nedelsky J. Law's relations: a relational theory of self, autonomy, and law. Oxford University Press; 2011.
17. Ho A. Relational autonomy or undue pressure? Family's role in medical decision-making. Scand J Caring Sci. 2008;22(1):128–35. https://doi.org/10.1111/j.1471-6712.2007.00561.x.
18. Gilbar R. Family involvement, independence, and patient autonomy in practice. Med Law Rev. 2011;19(2):192–234. https://doi.org/10.1093/medlaw/fwr008.
19. Hardwig J. Is there a duty to die? Hast Cent Rep. 1997;27(2):34–42. https://doi.org/10.2307/3527626.
20. Nelson JL. Taking families seriously. Hast Cent Rep. 1992;22(4):6–12. https://doi.org/10.2307/3563016.
21. Schram AW, Hougham GW, Meltzer DO, Ruhnke GW. Palliative Care in Critical Care Settings: a systematic review of communication-based competencies essential for patient and family satisfaction. Am J Hosp Palliat Med. 2017;34(9):887–95. https://doi.org/10.1177/1049909116667071.
22. Baker FX, Gallagher CM. Identifying and managing undue influence from family members in end-of-life decisions for patients with advanced Cancer. J Oncol Pract. 2017;13(10):702, e857–e862. https://doi.org/10.1200/jop.2017.020792.
23. Seaman JB, Arnold RM, Scheunemann LP, White DB. An integrated framework for effective and efficient communication with families in the adult intensive care unit. Ann Am Thorac Soc. 2017;14(6):1015–0. https://doi.org/10.1513/annalsats.201612-9655OI.
24. Lilly CM, De Meo DL, Sonna LA, et al. An intensive communication intervention for the critically ill. Am J Med. 2000;109(6):469–75. https://doi.org/10.1016/s0002-9343(00)00524-6.

Chapter 40
Medical Missions to Developing Countries (Pro)

Claire Hoppenot

Abstract Access to surgical care is disparate across the world. Medical mission trips, or short-term experiences in global health (STEGH), send medical professionals from high-income countries (HIC) to low- and middle- income countries (LMIC) to provide medical or surgical care. We will explore the "pro" aspect of surgical missions to LMIC through an ethical lens guided by the four principles of clinical ethics: beneficence, justice, nonmaleficence, and autonomy. Surgery is particularly amenable to STEGH because it can provide a long-term intervention in a single time-point, as shown in obstetric fistula and cleft lip programs. However, for surgical missions to be successful, surgeons must know their limitations, prioritize community needs, and plan for local post-operative patient care. They must work in partnership with local community and avoid taking medical professionals away from LMIC. Individual patients must understand the risks, benefits, and limitations of surgery. Additionally, while many students and trainees benefit from participating in STEGHs, they must not overstep their level of training. Based on these ethical criteria and literature search, we propose considerations for ethical STEGH programs, and acknowledge that greater contributors to health, such as poverty, education, and nutrition, must be addressed to improve health throughout the world.

Keywords Short term global surgery · Ethics · Medical missions · Short-term experiences in global health (STEGH) · Obstetric fistula medical missions · Cleft palate medical missions

C. Hoppenot (✉)
Dan L Duncan Comprehensive Cancer Center, Baylor College of Medicine, Houston, TX, USA
e-mail: Claire.hoppenot@bcm.edu

© The Author(s), under exclusive license to Springer Nature Switzerland AG 2022
V. A. Lonchyna et al. (eds.), *Difficult Decisions in Surgical Ethics*, Difficult Decisions in Surgery: An Evidence-Based Approach,
https://doi.org/10.1007/978-3-030-84625-1_40

Case
Dr. M is an obstetrician/gynecologist in Houston. She went to medical school in Ethiopia, then came to Houston for her residency. After becoming a practicing physician, she created a partnership with her medical school in Ethiopia. She and her department chief initially spent 2 weeks with the Ethiopian physicians to determine what assistance they needed. The physicians noted a backlog of radical hysterectomies for cervical cancer and fistula procedures, as well as a need for ultrasound training for gynecologic evaluation. They have a new residency program, one of the first in the country, and Dr M noticed that the trainees have minimal involvement in the operating rooms. Dr M started traveling with alternating colleagues for 2 weeks every 3 months throughout the year to assist with the backlog of cases, provide training, and develop a surgical teaching curriculum with the Ethiopian physicians. For certain cases they are able to coordinate in advance and bring equipment or medications that would not otherwise have been available locally. They sometimes bring nurses, residents, fellows or anesthesiologists who want to help and are interested in learning about a different health care setting. After obtaining funding, the Ethiopian physicians and then the trainees came to Houston to participate in the yearly cadaver lab training. The American medical teams have found that they come home much more aware of the disparities in care not only internationally but within their own systems and apply time at home to advocate for local patients in need. Ethiopian medical teams have been able to expand their department, attract local physicians, and work on expanding their educational curriculum to other teaching institutions in the country.

40.1 Introduction

Access to surgical care is widely disparate throughout the world. While high-income countries (HIC) have more than 10,000 surgical procedures per 100,000 population, many low- and medium-income countries (LMIC) throughout Africa and Southeast Asia have fewer than 500 [1]. In Ghana, for example, the rate of surgery is about 869/100,000; 22% of these surgeries are performed in hospitals without fully trained surgeons [2]. Estimates from the World Bank Group suggest that as many as 1.8 million deaths could be prevented with better access to surgical care [3]. Disability-adjusted life years (DALYs), which take fatal and nonfatal burden of disease by considering years of life lost as well as the effect of disability, could show an even greater improvement with improvement in access to surgery.

Many health care professionals enter the profession to intervene on suffering and health out of a moral duty [4]. Although the sense of duty is more immediate towards patients who are geographically close, human suffering exists throughout the world [4]. Additionally, a history of imperialism and racism by HIC towards LMIC caused or worsened the disparities that exist today, augmenting the sense of responsibility of citizens of HIC [5]. One response to this sense of duty has been medical and

Table 40.1 Working group guidelines for trainees in global health [6, 8]

For programs:	• Develop a well-structured program with set expectations both for the traveling trainees and for the sending and host institutions
	• Provide formal training for trainees and host
	• Monitor costs to host institutions and compensate those who facilitate the trip
	• Establish methods of communication and feedback
	• Provide pre-trip training with trainees to set appropriate expectations
	• Establish who will provide supervision appropriate for the trainee's level of training
	• Collect data on outcomes and training experiences
	• Encourage bi-directional exchanges
	• Encourage sustainability
For the trainee:	• Follow the policies and laws of the country and host institution.
	• Follow local cultural, political and financial norms
	• Do not do procedures that you wouldn't do unsupervised in your home institution
	• Focus on the educational nature of the trip
	• Seek to learn about medical and cultural aspects of the host institution

surgical mission trips and short-term experiences in global health (STEGHs). STEGHs allow health care professionals to spend 1–30 days providing clinical care, public health education, or other forms of global health interventions in LMIC [6].

We will discuss the ethical issues inherent to STEGHs through the lens of Beauchamp and Childress' four principles of ethics: beneficence and nonmaleficence (including clinical, cultural and educational), autonomy (of the individual and the community), and justice [7]. We will argue that there is an ethical way to proceed with a STEGH, and that as the world simultaneously becomes smaller and more segregated, continuing to share our medical knowledge and community experiences across the world in an ethical manner can be beneficial for all parties involved (see Table 40.1).

40.2 Search Strategy

A PubMed search was performed with the key terms "Short term global surgery," "Ethics," "Medical missions," and "Short-term experiences in global health" from 1970 to today. References within these searches were used to find further references.

40.3 Discussion

40.3.1 Beneficence

A man was walking on a beach covered in starfish brought in by the tide. He noticed a small boy throwing the starfish back into the sea. "What are you doing? There are too many, you'll never be able to make a difference," he told the boy. The boy threw another starfish into the sea. "I made a difference to that one," he said. – Adapted from Loren Eiseley's "The Star Thrower" [9]

The primary purported goal of STEGHs is beneficence; that is, to decrease the surgical burden of disease within the host community. And indeed, STEGHs can provide much-needed assistance by providing surgical care or filling in the gaps in existing care [10]. As in the story of the star thrower, although the effort may seem inconsequential on a beach covered in starfish, an individual can make a difference to each starfish thrown back into the sea.

A general understanding of the political, structural and medical situation can maximize individual efforts, however. The World Bank group provides guidance on how to select procedures that efficiently provide the most benefit [1, 11]. They recommend prioritizing programs that provide high-quality cost-effective essential surgeries, defined based on cost-effectiveness and community impact in terms of DALYs, before committing resources to more specialized surgical care [1, 11]. These surgeries include procedures in obstetrics, trauma and the digestive tract. In particular, they suggest that global disease burden could be substantially decreased with an increase in surgeries for cataracts, congenital cardiac defects, cleft lip/palate, neural tube defects, and obstetric fistulas. These have been the targets for many STEGHs; we will focus on groups treating obstetric fistulas and cleft lips/palates as two examples of successful interventions.

Obstetric vesicovaginal fistulas are connections from the vagina to the bladder or rectum that create an incontinent passage of urine or stool through the vagina. They occur due to tissue necrosis from pressure as a sequela of obstructed labor. An estimated 3.5 million obstetric fistulas are diagnosed each year [12]. The continuous passage of urine and stool cause irritation of the labia and medial thighs, as well as a constant odor. As a result, women with a fistula are ostracized and unable to make a living [13]. Although continence can be achieved with vaginal or abdominal surgery in 70% of the cases [14], women who are able to have surgery wait on average 7 years between the diagnosis and treatment of an obstetric fistula [13]. This time frame suggests a lack of access, due to both distance and surgeon availability. The Fistula Foundation, based out of San Jose, US, has developed a program that combines local surgeons and STEGHs to amplify the local efforts for fistula repairs, and to bring surgery to more remote parts of the world. They have provided thousands of fistula repairs in 32 countries in Africa and Asia and continue to partner with and support local programs. Additionally, some of the programs that started off as STEGHs have developed into self-sustaining permanent local programs [13]. For example, Eritrea initially hosted STEGHs for a large part of their fistula repairs, but by 2012 they had developed a medical school and training program in obstetrics and gynecology, and 80% of the local fistula surgeries were done by local surgeons [13].

Operation Smile, based out of Virginia Beach, US, has repaired cleft palates and lips of more than 130,000 children and young adults in 80 countries throughout the world [15]. These surgeries can help prevent social ostracization and aspiration events [15, 16]. Although initially dominated by STEGHs, local hospitals and programs have developed to provide long-term care throughout the year [15]. The Guwahati Comprehensive Cleft Care Center (GCCCC) in India was initially a destination for STEGHs, but it now offers otolaryngology, speech therapy, dentistry, nutrition counseling, with most of the staff being local providers [11]. They continue to host STEGHs, but local surgeons provide surgery continuously throughout the year and have shown improved post-operative outcomes over the time of the transition and development of a permanent center [17]. In addition to clinical care, they seek to achieve collaboration and quality improvement, which requires a partnership with local governments as well as health and education systems.

These examples reveal the positive impact provided by STEGHs within a program that has a big picture of the local situation. Individually and as an organization, it is important to that the goal remain doing good for the local community. As more global health programs develop and institutions use these programs as a marketing tool, it is important to acknowledge the potential for career advancement to be a motivation factor [4, 12], in addition to beneficence [18]. Participants should also avoid becoming a medical tourist who collects experiences and stories about medical adventures abroad [4]. However, participants should acknowledge that there are also personal benefits to STEGHs, such as developing a new perspective on research, fulfilling a humanitarian passion, and putting a perspective on health care spending [19]. Medical and cultural exchange between host and traveling teams can inspire and empower both teams, but the primary goal should remain patient care as prioritized by the host community.

40.3.2 Justice

Many of the world's poorest countries are in areas, such as Africa or Southeast Asia, that have previously been colonized and exploited by European and American political powers [5]. Attempts to improve health care by colonizers frequently were misled and undermined local practices and communities without providing much health-related benefit [5]. In large part due to political mismanagement and poverty, billions of people still lack access to medical and surgical care [12]. Seventy percent of the world population lives in countries with less than $100 per capita spending of health care, but these countries only host a quarter of the operations performed annually world-wide [12]. Based on expert opinion, about 11% of the burden of disease world-wide could be treated with surgical intervention [1]. The avertable DALYs are greater with surgery than that of treatment of tuberculosis or malaria [1].

There is no inherent reason why a surgical procedure used routinely in many parts of the world, such as a cesarean delivery or repair of a cleft lip or a fistula, would not be provided everywhere. Surgeons who are willing and able to travel abroad can start building the surgical capacity of LMIC and slowly make a dent in the gaps in access to care [1]. While relocating to a LMIC completely may make the biggest strides towards justice, it can be a lot to ask for surgeons with family and professional ties. Short-term trips, ideally through an established organization with a long-term view and relationship, can provide a regular contribution. These contributions won't cause long-term systematic changes in global health disparities; this will require advocacy on the national level in health care systems, poverty, and education, which is outside the scope of training of many surgeons [1]. But, when done safely and ethically, these programs can provide assistance to individuals in their time of need.

40.3.3 Nonmaleficence

Unfortunately, medical trips can also cause unintended harm. These must be acknowledged and avoided. First, it is important for surgeons to remember their limits when faced with problems outside of their usual scope of practice [4]. A surgeon must say no to inappropriate surgery even when there is no good alternative, despite a desire to help people living in poverty they may not have previously encountered; doing something is not always better than doing nothing [18]. It is also important to have a plan for the management of postoperative complications, many of which will occur after the surgical team has left the country [10, 18, 20]. Postoperative rehabilitation and social support, such as for reintegration in the community after fistula surgery, must be available when setting up the STEGH for these issues.

STEGHs must also be careful not to adversely affect the local community. Partnering with the community is critical [18, 19]. Acting independently, STEGHs can run the risk of taking patients from local physicians, who depend on patients for their livelihood. Some of the poorest countries have less than 1 surgical specialist per 100,000 population; the Lancet Commission on Global Surgery, which consists of a group of surgical experts who assemble the best evidence on the state of global surgery and develop strategies to improve access to surgical care, recommends 20 specialists to adequately manage surgical disease [19]. Surgeons on STEGHs should help complement what local surgeons can provide for patients, and not compete with them. Local surgeons may also have the best overview of the local needs and will be the ones providing long-term and post-operative care.

There is also a risk that local surgeons will see connections with STEGHs as an opportunity to leave their community for a position abroad [4, 20, 21]. This is known as "brain drain." Millions of dollars are spent by African governments to train physicians who then go to practice in more stable, affluent countries [13]. Trainees selected for exchanges should be committed and encouraged to return to their home countries after the exchange [19, 20]. Additionally, supporting local programs by capacity-building can improve a surgeon's work conditions within the LMIC [16].

Most, if not all, of the harm done by medical missions is inadvertent. However, this is harm, nonetheless. Medical professionals developing and participating in STEGHs must remember the risks and ensure that the program can develop a partnership with the community to help mitigate the risks of harm.

40.3.4 Autonomy

Autonomy usually refers to an individual patient's ability to make decisions for themself. This requires a patient to understand the implications of the diagnosis and treatment offered, as well as its risks. Full understanding is difficult in the best of situations, but during STEGHs, language, cultural differences, and power dynamics make the conversation even more difficult [12, 15]. In a qualitative study of 10 patients in a medical mission setting, Sceats et al. showed that despite the use of translators, no patient was able to recall four risks discussed during the consent discussion, and most patients relied on vicarious experiences and discussions, and not the consent process with their surgeon, for medical decision-making [22]. Surgeons must be sensitive to barriers in communication and unrealistic expectations that a host community may have. Partnering with the local medical community is critical throughout the process [18, 19].

In the setting of a STEGH, respecting the autonomy of the local patients and caregivers also encompasses the cultural preferences and local treatment options within the host community. In addition to respecting host country laws [23], host community interests and practices should tower over mission interests [24]. The host communities should direct missions towards their needs and priorities and have a stake in the medical and social outcomes of developing the relationship [21]. These partnerships require STEGH participants to have cultural humility, defined as "lifelong commitment to self-evaluation and self-critique, redressing the power imbalances in the patient-physician dynamic, and to develop mutually beneficial and non-paternalistic clinical and advocacy partnerships with communities" [25]. Physicians hosting trainees on STEGHs have noted the importance of cultural humility and understanding the interaction between culture and medical care in traveling trainees [26], and these are the traits that allow traveling and host physicians to develop true partnerships [27].

40.3.5 Surgery as a Special Case

Surgery can provide short-term interventions that have long-lasting effects. The repair of a vesicovaginal fistula allows a woman to return to a productive life within her village [13, 28]. The closure of a cleft palate can prevent aspiration pneumonia and ostracization of a child due to disfigurement [15, 18]. Training physicians and physician extenders on cesarean deliveries has decreased maternal mortality from obstructed labor [19]. Concerns regarding postoperative complications and needs outside of the scope of the medical trip must be addressed and planned for, but unlike medical management of chronic medical problems, surgery is frequently a single point of intervention that can provide lifelong benefit.

Additionally, surgical interventions are cost-effective. Analyses of cleft lip and cleft palate repairs based on Operation Smile costs that included operating overhead, salaries, travel expenses, and training were found to be cost-effective, as were cesarean deliveries for obstructed labor [11]. Even the most expensive STEGH surgeries in the literature, neurosurgeries, were overall cost-effective in retrospective analyses [29].

40.3.6 STEGHs for surgical trainees

Many medical schools and residency programs have developed global health programs, in large part due to interest by trainees. Many trainees hope to be useful at a time of imbalance between a desire to help people and limitations of their status as trainees [20]. However, it is important to remember that traveling abroad does not change the status of "trainee."

Medical students and residents receive many benefits from STEGHs. STEGHs provide exposure to types of surgeries they may not otherwise see in their training program [20]. Trainees learn to work in a multi-cultural setting, develop comfort in communication, and come home with increased cultural sensitivity [30, 31]. They are more likely to work in primary care specialties and underserved communities [6, 30, 31]. Ultimately, for medical students, STEGHs should be viewed not as service, but as a learning opportunity. There is a lot to be learned both in terms of medicine and culture, and medical students should have a similar role in clinics in LMIC as in their country of origin. In a survey, host institutions were interested in hosting trainees, and they equally prioritized teaching about local medicine and local culture [26]. Most host physicians felt that trainees got more out of the trip than they gave. Programs could also consider a bi-directional exchange could provide that benefit to LMIC trainees.

A working group on ethics guidelines for global health training makes recommendations presented in Table 40.1 [6, 8]. They highlight that these trips are educational, not service oriented. Clear guidelines should be provided for hosts and participants, and that participants should behave as they would in their country in terms of following the law and having adequate supervision. They suggest thorough pre-trip training and having a clear agreement and ongoing communication with the host institution.

40.3.7 STEGH Frameworks

An ethical STEGH program must be sensitive to potential pitfalls in beneficence, nonmaleficence, autonomy and justice (see Table 40.2). Multiple frameworks have been suggested for STEGHs to provide a long-lasting impact while causing minimal burden. Because visiting teams generally cannot commit to spending a large

Table 40.2 Recommendations for an ethical STEGH program

Principles of ethics	Application of ethical principles to STEGH
Beneficence	Prioritize needs of the host communities (particularly over the desires of STEGH participants). [18, 24]
	Assess disease burden and the ability of surgery to improve it with a STEGH. [1, 24]
	Focus on nonemergent problems that cannot be taken care of by local surgeons. [18]
	Assess outcomes. [6, 10, 19]
	Teach. [18]
	Create long-term relationships. [18]
Autonomy	Engage the local community [6, 21]
	A single STEGH without a local partner is rarely ethically justified. [24]
	In addition to clinical care, focus on capacity-building to develop a local permanent program with resources available locally. [19]
Nonmaleficence	Know your limits (you have the option to decline surgery). [10]
	Follow host country laws, and work with programs in both countries that follow host country laws. [23]
	Consider creating certification programs for STEGHs to create oversight. [23]
	Start with capacity-assessment to establish what you need before the trip, and work within the limitations of the host resources. [10, 24]
Justice	Advocate locally and internationally to remove barriers to access to surgical care. [19]
	Commit to reciprocity and mutual benefit. [6]

portion of the year in LMIC, coordinating multiple visiting teams with a single local partner can provide continuity with the community and local medical teams [24]. Collaboration between multiple academic centers with a commitment to one LMIC institution can provide stability independent changes in faculty interest or funding that a single institution may have; such a program could envision having surgeons and residents join the department of a host institution for the month to help provide surgical volume as well as education [12]. These relationships can be formed with institutions or with programs such as the Fistula Foundation or Operation Smile, which have oversight and a history as well as continuity within many communities. The key is to develop accountability, continuity, and long-lasting exchanges with host communities.

40.4   Concluding Remarks

I benefitted from traveling on STEGHs as a student; the trips helped me to develop an interest in medicine, understand differences in medical systems and hone language skills that I use every day. These were learning opportunities, not service. Now, as a practicing gynecologic oncologist at a county hospital, I notice many disparities both in local patients and those who have traveled internationally. I acknowledge that there is a global burden of disease, including gynecologic cancers, that can be treated with surgery, and I have the skills to do so. STEGHs are appealing because our training is in medicine; we can take a history (even with a translator), do an exam, make a surgical plan weighing risks and benefits, and execute it. STEGHs provide the opportunity to help those in need throughout the world, while staying within the scope of our profession. Greater contributors to health, including poverty, education, and nutrition, are outside of our training and therefore feel less accessible. Meanwhile, people are suffering, and we have the skills to help. The key is to be sure that what we do is beneficial, and I hope that the guidelines described in this chapter can assist in assessing the ethical basis of STEGH programs.

Surgical medical missions will and should continue, and they can be done ethically. In particular, we need to focus on mutual respect, the development of a long-term relationship, investment in infrastructure, respect for local laws, and ensuring surgical cases are appropriate for the follow up care and surgeons involved. The world is only getting smaller, and interactions across cultures and medical systems are important for both students and practicing physicians. STEGHs during medical school should be considered educational, rather than providing a clinical contribution. And close oversight of medical outcomes and professional behavior of all medical teams must be established when developing these programs. However, STEGHs will not solve LMIC's long-term health care challenges. Developing venues for motivated participants to contribute to fighting disparities in health care, education, and wealth on a local and global scale between STEGHs could provide long-term systemic benefit.

40.5 Selected References

- Mock CN, Donkor P, Gawande A, Jamison DT, Kruk ME, Debas HT. Essential surgery: key messages of this volume. In: Debas HT, Donkor P, Gawande A, Jamison DT, Kruk ME, Mock CN, editors. Essential surgery: disease control priorities. vol. 1. 3rd ed. World Bank; 2015. https://doi.org/10.1596/978-1-4648-0346-8.

    – World Bank publication balancing effectiveness with cost, on a global and personal scale, of surgical interventions to address disease burden in low- and middle-income countries.

- Sznajder KK, Chen MC, Naughton D. How should mission trips be administered? AMA J Ethics. 2019;21(9):E722–8. https://doi.org/10.1001/amajethics.2019.722.

    – AMA journal of ethics publication highlighting the importance of respect, beneficence and justice in trainee global health experiences.

- Beauchamps TL, Childress JF. Principles of biomedical. 8th ed. Oxford University Press; 2019.

  - Textbook on biomedical ethics that forms the basis of many current approaches to clinical medical ethics.

- Mock C, Debas H, Balch CM, Brennan M, Buyske J, Cusack J, et al. Global surgery: effective involvement of US academic surgery: report of the American Surgical Association Working Group on global surgery. Ann Surg. 2018;268(4):557–63. https://doi.org/10.1097/sla.0000000000002934.

  - Working group report from the American Surgical Association addressing how US academic surgery can best decrease surgical disease burden in low- and middle-income countries. They highlight focusing on surgically treatable conditions, emphasizing cost-effective feasible, and harmonization with local priorities and existing world health initiatives.

- Rowthorn V, Loh L, Evert J, Chung E, Lasker J. Not above the law: a legal and ethical analysis of short-term experiences in global health. Ann Glob Health. 2019;85(1):79, 1–12. https://doi.org/10.5334/aogh.2451.

  - A call for participants in STEGHs to follow the law, both local and international, and to comport themselves ethically. They encourage participants through program to also ensure that the programs are following host country laws and procedures.

References

1. Mock CN, Donkor P, Gawande A, Jamison DT, Kruk ME, Debas HT. Essential surgery: key messages of this volume. In: Debas HT, Donkor P, Gawande A, Jamison DT, Kruk ME, Mock CN, editors. Essential surgery: disease control priorities, vol. 1. 3rd ed. World Bank; 2015. https://doi.org/10.1596/978-1-4648-0346-8.
2. Gyedu A, Stewart B, Gaskill C, et al. Improving benchmarks for global surgery: nationwide enumeration of operations performed in Ghana. Ann Surg. 2018;268(2):282–8. https://doi.org/10.1097/sla.0000000000002457.
3. Bickler SN, Weiser TG, Kassebaum N, et al. Global burden of surgical conditions. In: Debas HT, Donkor P, Gawande A, Jamison DT, Kruk ME, Mock CN, editors. Essential surgery: disease control priorities, vol. 1. 3rd ed. World Bank; 2015. https://doi.org/10.1596/978-1-4648-0346-8.
4. Stapleton G, Schroder-Back P, Laaser U, Meershoek A, Popa D. Global health ethics: an introduction to prominent theories and relevant topics. Glob Health Action. 2014;7:23569. https://doi.org/10.3402/gha.v7.23569.
5. Tilley H. Medicine, empires, and ethics in colonial Africa. AMA J Ethics. 2016;18(7):743–53. https://doi.org/10.1001/journalofethics.2016.18.7.mhst1-1606.
6. Sznajder KK, Chen MC, Naughton D. How should mission trips be administered? AMA J Ethics. 2019;21(9):E722–8. https://doi.org/10.1001/amajethics.2019.722.
7. Beauchamps TL, Childress JF. Principles of biomedical ethics. 8th ed. Oxford University Press; 2019.

8. Crump J, Sugarman J, Working Group on Ethics Guidelines for Global Health Training (WEIGHT). Ethics and best practice guidelines for training experiences in global health. Am J Trop Med Hyg. 2010;83(6):1178–82. https://doi.org/10.4269/ajtmh.2010.10-0527.
9. Eiseley L. The star thrower. Mariner Books; 1979.
10. Wall AE. Ethics in global surgery. World J Surg. 2014;38(7):1574–80. https://doi.org/10.1007/s00268-014-2600-5.
11. Alkire BC, Vincent JR, Meara JG. Benefit-cost analysis for selected surgical interventions in low- and middle-income countries. In: Debas HT, Donkor P, Gawande A, Jamison DT, Kruk ME, Mock CN, editors. Essential surgery: disease control priorities, vol. 1. 3rd ed. World Bank; 2015. https://doi.org/10.1596/978-1-4648-0346-8.
12. Schecter WP. Academic global surgery: a moral imperative. JAMA Surg. 2015;150(7):605–6. https://doi.org/10.1001/jamasurg.2015.0408.
13. Polan ML, Sleemi A, Bedane MM, Lozo S, Morgan MA. Obstetric fistula. In: Debas HT, Donkor P, Gawande A, Jamison DT, Kruk ME, Mock CN, editors. Essential surgery: disease control priorities, vol. 1. 3rd ed. World Bank; 2015. https://doi.org/10.1596/978-1-4648-0346-8.
14. Arrowsmith SD, Barone MA, Ruminjo J. Outcomes in obstetric fistula care: a literature review. Curr Opin Obstet Gynecol. 2013;25(5):399–403. https://doi.org/10.1097/gco.0b013e3283648d60.
15. Ott BB, Olson RM. Ethical issues of medical missions: the clinicians' view. HEC Forum. 2011;23(2):105–13. https://doi.org/10.1007/s10730-011-9154-9.
16. Farmer D, Sitkin N, Lofberg K, Donkor P, Ozgediz D. Surgical interventions for congenital anomalies. In: Debas HT, Donkor P, Gawande A, Jamison DT, Kruk ME, Mock CN, editors. Essential surgery: disease control priorities, vol. 1. 3rd ed. World Bank; 2015. https://doi.org/10.1596/978-1-4648-0346-8.
17. Park E, Deshpande G, Schonmeyr B, Restrepo C, Campbell A. Improved early cleft lip and palate complications at a surgery specialty center in the developing world. Cleft Palate Craniofac J. 2018;55(8):1145–52. https://doi.org/10.1177/1055665618762881.
18. Meier DE, Fitzgerald TN, Axt JR. A practical guide for short-term pediatric surgery global volunteers. J Pediatr Surg. 2016;51(8):1380–4. https://doi.org/10.1016/j.jpedsurg.2016.05.016.
19. Mock C, Debas H, Balch CM, Brennan M, Buyske J, Cusack J, et al. Global surgery: effective involvement of US academic surgery: report of the American Surgical Association Working Group on global surgery. Ann Surg. 2018;268(4):557–63. https://doi.org/10.1097/sla.0000000000002934.
20. Steyn E, Edge J. Ethical considerations in global surgery. Br J Surg. 2019;106(2):e17–9. https://doi.org/10.1002/bjs.11028.
21. Bioethics GNoWCCf. Global health ethics: key issues. World Health Organization; 2015.
22. Sceats LA, Morris AM, Narayan RR, Mezynski A, Woo RK, Yang GP. Lost in translation: informed consent in the medical mission setting. Surgery. 2019;165(2):438–43. https://doi.org/10.1016/j.surg.2018.06.010.
23. Rowthorn V, Loh L, Evert J, Chung E, Lasker J. Not above the law: a legal and ethical analysis of short-term experiences in global health. Ann Glob Health. 2019;85(1):79, 1–12. https://doi.org/10.5334/aogh.2451.
24. Loh LC, Cherniak W, Dreifuss BA, Dacso MM, Lin HC, Evert J. Short term global health experiences and local partnership models: a framework. Global Health. 2015;11:50. https://doi.org/10.1186/s12992-015-0135-7.
25. Tervalon M, Murray-Garcia J. Cultural humility versus cultural competence: a critical distinction in defining physician training outcomes in multicultural education. J Health Care Poor Underserved. 1998;9(2):117–25. https://doi.org/10.1353/hpu.2010.0233.
26. Cherniak W, Latham E, Astle B, et al. Visiting trainees in global settings: host and partner perspectives on desirable competencies. Ann Glob Health. 2017;83(2):359–68. https://doi.org/10.1016/j.aogh.2017.04.007.

27. Shah S. How should academic medical centers administer students' "domestic global health" experiences? AMA J Ethics. 2019;21(9):E778–87. https://doi.org/10.1001/amajethics.2019.778.
28. Browning A, Patel TL. FIGO initiative for the prevention and treatment of vaginal fistula. Int J Gynaecol Obstet. 2004;86(2):317–22. https://doi.org/10.1016/j.ijgo.2004.05.003.
29. Punchak M, Lazareff JA. Cost-effectiveness of short-term neurosurgical missions relative to other surgical specialties. Surg Neurol Int. 2017;8:37. https://doi.org/10.4103/sni.sni_199_16.
30. Drain PK, Primack A, Hunt DD, Fawzi WW, Holmes KK, Gardner P. Global health in medical education: a call for more training and opportunities. Acad Med. 2007;82(3):226–30. https://doi.org/10.1097/acm.0b013e3180305cf9.
31. Shah S, Wu T. The medical student global health experience: professionalism and ethical implications. J Med Ethics. 2008;34(5):375–8. https://doi.org/10.1136/jme.2006.019265.

Chapter 41
The Ethics of Medical Missions (Con)

Alberto R. Ferreres ⓘ

Abstract The access to surgical healthcare of adequate quality is characterized by inequity and unfairness worldwide, this situation tends to worsen in low- and middle-income countries. As a remedy to this situation, surgical missions sponsored by non-government organizations or academic institutions have become more popular, in particular for young trainees. Although these humanitarian efforts should be commended, the local impact of medical missions is many times compromised by different circumstances as well as by ethical challenges. The delivery of high- quality surgical services framed by the ethical principles of respect for patient autonomy, beneficence, nonmaleficence and justice should be the main concern of the surgical community worldwide. It is in the benefit of all those involved, and in particular, the patients, to understand and clarify these ethical challenges to better serve this population in low- and middle-income countries.

Keywords Global surgery · Surgical health care · Surgical ethics · Equity Fairness · Surgical health care · Surgical missions

A. R. Ferreres (✉)
Department of Surgery, University of Buenos Aires, Buenos Aires, Argentina

Department of Surgery, University of Washington, Seattle, WA, USA
e-mail: aferre17@uw.edu

© The Author(s), under exclusive license to Springer Nature
Switzerland AG 2022
V. A. Lonchyna et al. (eds.), *Difficult Decisions in Surgical Ethics*, Difficult
Decisions in Surgery: An Evidence-Based Approach,
https://doi.org/10.1007/978-3-030-84625-1_41

Case

Dr. Tourek Mas Ilayan is a foreign medical graduate who has risen to Associate Professor of Surgery at a medical school where he is also the Cardio-Thoracic Division chief. Every year, together with a group of seven to eight of his surgical and anesthesia colleagues and some residents, he organizes medical missions to underserved locations in his home country, him being the sole individual fluent in the local language. These trips last about one week. Plenty of cases are set up by local people and organizations, and patients from adjacent locations rush into the facility where this activity takes place and have access to these surgeries. Many of the surgical procedures, although within the range of their training, are mostly out of the regular scope of practice of the travelling specialists. Local support is mostly represented by nurses and surgical assistants; in few cases local physicians or surgeons are involved. Local physicians' organizations have complained about the trips, and emphasized the burden of postoperative complications, which require management by local surgeons. However, Dr. Mas Ilayan considers that he is providing care for patients which otherwise would be neglected and plans to continue with his humanitarian efforts, if not in his home country, then in a neighboring one.

41.1 Introduction

Surgical conditions and their unmet solution represent a major and significant contributor to the global burden of disease and are particularly prevalent and suffered by the population in low- and middle-income countries (LMIC), originally the so called Third World [1].

Several challenges to the ethical principles may be encountered during the achievement of these missions worldwide. The four Ethical Principles were collated by Beauchamp and Childress, based on the original prima facie principles, described by Sir David Ross in 1930 [2]. They represent a systematic approach to Medical Ethics and an aid for problem- solving conflicts [3]. The principlist approach offers a worksheet of moral and ethical parameters to assess and solve ethical conflicts in everyday surgical care. Each principle may be linked to different aspects in the field of global surgery and thus develop a typology, as appreciated in Table 41.1 and will serve as a guideline for discussion.

A typical challenge, confronted to all the four ethical principles, is represented by the establishment of an effective communication between both sides of the dyadic patient- surgeon relationship. The language barrier between the surgical manpower and the patients and the local human resources is a very important fact to consider, although the leader is a national. The communication factor also involves a proper acknowledgement by the visiting team of the local culture and values. The communication process between the surgeon in charge and the patient and his or her

Table 41.1 Typology of ethical topics in Global Surgery

Principle	Topics
Justice	• Licensing/authorization to perform surgery • Professional liability issues • Working in an unusual environment/ setting, with lack of resources and/or supplies • Participation of surgeons not adequately trained to perform the requested procedures • Performing procedures out of the scope of usual practice • Replacement of the government duty to offer adequate surgical care • Observance of human rights • Cultural and values' differences • Communication issues
Respect for patient autonomy	• Surgical informed consent process • Language barriers • Disclosure of the surgeon own experience • Recognition of patients' requests • Communication issues
Beneficence	• Surgical diligence and expertise • Appropriate and reliable judgment • Professionalism/ professional traits • Supervision of postoperative course • Communication issues • Participation of surgeons not adequately trained to perform the requested procedures • Performing procedures out of the scope of usual practice • Accountability
Non-maleficence	• Surgical diligence and expertise • Appropriate and reliable judgment • Recognition of the limits of one's professional domain • vDisclosure and discussion of the surgeon own experience, risks, complications and errors • Communication issues

family may probably be compromised from the start, no matter the presence of a translator. This situation will affect the whole communication process: a valid surgical informed consent, shared decision making and alarms regarding risks and potential complications as well as truthfulness and disclosures. Within the latter, concern is raised about the complete disclosure of the surgeon' expertise and comfort in some of the procedures to be performed (e.g. general surgeon performing a cesarean section or an endocrine surgery fellow performing hernia repairs).

Added to the language barrier, and since the patients are usually suffering from chronic surgical conditions unresolved by the local government, the issue of patients' freedom and the respect of the visiting surgical team for patient autonomy may collide. Usually, surgical missions overseas tend to last no more than 7 to 10 days, with a very tight schedule, which may prevent taking care of all the patients in need of surgical care. In addition, there is the question of who will be in charge of postoperative follow-up with an emphasis on managing complications.

The starting point of the relationship between the patients and the participant in the surgical mission is one of unfairness, or justice, in which their basic human rights are violated due to their lack of access to adequate health care, including surgical care. In summary all of the four ethical principles, as well as the patients taken care, may suffer some type of impairment through the surgical care provided by international global missions to LMIC.

41.2   Search Strategy

A search using the following MeSH terms (ethics, surgical ethics, global surgery, surgical missions, ethical challenges) was performed in these databases: Pubmed, Medline and LiLacs between the years 1995–2020. References included within the retrieved publications were further assessed and those considered the most appropriate have been included in the chapter's list of references.

41.3   Discussion

Access to adequate medical care should be considered a human right all over the world. In that sense, the United Nations' 1948 Universal Declaration of Human Rights states in article 25, first part:

> Everyone has the right to a standard of living adequate for the health and well-being of himself and of his family, including food, clothing, housing and medical care and necessary social services, and the right to security in the event of unemployment, sickness, disability, widowhood, old age or other lack of livelihood in circumstances beyond his control [4].

The right to health is further defined in Article 12 of the 1966 International Covenant on Economic, Social and Cultural Rights [5]. In addition to this document the United Nations Office of the High Commissioner for Human Rights has described the entitlements of the right to health, which include:

- The right to a system of health protection providing equality of opportunity for everyone to enjoy the highest attainable level of health
- The right to prevention, treatment and control of diseases
- Access to essential medicines, maternal, child and reproductive health
- Equal and timely access to basic health services
- The provision of health-related education and information
- Participation of the population in health- related decision-making at the national and community levels
- All services, goods and facilities must be available, accessible, acceptable and of good quality [6]

In compliance with these documents, there should be both a duty and an obligation by governments to guarantee and provide these services; to comply with the above-mentioned requirements, no matter their political sign or inclination, on a timely and adequate basis, and not to depend on the good will of foreign third-party providers. While an obligation is a "must", a duty is "ought", which evidences the moral strength of these duties. Most of these LMICs are managed by inefficient and sometimes corrupt systems, to whom public health is not a priority and so the UN guidelines remain mostly unfulfilled for the vast majority of nationals in those countries, especially those in vulnerable situations. Besides, many African countries do not lack in natural resources, such as diamonds, minerals and oil [7].

Although in LMIC the number of physicians and surgeons is low, the governments, usually characterized by unfairness, utterly indolence and lack of transparency, have not taken measures to solve the overall situation. In addition, the Institute of Medicine (today the National Academy of Medicine) has defined the quality of care as the "provision of care that is safe, effective, efficient, timely and patient centered for all those who are in need" [8]. In 1997, the Institute of Medicine stated that "America has a vital and direct stake in the health of the people around the globe, and this interest derives from both America's long and enduring tradition of humanitarian concern and compelling reasons of enlightened self-interest" [9].

Current surgical missions to LMIC are considered by some authors as a new form of colonialism and/or imperialism. Some of the first US health campaign overseas were rooted in a concept of colonialism and profit and not pure altruistic goals. Two situations exemplify this assertion. The first is the work of Chief Sanitary Officer William Gorgas in the construction of the Panama Canal (1904–1914) whose goal was keeping the workers free of malaria and yellow fever [10]. The second was the Rockefeller Foundation's first campaign rooted in the mission "to promote the well-being of humanity throughout the world", really pursued the eradication of hookworm in South America, which affected the productivity of their workers [11].

There are several approaches to the concept of global surgery and the matters it involves. Global surgery generally refers to the provision of surgical care in low-resource settings, mostly LMIC, usually performed by non-local physicians. It is usually characterized by the fact of placing medical and/or surgical volunteers in a context of unfamiliar places, with different languages and cultural bonds and severe constraints regarding infrastructure and resources. Although surgery should be considered an indivisible and indispensable part of health care, the global disparity to surgical care between rich and poor is astounding, not only within countries but between individuals of different countries.

Meara et al. [12] informed these facts:

5 billion people lack access to safe, affordable surgical and anesthesia care when needed
43 million additional surgical procedures are needed each year to save lives and prevent disability
33 million individuals face catastrophic health expenditures due to payment for surgery and anesthesia each year

Many Third World countries are open to foreign surgical labor force, in contrast to the US and most western countries which tend to be much more stringent in receiving foreign physicians, who are usually well trained in their countries. This may be due to many reasons, one of them professional liability issues. It is clear, however, that surgical missions to LMIC will not solve the inequity and failure of the implemented health care systems in those countries.

Bath et al. consider global surgery as the enterprise of providing improved and equitable surgical care to the world's population [13]. Dare et al. define global surgery as an area of study, research, practice and advocacy that seeks to improve health outcomes and achieve health equity for all people who require surgical care, with a special emphasis on underserved populations and populations in crisis. It uses collaborative, cross-sectorial and transnational approaches, and is a synthesis of population-based strategies with individual surgical care [14].

The most common and usual model for surgical intervention in LMIC settings is represented by the one week to ten-day short-term surgical mission consisting of a group of providers from a developed country going to a LMIC where they provide as many surgical procedures as they and the local setting are able to manage. This type of mission provides much needed surgical interventions but does not address the core of the chronic lack of surgical care in the local communities. They also usually fail in the management of perioperative care, adequate follow-up, potential complications, and poor communication with the local medical practitioners and health care staff and personnel.

There are some benchmarks which may assist in the goal of defining the ethical implications of a global mission as in the case. Since the main goal of these missions is represented by the offering and performance of surgical procedures to a limited number of patients, due to the short time of the activity, the following conundrums should undergo detailed scrutiny:

- Surgical competence and diligence of the visiting surgeons: related to the training and focus of the participants in the field of practice which will be requested and required during their trip. What may happen if a foreign trainee is asked to perform a procedure which lies outside their comfort zone or previous experience?
- Partnership with local human resources and organizations is of paramount importance and may lead to the teaching and training of the local physicians.
- Sustainability and continuity of care, represented by the question "What happens when the team leaves?"
- Outcomes monitoring

In the introductory vignette, it seems clear that the group headed by Dr. Mas Ilayan does not comply with the mentioned salient points. Since the surgical mission lasts a maximum of ten days, late complications and sequelae may eventually request the care of another team, if available. And there is no accountability of the activity displayed by the travelling group.

41.4 Justice

Aristotle first conceptualized justice as the "rendering to each individual of what is due to him or her" [15] and in the health care arena, refers to the achievement of fairness and equity. It is only fair to provide patients in LMIC's with the same application of the morally accepted laws as happens in their home countries and settings. Respect for patients' individual rights should be a priority. A final consideration regarding the concept of social justice, which encompasses these overseas humanitarian undertakings, should be made. Many times the trips are justified by the common good, which consists of the ultimate realization of individual and social capabilities. These aims are shared by both the individual and the collective. Social justice pursues the common good, which should be characterized by the social coexistence of human dignity, altruism, and solidarity with a particular focus for those in civil society with the greatest needs and the least advantages. In order to comply with this principle, medical missions overseas should be in accordance with the following provisions: (1) these ventures should be part of local initiatives aimed at the implementation, organization, development and strengthening of local healthcare resources, (2) the agenda of healthcare issues and priorities should be established by the local community or government bodies preventing paternalistic, colonial or imperialistic approaches, (3) the missions should nurture harmony between treatment provided by the visitors and a more comprehensive promotion of health, (4) follow up and thus continuity of care should be assured, (5) attention should be paid not only to healthcare issues but to many other social determinants (education, employment, social infrastructure, among others), and in this aspect non-government-organizations and academic and foreign institutions play a role in controlling local state governments, (6) Critical evaluation and assessment of each health mission is mandatory for improvement and empowerment of the local communities [16].

As shown in Table 41.1 I, there are several topics which compromise the ethical principle of justice in this mission, and which emerge clearly.

One of the initial aspects to guarantee the safety of the mission and patients is compliance with local licensing procedures and/or authorizations and health standards so as to prevent any clash with regulatory issues and professional liability issues. Have the members of this mission or Dr. Mas Ilayan requested due authorization to local authorities for the performance of the surgical procedures in accordance with local regulations? Was this authorization granted? Working under limited resources' conditions may impose also additional risks to the patients, because many practitioners are not used to those settings in their home institutions, and many times they perform procedures which are not within their usual scope of practice. This may compromise not only the quality of the provided care but may also have unintended consequences. The volunteer surgeon needs to have a high level of skill and empathy to adapt to these types of settings, and that is not typically the situation of the surgical residents involved in the mission. Gil et al. describe that only 70% of hernia repairs performed in Africa used electrocoagulation due to the lack of this equipment in operating rooms [17]. Howe considers that many times volunteers perform operations in less optimal conditions that they are used to in their native settings [18] and Bernstein describes the medical and moral unease of performing surgery with equipment and assistance so inferior to that back at his hospital [19]. Frequently, patients in developing countries often suffer from conditions that are not known, infrequent or not prevalent in the developed world. This represents a challenge for surgical volunteers, who encounter patients with more advanced disease than they are accustomed to due to delayed or lack of available healthcare which adds to the difficulty of performing the procedure itself.

Another important challenge to the principle of justice is the observance of the human rights of the patients, who are in a vulnerable situation, based on being placed into a situation where to choose with freedom is unthinkable and condemned by their social status. Of course, the contrast in culture and values, added to the language barrier magnifies communication barriers which prevent open discussion of the surgical indication, risk/benefits ratios and shared decision-making process. As an example of language barriers preventing effective communication, Groen reported that fourteen official languages exist in Sierra Leone [20]. In the depicted case, only Dr. Mas Ilayan is fluent in the local language, while the rest of the members are only fluent in English, preventing sound, safe and reliable communication, since additional translators are not available.

Last, but not the least, the usual criticism to short surgical global missions is represented by the dictum "You can't carry out medical programs in episodes", reflecting the lack of real programs, and not just actions, to strengthen local resources and support the training of the local surgical and medical manpower. Although Dr. Ilayan has travelled to this country several times, his relationship with local physicians and health organizations is not smooth.

41.5 Beneficence and Non-Maleficence

Beneficence is represented by acts of mercy, kindness, and charity and involves the principle of acting with the best interest of the other in mind. Positive beneficence supports the disposition of moral duties: to protect and defend the rights of others and imposes positive requirements of action. Non-Maleficence is based on the dictum "Primum non nocere" ("First, do no harm") and requests intentionally refraining from actions that would cause harm. It includes not only the duty not to inflict harm but also the duty not to impose a risk of harm. It is worth remembering Jonsen's editorial regarding the first conflict every physician encounter: "altruism vs self-interest" [21]. Despite the general idea of altruism surrounding overseas medical missions, the self-interest of the participants, which may range from hands-on expertise with difficult and/or uncommon cases to tax benefits, should be thoroughly explored.

Providing surgical care to at least some patients who lack access, either as a result of financial, geographical or other reasons, has been traditionally seen as a virtue in medical practice. Many pursue this virtue by providing care to unfunded patients in their local practice area, without the need to travel overseas. Many authors emphasized the potential for unintentional harm to the intended beneficiaries of this type of provider care [22]. Nonetheless, and according to the facts presented earlier, the impact of these missions on global underserved surgical needs is not significant. In the case presented, about 100 to 120 cases are performed during the week of the mission led by Dr. Mas Ilayan. While this is a large number of cases to the visiting surgeons it does not begin to address the needs of the community they visit.

Another issue is the surgical diligence and expertise of the surgeons in the diseases they are going to take care and operate upon. Is it fine for a transplant surgeon to operate large incarcerated inguinal hernias in a completely different setting? Is it ok for a PGY4 to perform or assist a huge goiter expanding to the upper mediastinum? Probably the question in adequate conditions should be a no. These issues should be included in a wider discussion regarding the accountability of the whole mission and its real impact on the life and welfare to the population [23]. Another Achilles' heel of these overseas missions is the lack of appropriate professional conduct, and an example is the relationship with the local health force, that in the case in discussion seems to be uncertain. The only way to prevent this from happening is to connect and partner with local physicians and/or institutions in order to build a local surgical force grounded on the education and training provided, a fact that Dr. Mas Ilayan has not given enough attention. Record keeping can be an issue in these settings and thus may also be compromised, quite opposite to what happens in the home settings, where there is a compelling duty to comply with regulations regarding the documentation of physicians' involvement and practice.

Another matter of concern is the management of the postoperative course after the surgical team deploys and the situation returns to normal, with no available and immediate care, forcing the population to move to another town to seek surgical care. These circumstances place patients at a higher risk for complications than would be accepted at home, and clash with the ethical duties of a surgeon, whose mission is to perform the procedure and supervise the postoperative course until full medical release.

At times the motivation for missions may benefit the provider of short-term aid more than the intended recipient. As an example, residents or medical students may be given the opportunity to gain experience doing procedures on a population where there is less emphasis on supervision and informed consent than would take place at their home academic institutions. These circumstances will undoubtedly give them access to patients and situations that they would not otherwise have [24]. One of the main reasons for surgeons in training to travel to South Africa, for example, was to gain experience and training in the management of trauma patients in settings with a high incidence of mass casualties [25].

41.6 Respect for Autonomy

This principle underlies the individual decision-making in health care and research, as patients and as subjects, throughout the whole health care process. There are two conditions which are essential for the achievement of this principle: liberty (freedom from external controlling forces or influences) and agency (the capacity and capability for intentional action). The basic paradigm of autonomy in health care is represented not only by the informed consent process, but also by the freedom to choose and a shared decision-making process. It also requires that patients are not deceived by the behavior of their physicians. In many global missions, this principle is at risk in many ways. Language and cultural barriers are a challenge for a sound and valid informed consent process, foreign doctors in communities with low and very low health literacy level may be seen as having a special or higher authority. These flaws surely would not be accepted in other settings, making these communities more prone to abuses and paternalistic approaches. Many times, as in the above case, most participants are performing beyond their scope of training, increasing risks of physician care, errors and harm to the patients. In summary, the following issues should be given proper attention:

- Do patients have the right to choose treatment based on informed consent?
- Patients should not be deceived or given false expectations.
- How are language, communication and cultural barriers/issues given proper and adequate attention?
- How are patients gathered if no contact with local physicians has been established?

It seems very clear that the principle of autonomy is compromised most times, due to the vulnerability and low health literacy of the population, as well as the language barriers.

Lasker et al. defined six core consensus principles to assure effective and ethical short-term health activities. They include: (1) appropriate recruitment, preparation and supervision of volunteers, (2) the host partner, either a non-government organization, medical organization, hospital, charity, who defines the program and their role in it, (3) the sustainability and the continuity of programs, (4) espect for governance and compliance of legal and ethical standards, (5) regular evaluation and audit of programs and outcomes for the assessment of their impact and (6) mutuality of learning, training and respect for local health professionals (Table 41.2). But, regretfully, little compliance with these guidelines have been achieved [26].

Table 41.2 The six core principles for effective and ethical short term medical missions [26]

1. Appropriate recruitment, preparation and supervision of volunteers
2. The host partner, either a non-government organization, medical organization, hospital, charity, who defines the program and their role in it
3. The sustainability and the continuity of programs
4. Respect for governance and compliance of legal and ethical standards
5. Regular evaluation and audit of programs and outcomes for the assessment of their impact
6. Mutuality of learning, training and respect for local health professionals

Welling, et al. provide a valuable and illustrative overview of many of these criticisms by describing the "seven sins of humanitarian medicine", which may serve as a guiding template for assessment and evaluation of medical and surgical global missions [27]. These include:

1. Leaving a mess behind, with special emphasis on complications and undesired outcomes
2. Failing to match technology to local needs
3. Failure of non-governmental organizations to cooperate and help each other, and accept help from military organizations
4. Failing to have a follow-up plan
5. Allowing politics, training, or other distracting goals to trump service, while representing the mission as service-oriented
6. Going where we are not wanted or needed and/or being poor guests
7. Doing the right thing for the wrong reason

This includes going on an unusual vacation, doing a "first" case, performing a large number of complex/unusual cases in a quick fashion and without the requirements of informed consent process, adequate monitoring, follow up, without the need to train local surgeons, and to achieve fame or recognition.

A unifying theme underlying many of these sins is a systemic failure to consult or cooperate with the local population and healthcare providers, or other international groups operating in the same location. Another common topic is the usual lack of sustainability of these missions which are, many times, characterized by: a) lack of continuity of care, in order to avoid an operation as an isolated event, b) the guarantee of an adequate follow-up care and precise management of long-term complications, c) weak collaboration in teaching and training local human providers and d) lack of information regarding outcomes' measurement. All these traits can be easily identified in Dr. Mas Ilayan's mission.

41.7   Case Conclusion

In summary, the surgical mission led by Dr. Mas Ilayan should comply with the following issues to be considered ethically and morally sound:

- Are the professional goals of Dr. Mas Ilayan and his team clarified and aligned with the hosts' goals?
- Which are the real reasons for his enterprise? Is it just beneficence? Or is there any hidden benefit for all those participants? (e.g. benefits in tax revenue)
- Is there an established partnership between organizations/ academic institutions supervising the surgical mission?
- Has there been preparation standards established in partnership between the ongoing team and the local organization?
- Who is/are the one/s responsible/s for defining the scope of the surgical procedures which will be performed?

- Which will be the standards of care to abide for?
- Who will be held accountable for the surgical indication in each particular case?
- What type of available infrastructure will the team rely upon?
- Are there enough and adequate supplies and/or resources?
- Is the team bringing with them supplies? What type or kind of them? How will they clear customs?
- What about local licensing or permits to perform surgery?
- Who will look and take care for patients after the team deploys from the area?
- What type of relationships with local physicians/ medical associations will be established and nurtured?
- What type of learning/ training will the local physicians receive?

Regarding the appropriateness of direct care delivery, one should be stringent in the sense that the ethical goal of any medical humanitarian mission is "ensuring the right surgeon performs the right procedure on the right patient with the right resources" [28], and this has not happened in the case under discussion.

41.8   Concluding Remarks

- There is no doubt that global surgical care programs may address disparities in health and surgical care worldwide, but their significance and impact are controversial. Nonetheless, strong demands to the local governments should be made to prevent serious omissions in health care and corruption
- Medical humanitarian missions should be ethical, safe and responsible. A key component includes planning, follow-up and sustainability
- These programs present a unique set of ethical challenges, that should be addressed by the participants and leaders of these missions
- Is still the safety and well-being of the patients at the core of these modalities, or it is only beneficial to the moral conscience of the physicians involved in the sense that "they are doing something good"?
- These modalities should be under close scrutiny in order to achieve a better knowledge of their outcomes
- It is important to develop and hone partnerships with local physicians, surgeons, and institutions in order to guarantee the training of local resources and thus, that follow-up is ensured
- The ultimate goal should be to convince the local governments about the benefits of establishing adequate standards of health and surgical care as well as referral and counter referral networks.
- Global surgical missions should not be an example of itinerant surgery, and if performed in that fashion should be condemned and avoided
- If global surgical missions are to be ethically sound, they need to heed Welling's advice so as to prevent the commission of any sins [27].

41.9 Selected References

- Scheiner A, Rickard JL, Nwomeh B, et al. Global surgery pro-con debate: a pathway to bilateral academic success or the bold new face of colonialism? J Surg Res. 2020;252:272–280. doi:https://doi.org/10.1016/j.jss.2020.01.032

  - A pro-con analysis of global surgery. Among the pro are: the possibility of establishing bilateral a partnership, which is mutually beneficial as well as mentorship processes. And among the con are: elements of colonialism/imperialism; pitfalls of the surgical missions in the fields of continuous care, surgical education and research.

- Grant CL, Robinson T, Al Hinai A, Mack C, Guilfoyle R, Saleh A. Ethical considerations in global surgery: a scoping review. BMJ Global Health. 2020;5:e002319. doi:https://doi.org/10.1136/bmjgh-2020-002319

  - A scoping review of different relevant databases identifying literature pertaining to the topic of ethics in global surgery in four domains: clinical care and delivery; research, monitoring and evaluation; engagement in collaboration and partnerships.

- Welling DR, Ryan JM, Burris DG, Rich NM. Seven sins of humanitarian medicine. World J Surg. 2010;34: 466–470. doi:https://doi.org/10.1007/s00268-009-0373-z

  - The authors list concerns, mistakes that are common and challenge the success of humanitarian missions. Some are: (1) leaving a mess behind, (2) failing to match technology to local needs and abilities, (3) failure of non-government-organizations to cooperate and help each other, (4) failing to have a follow-up plan, (5) allowing politics, training, or other distracting goals to trump service, while representing the mission as service, (6) going where we are not wanted, or needed and/or being poor guest and (7) doing the right thing for the wrong reason.

References

1. Farmer PE, Kim JY. Surgery and Global Health: a view from beyond the OR. World J Surg. 2008;32:533–6. https://doi.org/10.1007/s00268-008-9525-9.
2. Ross WD. The right and the good. Oxford University Press; 1930.
3. Beauchamp TL, Childress JF. Principles of biomedical ethics. 8th ed. Oxford University Press; 2019.
4. United Nations. Universal Declaration of Human Rights.1948. Accessed December 13, 2020. https://www.ohchr.org/EN/UDHR/Documents/UDHR_Translations/eng.pdf.
5. International Covenant on Economic, Social and Cultural Rights, 993 UNTS 3, entered into force 3 January 1976. Accessed December 13, 2020 https://www.ohchr.org/Documents/ProfessionalInterest/cescr.pdf.
6. Office of the United Nations High Commissioner for Human Rights and World Health Organization. The Right to Health. Fact Sheet No. 31. Accessed December 13, 2020. https://www.ohchr.org/Documents/Publications/Factsheet31.pdf.

7. Scheiner A, Rickard JL, Nwomeh B, et al. Global surgery pro-con debate: a pathway to bilateral academic success or the bold new face of colonialism? J Surg Res. 2020;252:272–80. https://doi.org/10.1016/j.jss.2020.01.032.

8. Institute of Medicine Committee on Quality of Health Care in America. *Crossing the quality chasm: a new health system for the 21st century.* National Academy Press; 2001.

9. Institute of Medicine Board on International Health. *America's vital interest in global health: protecting our economy, and advancing our international interest.* National Academy Press; 1997.

10. Harrison MA. A global perspective: reframing the history of health medicine, and disease. Bull Hist Med. 2015;89:639–89. https://doi.org/10.1353/bhm.2015.0116.

11. Palmer S. Toward responsibility in international health: death following treatment in Rockefeller hookworm campaigns 1914–1934. Med Hist. 2010;54:149–70. https://doi.org/10.1017/s0025727300000223.

12. Meara JG, Leather AJM, Hagander L, et al. Global surgery 2030: evidence and solutions for achieving health, welfare and economic development. Lancet. 2015;386:569–624. https://doi.org/10.1016/s0140-6736(15)60160-x.

13. Bath M, Bashford T, Fitzgerald JE. What is global surgery? Defining the multidisciplinary interface between surgery, anaesthesia and public health. BMJ Glob Health. 2019;4:e001808. https://doi.org/10.1136/bmjgh-2019-001808.

14. Dare AJ, Grimes CE, Gillies R, et al. Global surgery: defining an emerging global field. Lancet. 2014;384:2245–7. https://doi.org/10.1016/s0140-6736(14)60237-3.

15. Aristotle. *Nicomachean Ethics.* Translated by Terence Irwin. 2nd ed. Hackett; 1999:67–74.

16. Vicini A. Social justice and the promotion of the common good in medical mission to low-resourced countries. Ann Global Health. 2019;85(83):1–2. https://doi.org/10.5334/aogh.2519.

17. Gil J, Rodriguez JM, Hernandez Q, et al. Do hernia operations in African international cooperation programmes provide good quality? World J Surg. 2012;36:2795–801. https://doi.org/10.1007/s00268-012-1768-9.

18. Howe KL, Malomo AO, Bernstein MA. Ethical challenges in international surgical education, for visitors and hosts. World Neurosurg. 2013;80(6):751–8. https://doi.org/10.1016/j.wneu.2013.02.087.

19. Bernstein MA. Ethical dilemmas encountered while operating and teaching in a developing country. Can J Surg. 2004;47:170–2. 15264377.

20. Groen RS, Kamara TB, Dixon-Cole R, et al. A tool and index to assess surgical capacity in low income countries: an initial implementation in Sierra Leone. World J Surg. 2012;36:1970–7. https://doi.org/10.1007/s00268-012-1591-3.

21. Jonsen A. Watching the doctor. N Engl J Med. 1983;308:1531–5. https://doi.org/10.1056/nejm198306233082571.

22. Zientek D, Bonnell R. When international humanitarian or medical missions go wrong: an ethical analysis. HEC Forum. 2019; https://doi.org/10.1007/s10730-019-09392-6

23. Grant CL, Robinson T, Al Hinai A, Mack C, Guilfoyle R, Saleh A. Ethical considerations in global surgery: a scoping review. BMJ Glob Health. 2020;5:e002319. https://doi.org/10.1136/bmjgh-2020-002319.

24. Crump JA, Sugarman J. Ethical considerations for short-term experiences by trainees in global health. JAMA. 2008;300:1456–8. https://doi.org/10.1001/jama.300.12.1456.

25. Steyn E, Edge J. Ethical considerations in global surgery. BJS. 2019;106:e17–9. https://doi.org/10.1002/bjs.11028.

26. Lasker JN, Aldrink M, Balasubramaniam R, et al. Guidelines for responsible short-term global health activities: developing common principles. Glob Health. 2018;14:18. https://doi.org/10.1186/s12992-018-0330-4

27. Welling DR, Ryan JM, Burris DG, Rich NM. Seven sins of humanitarian medicine. World J Surg. 2010;34:466–70. https://doi.org/10.1007/s00268-009-0373-z.

28. Asgary R, Junck E. New trends of short-term humanitarian medical volunteerism: professional and ethical considerations. J Med Ethics. 2013;39:625–31. https://doi.org/10.1136/medethics-2011-100488.

Chapter 42
Invited Commentary: Medical Missions to Developing Countries

Amy G. Lehman

Abstract As a practitioner who transitioned from working in a tertiary care academic medical center in a major metropolitan city in the United States, to the founder of an organization working in health systems-building in one of the most operationally difficult countries in the world, my views about short-term experiences in global health (STEGH) certainly run deep. Starting out, I focused on immediate and pressing health issues in the Lake Tanganyika basin in East/Central Africa—one of which was maternal morbidity and mortality, and thus obstetric fistula formation.

More recently, I am addressing upstream health-system related problems rather than on diseases per se (surgical and otherwise)—most specifically on improving the flow of community-level public health data. First and foremost, we need reliable data on the incidence of common health challenges.

Keywords Short-term experiences in global health (STEGH) · Lake Tanganyika Floating Health Clinic (LTFHC) · Health justice · Population health · Obstetric fistula formation · Maternal and fetal death

As a practitioner who transitioned from working in a tertiary care academic medical center in a major metropolitan city in the United States, to the founder of an organization working in health systems-building in one of the most operationally difficult countries in the world, my views about short-term experiences in global health (STEGH) certainly run deep [1]. I loved, and often miss, being in a well-equipped operating room, participating in complex operations where we have all the benefits of science and technology, where it was natural to take for granted enough supplies, masks, gowns, gloves—and where electricity and clean running water are givens.

A. G. Lehman (✉)
The Lake Tanganyika Floating Health Clinic, Chicago, IL, USA

Iroko Health, Kalemie, Democratic Republic of the Congo
e-mail: amy@floatingclinic.org

© The Author(s), under exclusive license to Springer Nature Switzerland AG 2022
V. A. Lonchyna et al. (eds.), *Difficult Decisions in Surgical Ethics*, Difficult Decisions in Surgery: An Evidence-Based Approach,
https://doi.org/10.1007/978-3-030-84625-1_42

Why make this transition? Of course, my actual journey is more complex, but the essence of this answer is simple: a deep commitment to health justice and equity. I did not participate in STEGH during my training, and, frankly, there weren't many opportunities for the previous generation of trainees. Therefore, much of my journey was based on long-time individual interests and relationships that I had developed over the course of my secondary and post-secondary education. And when I transitioned from one role to a very different one, I had to re-learn and re-analyze different problem sets, expand my knowledge base in population health and infectious diseases, and confront some of the issues that had always nagged at me in surgical training: Is there really strong evidence for all the operations and interventions we are doing? For all our practices? Could we achieve good results with other/ different means under more financially constrained conditions?

Starting out, I focused on immediate and pressing health issues in the Lake Tanganyika basin in East/Central Africa—one of which was maternal morbidity and mortality, and thus obstetric fistula formation [2]. This is a common problem where health systems are extremely weak, and basic prenatal and delivery care is hard to access. In my catchment area, the lack of roads/other basic municipal infrastructure, the lack of 3G and above signal coverage, plus challenges of physical insecurity, significantly amplify the risk of maternal and fetal death, and fistula injury. Many people are aware of Nobel Peace Prize winner, Dr. Denis Mukwege's excellent work at the Panzi Hospital outside Bukavu in South Kivu—however, it's one of only two well-supported, skilled high-volume centers in a country that is the size of western Europe (and they are both on Lake Kivu) [3]. Women often have to wait several months, living on the hospital compound, before they are able to receive surgical care. And for the majority of women, the distances and costs of travel are simply too great to overcome. We recognized that fistula care capacity had to be expanded to other areas of the Democratic Republic of Congo (DRC), so when we organized a surgical outreach, we included several Congolese health care workers, from doctors to nurses to community health volunteers. While we understood that developing high-quality surgical care would take a significant amount of time and resources, we believed we could make inroads around satellite services that might decrease the incidence and severity of fistulas, and in the meantime provide care to women who had been waiting years for treatment. For a snapshot of our work in this area, please view these short documentaries [2, 4].

As the years have passed, I have focused much of my energy on trying to address upstream health-system related problems rather than on diseases per se (surgical and otherwise)—most specifically on improving the flow of community-level public health data [1]. In weak systems, nothing can be taken for granted. First and foremost, do we even have reliable data on the incidence of common health challenges? If we don't, then how do we know how to design effective interventions? Through our own data collection work at the household level in South Kivu, we estimate that only twenty-five percent of community-level public health indicators actually flow to the first level of supervision in the Ministry of Health from fragile and difficult to access locations (Fig. 42.1).

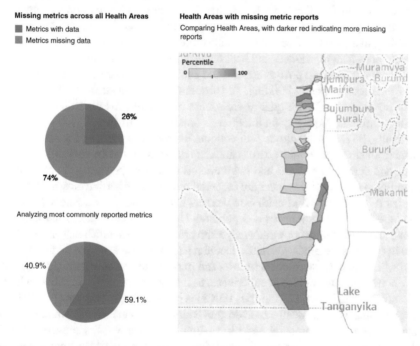

Fig. 42.1 Missing metrics across health areas of Lake Tanganyika. (Source: With permission from the Lake Tanganyika Floating Health Clinic)

In the age of the novel coronavirus pandemic, this has deep and consequential implications for global disease surveillance and security [5]. The world has learned the hard way that global health inequities can have a profound and potentially negative effect on more developed systems. Ultimately, we all have to care about global health systems particularly with regard to transmissible diseases [6].

Because of the complexity of our catchment area which includes a fluid human security element, we rarely, if ever, host STEGH outreaches with outside institutions. If we were to host, we would conduct extensive discussions with potential partnering organizations and screen participants for skill sets, experience with travel in fragile contexts, and motivations for participation, and be very transparent about inherent risks. Having said that, I believe that participation in appropriately designed and executed STEGH is incredibly enriching to medical trainees of all kinds, inclusive of surgical trainees, as well as people well into their professional practice. The key is to responsibly design STEGH.

As both authors appropriately point out, STEGH participation requires a stringent set of requirements to be met in order to maximize benefits and minimize harms or unintended consequences to all involved (most importantly, to patients and host health systems). Visiting programs have a set of responsibilities that include: partnership and familiarity with host health systems and practitioners; obtaining credentials (including temporary licensure); ensuring feasible continuity of care, including availability of supplies; establishing program length of time to accommodate both patient, trainee, and host country needs; risk-stratification and education of patients pre-and post-treatment; and general program design that enables and prioritizes local capacity building, and absolutely does not stress the local system. Respect, safety, and high-quality care must be ensured for all patients who are treated, which includes having interpreters on-site at all times.

Ideally, STEGHs should be bidirectional learning experiences for medical providers/trainees. "Standard of care" can mean different things in very different contexts, and certain operations and interventions cannot be performed in all settings. Humility, patience, and respect are essential attributes of participants in STEGHs. The scope of practice for health care workers can traverse a wide range, dependent upon the host country's needs and policies. The flow of expertise is not unidirectional, and often indigenous knowledge and practice can establish new standards of care in certain specialties. Obstetric fistula repair is a good example of an operative field where expert practitioners in low- and middle-income countries (LMICs) can have a much greater wealth of experience, as the incidence of obstetric fistula in the US and other high-income countries (HICs) is comparatively very low [7]. STEGH programming should ideally include prevention and management strategies. For example, supporting prenatal and birth planning clinics reduces the overall incidence of obstructed labor and fistula formation, and a significant percentage of simple vesico-vaginal fistulas can be completely treated with catheter-based decompression of the bladder only, if they are appropriately identified at the time of injury (and, crucially, there is an adequate supply of indwelling catheters, and health care workers who can insert them, observe and educate patients about their care) [8]. Not all expensive and high-tech interventions are necessary, and particularly in surgery, a number of HIC practices are the result of custom and habit vs. rigorously tested and proven methodologies. Those visiting LMICs from HIC should strive to remember that.

The performance of LMIC's health systems can vary, and the "should," "why," and "how" of that performance is often very complex. Having worked for more than a decade in a resource-rich but fragile state, I believe penalizing patients due to national and international governance failures over which they have little to no control is inappropriate. However, participants in such contexts should be aware and capable of navigating challenging political and operational terrains [9]. Often private actors within dysfunctional states can deliver high-quality and rational preventive care as well as treatments—and indeed if we are to achieve the global, very ambitious, Sustainable Development Goals, that sort of engagement will be required alongside a commitment to health systems strengthening in general, which should include surgical capacity building.

Additionally, participation in STEGHs can help illustrate gaps in HIC training. What does it mean to be adequately trained in general surgery today? The answer may be more nuanced than those of us who have trained at HIC academic medical centers may initially think, where the pull of hyper-specialization is strong. How much experience with open cases and sharp dissection should a competent and versatile general surgeon have? Should a general surgeon be comfortable with performing caesarean sections? What percentage of the HIC surgical workforce should be broadly trained and competent across multiple domains, to be ready to work in rural and/or underserved areas [10]? This is the counterpoint in experience to the very real need to bring more specialized expertise and exposure to LMIC health systems.

References

1. Iroko Health. The challenge of obtaining community-level health data in the DRC. https://irokohealth.com. Accessed 11 April 2021.
2. LTFHC's Women's Reproductive Health Outreach. 2013. https://vimeo.com/57186390. Accessed 11 April 2021.
3. Sjoveian S, Vangen S, Mukwege D, Onsrud M. Surgical ourcome of obstetric fistula: a retrospective analysis of 595 patients. Acta Obstet Gynecol Scand. 2011;90(7):753–60. https://doi.org/10.1111/j.1600-0412.2011.01162.x.
4. Lake Tanganyika Floating Health Clinic. 2013. https://vimeo.com/56171735. Accessed 11 April 2021.
5. Mukwege D, Cadiere GB, Vandenberg O. COVID-19 response in Sub-Sahara low-resource setting: healthcare soldiers need bullets. Am J Trop Med Hyg. 2020;103(2):549–50. https://doi.org/10.4269/ajtmh.20-0543.
6. Congo Research Group. Ebola in the DRC: the perverse effects of a parallel health system. NYU Center on International Cooperation; 2020. http://congoresearchgroup.org/wp-content/uploads/2020/09/report-ebola-drc-the-perverse-effects-of-a-parallel-health-system.pdf. Accessed 11 April 2021.
7. Onsrud M, Sjoveian S, Mukwege D. Cesarean delivery-related fistulae in the Democratic Republic of Congo. Int J Gynec Obstet. 2011;114(1):10–4. https://doi.org/10.1016/j.ijgo.2011.01.018.

8. Pope R. A review of surgical procedures to repair obstetric fistula. Int J Gynec Obstet. 2020;148(Supp 1):22–6. https://doi.org/10.1002/ijgo.13035.

9. Kowene G. Denis Mukwege: UN guards DR Congo Nobel laureate after death threats. BBC News, September 10, 2020. https://www.bbc.com/news/world-africa-54100429. Accessed 11 April 2021.

10. Rickard J, Onwuka E, Joseph S, the Academic Global Surgery Taskforce. Value of global surgical activities for US academic health centers – a position paper by the Association for Academic Surgery Global Affairs Committee, Society of University Surgeons Committee on Global Academic Surgery, and ACS. J Am Coll Surg. 2018;227(4):455–66. https://doi.org/10.1016/j.jamcollsurg.2018.07.661.

Chapter 43
Ethics and National Health Policy Change: A Case Study of the Transplant System in China

Ashley Suah and Michael Millis (iD)

Abstract The evolution of China's sixty-year-old transplant system has had a global impact. For decades, China's ongoing scarcity of organs in the absence of regulation of the transplant program resulted in the accepted use of executed prisoners' body parts as the primary source of transplanted organs. International awareness exposed an associated rise in transplant tourism and the ensuing predicament of organ trafficking. As a result, worldwide attention was directed towards these unethical practices. Establishment of a legal framework in 2007 and persistence in partnership between China and transnational allies led to the abolishment of donation by execution and the harvesting of Chinese prisoners' organs in 2015.

Keywords Ethics · Transplantation · China · Health policy · Transplant tourism
Organ trafficking · Prisoner body parts

> **Case**
> Zhong Haiyuan was a young, female schoolteacher from Ganzhou City, Jingxi Provence who was sentenced to death for "counterrevolutionary" offenses after numerous articles and big character posters composed by one of her colleagues, were discovered in her possession. She was shot twice in the head during her execution on April 30, 1978. China does not recognize brain death, thus until her heart ceased circulation, she was considered alive. Her body was taken to an operating facility at the prison and both of her kidneys were removed. One of her kidneys was transplanted into the son of a high-ranking military official, who reportedly facilitated the logistics of the procurement on the prison grounds [1].

A. Suah · M. Millis (✉)
Department of Surgery, University of Chicago Medicine, Chicago, IL, USA
e-mail: ashley.suah@uchospitals.edu; mmillis@surgery.bsd.uchicago.edu

© The Author(s), under exclusive license to Springer Nature
Switzerland AG 2022
V. A. Lonchyna et al. (eds.), *Difficult Decisions in Surgical Ethics*, Difficult
Decisions in Surgery: An Evidence-Based Approach,
https://doi.org/10.1007/978-3-030-84625-1_43

43.1   Introduction

43.1.1   Evolution of Transplantation in China

China's organ transplant program commenced in the 1960s and consisted primarily of kidney transplants, performed with the aid of foreign medical consultants. It was not until 1974 that the program was formally announced, yet this announcement was met with poor clinical outcomes [1]. Consequently, the transplant system struggled for the next decade. The early 1980s however, represented a turning point for China's transplant program with 1983 bringing forth the inauguration of annual crime initiatives which resulted in an increased number of prisoners being subjected to capital punishment [1–4]. A law was passed in 1990 which permitted the procurement of executed inmates' organs for the purposes of transplantation, which often occurred without permission from these prisoners or their families [5]. The absence of informed consent and lack of transparency in the practice of using criminals' body parts as a viable source of transplantable organs was rationalized with the notion that through their execution, these convicted felons would be prolonging the lives of innocent victims of end-organ failure. Unfortunately, these new crime campaigns involved a broadening of offenses punishable by death and significant governmental pressures to meet arrest quotas. As a result, many Chinese citizens were subjected to unfair trials and wrongful executions [1, 6, 7].

43.2   Search Strategy

The medical literature from 1990 until 2020 was searched utilizing the databases of PubMed and Google Scholar. The search was conducted using the terms: transplantation in China, China health policy, international ethics in transplantation, organ procurement, prisoner body parts, organ trafficking, medical tourism. In addition, we utilized the official website of the State Council of The People's Republic of China for official health policy pronouncements. Greater than 400 hits were obtained when keywords were used independently; approximately 20–50 hits when two keywords were combined. All years were included initially, however, pertinence was decided based on a number of factors including number of citations and publisher.

43.3   Discussion

Autonomy—Incarcerated individuals are recognized as members of a vulnerable population due to the restrictive nature of imprisonment. Incarceration compromises one's ability to make independent decisions. The utilization of prisoners' organs for transplantation, especially without their permission, directly infringes upon the principle of autonomy. All persons, including prisoners, should *always* have control over their bodies and be permitted to make their own decisions without the influence or coercion of medical providers or other persons in power.

Beneficence—For decades, China's transplant system did not have standardized clinical guidelines or a legal framework in place to ensure the best outcomes for all organ donors and recipients. Thus, despite advancements in knowledge and techniques, until a centralized quality control mechanism was established, and the well-being of all patients was prioritized, the principle of beneficence was not met.

Non-Maleficence—Utilizing the organs of the disadvantaged in order to benefit the privileged, poses a major ethical dilemma. The performance of high-risk operations and procedures without clinical guidelines and practice regulations lead to poor outcomes during the initial phases of China's transplant system.

Justice—Reform of the Chinese transplant system led to holding providers accountable for complying with internationally referenced regulations, respecting and treating all patients equally, improving access to all patients in need of organ transplantation, banning organ trafficking, and ensuring objective organ recovery and allocation (see Table 43.1).

Table 43.1 The four principles of ethics as they relate to transplantation reform in China

Autonomy	• Incarcerated individuals are recognized as members of a vulnerable population due to the restrictive nature of imprisonment. • Incarceration compromises one's ability to make independent decisions. • The utilization of prisoners' organs for transplantation, especially without their permission, directly infringes upon the principle of autonomy. • People, including prisoners, should *always* have control over their bodies and be permitted to make their own decisions without the influence or coercion of medical providers or other persons in power.
Beneficence	• For decades, China's transplant system did not have standardized clinical guidelines or a legal framework in place to ensure the best outcomes for all organ donors and recipients. • Thus, despite advancements in knowledge and techniques, until a centralized quality control mechanism was established, and the well-being of all patients was prioritized, the principle of beneficence was not met.
Non-Maleficence	• Utilizing the organs of the disadvantaged in order to benefit the privileged, poses a major ethical dilemma. • The performance of high-risk operations and procedures without clinical guidelines and practice regulations lead to poor outcomes during the initial phases of China's transplant system.
Justice	Reform of the Chinese transplant system led to: • Holding providers accountable for complying with internationally referenced regulations • Respecting and treating all patients equally, improving access to all patients in need of organ transplantation • Banning organ trafficking, and • Ensuring objective organ recovery and allocation

43.3.1   The Cyclosporine Age

China's introduction to Cyclosporine A in the 1980s resulted in an improvement in graft outcomes with first-year recipient survival rising from 50 to 80 percent by 1987 and as high as 90 percent by 1991 [1, 5]. The use of organs from executed prisoners afforded a reliable source of transplantable organs for programs to take advantage of the technical and scientific advances. Further, China's economy was transitioning from a command economy to a market economy with a concomitant decrease in state funding for health care. Thus, a primary motivation for hospitals to establish transplant programs became financial gain and initiating and growing a transplant program provided a positive financial incentive to hospitals. Wealthy Chinese government officials and affluent foreigners (transplant tourists) were prioritized as recipients. Without regulation of China's developing transplant system, and no regard for the protection of prisoners' rights, massive transplant tourism ensued. The 1995 Ordinance from the Chinese Ministry of Health aimed to prohibit commercial trading of human organs and promote the regulation of living donor transplantation; however, this decree was not legally binding, and thus, not enforceable. China would continue down this path another eleven years before a legal framework for Transplantation was established.

43.3.2   Source and Rights of the Organ Donor

One of the most significant issues regarding the use of executed felons' organs was the disregard of autonomy with lack of written consent from the prisoners or their families. Although required by law; consent was rarely obtained [1]. Often, inmates and their families were not even informed that organs would be harvested. Occasionally, when consent was obtained, China's legal system encouraged the reciprocation of familial financial compensation. Traditional Chinese culture favors inhumation; however, more recently, the deceased are often cremated, rather than buried, especially in large Chinese cities [7]. The practice of cremation immediately after execution gave inmates' family members no certainty whether or not organs were removed from their loved ones [7, 8].

Although involvement of Chinese physicians in the execution process is a direct violation of international standards of medical ethics [9], many of the Chinese transplant centers had exclusive relationships with prisons. Physicians were noted to be on prison grounds the day prior to execution to perform examinations and collect blood tests in order to confirm matching of donors and recipients [10]. Although transplant surgeons were not involved with the actual execution, they were readily available on prison grounds to procure organs immediately after death. Often, execution dates were scheduled based on recipient needs, rather than the strict requirements of legal due process [1].

In order to optimize conditions for organ harvesting, it has been reported that execution protocols were allowed to be violated or intentionally abused to ensure that prisoners still had some level of circulatory activity after execution, as their organs were removed [1, 11]. More than half of the prisoner donors were young, healthy men between eighteen and twenty-five years old [1].

Beginning in 1949, the practice of execution in Mainland China was carried out by a firing squad with gunshot wounds to the head, unless organs such as eyes were needed, in which case, a gunshot wound to the heart was utilized [1, 7, 12]. Officials in other parts of China began using lethal injection to provide a more respectful death for prisoners. The use of lethal injection in China was formally accepted in 1996 and became the primary form of capital punishment in 2010 [12].

43.3.3 Regulation of Quality and Reform

China became the second largest transplant program worldwide (only behind the United States in number of organs transplanted annually) with 11,000 transplants performed between 2005 and 2006 [3]. The US performed 29,000 transplants in 2006 [13]. Nearly all of these Chinese organs were sourced from executed prisoners, and many were transplanted into foreign nationals. This robust volume of cases provided by an expeditious and affordable access to organs, resulting in an inundation of tourists traveling to China for performance of kidney and liver transplants [1–3].

Organ trafficking and transplant commercialism in China were the unfortunate consequences of global organ shortage and under-regulated growth of China's transplant system [2–4]. The internet and other virtual communication modalities facilitated making transplant tourism a global issue. Chinese hospitals were recognized as major destinations for wealthy and well-insured transplant tourists from around the world and frequently paid for by their respective Ministries of Health. The sale of executed prisoners' organs and the transplantation of living donors' organs into foreign patients was a direct violation of the ethical principle of justice. The rights of the donors, both deceased and living, were not valued as highly as those of the paying recipients. An unjust allocation of organs compromised the needs of vulnerable Chinese citizens for the benefit of privileged foreign nationals. Disadvantaged Chinese patients in need of life-saving transplantation were disregarded [1–3]. The process of securing donors was plagued with corruption. Additionally, a lack of regulation governing transplant quality, placed living donors and recipients at increased risk of possible complications related to the operations. This subjected transplanted patients to unnecessary harm, violating the principles of beneficence and non-maleficence.

In 2006, there were more than 600 Chinese hospitals performing solid organ transplants with 95% of transplanted organs recovered from executed prisoners [5–8]. Compensation for aggrieved parties continued to be encouraged by the

Chinese legal system and transplant tourism became widespread. That same year, the international press began to focus on the corruption within the Chinese transplant system and as a result, transparency led to reform. The Interim Provision on the Administration of Clinical Application and Management of Human Organ Transplantation was issued March 2006, detailing China's requirement to meet the technical and systemic demands of a robust transplantation program [14, 15]. In April 2006, the Committee on Organ Transplantation developed clinical protocols in an effort to standardize practice across all programs. These changes were announced at the National Summit of Transplant Centers in November 2006 and in May 2007, the state council passed the Human Organ Transplant Regulation to endorse legal regulation of solid organ transplantation in China [15]. The Ministry subsequently reduced the number of transplant hospitals from greater than 600 to 169, issuing new laws restricting the transplantation of foreign patients and prioritizing Chinese citizens [15]. As a result, medical institutions were expected to meet established requirements prior to proceeding with transplantations. From 2006 to 2007, with enactment of these regulations, the number of transplant institutions with full approval from the Ministry to perform transplantation decreased even further to only 87 centers [3, 5]. The Chinese government addressed the dilemma of financial compensation for organ donors by prohibiting this activity with severe and substantial penalties and in 2007, the Ministry issued a notice that ensured Chinese citizens would be given priority for receipt of an organ [3–5]. Deceased donor transplants decreased by more than threefold and living donor related transplants doubled [15].

To prevent exploitation of the incarcerated and protect donors' rights, in 2010 the Chinese government required analysis of all death sentences by the Supreme People's Court; written consent from donors prior to retrieval of organs; and restricted involvement of the transplant team until death had been declared [3, 4]. In an effort to promote alternative sources of organ donation, the Red Cross participated by advertising the need for organ donation. The Ministry also promoted organ-donating policies which allowed citizens to express their wishes on their driver's licenses [3, 5, 6]. The Ministry also encouraged initiatives to educate Chinese physicians and attempts to standardize diagnostic criteria for brain death [1, 3]. China's non-recognition of the brain death standard continues to greatly limit potential deceased, non-prisoner donors who arrive to the hospital after sustaining devastating intracranial injuries.

In response to increased awareness related to transplant commercialism, many non-governmental organizations, such as the Declaration of Istanbul Custodial Group, the Transplant Society, Amnesty International, and Human Rights Watch have taken an unequivocal stance against the practice of "donation by execution" and banning transplant tourism. These organizations have assisted in developing laws and guidelines opposing organ trafficking, while promoting alternatives in an attempt to bolster national self-sufficiency in organ donation [1–4]. The Declaration of Istanbul was developed in 2008 through the partnership of the two leading international professional organizations for transplantation and nephrology: the Transplantation Society and the International Society of Nephrology. The

Declaration of Istanbul Custodial Group is thus the collaboration of these two societies in concert with additional experts who share a unified focus of addressing human organ commercialization. Specifically, the Declaration of Istanbul Custodial Group sought to tackle the unjust treatment of disadvantaged people whose organs were being sourced the most, including executed criminals in China, deceased donors in Colombia, and indigent populations in India, Pakistan, Egypt, and the Philippines [2].

In collaboration with the World Health Organization, the Declaration of Istanbul Custodial Group organized an international forum, joining numerous specialists from 78 countries in Istanbul in 2008. At the meeting, a standardized set of guidelines was created to address deficiencies in practices of transplant programs worldwide, and more specifically, to shed more light on the issues of organ trafficking [2]. Versions of the Declaration of Istanbul on Organ Trafficking and Transplant Tourism were published in multiple journals in 2008, including Transplantation, International Society of Nephrology, the American Society of Nephrology, and The Lancet [2–5]. Through this promotion of transparency, advocacy, education, and accountability in transplantation practices, the Declaration of Istanbul led to the restriction of academic recognition when research or clinical practices involved executed prisoners [1–4]. Collaboration and partnership with academic societies, journal editors, and research funding agencies resulted in the withdrawal of abstract submissions, and restriction of the presentation or publication of data involving prisoners or other commercially obtained organs [2].

Partnership with institutions in developed countries formed in response to China's desire to ameliorate its transplant system. In 2006, Vice Minister Jiefu Huang, a transplant surgeon himself and faculty member at Peking Union Medical College, determined that China's transplant system must change. He sought the funding and guidance of the China Medical Board (grant to Peking Union Medical College), and transplant surgeon ethicist (Michael Millis) at the University of Chicago. It should be noted that John D. Rockefeller provided the initial endowment in 1910 for the Peking Union Medical College, the China Medical Board and the University of Chicago (1892). The purpose of this grant and the subsequent renewal was to address the inadequate legal, regulatory, and quality assessment of transplantation in China.

43.3.4   New Ethical System

At the China National Transplant Congress in October 2014, the Chairman of the National Organ Donation and Transplant Committee, Jiefu Huang, announced that "all hospitals are required to stop using organs from executed prisoners immediately and the sole source for organ transplant will be civilian organ donation system." This legislative decree was supported by the People's Republic of China's Premier, Li Keqiang and President, Xi Jinping. The use of executed prisoners' organs was officially banned on January 1, 2015 [10].

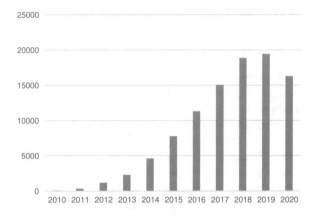

Fig. 43.1 Total number of transplants in China per year (non-prisoner). Use of organs from executed prisoners was banned in Jan 2015. 2020 data only through November

With the reformation of China's Transplant system came condemnation of transplant tourism, urgency to focus on the prevention of organ failure, and provision of organs to meet the needs of the citizens within resources from donors within the general population or through regional collaboration. While altruism and voluntary donation were encouraged, an emphasis was placed on prioritizing and maximizing deceased donor transplantation to relieve some of the burden of living donors [2–4]. Western transplant professionals were allowed to visit the Chinese Transplant centers to assist with the establishment of the organ procurement organization process and evaluate compliance with international standards. This important collaboration was paramount in affirming the relevant health system infrastructure and alleviating misconceptions and fears related to donor transplantation.

With this unified front against organ trafficking and focus on increased use of voluntary deceased donor organs, the number of deceased donor transplantations has increased significantly in the last 5 years [10]. With the implementation of the new voluntary system, 11,300 deceased donor organs were transplanted in 2016; a substantial increase from the 7,393 deceased donor organs transplanted in 2015 (see Fig. 43.1). As of 2016, 2.9 million citizens were recognized as organ donors, which is a 120-fold increase from the 24,000 donors recognized in 2010.

43.4 Concluding Remarks

In order to maintain the progress that has occurred over the last 15 years, the Chinese transplant system infrastructure must be continuously scrutinized and strengthened. International support in concert with unity amongst national and local governments is paramount. Chinese cultural perspectives and values must be respected; patient and family's wishes must be honored. Complete transparency with organ donation, recovery, allocation, and recipient selection cannot be compromised. Comprehensive data collection, inclusive of donor and recipient demographics, is critical. Finally, efforts to eliminate capital punishment in China are ongoing [12]. Capital punishment, carried out by lethal injection or gun shot, continues to be recognized as a legal penalty for murder and drug trafficking in China [11, 12]. Until the death penalty no longer exists, unwavering persistence to protect the incarcerated and determination to dissociate transplantation from prison systems must continue.

43.5 Selected References

- Danovitch GM, Chapman J, Capron AM, et al. Organ trafficking and transplant tourism: the role of global professional ethical standards—the 2008 Declaration of Istanbul. Transplant. 2013;95:1306–1312. https://doi.org/10.1097/tp.0b013e318295ee7d
- Steering Committee of the Istanbul Summit. Organ trafficking and transplant tourism and commercialism: the Declaration of Istanbul. Lancet. 2008;372:5–6.
- Participants in the International Summit on Transplant Tourism and Organ Trafficking Convened by the Transplantation Society and International Society of Nephrology in Istanbul, Turkey, April 30–May 2, 2008. The declaration of Istanbul on organ trafficking and transplant tourism. Clin J Am Soc Nephrol. 2008; 3(5): 1227–1231. https://doi.org/10.2215/cjn.03320708

  - Through promotion of transparency, advocacy, education, and accountability in transplantation practices, the Declaration of Istanbul led to the restriction of academic recognition when research or clinical practices involved executed prisoners.

References

1. Organ procurement and judicial execution in China. Human Rights Watch/Asia. August 1, 1994;6(9). https://www.hrw.org/report/1994/08/01/organ-procurement-and-judicial-execu-tion-china. Accessed 15 Apr 2021.
2. Danovitch GM, Chapman J, Capron AM, et al. Organ trafficking and transplant tourism: the role of global professional ethical standards—the 2008 Declaration of Istanbul. Transplantation. 2013;95:1306–12. https://doi.org/10.1097/tp.0b013e318295ee7d.
3. Steering Committee of the Istanbul Summit. Organ trafficking and transplant tourism and commercialism: the declaration of Istanbul. Lancet. 2008;372:5–6.
4. Participants in the International Summit on Transplant Tourism and Organ Trafficking Convened by the Transplantation Society and International Society of Nephrology in Istanbul, Turkey, April 30–May 2, 2008. The declaration of Istanbul on organ trafficking and transplant tourism. Clin J Am Soc Nephrol. 2008;3(5):1227–31. https://doi.org/10.2215/cjn.03320708.
5. Huang J, Mau Y, Millis M. Government policy and organ transplantation in China. Lancet. 2008;372:1937–8. https://doi.org/10.1016/s0140-6736(08)61359-8.
6. Huang J. Ethical and legislative perspectives on liver transplantation in the People's Republic of China. Liver Transpl. 2007;13:193–6. https://doi.org/10.1002/lt.21081.
7. Guttmann RD. On the use of organs from executed prisoners. Transplant Rev. 1992;6:189–93. https://doi.org/10.1016/s0955-470x(10)80004-7.

8. Sui W, Yan Q, Xie S, et al. Successful organ donation from brain dead donors in a Chinese organ transplantation center. Am J Transplant. 2011;11:2247–9. https://doi.org/10.1111/j.1600-6143.2011.03694.x.
9. Tibell A. The Transplantation Society's policy on interactions with China. Transplantation. 2007;94:292–4. https://doi.org/10.1097/01.tp.0000275181.33071.07.
10. Wang H. New era for organ donation and transplant in China [interview]. Bulletin WHO. 2012;90:802–3. https://doi.org/10.2471/blt.12.031112.
11. Shi BY, Chen LP. Regulation of organ transplantation in China: difficult exploration and slow advance. JAMA. 2011;306(4):434–5. https://doi.org/10.1001/jama.2011.1067.
12. Zhang L. China's death-penalty debate. The New York Times. December 29, 2014. https://www.nytimes.com/2014/12/30/opinion/chinas-death-penalty-debate.html?searchResultPosit ion=1. Accessed 1 Sep 2020.
13. National Data. Organ Procurement and Transplantation Network. US Dept Health Human Services. https://optn.transplant.hrsa.gov/data/view-data-reports/national-data/#. Accessed 12 Dec 2020.
14. Cameron JS, Hoffenberg R. The ethics of organ transplantation reconsidered: paid organ donation and the use of executed prisoners as donors. Kidney Int. 1999;55:724–32. https://doi.org/10.1046/j.1523-1755.1999.00286.x.
15. Huang JF, Wang HB, Zheng SS, et al. Advances in China's organ transplantation achieved with the guidance of law. Chin Med J. 2015;128(2):143–6. https://doi.org/10.4103/0366-6999.149183.

Part XI
Covid-19 Pandemic of 2020

Chapter 44
COVID-19 Caught the World Unprepared

Boris D. Lushniak (iD)

Abstract Public health plays a key role in assuring the health of communities and this mission becomes even more apparent in the midst of public health emergencies, such as pandemics. The COVID-19 pandemic is the fifth pandemic that the global population has experienced in the last 100 years. It is unique in that it is the first pandemic caused by a coronavirus and not by an influenza virus and therefore has distinctive epidemiological features. As a novel virus and a novel pandemic, the learning curve has been steep. The timeline over this past year shows an eruptive spread of the pandemic from Asia to Europe, to the Americas. The approaches of fighting this pandemic vary and have shown both successful results and disastrous paths. The world is presented with many issues that have become apparent in the midst of this public health crisis. Optimism, however, is a critical feature as science progresses with new approaches on public health interventions, therapeutic modalities, and vaccine development and distribution.

Keywords Pandemic · COVID-19 · Coronavirus · SARS-CoV-2 · Epidemiology Public health

44.1 Introduction

44.1.1 Public Health

In CEA Winslow's classic definition from 1921, public health is defined as "the science and art of preventing disease, prolonging life and promoting physical health" [1]. Public health has certainly evolved with time, but the basic premises of the

B. D. Lushniak (✉)
University of Maryland School of Public Health, College Park, MD, USA
e-mail: lushniak@umd.edu

© The Author(s), under exclusive license to Springer Nature
Switzerland AG 2022
V. A. Lonchyna et al. (eds.), *Difficult Decisions in Surgical Ethics*, Difficult
Decisions in Surgery: An Evidence-Based Approach,
https://doi.org/10.1007/978-3-030-84625-1_44

617

"three p's"—preventing disease and injury, promoting health (physical, mental, and social well-being), and prolonging a high quality life—have held over the course of a century.

The public health model includes important pathways to achieve the goal of the "three p's". This model consists of four major steps: (1) Surveillance—what is the problem? (2) Risk factor identification—what is the cause? (3) Intervention and evaluation—what works to prevent or decrease the problem? and, (4) Implementation—how do you do it? (see Fig. 44.1) [2]. The goal of public health is to get to that last stage, which includes the implementation of policies, regulations, and initiatives which would have a positive impact on the health of the population. However, we don't get to that last stage without robust and scientifically valid information and data from the first three steps.

With this approach public health has had incredible achievements. Over the course of the twentieth century the world has changed for the better as a result of public health actions. These include achievements and progress in vaccinations, motor-vehicle safety, safer workplaces, heart disease and stroke, safer and healthier foods, healthier mothers and babies, family planning, fluoridation of water, recognition of tobacco as a health hazard, and control of infectious diseases [3].

The definition of public health and the public health model applies in the varied essential services of public health, which broadly include assessment, policy development, and assurance (see Table 44.1) [4]. Public health, in its day-to-day work, deals with chronic diseases, substance abuse, common infectious disease, and other physical, mental, and environmental health issues that affect our communities. But the public health approach becomes even more vibrant and critical during public health crises, where the "three p's" are tested in the midst of rapidly evolving scenarios, marked uncertainty, and many unknown variables. New approaches, new strategies, and new data sources need to be recognized and highlighted for an effective response as part of an emergency public health mission.

The need for public health action is certainly apparent in the midst of infectious disease disasters, which are events during which a biological agent can result in mass casualties. Infectious disease disasters require actions that include the four

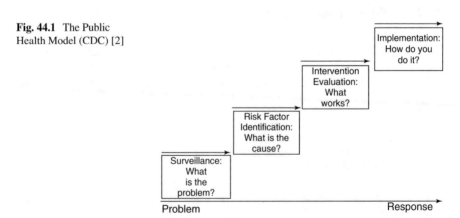

Fig. 44.1 The Public Health Model (CDC) [2]

Table 44.1 Essential Public Health Services (CDC, revised 2020) [4]

1.	Assess and monitor population health status, factors that influence health, and community needs and assets
2.	Investigate, diagnose, and address health problems and hazards affecting the population
3.	Communicate effectively to inform and educate people about health, factors that influence it, and how to improve it
4.	Strengthen, support, and mobilize communities and partnerships to improve health
5.	Create, champion, and implement policies, plans, and laws that impact health
6.	Utilize legal and regulatory actions designed to improve and protect the public's health
7.	Assure an effective system that enables equitable access to the individual services and care needed to be healthy
8.	Build and support a diverse and skilled public health workforce
9.	Improve and innovate public health functions through ongoing evaluation, research, and continuous quality improvement
10.	Build and maintain a strong organizational infrastructure for public health

principles of emergency management—specialized mitigation, preparedness, response, and recovery. Infectious disease disasters include bioterrorism attacks (e.g., anthrax 2001), outbreaks of emerging or reemerging infectious diseases (e.g., Ebola 2015), and pandemics (e.g., influenza, COVID-19).

44.1.2   Pandemics

The World Health Organization (WHO) loosely defines a pandemic as an epidemic occurring worldwide which crosses international boundaries and usually affects a large number of people [5]. Three conditions must exist for a pandemic to occur—1) the population is exposed to a novel pathogen and therefore has no or limited immunity to that pathogen; 2) infection with the pathogen results in serious illness with high levels of morbidity and/or mortality; and, 3) the pathogen is transmitted efficiently from person to person.

In the last 100 years, the world has seen four pandemics (see Table 44.2). All were the result of novel influenza strains that spread to humans from the animal world, usually from swine or birds. The most infamous pandemic occurred a century ago. Incorrectly termed "the Spanish influenza", it spread across the globe in 1918–19, resulting in over 50 million deaths, including over 675,000 deaths in the US. Subsequent pandemics in 1957–58, 1968–69, and most recently in 2009–10 were milder in comparison but still deeply affected the health of the global population [6].

The potential for pandemics has become a matter of more concern in our modern society. The global population has become larger and more urbanized, yet, through the one health concept, is still interconnected with the animal world. Through the advancement of high-speed air travel, the level of international connectedness has increased, and the globe has become a smaller place. In addition, with medical and

Table 44.2 Past Pandemics (WHO) [6]

	1918–19	1957–58	1968–69	2009–10
Type	H1N1 Spanish flu	H2N2 Asian flu	H3N2 Hong Kong flu	H1N1 Swine flu
World deaths	50 million plus	1–2 million	700,000	151,000–575,000
US deaths	675,000	70,000 plus	34,000 plus	12,469
High risk groups	Young adults	Infants, elderly	Infants, elderly	Children, working adults
Other info	20–40% of global population infected	Spread to US in 4–5 months; global spread in 8 months	Spread to US in 2–3 months	US with 60.8 million cases; 274,000 hospitalized

public health advancements, the population of higher risk individuals, including the elderly and those with chronic diseases has increased. With these transitions, public health has focused on a "not if, but when" pandemic scenario and pandemic preparedness has become a key component of the public health mission. Former US Secretary of Health and Human Services Michael Leavitt stated in 2007 that: "Everything we do before a pandemic will seem alarmist. Everything we do after a pandemic will seem inadequate. This is the dilemma we face, but it should not stop us from doing what we can do to prepare. We need to reach out to everyone with words that inform, but not inflame. We need to encourage everyone to prepare, but not panic." [7]

Global health security is a key feature of pandemic preparedness and in 2019 the first comprehensive index of global health security capabilities of 195 nations was published [8]. Experts assessed various categories and indicators of a nation's preparedness which included: prevention of the emergence, release, or spread of pathogens; detection and reporting of epidemics; rapid response to the spread of an epidemic and its mitigation; health system capabilities to treat the sick and protect healthcare workers; commitments to improving national capacity, addressing gaps, and compliance with international norms; and, the overall risk environment and vulnerability. The assessment concluded that on a global scale national health is fundamentally weak and no country is fully prepared. Globally the average score was 40.2 out of a 100-point scale. Sixty high income nations had an average score of 51.9 but 116 high- and middle-income nations did not score above 50. The US was ranked first in the world with a score of 83.5.

44.2 Discussion

44.2.1 Coronaviruses and COVID-19

Coronaviruses are a large family of RNA viruses which infect many species in the animal world. Until late 2019 there were six known coronaviruses which infected humans, four of which were common cold viruses (OC43, HKU1, 229E, NL63) [9].

Two others were new 'emerging' viruses of the twenty-first century which caused Severe Acute Respiratory Syndrome (SARS) and Middle East Respiratory Syndrome (MERS). SARS was first reported in Asia in 2003 and was caused by a new pathogen, SARS-CoV. Initially the outbreak of this novel virus caused international concern, ultimately infecting 8098 people (8 in the US) in 24 nations with 774 deaths (crude mortality rate of 9.5%). The virus ultimately disappeared. MERS was first reported in Saudi Arabia in 2012, was caused by another novel virus, MERS-CoV, and infected 2494 people (2 in the US) in 27 nations with 858 deaths (crude mortality rate of 34.4%). MERS continues to linger, but with only a handful of cases each year.

On December 31, 2019, the Wuhan Municipal Health Commission in China reported a cluster of cases of pneumonia of unknown cause [10]. Retrospectively, cases may already have been present in early December, but this was the first report to the WHO, of what was the initial steps of an unfolding, worldwide, public health crisis. What followed was an incredibly quick timeline of pathogen identification, attempts at containment and control, global spread, and included the advancement of scientific knowledge and the difficulties of the public health response (see Table 44.3) [11]. By January 4, 2020, WHO reported on social media that there was a cluster of 44 suspected pneumonia cases, with no deaths, in Wuhan, Hubei province, and by the next day published further information on the new virus and the outbreak. Guidance and advice were issued to all nations on how to detect, test and manage potential cases, based on what was known about the virus at the time. With the past experiences with SARS and MERS, infection control guidance was published recommending droplet and contact precautions.

Twenty-first century science moved quickly. How different life was 100 years previously when the nature of the 1918 influenza was for the most part unknown. By January 7, a novel pathogen was discovered to be the likely source of the disease, the first key criteria of a potential pandemic. By January 11, the first death was reported in China, indicating that the new virus caused a serious illness, another factor in the developing pandemic. By January 12, China publicly shared the genetic sequence of a novel virus, ultimately designated as SARS-CoV-2, which caused a new disease, COVID-19.

Although Wuhan was the initial epicenter of the outbreak, spread across international borders occurred quickly and by January 13 a case was confirmed in Thailand, then later in Japan and South Korea. By January 14, WHO acknowledged that there may have been human to human transmission, a third key component of the potential of a pandemic, and this was confirmed by January 21. Also, on January 21 the US reported its first case, with other cases reported in subsequent days in Australia, France, Italy, Malaysia, and Canada (see Chaps. 46 and 47). On January 23 Wuhan implemented drastic public health measures by shutting down the city—at the time there were 580 cases and 17 deaths. By January 30 WHO determined that the outbreak constituted a Public Health Emergency of International Concern and on January 31 the US declared a public health emergency.

What followed was a "runaway train" of a pandemic spreading across the globe. By February 10 there were over 900 deaths worldwide, surpassing the death tolls of both SARS and MERS. On February 25 a Centers for Disease Control and Prevention

Table 44.3 COVID-19 Timeline December 2019–December 2020 (ThinkGlobalHealth) [11]

• Dec 31—WHO office in China informed of pneumonia cases with unknown cause
• Jan 7—Novel coronavirus identified
• Jan 11—First death reported in China
• Jan 12—Genetic sequence of virus shared
• Jan 21—WHO confirms human to human transmission; first US case
• Jan 30—WHO declares public health emergency of international concern
• Jan 31—US declares public health emergency; US bans entry from China
• Feb 6—First death reported in US
• Feb 26—Brazil case (all continents); more new cases reported outside of China than in China
• Mar 7— > 100,000 cases in over 100 nations (took 3 months)
• Mar 11—WHO declares a pandemic; US restricts EU travel
• Mar 13—Europe is epicenter; US national emergency; US school closures begin
• Mar 17—Seen in all 50 US states
• Mar 19— > 200,000 cases globally (12 days since 100,000); Wuhan no new cases
• Mar 22— > 300,000 cases globally (3 days since 200,000)
• Mar 24— > 400,000 cases globally (2 days since 300,000); Olympics postponed
• Mar 26—US is epicenter with >82,000 cases and 1100 deaths
• April 10—For the first 100 days >100,000 global deaths
• April 27—3 million cases globally; 1 million in US
• May 28—100,000 deaths in US
• June 28—500,000 global deaths; 10 million global cases
• July 7—WHO acknowledges emerging evidence of airborne spread
• August 13—WHO reports cost to global economy of pandemic is $375 billion/month
• August 24—First case of reinfection in Hong Kong
• September 2—COVID cases in Europe almost back to March levels
• October 2—President Trump and others at White House test positive
• November 8— > 50 million cases globally
• November 19—250,732 deaths in US
• December 8—UK identifies new more infectious strain; UK begins immunization campaign
• December 11—US FDA issues EUA for Prizer-BioNTech vaccine
• December 18—US FDA issues EUA for Moderna vaccine
• December 23—US administers first 1 million vaccines; first case reported in Antarctica
• January 1—US surpasses 20 million cases with over 100,000 hospitalizations/day in December   —83,572,007 global cases; 1,820,841 global deaths; 345,844 deaths in US

(CDC) official caused a political storm by stating that "this might be bad." On February 26 a case in Brazil solidified the fact that the disease had spread to all six populated continents and now more cases were reported outside China than in China. On March 11, WHO declared a pandemic—the second pandemic of the twenty-first century and the first in the previous 100 years that was not caused by an influenza virus.

By mid-March the epicenter shifted from Asia to Europe, with Italy initially most severely affected. In the US, schools began closing, sporting and other mass-gathering events cancelled, and all 50 states reported cases. Globally, it took three months for the first 100,000 confirmed cases in 100 nations. The next 100,000 people were infected in 12 days, the next 100,000 in three days, the next in two days. By late March, the epicenter switched from Europe to the US, with New York and New Jersey being the US hotspots (see Chap. 46).

By April, over a million cases were diagnosed worldwide with over 51,000 deaths. At the time the global economic impact was estimated to be between $2–4 trillion and almost 90% of students worldwide were affected by school closures. After the first 100 days of the pandemic, the world saw over 100,000 deaths.

But there was also some promising news at this stage. After a 76-day lockdown, the city of Wuhan reopened. The measures of aggressive testing, treating, contact tracing, isolation and quarantine in conjunction with the non-pharmaceutical interventions of mask wearing, hand washing, and limiting contact through physical distancing worked.

Throughout the summer of 2020, we saw the full spectrum of the pandemic. Some nations took on the pandemic aggressively through public health measures and saw slow but steady improvement in the spread of the disease. Others, such as Sweden, took less drastic approaches, and although with some initial success, saw a flash of increased mortality as the disease spread in vulnerable populations. Other nations saw initial successes being tempered by returning hotspots and surges that were usually associated with society opening up and public health measures being dropped prematurely.

On the other extreme of the spectrum were nations like the US. The US was the highest ranked nation in the Global Health Security Index (GHSI) and yet the pandemic continued to spread unabated. Other countries which had ranked high in the GHSI, such as South Korea and Thailand, have been more successful in fighting COVID-19 [12].

In general, through the summer, nations of the European Union and in other regions of the world successfully "flattened the curve" of the number of cases and deaths and then further decreased this curve. The US "flattened the curve" at a relatively high level and then saw a steady rise of both cases and deaths as the summer waned on (see Fig. 44.2) [13].

By mid-October, there were over 40 million cases globally with over eight million of those in the US. The tragic deaths from COVID-19 now numbered over one million globally with over 221,000 deaths in the US. Regional public health measures in the initial US hotspots of New York and New Jersey had been successful, but other regions later became the new US hotspots, as public health measures were inconsistently implemented. Along with India and Brazil the US remained the epicenter of the pandemic well into the late stages of 2020 [14]. The fall and winter brought with it a new wave in Europe and in the US (see Fig. 44.2) [13]. This resurgence can be attributed to multiple causes including the further relaxation of public health measures and the influx of cooler weather, which led to a switch to more indoor gatherings.

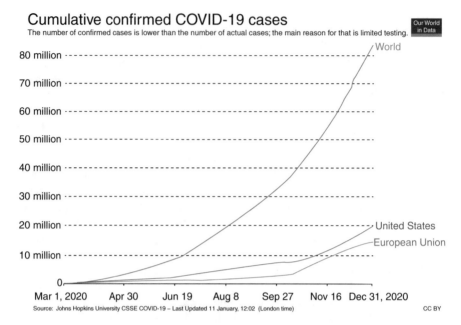

Fig. 44.2 Confirmed Covid-19 Cases Comparing the World, US, and EU [13]

By the end of 2020, as we approached the one-year mark of the pandemic, there were over 80 million cases worldwide and over 20 million in the US. Global deaths surpassed 1.75 million with nearly 350,000 deaths in the US. New strains of the virus appeared, some being more contagious. We entered 2021 under very bleak circumstances.

Yet there was a new hope. With the advancements of twenty-first century medical science and biotechnology, the promise of safe and effective vaccines entered the picture.

44.2.2 The Issues

Not since the influenza pandemic of 1918–19 has our society been so stressed in the midst of a public health crisis. There are many reasons which have led to a failure of control and containment of the virus. In the US, a lack of a national strategy and ineffective national leadership, politics getting in the way of science, an overtaxed public health system, a failure of diagnostic testing, a shortage of medical supplies including personal protective equipment (PPE) for health care workers, confusion in implementing and enforcing public health recommendations caused by mixed messaging, misinformation and distrust in science, and economic concerns affecting the implementation of public health measures, all played a role.

With the lack of national leadership and a national strategy in the US, decision-making fell into the realm of state and local political leaders. The public health response became a local and state responsibility. Testing, tracing, isolation, and quarantine taxed a public health infrastructure that had not been supported over the years and was severely understaffed and under-resourced. In 2017, of the $3.3 trillion spent annually on healthcare only 3% went to public health and since 2008 local health departments had eliminated over 55,000 jobs because of hiring freezes or budget cuts [15]. **Public health was not prepared for this pandemic.**

The failure of diagnostic testing in the US has proven to be one of the early lightning rods of this crisis. Globally, the first diagnostic test was released by the Germans in mid-January. In the US the CDC prepared a diagnostic test and the Food and Drug Administration issued an Emergency Use Authorization (EUA) for this diagnostic on February 2, 2020. The test was initially very problematic as reagent issues resulted in an inaccurate tool at a critical point of the pandemic. Add to that the shortages of lab supplies and oversaturation of laboratory capabilities, the diagnostic test crisis continued well into the fall of 2020. This occurred despite the involvement of a wide range of public health and academic labs, clinical labs, and the private sector. Development of rapid tests, point of care tests, and antigen tests has been slow but remains crucial in the next stages of the pandemic. Serological antibody tests (IgG, IgM) have been developed but remain problematic, and have been tainted with quality control issues, inadequate levels of sensitivity and specificity, and the uncertainty of test relevance and the role of antibodies in this disease.

Personal protective equipment (PPE) issues also surfaced at the beginning stages of the pandemic. Shortages of medical PPE (N95 masks and surgical masks) led to a pathway of once unheard of practices of reuse and disinfection of these critical tools. For the general public the use of cloth masks/face coverings became controversial and politicized. Similar to the situation a century ago, in addition to mask wearing, the other non-pharmaceutical interventions of social/physical distancing and handwashing became the key tools. Lack of consistent approaches, implementation and enforcement were problematic to say the least.

The medical care response was hampered by an overtaxed medical care system especially in hotspot areas, and this resulted in a human toll, affecting both the physical and mental health of health care workers. Issues of surge capacity of bed space, critical care units, ventilators, and other resources, pointed out the ineffectiveness of our nation's emergency preparedness and brought into question the vulnerabilities of the medical supply chain.

Messaging about the pandemic, from the highest levels of the US government, failed to take into account scientifically based approaches and the basics of health communication and health literacy. Mixed messages and misinformation remain rampant and lead to confusion in the population. One viewpoint is that despite the high ranking in GHSI the US had received a low score on a key factor—public confidence in government, which can be a factor in whether individuals follow disease-control recommendations, even if the message was clear and consistent [12]. The roles of the press and news networks in messaging, especially in a politically charged environment, continue to unfold.

The worldwide economic impact is overwhelming. We suffer through historic levels of unemployment, stock market variability, and consumer product shortages. There are drastic effects on the education system, social gatherings and large-scale events, and on travel. The pandemic is by definition a global event. National and international politics, travel restrictions, racism and nationalism, the role of the WHO and China, leads to a world searching for blame.

And in the midst of all this, we still need to deal with a novel virus that seems to surprise us at every turn. It is "novel" in not only being new and unique, but also in portraying its storyline as a "novel", with unforeseen twists and turns. But, alas, this is a non-fiction tragedy. The scientific world is learning about the virus at an incredible pace, and this can lead to the premature release of information, and at times contradictory and confusing conclusions. These stem, in part, from a break in the traditional scientific process, especially the role of time-consuming, but necessary, scientific peer review. This resulted in further confusion surrounding the retraction of some published papers, even in the most prestigious medical journals, such as the Lancet and the New England Journal of Medicine.

Without a doubt the SARS-CoV-2 virus is a tough foe. The symptoms of COVID-19 are not specific and mimic other respiratory diseases, such as influenza. Many people carry the virus with either mild or no symptoms. Even the knowledge of the routes of transmission of the virus have evolved. We've gone from a world that emphasized recommendations that protected us from large droplets during close contact with symptomatic people (masks only for health care workers) and fomites (disinfecting surfaces), to now including the role of airborne aerosols (masks for all and evaluations of ventilation and filtering systems). New information keeps appearing and stirring new controversies.

There are many unknowns. We do not know why some heathy adults and children develop serious illness. We do not know the long-term repercussions of the disease or the status of the immune system post-infection. We do not know how new strains of the virus will influence the pandemic. We continue to learn more about the COVID-19 disease, with the uncertainties of immunity and recurrent disease, and complications such as neurological manifestations, hyper-inflammation, acute respiratory distress syndrome, cardiac dysfunction, hypercoagulability, acute kidney injury, pediatric multi-system inflammatory syndrome, and other potential long-term effects.

We do know that mortality and severity of illness increases in higher age groups and those with underlying chronic diseases and obesity. We see stark health disparities and outcomes in populations of color, especially the Black, Latinx/Hispanic, and the indigenous/Native American populations. As the pandemic spread through our communities it uncovered our larger societal issues. Key features became quite apparent as communities suffered—health disparities, health equity, systemic racism, medical care access, and the association of health with social determinants [16].

We seek old and new approaches to the treatment of COVID-19. The "Solidarity" clinical trial, an international endeavor enrolling 12,000 patients in

500 hospital sites in over 30 nations, is investigating over 30 drugs as potential treatments [17]. Remdesivir (EUA on 5/1/20) is a new antiviral, which showed some initial potential in shortening the course of illness and decreasing mortality for the severely ill. Yet, recent data from "Solidarity" are not encouraging. Treatment and prevention using hydroxychloroquine (EUA withdrawn on 6/15/20) became quite controversial and proved ineffective. Lopinavir/ritonavir and interferon also had no effect on mortality or the course of serious illness. Thus far only steroids (dexamethasone) have been proven to be effective against severe COVID-19. The use of convalescent plasma, monoclonal antibodies, 100% oxygen as opposed to intubation, and patient positioning have been introduced as new approaches with mixed results.

Work continues on vaccines using novel approaches to provoke an immune response. These new approaches introduce the potential to develop vaccines through various pathways—genetic vaccines (use one or more coronavirus genes); viral vector vaccines (use a virus to deliver genes into cells); protein-based vaccines (use a coronavirus protein or fragment); whole-virus vaccines (use a weakened or inactivated coronavirus); and, re-purposed vaccines (e.g., BCG vaccine).

As we enter 2021, there are well over 100 vaccine candidates in the pipeline with at least 85 in a preclinical stage (animal studies); 43 in phase I trials (safety and dosage trials in small numbers of volunteers); 21 in phase II (expanded safety trials in hundreds of volunteers); 20 in phase III (large scale efficacy trials in thousands of volunteers) [18]. On June 25, 2020, a Chinese vaccine (Ad5-nCoV, Beijing Institute of Biotechnology and CanSino Biologics) was approved for limited use under "military specially needed drug approval". On August 11, Russia announced the approval of its own vaccine (Gam-Covid-Vac Lyo, The Gamaleya Research Institute). On November 9, 2020, Pfizer and BioNTech presented preliminary findings on their vaccine (Comirnaty/tozinameran/BNT162b2) showing an astounding 95% effectiveness. On December 11, 2020 the US Food and Drug Administration granted an EUA for this vaccine. Moderna and NIH announced preliminary data for their vaccine (mRNA-1273) with a similar effectiveness on November 19 and an EUA was granted on December 18. These vaccines will be "game-changers" and other vaccines will potentially be granted EUAs in early 2021.

We are now in the midst of a vaccine race, reminiscent of the space race of the last century. This warp-speed marathon to find more vaccines leads us down a path of multiple difficulties and issues: assuring safety and efficacy; properly designing placebo-controlled phase III trials as well as potential challenge trials; inclusion of all demographic groups in clinical trials; solving the issues of vaccine health communication and dealing with vaccine hesitancy; determining population prioritization for receiving vaccines; and, securing high quality manufacturing and efficient and equitable distribution to assure global availability. The initial distribution of the vaccines in the US has been a challenge from issues of specifying priority groups to the logistics of a massive and unprecedented national vaccination program to the issue of limited vaccine supplies. Nothing will be easy here.

44.3   Conclusion

In public health we need to be optimists. It has been over 100 years since the global population has experienced a public health crisis of this magnitude. However, we have never had this overlap of a severe, global public health crisis with the advanced state of medical science. This is the source of my optimism.

In the meantime, we need to control COVID in our communities. "Test, trace, isolate" is key. We need to adhere to the three W's: Wear a mask, Watch your distance, Wash your hands (see Fig. 44.3) [19]. We need to monitor and respond to the fluid landscape of this pandemic—monitor conditions and immediately take steps to limit and mitigate any rebounds or outbreaks. We need to assure a successful and timely vaccination program.

In the words of Dr. Anthony Fauci, the director of the National Institute of Allergy and Infectious Diseases: "Now we have something that turned out to be my worst nightmare…it has devastated the world [20]." There remains an incredible challenge ahead of us: "This is something that is quite problematic, and to say it's challenging is to really say the least [21]."

44.4   Selected References

- CDC. Ten essential public health services. Accessed 13 Jan 2021. https://www.cdc.gov/publichealthgateway/publichealthservices/essentialhealthservices.html.

   - Provides a great overview of public health and its mission in our communities.

- Johns Hopkins University. Coronavirus resource center. Accessed 13 Jan 2021. https://coronavirus.jhu.edu/map.html.

   - Up to date data on the pandemic with accurate global and country specific information.

Fig. 44.3 The Three W's of COVID Prevention (CDC) [19]

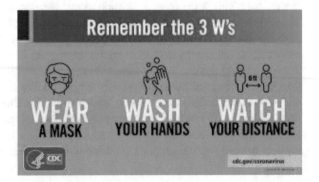

References

1. Winslow CEA. The widening fields of public health. Hospital (Lond 1886). 1921;70:178. Accessed 13 Jan 2021. https://www.ncbi.nlm.nih.gov/pmc/articles/PMC5247976.
2. CDC. Public health model. Accessed 13 Jan 2021. https://www.cdc.gov/training/publichealth101/documents/introduction-to-epidemiology.pdf.
3. CDC. Ten great public health achievements – US 1900–1999. MMWR. 1999;48:241–243.
4. CDC. Ten essential public health services. Accessed 13 Jan 2021. https://www.cdc.gov/publichealthgateway/publichealthservices/essentialhealthservices.html.
5. Heath K. The classical definition of a pandemic is not elusive. Bull World Health Organ. 2011;89:540–1. https://doi.org/10.2471/blt.11.089086.
6. WHO. Past pandemics. Accessed 13 Jan 2021. https://www.euro.who.int/en/health-topics/communicable-diseases/influenza/pandemic-influenza/past-pandemics.
7. Schnirring L. HHS hears community leaders' ideas on pandemic readiness. CIDRAP News. June 14, 2007. Accessed 13 Jan 2021. https://www.cidrap.umn.edu/news-perspective/2007/06/hhs-hears-community-leaders-ideas-pandemic-readiness.
8. GHS Index. 2019 global health security index. Accessed 13 Jan 2021. https://www.ghsindex.org.
9. NIH/National Institute of Allergy and Infectious Diseases. Coronaviruses. Accessed 13 Jan 2021. https://www.niaid.nih.gov/diseases-conditions/coronaviruses.
10. WHO. WHO timeline – COVID-19. Accessed 13 Jan 2021. https://www.who.int/news-room/detail/27-04-2020-who-timeline%2D%2D-covid-19.
11. ThinkGlobalHealth. Timeline of the coronavirus. Accessed 13 Jan 2021. https://www.thinkglobalhealth.org/article/updated-timeline-coronavirus.
12. Nuzzo JB, Bell JA, Cameron EF. Suboptimal US response to COVID-19 despite robust capabilities and resources. JAMA. 2020;324:1391–2. https://doi.org/10.1001/jama.2020.17395.
13. Our World in Data. Coronavirus (COVID-19) cases. Accessed 13 Jan 2021. https://ourworldindata.org/covid-cases.
14. Johns Hopkins University. Coronavirus resource center. Accessed 13 Jan 2021. https://coronavirus.jhu.edu/map.html.
15. Trust for America's Health. A funding crisis for public health and safety. Accessed 13 Jan 2021. https://www.tfah.org/report-details/a-funding-crisis-for-public-health-and-safety-state-by-state-and-federal-public-health-funding-facts-and-recommendations.
16. CDC. Health equity considerations and racial and ethnic minority groups. Accessed 13 Jan 2021. https://www.cdc.gov/coronavirus/2019-ncov/community/health-equity/race-ethnicity.html.
17. WHO. Solidarity clinical trial for COVID-19 treatments. Accessed 13 Jan 2021. https://www.who.int/emergencies/diseases/novel-coronavirus-2019/global-research-on-novel-coronavirus-2019-ncov/solidarity-clinical-trial-for-covid-19-treatments.
18. Zimmer C, Corum J, Wee SL. Coronavirus vaccine tracker. *The New York Times*. March 5, 2021. Accessed 7 March 2021. https://www.nytimes.com/interactive/2020/science/coronavirus-vaccine-tracker.html.
19. CNN. Dr. Anthony Fauci's 'worst nightmare' is Covid-19. Accessed 13 Jan 2021 https://www.cnn.com/2020/06/09/health/fauci-coronavirus-worst-nightmare/index.html.
20. CDC. 3 W's of COVID prevention. Accessed 13 Jan 2021. https://twitter.com/cdcemergency/status/1303333560472961024.
21. CNBC. Dr. Fauci warns the US will see a 'surge upon a surge' of COVID cases following the holidays. Accessed 13 Jan 2021. https://www.cnbc.com/2020/12/01/dr-fauci-warns-the-us-will-see-a-surge-upon-a-surge-of-covid-cases-following-the-holidays.html.

Chapter 45
The Panic of the Pandemic: Who Lives, Who Dies

Piroska Kopar ⓘ, Douglas Brown, and Peter Angelos ⓘ

Abstract The COVID-19 pandemic has fiercely altered the landscape for allocating scarce medical resources in the United States and internationally. This chapter compares and contrasts the ethical frameworks that guide triaging paradigms across countries and institutions. Grounding ethical imperatives and their actualization into allocation guidelines is examined in detail, with consideration given to special populations. Public trust and the socioeconomic factors that influence clinical outcomes are discussed in light of ethical norms. The pandemic's effects on the ethical practice of surgery are outlined. The chapter closes with guidance for future health care crises based on lessons learned during this pandemic.

Keywords Scarce resource allocation · Prioritization · Rationing · Triage Utilitarian healthcare · Surgical ethics · COVID-19

Case

Mr. M is a 72-year-old male with COPD and NYHA Class III heart failure who was admitted to the intensive care unit with COVID-19 pneumonia five days ago. Initially, he was given supplemental oxygen by high flow nasal cannula, but after he became hypoxic, he was intubated on hospital day one. Since that time, he has remained on high ventilator settings with no

P. Kopar (✉) · D. Brown
Department of Surgery, Center for Humanism and Ethics in Surgical Specialties, Washington University in St. Louis School of Medicine, St. Louis, MO, USA
e-mail: pkopar@wustl.edu; debrown@wustl.edu

P. Angelos
Department of Surgery and MacLean Center for Clinical Medical Ethics, The University of Chicago, Chicago, IL, USA
e-mail: pangelos@surgery.bsd.uchicago.edu

© The Author(s), under exclusive license to Springer Nature Switzerland AG 2022
V. A. Lonchyna et al. (eds.), *Difficult Decisions in Surgical Ethics*, Difficult Decisions in Surgery: An Evidence-Based Approach,
https://doi.org/10.1007/978-3-030-84625-1_45

improvement in his respiratory status either clinically or on imaging. The patient's wife, acting as his surrogate decision maker, has explained to the medical team that the patient would want to pursue all available aggressive measures. Meanwhile, Ms. A, a healthy 38-year-old woman, has presented to the emergency department of the hospital with severe gallstone pancreatitis complicated by acute respiratory distress syndrome requiring intubation. No ICU beds are available, and no transfer options are available to her. The emergency department physician requests the ICU to "make a bed" for her as soon as possible as the ED is overwhelmed by COVID patients. Under what circumstances (if any) is it ethically justified to redistribute scarce patient care resources from one patient to another patient?

45.1 Introduction

The COVID-19 pandemic rapidly and forcefully upset the practice of clinical medicine in the United States starting in March 2020 [1]. Cautious concern quickly gave way to widespread panic among patients and providers alike. ICUs were overwhelmed by both the number of patients and the severity of their illnesses, a situation significantly exacerbated by the palpable fear of the staff as they were putting their own lives on the line. During the following year, concerns transitioned from focusing on not enough available personal protective equipment (PPE) to focusing on the lack of readily available ventilators to focusing on the administration of experimental medications to focusing on vaccine development and dissemination, all while daily learning new information about the disease and its spread [2]. Scientific information and medical approaches became entangled with political sympathies [3]. Social isolation and the world's collective anxiety gave way to conspiracy theories that diminished trust in our academic and medical institutions [4]. The pace and energy of the surgical field were halted as elective and semi-elective cases were canceled for fear of spreading infection and taking up valuable resources [5]. All resources, in fact, became either completely or relatively scarce, a problem rarely encountered in high income countries. In this chapter, we examine the ethical dimensions of our response to the pandemic's ubiquitous question: 'Who will live and who will die?' We will begin by exploring the relevant ethical considerations and then study the particulars of resource allocation ethics, examining common themes and points of divergence. Finally, we will discuss the application of such guidance to the specialty of surgery and close with factors to consider under similar circumstances in the future.

45.2 Search Strategy

We conducted a search of PubMed and SCOPUS using the following terms: ethics OR moral AND resource allocation OR supply allocation OR equipment allocation OR resource management AND COVID-19 OR SARS CoV2 OR 2019-nCoV. Full text articles available via PubMed that were published in English in 2020–2021 were reviewed. Thirty-five articles addressing ethical considerations associated with resource allocation decisions in clinical practice both in the United States and abroad were identified and included in our synthesis.

45.3 Discussion

The most significant and characteristic ethical shift in the practice of medicine in the United States (and other developed countries) during the COVID-19 pandemic was a transition from primarily prioritizing individualized deontology-based care to a largely utilitarian healthcare delivery framework in which the objective is to save the most lives [6–13]. Multiple other ethical imperatives influenced this utilitarian sentiment variably across hospitals, states, and nations. The degree to which these other ethical norms balanced the primary objective to save the most lives possible resulted in a landscape of similar but divergent paradigms for the allocation of scarce resources, with few examples exactly alike [8, 14–16].

45.4 Competing Ethical Norms

Patient autonomy is widely considered as the medical ethical principle with the most weight. As the pandemic reframed our practice from a series of individual patient encounters to a public health emergency, the ethical priorities of public health reshaped our professional alliances [6–13]. Ethical considerations (see Table 45.1), as outlined by the Hastings Center in March 2020, included the duty to

Table 45.1 Competing ethical principles in resource allocation during a pandemic

Ethical principle	Toward the patient	Toward others (Medical and Support Staff)
Beneficence	Obligation to treat	Obligation to prioritize the 'common good'
Non-maleficence	Obligation to avoid inflicting additional pain or injury	Obligation to minimize risk to caregivers
Autonomy	Obligation to respect patient's self-determination	Obligation to respect the self-determination of other patients, professionals and institutions.
Justice	Obligation to guide without bias/discrimination	Obligation to equalize access to and to fairly distribute limited resources

treat/care, the duty to safeguard, and the duty to guide. The duty to treat has traditionally been a cornerstone of physicians' Hippocratic obligation and an implied principle upon which the covenant of trust is established between patient and doctor, and the duty to guide is evident in the priority assigned benefitting patients [17]. Usually, however, the physician's health is not itself at risk when providing care to a patient. The ethical principle of beneficence, therefore, is now tempered by both physician autonomy and the duty to safeguard our personnel resources in order to minimize harm (i.e., non-maleficence) [1]. Professional societal guidelines and ethics texts accept a certain degree of risk to providers, but warn against "suicide missions" in patient care [18]. Finally, by providing a framework for the allocation of scarce resources, the duty to guide embodies the principle of justice and emphasizes systematic, transparent, and thoroughly considered paradigms [19].

45.5 Tragic Choices and Frameworks for Allocation of Resources

Ethical dilemmas, by definition, present mutually exclusive options and, therefore, cannot satisfy every ethical imperative. Even if and when the wrath of the pandemic fades, over three million COVID deaths to date worldwide remind us of our astounding losses as the human race. Choices may be better or worse, but tragedy remains. Still, it is our ethical duty to choose the 'least bad' option and minimize loss [20]. The concepts of rationing and prioritization are not new to certain aspects of healthcare and a number of ethical frameworks have been proposed for the allocation of (temporarily) finitely scarce resources [8]. Most notably, the allocation of organs for transplantation follow strict rules about which previous debate has informed prioritization systems during the pandemic [21].

Approaches to prioritization frameworks include maximizing benefit/utilitarianism, favoring the worst-off, egalitarianism, and promoting social usefulness. A utilitarian approach aims to save the largest number of lives or life-years depending on the particular iteration of the framework and whether fair-innings are considered in the calculus. The concept of fair innings refers to the notion that people ought to have the chance to experience all life cycles and, therefore, a younger person should take priority over an older person. The worst-off approach finds its theoretical basis in the concept that a given quantity of improvement in one's life is relatively larger to one who is otherwise worse off. The same amount of excess, it is argued, would only provide an incremental benefit to one who is well off but may raise the quality of life of someone not well off significantly in comparison. This approach favors allocation of resources to the sickest first or possibly the youngest if fair-innings are considered [13–14].

An egalitarian approach, or treating people equally, makes no distinction about life stages, access to care, or social inequities. Most importantly, an egalitarian approach does not take into account a patient's prognosis for survival [13–14]. First

Table 45.2 Ethical Frameworks used for Scarce Resource Allocation

Frameworks	Ethical intent	Prioritized group
Maximizing benefit	Save most lives/life-years	Best likelihood of short term and long-term survival
Favoring worst-off	Maximize relative benefit	Sickest patients
Fair innings	Ensure equal opportunity to experience all life stages	Youngest patients
Lottery	Treat all people equally	Selected by chance
First come first serve	Treat all people equally	Selected chronologically and influenced by access to care
Instrumental value	Save the lives of those whose work will save more lives	Essential workers
Reciprocity	Save the life of those who put themselves at risk in order to save others	Patients who contracted disease while performing essential functions

come first served is the most common application of this approach, which is frequently used in ICU bed allocations during non-crisis circumstances and has been previously espoused by the American Thoracic Society [22]. The lottery is another version of the same foundational concept, leaving decisions to chance rather than to other factors. Social usefulness prioritizes an individual's contribution to society, either based on one's habits, instrumental value, or the idea of reciprocity. Due to unclear causal relationships and social and cultural complexities, no current framework takes lifestyle habits into account when making resource allocation decisions. Instrumental value is more readily accepted and refers to the situation in which someone who, through special skills or abilities, has the ability to save more lives than his own. Because saving such a person's life translates into saving a greater number of lives altogether, a person who has instrumental value is thus prioritized. Reciprocity, on the other hand, proposes to allocate resources to those who contract the disease by performing their duties and putting themselves in harm's way in order to care for patients [13–14]. These approaches to allocation of finite resources are summarized in Table 45.2.

45.6 Common Trends in Ethical Guidelines

Approaches to allocation of scarce resources have been synthesized with varying combinations. Common across institutions, nations, and continents has been the importance of stressing that standards of care have been altered into crisis standards temporarily and with the expectation of returning to normal [7, 9, 23–25]. Situational awareness by means of regular review of circumstances by the healthcare entities who put such crisis standards in place was thought to be critical to the ethical integrity of any ethical framework. Providers and institutions were warned not to preemptively alter their patient-centered practice in anticipation of a crisis situation until crisis circumstances were in fact confirmed [10, 26]. Once a hospital did reach this threshold, resource allocation schemes were to be enacted with transparency and consistency. In order to avoid ad hoc bedside rationing and reduce the moral distress of bedside clinicians, institutions were encouraged to develop triaging guidelines and triaging teams to aid the execution of difficult decisions [16, 19]. It has also been uniformly accepted that resource allocation guidelines should treat COVID+ and non-COVID+ patients in need of the same resources as ethically equally deserving of them [25].

A systematic examination of large-scale state, national, or transnational allocation paradigms in several developed countries found that all nine countries favored an approach grounded in a utilitarian strategy. [16] Similarly, a study evaluating hospital protocols for ventilator allocation found that the most common ethical imperative among twenty-six hospitals was justice [27]. Four other common themes identified in the same evaluation were transparency, stewardship, duty to care, and duty to prevent. Stewardship is analogous to the duty to safeguard. The duty to care describes an institution's obligation to not abandon patients even when the capacity to actively treat them has been exhausted. Most authors agree that a first come first served approach is never ethically optimal as those without easy access to medical care are disproportionally harmed. Similarly, wealth should not override allocation decisions. Lottery is recommended only as a tiebreaker when clinical aspects are equal [10, 13, 25]. Several articles have called for a clear distinction between declining to provide certain treatments because of medical futility and not providing care due to rationing [11, 28]. Interestingly, most narrative preambles to ethical frameworks avoid using the term 'ration' in favor of 'prioritizing' and 'resource allocation.' [16] Many texts commented on the importance of proper process, stressing that the opportunity to appeal a resource allocation decision plus systematic accountability are paramount to any paradigm's ethical merit [9, 12, 14, 20].

45.7 Differences in Ethical Guidelines

A key difference among institutional guidelines stems from the variations in the interpretations of the concept of patient autonomy. Virtually all frameworks in the US recognize individual patient rights as the de facto primary principle in medical ethics under normal circumstances, with the caveat that prioritizing patient autonomy may be altered for a limited time during a crisis of pandemic magnitude [2, 11]. In contrast, non-US authors do not consider patient autonomy to be an a priori right and approach the question with the intent to balance ethical principles even during non-crisis circumstances, albeit with fewer restrictions. Newdick, a scholar from the United Kingdom, is quite explicit about this difference as he asserts that individual rights are meaningless in the absence of a community and, therefore, cannot possibly be considered as primary [20].

Practical applications of these ideological differences manifest themselves in 'second-tier' triaging. Once a patient is identified as someone who is likely to benefit clinically from treatment (e.g., testing, ICU bed, ventilator, hospitalization, medications) based on local criteria, a second layer of allocation may be necessary depending on readily available resources [24]. It is within this second layer that variation is most often introduced into triaging algorithms and differences become a function of the approach to prioritization an institution adopts from among the options described above and summarized in Table 45.2 once efforts to save the most lives are exhausted. Below are second-tier triaging approaches that remain subjects of much debate.

45.8 Special Considerations: The Elderly

Italy and Spain in particular were sharply criticized as ageist in their initial policies for withholding interventions from older patients. The age limit varied between 80 and 85 years old, depending on the rates of infection at any given time [23, 29]. Other Western guidelines pointed to age as a clinically and not an ethically relevant element of decision making. These guidelines argued that a patient's age needs to be incorporated into the medical calculus. Critics of this line of reasoning highlighted evidence from prior clinical data to advocate for replacing age with functional status. The Frailty Score, they have asserted, is a validated instrument to guide clinical decisions of older patients [30–31]. Emanuel, however, proposed that age is ethically relevant, but limited its consideration to being a tiebreaker when otherwise similar patients are competing for the same resources. This argument is based on life-years saved when the saving of lives would otherwise be similar [13].

45.9 Special Considerations: Children

Most authors have not addressed the application of ethical guidelines to the triaging of pediatric patients. Laventhal et al. introduced the concept of children as subjects of triage protocols and noted that it is extremely unusual for pediatric patients to be unilaterally declared as having the status of 'do-not-resuscitate.' They called attention to the moral as well as ethical nature of this possibility; a distinction that is less palpable among adult patients. They made special mention of the ethical struggle present in the juxtaposition of an otherwise healthy young adult patient with a good prognosis alongside a sick child. Fortunately, children as a demographic, have been less susceptible to COVID and, as a result, few difficult decisions involving children were needed to be made [32].

45.10   Special Considerations: Healthcare Workers

Whether based on the concept of reciprocity or of instrumental value, prioritizing treatment of patients who themselves are healthcare workers is not infrequent in allocation algorithms [16]. When implemented with the intent to save more lives by saving more healthcare workers, this step-in paradigm is simply an extension of the overall imperative guided by utilitarian principles. However, prioritizing the care of a healthcare worker based on reciprocity even if her prognosis is otherwise poor represents a philosophically separate proposal [14]. Reciprocity can be said to inspire future action in that healthcare providers may be assured that they will be treated should they become infected. In this manner, reciprocity can be thought of as utilitarian. In the moment of decision-making, however, reciprocity runs the risk of 'paying a due' instead of promoting the current salvage of as many lives as possible, a sentiment that is more reminiscent of deontological views than of utilitarian ones. Notably, reciprocity has not been reported for the treatment prioritization of essential non-healthcare workers.

45.11   Special Considerations: Residents and Fellows in Training

Trainees' duty to care for patients during the pandemic has been argued to be both equivalent to and less than those of attending physicians [1, 33–34]. In practice, on the other hand, some institutions relied more heavily on the frontline work of residents and fellows than on attendings themselves. Proponents of resident and fellow obligation to deliver care point to the public oaths of physicians to promote patient benefit they are expected to internalize by the time they graduate from medical school. Critics call attention to the fact that trainees are socioeconomically worse off than attendings and, therefore, should be relatively protected from being exploited. In addition, the non-monetary compensation for their work largely provided in the form of daily education—formal and informal—on rounds, in the operating rooms, and in classrooms, were, at the time of the worst of the pandemic, almost entirely absent. The hierarchy separating surgical faculty and residents with the resulting power discrepancy led not just to compromised educational opportunities, but also to a certain loss of trust [35].

Several initiatives have been introduced to restore trust between surgical faculty and residents—e.g., (1) facilitating open dialogue between residents and faculty, (2) bolstering peer support groups within residency, (3) reintegrating residents into the preoperative decision-making process, (4) adjusting faculty teaching to address when surgery is medically necessary and times-sensitive for each patient on the OR schedule, (5) soliciting resident feedback on COVID safety protocols, (6) empowering residents to engage in informed consent discussions with patients and address advance directives when appropriate, (7) allowing residents who refused involvement in an operation the protection to explain their reasons since they may be signaling moral or physical distress that needs to be further addressed outside of patient care settings [35].

45.12   Public Perception and Trust

Transparency, consistency, asking for public input, and systematic review of processes have all been embraced as necessary elements to gaining the trust of patients [1]. In fact, one of the arguments against endorsing the prioritization of healthcare workers centers on the negative effects that such a practice would potentially incite among patients, ultimately eroding their trust in their caregivers [36]. Although it has not been formally studied, one might expect that the current variations in allocation paradigms among institutions may diminish public trust. Devereax et al. described their experience in creating a regional network for institutional consistency in the same geographic region successfully orchestrated by a single command center [37]. Other authors have also praised regional, rather than national, uniformity in allocation decisions in order to garner local trust and buy-in [38]. Vaccination, in particular, has been the subject of much public distrust fueled by a combination of political, cultural, and scientific factors [39]. The public's attitude towards vaccination is a complex problem, the discussion of which is beyond the scope of this chapter.

Public perception regarding the ethical merit of allocation guidelines has been better studied in Europe than in the United States [40–41]. While significant heterogeneity in preferences were found in hypothetical scenarios, people tended to prioritize based on medical prognosis as well as on being worse off. This latter consideration, in particular, is in sharp contrast to the expert recommendations of most pandemic ethicists, as they see the allocation of scarce resources to the patients who are worst off to be completely contrary to the agreed upon utilitarian approach to save the most lives. The public, nevertheless, has been found to identify this approach as second best in at least two published articles [36, 42]. A potential reason for this seeming contradiction is patients' fear of abandonment in the absence of treatment; a concern that many guidelines address with palliative recommendations [16]. The same studies have also shown the public's rejection of prioritizing based on lottery or reciprocity. While data on the public's answers to hypothetical decisions are available, no studies have addressed public understanding and insight into institutions' actual guidelines or their implementation.

45.13   The Socioeconomic Divide

Socioeconomic differences that translate into less readily available access to care and worse clinical outcomes exist nationally and internationally. Among developed nations, despite some cultural variation, there have been no salient departures from Western medical ethical approaches to resource allocation. In low-income countries, however, the allocation paradigms espoused in high-income countries are often meaningless. The very notion of any critical care, for example, is entirely absent from low-income Sub-Saharan nations, making distinctions of resource allocations rather abstract and academic. Given the stark differences in available medical options in these countries, Moodley has proposed the establishment of regionally tailored medical guidance to local physicians that include prioritizing the care of those patients who are likely to survive with treatments outside of hospitals [43].

For more diverse countries such as the United Kingdom and the United States, studies have found disturbing differences in the medical outcomes of ethnic minorities and those with low socioeconomic status [44–45]. This consequence is true in the UK despite the country's national health-care system [42]. The divide is even more sharply pronounced in the United States [46]. The challenges have been as specific as inability to maintain social distancing on public transportation and in many household environments. The ethical question arises, therefore, whether socioeconomic status ought to be weighed in prioritization decisions in order to raise public trust and to ensure fairness. While the problem is well-documented and public opinion in the United Kingdom supports the adoption of a system that would factor in patients' socioeconomic status into decision making, no systematic guidelines have transformed this scheme into practice [42].

45.14   The Pandemic's Effect on Surgery

Following state directives and American College of Surgery guidelines, many centers suspended elective and semi-elective operations in March 2020. This action resulted in tremendous stress on medical centers, surgical residents, and surgical departments. Clinics were closed and surgeons were instructed to remain at home unless needed at the hospital to assist with the care of COVID-19+ patients. The paradigm shift in focusing on the health of the population imposed by the coronavirus pandemic caused significant moral distress among surgeons. Telling patients who had been scheduled for surgery that their surgeries had to be postponed indefinitely took an emotional toll on surgeons who could not accommodate patient wishes even when the patients were willing to accept the risks, inserting an awkward level of paternalism into the surgeon-patient relationship most surgeons had not previously experienced in their practices [5].

In such a crisis setting, surgeons were predictably tempted to conflate 'elective' with 'optional' when discussing surgical procedures with patients. It should be noted that 'elective' means the acuity of the condition being surgically treated allows the surgeon and the patient to elect the timing and scheduling of the surgery without negative impact on outcomes. The coronavirus pandemic forced hospitals to curtail surgeries in order to offload the inpatient census, to preserve personal protective equipment, and to redistribute limited personnel. It quickly became evident that a tool was needed that would guide the systematic integration of novel factors such as resource limitations and COVID-19 transmission risk into

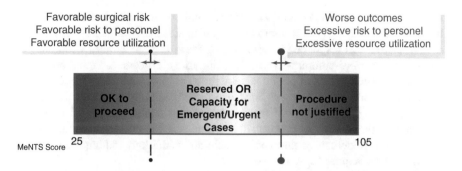

Fig. 45.1 The Medically Necessary Time-Sensitive (MeNTS) score [47]. Use of the cumulative medically necessary time-sensitive (MeNTS) score. Upper and lower threshold MeNTS scores can be assigned and dynamically adjusted to respond to the immediate and anticipated availability of resources and local conditions while preserving operating room capacity for trauma, emergency, and highly urgent cases

pre-existing processes. Such a tool would systematically score cases across specialties in order to improve efficiency and equitability while also reducing the emotional and ethical burdens on caregivers. Prachand, Milner, Angelos, et al. proposed the MeNTS Scoring System (see Fig. 45.1) [47]. By assigning values to each factor, the MeNTS Scoring System had a "forcing function" that compelled surgeons to consider additional factors they were not generally required to consider apart from the pandemic [48].

The question also arises regarding how surgical informed consent may have been modified under pandemic circumstances given limitations on preoperative in-person visits and discussions and the uncertainty inherent in the risk of contracting COVID-19 while in the hospital or undergoing an operation once infected [49]. Multiple studies on informed consent in surgery have shown that patients frequently make decisions based less on the complex medical and surgical information explained to them preoperatively, but rather based on the trust that the surgeon is able establish with his patient [50–51]. The consequences of the limit that crisis conditions placed on the preoperative bonding of patient and surgeon have not yet been studied.

45.15 After the Pandemic

Several essential lessons from the pandemic should better prepare us for future public health crises. Throughout the pandemic, but especially in the earliest phase, clinicians quickly assumed the role of triaging officers while providing direct patient care. There was a widespread sense of urgency and panic that translated into inconsistent and at times ad hoc bedside rationing. Although providers were clearly well-intentioned, physician-to-physician variation in the allocation of scarce resources is never ethically favorable. It is much preferred to follow guidelines that have been composed by taking all stakeholders into account and that are devoid of the emotional toll that denying certain treatments to a patient is likely to take. Almost immediately, institutions responded by establishing these very guidelines, with many of them forming triage committees or appointing triage officers. A limitation of this process has been the lack of public input at most hospitals and the dearth of openly accessible paradigms and descriptions of the deliberations that led up to them. Future guidelines would benefit from incorporating public values and providing transparency throughout the process. In addition, periodic evaluation of the relative success of the guidelines ought to occur, facilitating additions and improvements as new data might require [6, 9, 12, 16].

Another pitfall of institutional guidelines for the allocation of scarce resources during the pandemic has been their implementation in practice. As Dawson has observed, implicit and explicit triaging exist in parallel dimensions. Clinicians are well accustomed to routine triaging of non-finite resources, such as the timing of a particular test or intervention, or the admission to an ICU that is not actually full. Physicians make resource decisions daily as they select less-expensive medications for their patients or use a reusable instrument during an operation. Explicit rationing, however, is applied to finitely scarce resources, such as organs for transplantation or scarce resources during the pandemic. The challenge—both on an individual and on an institutional level—is to refrain from explicit triaging on an individual level. This discipline is mandatory to maintaining the ethical allocation of resources by ensuring fairness through consistency [12, 26]. An important lesson learned during the pandemic may be that uncritical procedure-driven efforts to prolong life at all costs is sometimes inappropriate. Although this objection is not a novel ethical concept, its practice is often limited by not considering palliative options among the armament of clinical choices [52]. It is imperative, however, as we slowly transition away from crisis standards of care, that no reflexive triage decisions are made without reinstalling the goals and values of individual patients as front and center in our care of patients.

45.16   Case Conclusion

In addressing the difficult situation of whether to remove life supporting treatment from one patient in favor of another, the first step is to clarify whether the treatment currently provided to Mr. M is in fact medically beneficial. The ICU physician should address the specific goals and values of Mr. M with his wife beyond the initial blanket statement of "do everything." The likely medical outcome must be discussed in detail along with the quality of life and supportive measures that will likely be necessary should the patient survive. If the patient has no meaningful chance of survival, then this must be explained to his family and non-beneficial care should not be offered in neither normal, nor crisis settings.

In the event that Mr. M has a reasonable chance of survival to a quality of life that would be acceptable to him, crisis circumstances enter allocation considerations. It is imperative that this approach is only taken if there is a true lack of other resource options. The care of Ms. A, even in this case, should only be prioritized if she has a better prognosis than Mr. M. Age alone should not be a factor in favoring Ms. A, but functional status should be. Any withdrawal of care of Mr. M much be accompanied by the provision of palliative measures, social support for his family, crystal clear communication and transparency.

45.17 Selected References

- Kramer JB, Brown DE, Kopar PK. Ethics in the Time of Coronavirus: Recommendations in the COVID-19 Pandemic. J Am Coll Surg. 2020;230(6):1114–1118. doi:https://doi.org/10.1016/j.jamacollsurg.2020.04.004

  - Early in this pandemic, the authors, using experience from the HIV/AIDS epidemic, address the ethical problems of who shall treat and be treated, who will be tested, how scarce resources are to be allocated, how end of life issues are to be addressed, and how confidentiality is to be maintained.

- Emanuel EJ, Persad G, Upshur R, et al. Fair Allocation of Scarce Medical Resources in the Time of Covid-19. N Engl J Med. 2020;382(21):2049–2055. doi:https://doi.org/10.1056/nejmsb2005114

  - Ethicists discuss using ethical values in guiding the rationing of scarce medical resources during this pandemic.

- American Thoracic Society. Fair Allocation of Intensive Care Unit Resources. Am J Respir Crit Care Med. 1997;156:1282–1301. doi:https://doi.org/10.1164/ajrccm.156.4.ats7-97

  - Principles of fair allocation of ICU resources and the position of the ATS towards these allocations as thought out and discussed almost a quarter of a century before the current pandemic, whose precepts hold true today.

References

1. Kramer JB, Brown DE, Kopar PK. Ethics in the time of coronavirus: recommendations in the COVID-19 pandemic. J Am Coll Surg. 2020;230(6):1114–8. https://doi.org/10.1016/j.jamacollsurg.2020.04.004.
2. Sprung CL, Joynt GM, Christian MD, Truog RD, Rello J, Nates JL. Adult ICU triage during the coronavirus disease 2019 pandemic: who will live and who will die? Recommendations to improve survival. Crit Care Med. 2020;48(8):1196–202. https://doi.org/10.1097/ccm.0000000000004410.
3. Adolph C, Amano K, Bang-Jensen B, Fullman N, Wilkerson J. Pandemic politics: timing state-level social distancing responses to COVID-19. J Health Polit Policy Law. 2021;46(2):211–33. https://doi.org/10.1215/03616878-8802162.

4. Udow-Phillips M, Lantz PM. Trust in Public Health is Essential amid the COVID-19 pandemic. J Hosp Med. 2020;15(7):431–3. https://doi.org/10.12788/jhm.3474.

5. Angelos P. Surgeons, ethics, and COVID-19: early lessons learned. J Am Coll Surg. 2020;230(6):1119–20. https://doi.org/10.1016/j.jamcollsurg.2020.03.028.

6. Kim SYH, Grady C. Ethics in the time of COVID: what remains the same and what is different. Neurology. 2020;94(23):1007–8. https://doi.org/10.1212/wnl.0000000000009520.

7. Kirkpatrick JN, Hull SC, Fedson S, Mullen B, Goodlin SJ. Scarce-resource allocation and patient triage during the COVID-19 pandemic: JACC review topic of the week. J Am Coll Cardiol. 2020;76(1):85–92. https://doi.org/10.1016/j.jacc.2020.05.006.

8. Mannelli C. Whose life to save? Scarce resources allocation in the COVID-19 outbreak. J Med Ethics. 2020;46(6):364–6. https://doi.org/10.1136/medethics-2020-106227.

9. Marckmann G, Neitzke G, Schildmann J, et al. Decisions on the allocation of intensive care resources in the context of the COVID-19 pandemic: clinical and ethical recommendations of DIVI, DGINA, DGAI, DGIIN, DGNI, DGP, DGP and AEM. Med Klin Intensivmed Notfmed. 2020;115(Suppl 3):S115–22. https://doi.org/10.1007/s00063-020-00709-9.

10. Binkley CE, Kemp DS. Ethical rationing of personal protective equipment to minimize moral residue during the COVID-19 pandemic. J Am Coll Surg. 2020;230(6):1111–3. https://doi.org/10.1016/j.jamcollsurg.2020.03.031.

11. Chan PS, Berg RA, Nadkarni VM. Code blue during the COVID-19 pandemic. Circ Cardiovasc Qual Outcomes. 2020;13(5):e006779. https://doi.org/10.1161/circoutcomes.120.006779.

12. Dawson A. Building an ethics framework for COVID-19 resource allocation: the how and the why. J Bioeth Inq. 2020;17(4):757–60. https://doi.org/10.1007/s11673-020-10022-x.

13. Emanuel EJ, Persad G, Upshur R, et al. Fair allocation of scarce medical resources in the time of Covid-19. N Engl J Med. 2020;382(21):2049–55. https://doi.org/10.1056/nejmsb2005114.

14. Sese D, Ahmad MU, Rajendram P. Ethical considerations during the COVID-19 pandemic. Cleve Clin J Med. 2020 Jun.; https://doi.org/10.3949/ccjm.87a.ccc038.

15. Fiest KM, Krewulak KD, Plotnikoff KM, et al. Allocation of intensive care resources during an infectious disease outbreak: a rapid review to inform practice. BMC Med. 2020;18(1):404. https://doi.org/10.1186/s12916-020-01871-9.

16. Tyrrell CSB, Mytton OT, Gentry SV, et al. Managing intensive care admissions when there are not enough beds during the COVID-19 pandemic: a systematic review. Thorax. 2021;76(3):302–12. https://doi.org/10.1136/thoraxjnl-2020-215518.

17. Berlinger N, Wynia M, Powell T, et al. Ethical framework for health care institutions & Guidelines for Institutional Ethics services responding to the Coronavirus Pandemic: Managing uncertainty, safeguarding communities, guiding practice. The Hastings Center. March 16, 2020. Accessed May 13, 2021. https://www.thehastingscenter.org/ethicalframeworkcovid19/.

18. Angoff NR. Do physicians have an ethical obligation to care for patients with AIDS? Yale J Biol Med. 1991;64(3):207–46. 1788990.

19. Gorovitz S. Ventilators, guidelines, judgment, and trust. Hast Cent Rep. 2020;50(3):5–6. https://doi.org/10.1002/hast.1117.

20. Newdick C, Sheehan M, Dunn M. Tragic choices in intensive care during the COVID-19 pandemic: on fairness, consistency and community. J Med Ethics. 2020;46(10):646–51. https://doi.org/10.1136/medethics-2020-106487.

21. Persad G. Will more organs save more lives? Cost-effectiveness and the ethics of expanding organ procurement. Bioethics. 2019;33(6):684–90. https://doi.org/10.1111/bioe.12587.

22. American Thoracic Society. Fair allocation of intensive care unit resources. Am J Respir Crit Care Med. 1997;156:1282–301. https://doi.org/10.1164/ajrccm.156.4.ats7-97.

23. Vergano M, Bertolini G, Giannini A, et al. Clinical ethics recommendations for the allocation of intensive care treatments in exceptional, resource-limited circumstances: the Italian perspective during the COVID-19 epidemic. Crit Care. 2020;24(1):165. https://doi.org/10.1186/s13054-020-02891-w.

24. Savulescu J, Vergano M, Craxì L, Wilkinson D. An ethical algorithm for rationing life-sustaining treatment during the COVID-19 pandemic. Br J Anaesth. 2020;125(3):253–8. https://doi.org/10.1016/j.bja.2020.05.028.
25. Vincent JL, Creteur J. Ethical aspects of the COVID-19 crisis: how to deal with an overwhelming shortage of acute beds. Eur Heart J Acute Cardiovasc Care. 2020;9(3):248–52. https://doi.org/10.1177/2048872620922788.
26. Dawson A, Isaacs D, Jansen M, et al. An ethics framework for making resource allocation decisions within clinical care: responding to COVID-19. J Bioeth Inq. 2020;17(4):749–55. https://doi.org/10.1007/s11673-020-10007-w.
27. Cheung ATM, Parent B. Mistrust and inconsistency during COVID-19: considerations for resource allocation guidelines that prioritise healthcare workers. J Med Ethics. 2021;47(2):73–7. https://doi.org/10.1136/medethics-2020-106801.
28. Spector-Bagdady K, Laventhal N, Applewhite M, et al. Flattening the rationing curve: the need for explicit guidelines for implicit rationing during the COVID-19 pandemic. Am J Bioeth. 2020;20(7):77–80. https://doi.org/10.1080/15265161.2020.1779409.
29. Herreros B, Gella P. Real de Asua. D. triage during the COVID-19 epidemic in Spain: better and worse ethical arguments. J Med Ethics. 2020;46(7):455–8. https://doi.org/10.1136/medethics-2020-106352.
30. Farrell TW, Francis L, Brown T, et al. Rationing limited healthcare resources in the COVID-19 era and beyond: ethical considerations regarding older adults. J Am Geriatr Soc. 2020;68(6):1143–9. https://doi.org/10.1111/jgs.16539.
31. Montero-Odasso M, Hogan DB, Lam R, et al. Age alone is not adequate to determine health-care resource allocation during the COVID-19 pandemic. Canadian Geriatrics J. 2020;23(1):152–4. https://doi.org/10.5770/cgj.23.452.
32. Laventhal N, Basak R, Dell ML, et al. The ethics of creating a resource allocation strategy during the COVID-19 pandemic. Pediatrics. 2020;146(1):e20201243. https://doi.org/10.1542/peds.2020-1243.
33. Hai S, Baroutjian A, Elkbuli A. Challenges and ethical considerations for trainees and attending physicians during the COVID-19 pandemic [letter]. J Am Coll Surg. 2020;231(2):301–2. https://doi.org/10.1016/j.amcollsurg.2020.05.009.
34. Kramer JB, Brown DE, Kopar PK. Ethics in the time of coronavirus: engaging the conversation: in reply to Hai and colleagues [letter]. J Am Coll Surg. 2020;231(2):302–3. https://doi.org/10.1016/j.amcollsurg.2020.05.008.
35. Tseng J, Roggin KK, Angelos P. Should this operation proceed? When residents and faculty disagree during the COVID-19 pandemic and recovery. Ann Surg. 2020;272(2):e157–8. https://doi.org/10.1097/sla.0000000000004080.
36. Buckwalter W, Peterson A. Public attitudes toward allocating scarce resources in the COVID-19 pandemic. PLoS One. 2020;15(11):e0240651. https://doi.org/10.1371/journal.pone.0240651.
37. Devereaux A, Yang H, Seda G, et al. Optimizing scarce resource allocation during COVID-19: rapid creation of a regional health-care coalition and triage teams in San Diego County. California Disaster Med Public Health Prep. 2020:1–7. https://doi.org/10.1017/dmp.2020.344.
38. Hertelendy AJ, Ciottone GR, Mitchell CL, Gutberg J, Burkle FM. Crisis standards of care in a pandemic: navigating the ethical, clinical, psychological and policy-making maelstrom. Int J Qual Health Care. 2021;33(1):mzaa094. https://doi.org/10.1093/intqhc/mzaa094.
39. Bajaj SS, Stanford FC. Beyond Tuskegee – vaccine distrust and everyday racism. N Engl J Med. 2021;384(5):e12. https://doi.org/10.1056/nejmpv2035827.
40. Grover S, McClelland A, Furnham A. Preferences for scarce medical resource allocation: differences between experts and the general public and implications for the COVID-19 pandemic. Br J Health Psychol. 2020;25(4):889–901. https://doi.org/10.1111/bjhp.12439.
41. Fallucchi F, Faravelli M, Quercia S. Fair allocation of scarce medical resources in the time of COVID-19: what do people think? J Med Ethics. 2021;47(1):3–6. https://doi.org/10.1136/medethics-2020-106524.

42. Roadevin C, Hill H. How can we decide a fair allocation of healthcare resources during a pandemic? J Med Ethics Published online January. 2021;13 https://doi.org/10.1136/medethics-2020-106815.
43. Moodley K, Ravez L, Obasa AE, et al. What could "fair allocation" during the Covid-19 crisis possibly mean in sub-Saharan Africa? Hast Cent Rep. 2020;50(3):33–5. https://doi.org/10.1002/hast.1129.
44. Khanna N, Klyushnenkova EN, Kaysin A. Association of COVID-19 with race and socioeconomic factors in family medicine. J Am Board Fam Med. 2021;34(Suppl):S40–7. https://doi.org/10.3122/jabfm.2021.s1.200338.
45. Patel AP, Paranjpe MD, Kathiresan NP, Rivas MA, Khera AV. Race, socioeconomic deprivation, and hospitalization for COVID-19 in English participants of a National Biobank. Int J Equity Health. 2020;19:114. https://doi.org/10.1186/s12939-020-01227-y.
46. Muñoz-Price LS, Nattinger AB, Rivera F, et al. Racial disparities in incidence and outcomes among patients with COVID-19. JAMA Netw Open. 2020;3(9):e2021892. https://doi.org/10.1001/jamanetworkopen.2020.21892.
47. Prachand V, Milner R, Angelos P, et al. Medically necessary, time-sensitive procedures: scoring system to ethically and efficiently manage resource scarcity and provider risk during the COVID-19 pandemic. J Am Coll Surg. 2020;231:281–8. https://doi.org/10.1016/j.jamcollsurg.2020.04.011.
48. Prachand V, Tseng J, Milner R, Posner M, Matthews J. Web-based medically necessary, time-sensitive (MeNTS) procedure scoring worksheet: in reply to Ing and Ing [letter]. J Am Coll Surg. 2020;231(3):407. https://doi.org/10.1016/j.jamcollsurg.2020.05.016.
49. Angelos P. Interventions to improve informed consent: perhaps surgeons should speak less and listen more. JAMA Surg. 2020;155(1):13–4. https://doi.org/10.1001/jamasurg.2019.3796.
50. McKneally MF, Ignagni E, Martin DK, D'Cruz J. The leap to trust: perspective of cholecystectomy patients on informed decision making and consent. J Am Coll Surg. 2004;199(1):51–7. https://doi.org/10.1016/j.jamcollsurg.2004.02.021.
51. McKneally MF, Martin DK, Ignagni E, D'Cruz J. Responding to trust: surgeons' perspective on informed consent. World J Surg. 2009;33(7):1341–7. https://doi.org/10.1007/s00268-009-0021-7.
52. Kopar PK, Brown DE, Turnbull IR. Ethics of codes and codes of ethics: when is it ethical to provide cardiopulmonary resuscitation during the COVID-19 pandemic? Ann Surg. 2020;272(6):930–4. https://doi.org/10.1097/sla.0000000000004318.

Chapter 46
A System Overwhelmed by a Pandemic: The New York Response

Brian Mitzman (iD), Samantha Ratner (iD), and Barron H. Lerner

Abstract The COVID-19 pandemic struck several regions of the United States early, stretching health care systems to the brink without much warning. Seattle and New York City specifically were two of the first cities impacted and had minimal warning to properly prepare. Staff shortages became standard, as trained critical care specialists became scarce. While the lack of appropriate health care providers became a common headline in the media, the ethical principles associated with the swift solutions that were enacted at the height of the pandemic have yet to be thoroughly discussed.

Keywords COVID-19 · Coronavirus · Workforce · Personnel management
Pandemic · Health planning · Health resources · Strategic stockpile

> **Case**
>
> Two weeks into a major pandemic, the hospital census exceeded capacity with no decrease in the foreseeable future. Fortunately, non-clinical hospital space had been successfully converted into new intensive care units for incoming patients. As the senior intensivist, you were informed that critical-care board certified staff were not available to staff these new units. Administration stated that help was on the way, and there were several options for manning the ICU

B. Mitzman (✉)
Division of Cardiothoracic Surgery, University of Utah, Salt Lake City, UT, USA

Department of Cardiothoracic Surgery, NYU Langone Health, New York, NY, USA
e-mail: brian.mitzman@hsc.utah.edu

S. Ratner
University of Michigan, Ann Arbor, MI, USA

B. H. Lerner
Department of Medicine, NYU Langone Health, New York, NY, USA
e-mail: Barron.lerner@nyulangone.org

© The Author(s), under exclusive license to Springer Nature
Switzerland AG 2022
V. A. Lonchyna et al. (eds.), *Difficult Decisions in Surgical Ethics*, Difficult
Decisions in Surgery: An Evidence-Based Approach,
https://doi.org/10.1007/978-3-030-84625-1_46

to use at your discretion. These included rapidly recertified retired physicians, medical students scheduled to graduate in the coming months, and outpatient subspecialists. There was limited time to make a decision, as the new intensive care units were being filled.

46.1   Introduction

Healthcare institutions often train for mass casualty incidents, planning for hospital resources and staffing to be stretched for a defined short period of time with a set expected number of patients. SARS-CoV-2, or COVID-19, was a mass casualty incident that, at its first peak, lasted for over 8 weeks in New York with an unclear endpoint. Protocols and algorithms that were laid out for incidents anticipating a mass influx of inpatients would fail after just several days. Much of the media and literature focused on resource utilization in terms of bed allotment, ICU availability, and personal protective equipment (PPE), but the real limiting factor to appropriately caring for COVID-19 patients was medical professionals experienced in treating critically ill respiratory failure patients.

At the height of the pandemic, there were an average of 1500 hospitalizations per day in New York City. [1]. Due to the increased hospitalizations and the increased duration of ICU stays (average 14–21 days for SARS-CoV-2), hospitals had to make room for more beds. In addition, more doctors were needed to accommodate the increase in patients. Normally, in the ICU, staffing is one nurse for every two patients, but maintaining this ratio became more difficult as nurses became sick and hospitalizations increased [2]. Hospitals struggled to find enough intensivists to care for these patients.

Unique and intuitive methods of increasing medical staff without compromising patient care or employee well-being had to be developed. Four main categories of health care professionals were called up to assist in the pandemic in New York: retired physicians, out of town health care providers, outpatient specialists, and medical students. In the heat of the crisis, these were excellent opportunities to recruit enthusiastic experienced professionals to supplement critical care specialists [3]. Each, however, had its own set of ethical considerations.

Several ethical principles guided decision making during the pandemic (see Table 46.1). The most prevalent principle was justice, which refers to equitable distribution of resources based on need. This was important when dealing with shortages of ICU beds, PPE, and physicians during the height of the pandemic. Another principle was beneficence, acting in ways that benefit patients, which was utilized when inviting retired physicians, medical students, and specialists to work in order to address the physician shortage. Non-maleficence, not inflicting harm on a patient, was also critical when deciding how to train and supervise specialists and medical students so that they could treat patients without harming them.

Table 46.1 Ethical Principles during the pandemic.

Ethical Principle	
Beneficence	Many health care providers, including medical students and previously retired physicians volunteered to return to practice to alleviate staff shortages
Nonmaleficence	The risks of having an inexperienced physician managing intensive care units had to be weighed against the over exhaustion of the usual hospital intensivists
Respect for Autonomy	Not only did most patients and family members not have a say in who was providing their care, but most were unaware of the physician's credentials and experience
Justice	Despite an all-hands-on-deck environment, those with the least seniority often were forced into the riskiest environments

46.2   Search Strategy

A MEDLINE search was performed using the terms "COVID," "Coronavirus," "SARS-CoV-2," "Staffing," "Resources," and "New York." To supplement scientific articles, a manual Google News search was performed to find reputable articles from major news outlets relating to COVID-19 resource utilization. A timeframe of March 1 through August 1, 2020 was utilized for this search. A specific focus was placed on articles directly relating to New York.

46.3   Discussion

46.3.1   Retired Physicians

As the number of COVID-19 cases rapidly increased in the New York City area, Mayor de Blasio and Governor Cuomo put out a call for reinforcements. It became quickly evident that there was a group of medical professionals who likely had free time to participate and, also theoretically, had the skillset to provide experienced high-level care—retired physicians. In just 1 day at the onset of the outbreak, 1000 retired and private practice physicians volunteered to assist in the pandemic in NYC [4]. Similarly, the National Health Service of the UK proactively sent letters to 15,000 retired physicians asking them to return [5].

46.4   Age and Risk

The first major risk factor directly linked to mortality with COVID-19 was age [6]. Retired physicians are older and often even 'elderly.' By having retired physicians work on the frontlines, were we putting the highest risk population in an unnecessarily high-risk situation? On the other hand, even a single volunteer physician could increase the capacity of an already full intensive care unit, so doesn't that enormous benefit outweigh the risk to one physician? There were no easy answers, but creative solutions were possible.

Rather than working on the front lines, elderly physicians could contribute meaningfully in other lower risk ways. Telehealth has become a staple in the COVID physician's arsenal [7]. Retired physicians could be assigned to telehealth, thereby freeing up lower risk individuals to work on the front line [8]. These older physicians could also participate more in a supervisory role, offering advice to the younger staff, organizational problem solving, and utilization of resources [9].

While some older external physicians willingly returned from retirement, internally many practicing surgeons stated that they had no choice but to participate. Younger healthcare workers were asked to volunteer, sometimes well outside their usual position. On the other hand, more senior staff were given leeway, with age often used as rationale to not participate. Without an approved medical exemption, younger staff were left with limited options. This put an unfair burden on junior faculty and staff throughout hospitals, with no route for escalation. During COVID-19, the principle of 'justice' related not only to patients, but also directly to the health care providers treating them.

46.5   Credentialing

Licensure typically is the rate limiting step in practicing medicine in a specific stage. Each state has its own requirements [10], and when moving to a new state, the application process could take 3–6 months. Another hurdle is institutional credentialing, often complex and redundant to ensure that those practicing medicine without oversight at a given hospital truly have the skillset and credentials to do so. Through executive orders from Governor Cuomo and individual institutional policy changes [11], the credentialing process was modified essentially to an honor system. For medical licensure, any active state license outside of NY in good standing was deemed adequate. Any NY state license that was previously active but not currently registered could be reinstated. CME requirements were temporarily suspended. Were the physicians being brought back to the workforce adequately prepared to care for these patients? There was no evaluation of current skill set, or way of knowing if the health care provider was up to date on the latest treatment strategy.

46.6   Medical Students on the Frontlines

If retired physicians were on one end of a spectrum, medical students were on the other. Medical schools transitioned to online classes and canceled clinical rotations in hospitals in order to protect students and allow physicians to devote more time to the frontline. However, senior medical students represented an untapped resource for resolving the shortage of physicians.

On March 24, 2020, New York University Grossman School of Medicine became the first school to offer senior medical students the option of graduating early and joining the frontlines. Approximately half of the senior class chose to graduate early, and NYU gained 52 new physicians on the frontlines [12]. In response to the physician shortage in New York, Governor Cuomo issued an executive order on April seventh, which allowed medical students who would graduate in 2020 to graduate early and begin practicing medicine with supervision from a licensed physician [13].

The major ethical concern relating to early graduating medical students was patient safety. Graduation was only 2 months later, therefore students had completed most of their graduation requirements. Early graduates were not meaningfully less prepared than a typical medical school graduate [14]. If hospitals were allowing recently graduated medical students to provide medical care independently, that would be both unethical and unsafe as they would not have had enough training or experience. However, supervision from a licensed physician was necessary, so offering early graduation as an option for senior medical students was in the best interest of patients [15]. As one physician can supervise more than one recently graduated medical student, the addition of students allowed each intensivist to treat more patients and improved overall efficiency.

Concerns that medical students would be coerced into graduating early could be both unsafe and unethical. Early graduation should be unquestionably voluntary. Although senior medical students could make valuable contributions, they were not yet physicians. They did not have the same obligation to the medical community as those who had completed their training and were licensed. Graduating early involved assuming the risks that came with working on the frontlines and the responsibilities of being a doctor. At a time when there were more unknown than known facts regarding COVID-19, this risk was not small. Medical schools were responsible for ensuring that students were not volunteering for the wrong reasons such as guilt or fear of facing consequences [16]. Before making this decision, students had to be apprised of the risks and responsibilities that came with early graduation. In future situations, medical schools could offer alternative opportunities for those who do not want to graduate early. This could include continuing PPE collection drives or becoming contact tracers. Students could make valuable contributions even if they did not choose to graduate early. Offering alternatives also mitigated the potential influence of guilt on this decision. Students could monitor patients with mild COVID-19 symptoms who were not admitted; expedite care for admitted patients by reviewing charts, drafting notes, and ensuring tests were performed; and follow-up with patients after discharge [15]. While still requiring supervision, these tasks could take significant burden off of senior physicians managing the most critically ill.

As the University College of Dublin correctly pointed out, "In a crisis, healthcare services that are at a point of extreme strain may unwittingly exploit the inherent altruism of many medical students. This, coupled with a lack of pandemic preparedness education in medical school, could leave these student volunteers vulnerable to unnecessary risk" [17].

Senior medical students are experienced navigators of hospitals and hospital teams. Often, before a clinical rotation, they are given the advice that their main job is to "minimize the workload of the residents and attendings" [18]. This is where they can excel during a pandemic without undue risk. These students already have appropriate HIPAA training and hospital clearance and can function as the linchpin between the various pandemic teams.

Finally, students must be compensated for their work. Discussions of hazard pay, and tuition reimbursement have stalled in recent months. Most New York health systems offered the early/recently graduated medical students an intern-level salary [19].

46.7 Outpatient Sub-Specialists

46.7.1 Qualifications

The common pathway for an "intensivist" is to complete an internal medicine residency, followed by a pulmonary/critical care fellowship [20]. While many will choose employment that includes inpatient intensive care call, a large percentage may opt for outpatient practice only, often subspecializing in some element of pulmonary medicine. These specialists are technically qualified and board-certified in pulmonary/critical care medicine, but many have not worked in a hospital environment for years. This could leave them unprepared for a sudden shift to general care on the frontlines. Putting an unprepared physician on the frontline is not in the best interest of patients. However, is it better to have "more hands-on deck," or a larger cohort of physicians that includes those that are inexperienced?

In addition, because they are unprepared, these specialists must also be supervised. Would this necessary supervision do more harm than good? Could proficient physicians help more people if they did not have to supervise those without recent experience?

One major New York hospital came up with a tiered system for the care of COVID-19 patients and utilization of sub-specialists (see Table 46.2). Tier 1 included newly admitted acutely ill patients who needed a critical care setting. Tier 2 were the "chronically critically ill." These patients were either being weaned from a ventilator and progressing or pending a tracheostomy. Tier 3 were lingering patients who already received a tracheostomy or had a stable airway and unchanged vent settings. The sickest patients were put into the Medical Intensive Care Unit (converted entirely to a COVID-19 Unit). This was staffed only by experienced inpatient intensivists. Other less-critical Tier 1 patients were put into COVID-19 intensive care units that were built out in non-intensive care settings (the surgical recovery room, operating rooms, endoscopy suites, and the library). These were staffed by physicians who were not critical care board certified, but had significant experience managing patients in an intensive care setting. They had moderate supervision from a staff intensivist (see Fig. 46.1). Tier 2 were often located on previous telemetry floors that had been converted to negative pressure wings and were

Table 46.2 Tiered COVID-19 Patient Allocation System

TIER 1	
Type of Patient:	Newly admitted, Critical Care Setting Required
Primary Physician:	(a) PCCM-Certified Staff Intensivist (MICU)
	OR
	(b) Non-Certified Pulmonary Specialist with ICU Experience (oversight by PCCM physician)
Patient Status:	Unstable, frequent changes in treatment plan and ventilator settings
TIER 2	
Type of Patient:	"Chronically critically Ill" or stable non-ventilated newly admitted patients
Primary Physician:	Specialists without any recent critical care experience (Cardiology, Neurology, etc)
	(Oversight provided by PCCM Physician)
Patient Status:	Protocolized, no major changes in treatment plan or ventilator settings for >48 h
TIER 3	
Type of Patient:	Stable patients from Tier 2 that could not be extubated or discharged
Primary Physician:	Hospitalist without critical care experience
	(PCCM physician available for ventilator weaning questions and for changes in patient status)
Patient Status:	No critical care issues except for ventilator management (minimal settings without any changes required)

MICU Medical Intensive Care Unit, *PCCM* Pulmonary and Critical Care Medicine, *ICU* Intensive Care Unit

Supervised ICU Staffing Model for Tier-1 COVID-19 Patients

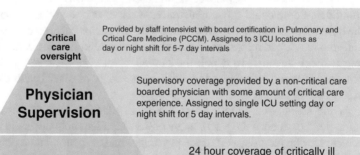

Critical care oversight — Provided by staff intensivist with board certification in Pulmonary and Critical Care Medicine (PCCM). Assigned to 3 ICU locations as day or night shift for 5-7 day intervals

Physician Supervision — Supervisory coverage provided by a non-critical care boarded physician with some amount of critical care experience. Assigned to single ICU setting day or night shift for 5 day intervals.

Primary Critical Care Coverage — 24 hour coverage of critically ill patients provided by in house redeployed nurse practitioners, physician's assistants, residents, and fellows

Fig. 46.1 Staffing model employed by major New York health system to provide adequate physician coverage of intensive care patients with appropriate board-certified critical-care oversight

managed by sub-specialists who may not have had any recent critical care experience. Most of these patients were protocolized and were stable. Physicians managing these units included cardiologists, outpatient pulmonologists, and neurologists. There was significant oversight in these units, with a single staff intensivist providing daily oversight of several of these units for any sudden changes in patient condition. Finally, Tier 3 were managed by hospitalists without any major critical care experience, but with intensivists available for questions relating to ventilator weaning. The non-COVID-19 floors were managed by healthcare providers of any specialty who did not feel comfortable participating in the care of COVID-19 patients.

46.8   Feelings of Unpreparedness

As with hospital-based junior faculty, many outpatient specialists were given two options: volunteer to work as a COVID hospitalist/intensivist or take unpaid leave.

Many were forced out of their comfort zone due to inexperience, but the financial repercussions for not volunteering were too great to consider the alternative. Although New York City urgently needed physicians, forcing inexperienced providers into situations that they have not been trained for is not in the best interest of patients, and can be considered a violation of the ethical principle of non-maleficence.

Specialization allows physicians to focus on and master the treatment of specific conditions, which is typically beneficial for patients. However, the COVID-19 pandemic turned specialization into a weakness. Focusing on a specific subset of conditions without exercising general care skills left specialists unprepared for general care on the frontlines [21].

Everyone should contribute to the situation, but not every doctor had to be on the frontlines. Some could do administrative work or take on other responsibilities in the hospital that limited exposure to COVID-19. Many PhD research scientists volunteered to work in roles such as unit clerks and patient liaisons. Similar to graduating medical students, lessening the burden of the critical care specialists was a priority and could be achieved by utilizing a variety of other health care providers in low-risk situations.

While hospital-based physicians often had adequate time off between COVID shifts (ie: 5 days on, 5 days off), many of the outpatient volunteers did not have that benefit. During their days off, these physicians had to focus on their outpatient practice. Physicians with an outpatient practice had to take on more responsibility and work longer hours.

What about medical sub-specialists that were very removed from inpatient acute medical care such as dermatologists, ophthalmologists, surgical subspecialists? Whose duty was it to ensure that these physicians were currently qualified to treat

COVID patients? While it was recommended that "medical boards and critical care associations must provide refresher training in various aspects of critical care to dermatologists," [22] this was left up to individual health care systems and critical care divisions to institute.

Further, many of these subspecialists were experts in their fields and often leaders in their specific sub-community of medicine. It was important to recognize that despite the potential feelings of being overwhelmed and over their head, they might not feel comfortable asking for help. It was important to foster open and honest communication when people were forced to do stressful jobs they were not prepared for.

46.9   The Silver Lining

For many specialists, the uncharted territory of general practice was a humbling, yet rewarding, experience that led to a greater sense of community [23]. They worked with and learned from physicians in other specialties. In addition, in the face of tragedy, physicians learned to focus on and celebrate the successes. For example, Long Island Jewish Medical Center played the song "Here Comes the Sun" by the Beatles whenever a patient was extubated [24]. This experience reminded some physicians of the oath they took and why they originally chose to pursue medicine: to help people [25].

46.10   Resolution

Before sending specialists to the ICU, hospitals should provide training. Fortunately for this disease process, much of the care could become protocolized and was similar from patient to patient. Once a patient's acute process was stabilized by an admitting intensivist, the tenants of treatment fell around three broad categories: ventilator management, treatment with experimental medications, and ventilator weaning/extubation. Virtual tutorials were recorded and provided to all physicians coming onto a COVID service. Hospitals could not reasonably expect specialists to smoothly transition to the frontlines without training [22].

As the Society of Critical Care Medicine aptly stated, "Therefore, our priority should focus not only on increasing the numbers of mechanical ventilators but on growing the number of trained professionals for both the near and long term who will be needed to care for the critically ill and injured with respiratory failure during crisis conditions" [26].

46.11   Case Conclusion

There was little time to plan and the new intensive care units filled overnight. All options discussed above were utilized for staffing, along with some additional resources. Retired physicians, outpatient specialists, locums' physicians, and graduating medical students were all included in the staffing schema in order to alleviate the burden on the hospital intensivists. Graduating fellows were given "war time promotions" to attending status. The principle of 'non-maleficence' took priority. There was more benefit than risk to having those with at least the most basic training managing patients, as opposed to having specialty trained intensivists who were stretched too thin to make proper decisions. The key to patient safety was appropriate supervision and teamwork by those with the most experience.

46.12   Concluding Remarks

COVID-19 stretched New York's healthcare resources to the brink of collapse. The limiting factor for continued expert care of these patients was experienced staffing. Several cohorts of health care professionals were able to be drafted during the height of the pandemic, but many normal regulations and methods of credential validation needed to be waved. At the time, it was important to get the appropriate staff in the door and provide the much-needed physical presence to care for these patients. We must now consider the ethical implications of each of our choices, including undue risk, utilization of the underqualified, and forced volunteerism, so that we can plan appropriately for the future.

46.13   Selected References

- Keeley C, Jimenez J, Jackson H, et al. Staffing Up For the Surge: Expanding the New York City Public Hospital Workforce During the COVID-19 Pandemic. Health Affairs. 2020;39:1426–1430. doi:https://doi.org/10.1377/hlthaff.2020.00904
    - Leadership in the NYC Health + Hospitals public health care system discuss the redeployment of staff to their eleven standing hospitals and three field hospitals.
- Orbey E. The Medical Students Who Joined the Battle Against the Coronavirus. *The New Yorker*. 6 May 2020. Accessed 3 August 2020. https://www.newyorker.com/science/medical-dispatch/the-medical-students-who-joined-the-battle-against-the-coronavirus

– Medical students from various health care systems in New York describe their experiences during the COVID-19 pandemic, and feelings of helplessness, imposter syndrome, and overall psychologic stress.

References

1. Almukhtar S, Aufrichtig A, Bloch M et al. New York City covid map and case count. The New York Times. 5 October 2020. https://www.nytimes.com/interactive/2020/nyregion/new-york-city-coronavirus-cases.html. Accessed 5 Oct 2020.
2. Hersher, R. Improvisation and retraining may be key to saving patients in New York's ICUs. NPR. 8 April 2020. https://www.npr.org/sections/health-shots/2020/04/08/830153837/improvisation-and-retraining-may-be-key-to-saving-patients-in-new-yorks-icus. Accessed 3 Aug 2020.
3. Keeley C, Jimenez J, Jackson H, et al. Staffing up for the surge: expanding the new York City public hospital workforce during the COVID-19 pandemic. Health Aff. 2020;39:1426–30. https://doi.org/10.1377/hlthaff.2020.00904.
4. Marsh, J. In one day, 1,000 NYC doctors and nurses enlist to battle coronavirus. New York Post. 18 March 2020. https://nypost.com/2020/03/18/in-one-day-1000-nyc-doctors-and-nurses-enlist-to-battle-coronavirus/. Accessed 3 Aug 2020.
5. Norman G. Britain asking 65,000 retired nurses and doctors to return to work to help fight coronavirus. Fox News. 20 March 2020. https://www.foxnews.com/world/britain-coronavirus-retired-nurses-doctors. Accessed 3 Aug 2020.
6. Liu K, Chen Y, Lin R, Han K. Clinical features of COVID-19 in elderly patients: a comparison with young and middle-aged patients. J Infect. 2020;80:e14–8. https://doi.org/10.1016/j.jinf.2020.03.005.
7. Hollander JE, Carr BG. Virtually perfect? Telemedicine for COVID-19. N Engl J Med. 2020;382:1679–81. https://doi.org/10.1056/nejmp2003539.
8. Senior Physician COVID-19 Resource Guide. American medical association. 28 March 2020. https://www.ama-assn.org/delivering-care/public-health/senior-physician-covid-19-resource-guide/. Accessed 3 Aug 2020.
9. Buerhaus PI, Auerbach DI, Staiger DO. Older clinicians and the surge in novel coronavirus disease 2019 (COVID-19). JAMA. 2020;323:1777–8. https://doi.org/10.1001/jama.2020.4978.
10. Federation of State Medical Boards. COVID-19 Related Legislation. https://track.govhawk.com/reports/Mwz7b/public. Accessed 3 Aug 2020.
11. Governor Andrew M. Cuomo. Executive order no. 202.5: continuing temporary suspension and modification of laws relating to the disaster emergency. New York State. 18 March 2020. https://www.governor.ny.gov/news/no-2025-continuing-temporary-suspension-and-modification-laws-relating-disaster-emergency/. Accessed 7 Dec 2020.
12. Orbey E. The medical students who joined the battle against the coronavirus. The New Yorker. 6 May 2020. https://www.newyorker.com/science/medical-dispatch/the-medical-students-who-joined-the-battle-against-the-coronavirus. Accessed 3 Aug 2020.
13. COVID-19 Pandemic and Professional Practice. Office of the professions. New York State Education Department. http://www.op.nysed.gov/COVID-19_EO.html. Accessed 7 Dec 2020.
14. Kinnear B, Kelleher M, Olson APJ, Sall D, Schumacher DJ. Developing trust with early medical school graduates during the COVID-19 pandemic. J Hosp Med. 2020;15:367–9. https://doi.org/10.12788/jhm.3463.
15. Miller DG, Pierson L, Doernberg S. The role of medical students during the COVID-19 pandemic. Ann Intern Med. 2020;173:145–6. https://doi.org/10.7326/m20-1281.
16. Khamees D, Brown CA, Arribas M, Murphey AC, Haas MRC, House JB. In crisis: medical students in the COVID-19 pandemic. AEM Educ Train. 2020;4:284–90.

17. O'Byrne L, Gavin B, McNicholas F. Medical students and COVID-19: the need for pandemic preparedness. J Med Ethics. 2020;46:623–6. https://doi.org/10.1136/medethics-2020-106353.
18. Stokes DC. Senior medical students in the COVID-19 response: an opportunity to be proactive. Acad Emerg Med. 2020;27:343–5. https://doi.org/10.1111/acem.13972.
19. Murphy B. COVID-19: states call on early medical school grads to bolster workforce american medical association. 31 March 2020. https://www.ama-assn.org/delivering-care/public-health/covid-19-states-call-early-medical-school-grads-bolster-workforce. Accessed 3 Aug 2020.
20. Halpern NA, Pastores SM, Oropello JM, Kvetan V. Critical care medicine in the United States: addressing the intensivist shortage and image of the specialty. Crit Care Med. 2013;41:2754–61. https://doi.org/10.1097/ccm.0b013e318298a6fb.
21. Cram P, Anderson ML, Shaughnessy EE. All hands on deck: learning to "un-specialize" in the COVID-19 pandemic. J Hosp Med 2020;15:314–315. https://doi.org/10.12788.jhm.3426
22. Bhargava S, Rokde R, Rathod D, Kroumpouzos G. Employing dermatologists on the frontline against COVID-19: all hands on deck [letter]. Dermatol Ther. 2020:e13420. https://doi.org/10.1111/dth.13420.
23. Seah KTM. Redeployment in COVID-19: old dogs and new tricks. Emerg Med J. 2020;37:456. https://doi.org/10.1136/emermed-2020-210052.
24. DePeralta DK, Hong AR, Choy C, et al. Primer for intensive care unit (ICU) redeployment of the noncritical care surgeon: insights from the Epicenter of the coronavirus disease 2019 (COVID-19) pandemic. Surgery. 2020;168:2215–7. https://doi.org/10.1016/j.surg.2020.05.010.
25. Sarpong NO, Forrester LA, Levine WN. What's important: redeployment of the orthopaedic surgeon during the COVID-19 pandemic: perspectives from the trenches. J Bone Joint Surg Am. 2020;102:1019–21. https://doi.org/10.2106/jbjs.20.00574.
26. Halpern NA, Tan KS. United States resource availability for COVID-19. Society of Critical Care Medicine. 12 May 2020. https://www.sccm.org/getattachment/Blog/March-2020/United-States-Resource-Availability-for-COVID-19/United-States-Resource-Availability-for-COVID-19.pdf. Accessed 15 Feb 2021.

Chapter 47
Cardiovascular Services in the COVID-19 Hot Zone: Italy

Gino Gerosa ⓘ, Nicola Pradegan ⓘ, and Assunta Fabozzo ⓘ

Abstract The epidemic of severe acute respiratory syndrome coronavirus-2 (SARS-CoV-2), the causative agent of coronavirus disease 2019 (COVID-19), represents the third introduction of the highly pathogenic coronavirus into the population. Italy was the first European nation to be affected by COVID-19 with 2,047,696 confirmed total cases and 71,925 deaths by December 27, 2020. On January 31, 2020, the first two COVID-19 cases were confirmed in visitors to Italy and the National Emergency was declared. As a way to contain the disease, the government established a stepwise strategy which ended in severe lockdown measures applied on the entire Country by March 9, 2020. The number of patients admitted to the emergency department for other causes dramatically dropped in that period, and although patients with cardiovascular disease are more predisposed to severe illness with COVID-19, there was a critical drop in admissions for acute cardiovascular conditions. With this chapter, the authors aim to describe clinical challenges and longitudinal trends in hospital admissions for emergent cardiac surgery cases during the COVID-19 pandemic worldwide and especially in northeast Italy.

Keywords COVID-19 · Cardiac surgery · Veneto · Italy · Emergencies · Hub Center

G. Gerosa (✉) · N. Pradegan · A. Fabozzo
Department of Cardio-Thoracic and Vascular Sciences and Public Health, Hospital-University of Padova, Padova, Italy
e-mail: gino.gerosa@unipd.it

© The Author(s), under exclusive license to Springer Nature
Switzerland AG 2022
V. A. Lonchyna et al. (eds.), *Difficult Decisions in Surgical Ethics*, Difficult
Decisions in Surgery: An Evidence-Based Approach,
https://doi.org/10.1007/978-3-030-84625-1_47

Cases

The Padova University Hospital is a leading center for surgical treatment of heart failure in Northern Italy. Since its beginning, the coronavirus disease 2019 (COVID-19) pandemic has involved all medical and surgical subspecialties, with different types of patients affected by this new infection. Patients with heart failure are usually fragile, and at major risk of complications secondary to infections. We previously reported [1] two positive COVID-19 patients, affected by multiorgan comorbidities and assisted with left ventricular assist device (LVAD), who favorably resolved.

Patient #1 was a 61-year-old male who was admitted in March 2020, 2 months after a HeartMate III implantation. His comorbidities included diabetes, chronic obstructive pulmonary disease and chronic kidney disease (CKD). He was admitted with a diagnosis of worsening heart failure and tested positive for the severe acute respiratory syndrome coronavirus-2 (SARS-CoV-2). He was asymptomatic, did not experience respiratory symptoms and was treated with acetaminophen. He finally recovered from his cardiac decompensation and was discharged in stable condition.

Patient #2 was a 72-year-old male who underwent a Jarvik 2000 implantation in 2016. He was admitted for an LVAD exit-site infection. He had multiple comorbidities: type 2 diabetes, CKD, atrial fibrillation, dyslipidemia, history of endocarditis and two cerebral ischemic strokes. Ten days before admission (in March 2020) he reported an episode of fever, treated at home with acetaminophen. During the hospitalization, his roommate developed COVID-19 and died. For this reason, our patient underwent a nasopharyngeal swab test that was positive for SARS-CoV-2. The exit-site infection was successfully treated with antibiotics (levofloxacin) and no other problems related to the device were found. He did not develop pulmonary symptoms and got well.

47.1 Introduction

The epidemic caused by SARS-CoV-2, the causative agent of coronavirus disease 2019 (COVID-19), represents the third introduction of the highly pathogenic coronavirus into the population. COVID-19 and the previous iterations (SARS coronavirus-1 in 2002 and Middle East respiratory syndrome -MERS- coronavirus in 2012) are RNA viruses transmitted from animals to humans that can cause a spectrum of respiratory symptoms, ranging from mild symptoms (cough, fever, malaise, anosmia, fatigue, and loss of appetite) to acute respiratory distress syndrome (ARDS) [2].

Italy was the first European nation to be affected by COVID-19 with 2,047,696 confirmed total cases and 71,925 deaths by December 27, 2020. At its beginning, the pandemic was mainly located in northern Italy [3].

47.2   Search Strategy

For this topic, a PUBMED search strategy was used. A single year search was applied, and the databases included those of our own data. Keywords used for search were COVID-19 and acute cardiovascular events/hospitalization.

47.3   Discussion

47.3.1   Lockdown of the Country

On January 31, 2020, the first two COVID-19 cases were confirmed in visitors to Italy and the National Emergency was declared. The first Italian patient with COVID-19 was identified only on February 21, 2020. The first two patients identified came from Wuhan and were isolated in Rome whereas the first Italian patient was identified in Codogno, a small city in the North of Italy. As a way to contain the disease, the government established a stepwise strategy starting with the complete lockdown of the initial foci in northern Italy (such as Codogno in Lombardy, and Vo' Euganeo in Veneto (see Fig. 47.1) on February 20, 2020, and subsequent

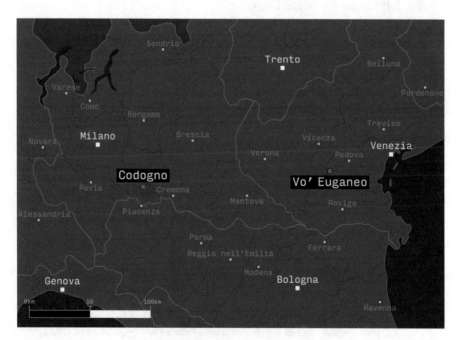

Fig. 47.1 Map showing the location of the two main coronavirus disease-19 (COVID-19) foci in the North of Italy by the end of February 2020

adoption of progressively more stringent lockdown measure of the entire nation as of March 9, 2020 [4].

The lockdown phase did not allow people to leave their homes except for essential reasons such as a key job, visiting a doctor or pharmacy, and buying groceries. Political restrictions focused on stay-at-home measures and appropriate physical distancing to mitigate transmission. These restrictions lasted until May 4, 2020, when, as a result of a favorable COVID-19 epidemiological regression trend, the Italian Government decided to start the so called 'phase two'. Public activities were gradually reopened, and people were allowed to meet each other again, with a progressive loosening of previous rules by means of additional decrees [5].

47.4 Healthcare System Reorganized

Health care systems have been reorganized to cope with the enormous increase in the number of acutely ill patients (see Table 47.1). The pandemic has also led to deferral or cancellation of nonessential procedures, in-person patient visits, and routine diagnostic evaluations.

47.5 Effect on Cardiac Services

Cardiac surgery services have been significantly affected by COVID-19 worldwide [6]. In response to the burden of the current pandemic, many elective cardiac surgery procedures have been delayed. The main reasons were the unquantifiable risk of acquiring COVID-19, and many of the intensive care resources have been redistributed to the care of the tremendous volume of COVID victims. A similar scenario

Table 47.1 Ethical principles applied during a pandemic

Principle	Application
Beneficence	Emergent and urgent surgeries (including heart transplantation and mechanical devices implantation for acute treatment of cardiogenic shock) must be guaranteed during a pandemic, and patients are treated as if infected until results of the molecular tests are known, to avoid the risk of infection of the health personnel
Non-maleficence	Elective surgeries may be delayed, based on patients' health conditions to avoid aggravating their infection
Autonomy	Telemedicine may be the main "at-distance" tool used to empower patient autonomy and keep the quality and the continuity of their healthcare at the highest level during COVID 19 pandemic
Justice	As the number of elective surgeries has been reduced, at least half of our ICU beds, ventilators and supplies were re-distributed to support care of COVID patients. Furthermore, almost a quarter of our staff, especially, OR and ICU nurses were referred to COVID wards

happened in northern Italy, where the Regional Authorities decided to delay elective procedures during the acute phase (March–April 2020), allowing only emergent surgeries [7].

Differently from the northwestern Lombardy region (in which 16 of the 20 cardiac surgical units discontinued services and all emergent/urgent cases were diverted to the remaining four 'hub' centers), the Italian northeast area did not establish a 'hub' center and all cardiac surgery units continued to individually manage the incoming emergent cases [7, 8].

Patients with cardiovascular disease seem to face an excessive risk of severe illness with COVID-19 [9]. However, there also is an indirect impact of the pandemic on these high-risk patients, even among those without direct viral infection or exposure. Several reports have identified a lower volume of hospital presentations for acute cardiovascular illnesses during the pandemic such as acute coronary syndromes and aortic dissections in developed countries (e.g., U.S. and Europe) [10–13].

These data have raised concerns that similar reductions may be seen across other life-threatening cardiovascular conditions that generally require early in-hospital evaluation and emergent surgical treatment. Emergency cases in cardiac surgery represent serious, unexpected, and often dangerous situations requiring immediate action. Each cardiovascular guideline defines emergent scenarios according to the timing of surgical treatment. The main list of emergencies in adult cardiac surgery is summarized in Table 47.2.

Table 47.2 Summary of emergencies in adult cardiac surgery.

Emergency	Definition
Acute thoracic aortic syndromes (AAS)	Type A aortic dissection Intramural hematoma (with pericardial effusion, periaortic hematoma, or large aneurysms) Type A penetrating aortic ulcer Aortic pseudoaneurysm Rupture of aortic aneurysm Traumatic aortic injury (free aortic rupture or large periaortic hematoma)
Acute coronary syndromes (ACS)	Non-ST-elevation ASC (very high-risk patients with ongoing ischemia or hemodynamic instability with an indication for coronary artery bypass grafting) ST-segment elevation myocardial infarction (STEMI) (selected STEMI patients with ongoing ischemia and large areas of jeopardized myocardium, unsuitable for percutaneous coronary intervention) Cardiogenic shock due to mechanical complications of myocardial infarction (papillary muscle rupture with severe mitral valve regurgitation, ventricular septal defect, free wall rupture, rupturedpseudoaneurysm)

(continued)

Table 47.2 (conitnued)

Emergency	Definition
Emergent valve surgery	Severe aortic regurgitation (in the setting of acute aortic syndromes or endocarditis) Severe mitral regurgitation (in the setting of ACS) Obstructive prosthetic valve thrombosis in critically ill patients without a contraindication to surgery
Emergent endocarditis	Aortic or mitral native or prosthetic valve with severe acute regurgitation, obstruction or fistula causing refractory pulmonary oedema or cardiogenic shock
Acute heart failure or cardiogenic shock (INTERMACS 1)	Short-term mechanical support systems, including percutaneous cardiac support devices, extracorporeal membrane oxygenation (ECMO), and paracorporeal ventricular assist device Heart transplantation in level-1 urgency status patients (Italy)
Cardiac tumors	Cardiac myxoma obstructing the mitral valve Acute cardiac tamponade or massive endocardial invasion requiring surgical management
Others	Acute penetrating cardiac trauma (e.g., stabbing, shotting) with hemorrhagic shock Massive pulmonary embolism Other forms of acute cardiac tamponade

Literature analysis based on the most recent evidence published worldwide on 'lockdown' politics confirms that the COVID-19 pandemic has caused a significant reduction in the number of patients presenting with emergent cardiovascular conditions. De Rosa et al. [11] and Mafham et al. [12], in Italy and England respectively, found a reduction between 40–50% of acute coronary syndrome (ACS) cases (either N-STEMI and STEMI) from February to March 2020 as well as when comparing March 2019 to March 2020, similar to our data. Furthermore, a preliminary study about the incidence of type A acute aortic dissections among cardiac surgical services in New York City recognized a significant drop in monthly surgical case volume of this life-threatening condition before and after March 1, 2020 [13].

Several hypotheses might explain this finding. First, a true population-level reduction in cardiovascular events necessitating healthcare attention is plausible: shifts in dietary patterns and reduced exposure to ambient air pollution (as during spring 2020 thanks to lockdown measures) may have contributed to reduced daily risks. However, the observation that the decline in emergent admissions had partly reversed by the end of May 2020, suggests that environmental changes were unlikely to be major contributors to the observed trends in cardiovascular emergencies in the current pandemic. Additionally, public health messages promoting social distancing and new reports focusing on the death toll associated with COVID-19, contributed to increased generalized anxiety in society.

Our preliminary data (yet unpublished) on the topic, collected in a high-volume Center, also a hub for the heart failure network in the Italian Northeastern Regions (see Fig. 47.2), demonstrated that the smallest weekly number of emergent admissions was found in the same week in which the northeast Italian area counted the

Fig. 47.2 Geographic distribution of the adult cardiac surgery centers involved in this study

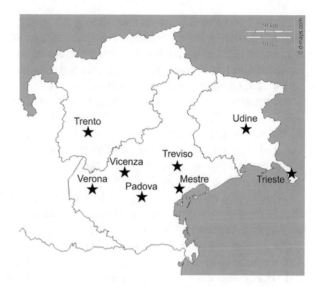

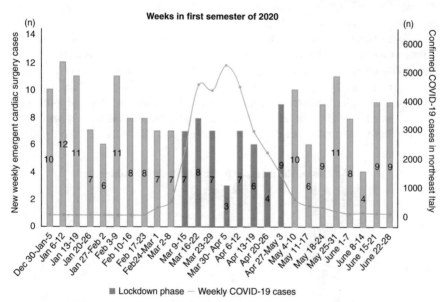

Fig. 47.3 Weekly emergent cardiac surgical cases between January 1, 2020 and June 30, 2020

highest number of COVID-19 cases during the first half of 2020 (see Fig. 47.3). From January 1 to June 30, 2020, 571 patients required an emergent admission and cardiac surgical procedure in the 8 cardiac surgical centers involved in our study. The total number of emergent cases admitted during the pre-lockdown and the lockdown period were 84 and 51, respectively, with a reduction of 39% in the number of cardiac surgical emergencies. Therefore, a significant reduction was found in the number of acute cardiac syndromes during the lockdown phase according to the national government decrees, although overall diagnosis for emergent conditions dramatically decreased but not the rate of in-hospital mortality.

To explain this finding, patient aversion to seeking care in medical centers that cared for documented or suspected patients with COVID-19 (a notion well captured in the lay media) certainly played a role. In Italy, the Lombardy region documented a 59% increase in the number of out-of-hospital cardiac arrests between February 21 through March 31, 2020 [14]. A similar study performed by the Emergency Department at the Padova University Hospital (a center in our study) did not find a significant increase in out-of-hospital cardiac arrests during lockdown when compared to the same period in 2019 [15].

Additionally, mechanical complications of myocardial infarction (e.g., papillary muscle rupture with severe mitral valve regurgitation, ventricular septal defect, free wall rupture, ruptured pseudoaneurysm) requiring emergent cardiac surgery significantly increased during 'phase two' when compared to the same period in 2019. This dramatic change in the type of patients admitted for emergent cardiac surgery had already been anticipated by a previously published case series, in which all 10 patients delayed seeking medical attention (despite being symptomatic for days) because of the fear of contracting SARS-CoV-2 [16].

Late manifestation of cardiovascular disease (such as those reported above) represent an indirect consequence of lockdown restrictions: in fact, stay-at-home messaging from major associations, governmental bodies, and media outlets, may have led to patients delaying or deferring hospital admission for acute cardiovascular conditions requiring emergent treatment. Therefore, an increase in the proportion of deaths related to acute heart failures requiring emergent cardiac surgery was found during phase two and gives pause for thought (see Fig. 47.4). In fact, patients

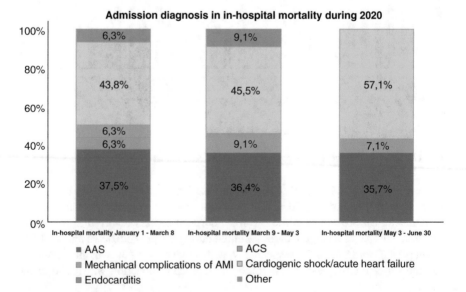

Fig. 47.4 Admission diagnosis of cases of in-hospital mortality during 2020

missing their outpatient consultations might have worsened their cardiac function to the point of developing acute heart failure requiring surgery, with a worse prognosis.

To this purpose, strategies concerning people's education and centralization of cardiovascular care toward 'protected' structures could restore the patient's confidence in going to the Emergency Departments at an early stage of symptoms and stem a phenomenon that could trigger an important increase in cardiovascular morbidity and mortality. Furthermore, additional resources such as telemedicine should be greatly increased (especially in the field of outpatient consultations) [17–19].

Among the 396 surviving heart transplant patients to date, six patients developed COVID-19 with two succumbing to the disease. This small series led us to develop a specific protocol to manage heart transplant patients both while on the waiting list, and at the time of donor heart availability and during follow-up [20, 21].

47.6 Guidelines at the Time of COVID-19

The European Society of Cardiology (ESC) in mid-2020 produced a guidance—not a formal guideline—regarding the COVID-19 pandemic [22]. The document suggests appropriate measures to prevent SARS-CoV-2 spread among Health Care Personnel (eg. use of appropriate protection masks, hand washing, body temperature monitoring and surveillance nasopharyngeal swabs). Regarding patient management, less invasive diagnostic tools and procedures are suggested whenever possible, but no significant changes have been applied to normal clinical and surgical practice. It encourages health care workers to educate patients in wearing masks, promoting social distancing and washing hands. The Italian Society of Cardiac Surgery, [7, 8] however, recommended that during the pandemic outbreak and in the presence of a high number of COVID-19 cases, it is preferable to postpone elective surgeries, permitting only admission to emergent/urgent cases [23]. When the SARS-CoV-2 status is unknown at the time of admission in these patients as well as in COVID-19 positive patients admitted for acute cardiovascular disease, two different pathways should be organized. Whenever possible, short intensive care unit and hospitalization length of stay should be favored. Patient follow-up (especially for management of chronic compensated disease) should be ensured by means of telemedicine tools.

47.7 A New Sunrise: 2021 and the Vaccination Era

After authorization of the Pfizer-BioNTech COVID-19 vaccine by the European Commission on December 21, 2020, Italy started its vaccination campaign on December 27, 2020. Health care and administrative personnel, together with guests and personnel of nursing homes have been the first people to be vaccinated. 1,072,086 vaccines have been administered by January 16, 2021, which means >1% of the Italian population. Despite an initial skepticism among health care workers, almost 80% of all the distributed doses have already been administered (demonstrating that health care workers trust in the new vaccination program and recognize its importance). Almost 60% of all vaccinated persons are between 40 and 60 years of age [24]. According to published data, Italy and Germany are currently the leading countries in EU for the number of vaccinated people [25]. The vaccination program in the general population has started, with the only limitation being vaccine availability (dependent upon Big Pharma delivery). Italy is aware that a rapid strategy of vaccination in addition to the current rules of hand washing, mask wearing, and social distancing are the only tools to lower the health and economic consequences of the COVID-19 pandemic. For this reason, the National Health Ministry is already recruiting physicians and nurses to administer vaccines among the population, starting with the oldest and the most fragile people.

47.8   Case Concluded

Our case series highlights the unpredictable behavior of SARS-CoV-2 infection. According to the current literature, SARS-CoV-2 has been more aggressive in fragile individuals and our patients were at extremely high risk due to their multiple comorbidities. However, the successful outcome of both patients might be the consequence of multiple factors: LVAD as a guarantee to maintain support of cardiovascular function, and anticoagulation therapy as a protective treatment against COVID-19 related thromboembolism. Regarding this second point, the anticoagulation/ antiaggregation levels was strictly monitored through serial thromboelastography and platelets aggregation tests and adjusted accordingly. We left unchanged our protocol which consists of oral anticoagulation with a target of 2.5–3.0 INR. Antiplatelet agents are added in HeartMate III patients according to aggregometry profiles, and in Jarvik 2000 patients due to its intrinsic negative action on platelets count. Consequently, no prophylactic modification to therapy was applied without clinical or laboratory evidence.

47.9   Conclusion

During the lockdown phase of the COVID-19 pandemic in the northeast area of Italy, there was a significant reduction in hospital admissions for cardiac surgery emergencies (with young male patients being the mostly involved group). However, during the recovery phase ('phase two') there was a significant surge in the number of late manifestations of cardiac disease (e.g., mechanical complications of myocardial infarction, acute heart failure), with an increase in the proportion of in-hospital deaths related to acute heart failure requiring surgical management. Although reasons for the observed decline in these hospital admissions are likely multifactorial, educational platforms and formal guidance for high-risk patients regarding when to seek emergency care are needed. Furthermore, this high-risk population should be longitudinally followed to determine the potential impact of COVID-19 pandemic on long-term cardiovascular health.

47.10   Selected References

- Bonalumi G, di Mauro M, Garatti A, Barili F, Gerosa G, Parolari A; for the Italian Society for Cardiac Surgery Task Force on COVID-19 Pandemic. The COVID-19 outbreak and its impact on hospitals in Italy: the model of cardiac surgery. Eur J Cardiothorac Surg. 2020;57(6):1025–1028. doi:https://doi.org/10.1093/ejcts/ezaa151
- Clerkin KJ, Fried JA, Raikhelkar J, et al. COVID-19 and Cardiovascular Disease. Circulation.   2020;141(20):1648–1655.   doi:https://doi.org/10.1161/circulationaha.120.046941
- Bhatt AS, Moscone A, McElrath EE, et al. Fewer Hospitalizations for Acute Cardiovascular Conditions During the COVID-19 Pandemic. J Am Coll Cardiol. 2020;76(3):280–288. doi:https://doi.org/10.1016/j.jacc.2020.05.038
- Parolari A, di Mauro M, Bonalumi G, et al. Safety for all: coronavirus disease 2019 pandemic and cardiac surgery: a roadmap to 'phase' 2. Eur J Cardiothorac Surg. 2020;58(2):213–216. doi:https://doi.org/10.1093/ejcts/ezaa187

  - These selected papers have been produced during the pandemic to highlight the indirect consequences of national lockdowns on hospital admissions for cardiovascular disease. They have also pointed out that a strong joint effort of multiple centers has been necessary to open a new, emergent, clinical path to face the pandemic with regard to the management of patients with cardiac disease.

References

1. Piperata A, Bottio T, Gerosa G. COVID-19 infection in left ventricular assist device patients. J Card Surg. 2020;35:3231–4. https://doi.org/10.1111/jocs.14969.
2. Guo YR, Cao QD, Hong ZS, et al. The origin, transmission and clinical therapies on coronavirus disease 2019 (COVID-19) outbreak—an update on the status. Mil Med Res. 2020;7(1):11. https://doi.org/10.1186/s40779-020-00240-0.
3. Dipartimento della Protezione Civile. COVID-19 Italia—Monitoraggio della situazione. [COVID-19 Italy—monitoring the pandemic]. https://opendatadpc.maps.arcgis.com/apps/opsdashboard/index.html#/b0c68bce2cce478eaac82fe38d4138b1. Accessed 16 Dec 2020.
4. Il Presidente Conte firma il Dpcm 9 marzo 2020. Governo Italiano Presidenza del Consiglio dei Ministri. 9 Marzo 2020. [The President signs the prime ministerial decree on March 9th 2020. Italian Governement]. http://www.governo.it/it/articolo/firmato-il-dpcm-9-marzo-2020/14276. Accessed 11 Nov 2020.

5. Visto il secrets del Presidente del Consiglio dei ministry. 26 aprile 2020. [Updates on the Prime Minister Decree. April 26th 2020]. http://www.governo.it/sites/new.governo.it/files/Dpcm_img_20200426.pdf. Accessed 11 Nov 2020.
6. Shafi AMA, Hewage S, Harky A. The impact of COVID-19 on the provision of cardiac surgical services. J Card Surg. 2020;35(6):1295–7. https://doi.org/10.1111/jocs.14631.
7. Bonalumi G, Di Mauro M, Garatti A, Barili F, Parolari A, Gerosa G. Pandemia da COVID-19 e Chirurgia Cardiaca: position paper della task force della Società Italiana di Chirurgia Cardiaca COVID-SICCH [COVID-19 outbreak and cardiac surgery: position paper from the COVID-SICCH task force of the Italian Society for Cardiac Surgery]. G Ital Cardiol (Rome). 2020;21(6):396–400. https://doi.org/10.1714/3359.33320.
8. Bonalumi G, di Mauro M, Garatti A, Barili F, Gerosa G, Parolari A, for the Italian Society for Cardiac Surgery Task Force on COVID-19 Pandemic. The COVID-19 outbreak and its impact on hospitals in Italy: the model of cardiac surgery. Eur J Cardiothorac Surg. 2020;57(6):1025–8. https://doi.org/10.1093/ejcts/ezaa151.
9. Clerkin KJ, Fried JA, Raikhelkar J, et al. COVID-19 and cardiovascular disease. Circulation. 2020;141(20):1648–55. https://doi.org/10.1161/circulationaha.120.046941.
10. Bhatt AS, Moscone A, McElrath EE, et al. Fewer hospitalizations for acute cardiovascular conditions during the COVID-19 pandemic. J Am Coll Cardiol. 2020;76(3):280–8. https://doi.org/10.1016/j.jacc.2020.05.038.
11. De Rosa S, Spaccarotella C, Basso C, for the Società Italiana di Cardiologia and the CCU Academy investigators group, et al. Reduction of hospitalizations for myocardial infarction in Italy in the COVID-19 era. Eur Heart J. 2020;41(22):2083–8. https://doi.org/10.1093/eurheartj/ehaa409.
12. Mafham MM, Spata E, Goldacre R, et al. COVID-19 pandemic and admission rates for and management of acute coronary syndromes in England. Lancet. 2020;396(10248):381–9. https://doi.org/10.1016/S0140-6736(20)31356-8.
13. El-Hamamsy I, Brinster DR, DeRose JJ, et al. The COVID-19 pandemic and acute aortic dissections in New York: a matter of public health. J Am Coll Cardiol. 2020;76(2):227–9. https://doi.org/10.1016/j.jacc.2020.05.022.
14. Baldi E, Sechi GM, Mare C, for the Lombardia CARe Researchers, et al. Out-of-hospital cardiac arrest during the Covid-19 outbreak in Italy. N Engl J Med. 2020;383(5):496–8. https://doi.org/10.1056/nejmc2010418.
15. Paoli A, Brischigliaro L, Scquizzato T, Favaretto A, Spagna A. Out-of-hospital cardiac arrest during the COVID-19 pandemic in the province of Padua, Northeast Italy. Resuscitation. 2020;154:47–9. https://doi.org/10.1016/j.resuscitation.2020.06.031.
16. Shah K, Tang D, Ibrahim F, et al. Surge in delayed myocardial infarction presentations: an inadvertent consequence of social distancing during the COVID-19 pandemic. JACC Case Rep. 2020;2(10):1642–7. https://doi.org/10.1016/j.jaccs.2020.07.004.
17. Molinari G, Molinari M, Di Biase M, Brunetti ND. Telecardiology and its settings of application: an update. J Telemed Telecare. 2018;24(5):373–81. https://doi.org/10.1177/1357633x16689432.
18. Parolari A, di Mauro M, Bonalumi G, et al. Safety for all: coronavirus disease 2019 pandemic and cardiac surgery: a roadmap to 'phase' 2. Eur J Cardiothorac Surg. 2020;58(2):213–6. https://doi.org/10.1093/ejcts/ezaa187.
19. Di Mauro M, Barili F, Bonalumi G, Garatti A, Parolari A, Gerosa G. Chirurgia cardiaca e pandemia COVID-19: note operative della task force COVID-SICCH per la fase 2 [cardiac surgery and COVID-19 outbreak: operative indications for the phase 2 by the COVID-SICCH task force]. G Ital Cardiol (Rome). 2020;21(8):589–93. https://doi.org/10.1714/3405.33890.
20. Caraffa R, Bagozzi L, Fiocco A, et al. Coronavirus disease 2019 (COVID-19) in the heart transplant population: a single-Centre experience. Eur J Cardiothorac Surg. 2020;58(5):899–906. https://doi.org/10.1093/ejcts/ezaa323.

21. Fiocco A, Ponzoni M, Caraffa R, et al. Heart transplantation management in northern Italy during COVID-19 pandemic: single-Centre experience. ESC Heart Fail. 2020;7(5):2003–6. https://doi.org/10.1002/ehf2.12874.
22. The European Society for Cardiology. ESC guidance for the diagnosis and management of CV disease during the COVID-19 pandemic. Updated 10 June 2020. https://www.escardio.org/The-ESC/Press-Office/Press-releases/ESC-Guidance-for-the-Diagnosis-and-Management-of-Heart-Disease-during-COVID-19. Accessed 7 Feb 2021.
23. Bagozzi L, Bottio T, Tarzia V, et al. Can patients be transplanted or undergo Ventricular Assist Device placement during the COVID-19 pandemic? Padova perspective. ASAIO. Online ahead of print. Jan 18, 2021. https://doi.org/10.1097/MAT.0000000000001400.
24. National health department: COVID-19 vaccination program. https://www.governo.it/it/cscovid19/report-vaccini/.
25. Harris C. COVID-19 vaccine rollout: how do countries in Europe compare? 02/14/2021. https://www.euronews.com/2021/02/14/covid-19-vaccinations-in-europe-which-countries-are-leading-the-way.

Part XII
Surgical Innovation/Research

Chapter 48
Ethical Questions of Surgical Trials

Lauren McLendon Postlewait and Puneet Singh (iD)

Abstract In surgical clinical trials, the pillars of medical ethics (beneficence, non-maleficence, justice, and autonomy) all play a role. During the conceptualization of a surgical study, there must be established doubt as to the value and/or role of the studied intervention (clinical equipoise) to ethically conduct the study (non-maleficence). Trial design must be carefully approached to minimize risks to participants (non-maleficence) while maximizing the clinical value of the outcomes to serve future patients and allow for the practice of evidence-based medicine (beneficence and justice). In trial enrollment, the surgeon must have appropriate conversations with patients about the understood risks and benefits of treatment arms, randomization, and the potential for non-therapeutic interventions if applicable. With appropriate informed consent, patients can voluntarily participate in studies (autonomy). There are many hurdles in conducting clinical trials in surgery, some of which present as ethical dilemmas. However, the failure to better understand the interventions we provide can ultimately lead to widespread patient harm. Thus, advancing knowledge by conducting or participating in surgical clinical trials supports a surgeon's ethical duty to both their patients and the field of surgery.

Keywords Ethics · Surgery · Clinical trials · Clinical equipoise · Human research Informed consent

L. M. Postlewait
Division of Surgical Oncology, Department of Surgery, Emory University School of Medicine, Atlanta, GA, USA
e-mail: lauren.postlewait@emory.edu

P. Singh (✉)
Department of Breast Surgical Oncology, Division of Surgery, University of Texas MD Anderson Cancer Center, Houston, TX, USA
e-mail: psingh6@mdanderson.org

© The Author(s), under exclusive license to Springer Nature Switzerland AG 2022

675

V. A. Lonchyna et al. (eds.), *Difficult Decisions in Surgical Ethics*, Difficult Decisions in Surgery: An Evidence-Based Approach,
https://doi.org/10.1007/978-3-030-84625-1_48

Case

A 55-year-old woman is currently being treated for breast cancer. She presented with a right-sided 3 cm triple negative (estrogen receptor, progesterone receptor, and HER-2 receptor negative) invasive ductal carcinoma with no concerning lymph nodes on ultrasound. She completed neoadjuvant chemotherapy, and subsequent imaging showed radiographic complete response. Vacuum-assisted biopsy of the tumor bed showed pathologic complete response, concordant with radiographic findings. She presents to surgery clinic to discuss options for next steps in therapy. National Cancer Care Network (NCCN) guidelines recommend sentinel lymph node biopsy in conjunction with mastectomy or with partial mastectomy and radiation as the next steps in her care [1]. However, there is debate within the breast surgical oncology community as to the benefit of surgical intervention in these exceptional responders to neoadjuvant therapy, such as this patient. To address this question, there is an ongoing surgical clinical trial assessing oncologic and survival outcomes of such patients who forgo surgical intervention and pursue breast radiation as the only local therapy [2]. She meets inclusion criteria to be enrolled in this trial. Yet, as her surgeon, there are certain ethical concepts that must be considered.

48.1 Introduction

In the transition from student to physician, when we accept the responsibility and privilege of wearing the long white coat and caring for the lives of other human beings, we have a ritual. We take an oath. Referencing the origins of medicine in Greece and the practice of Hippocrates, medical school graduates vow to uphold a certain standard in their work. These declarations emphasize the ethical principles of beneficence, non-maleficence, autonomy, and justice. Also, central to this oath is the idea of applying the scientific data attained by one's predecessors to patient care and then growing that body of knowledge to further the field [3, 4].

As such, from the beginnings of individual medical practice, we each find ourselves at the intersection of ethics, research, and clinical care. We have pledged to practice and contribute to evidence-based medicine, but how do we pursue this while balancing these ethical principles? This is especially pertinent in the field of surgery where, in an effort to heal, we take the knife to another's flesh. To take a patient's life into one's hands in this way, the surgeon must be confident in the outcomes. But how do we measure whether this confidence is justified? Further, how do we ethically perform surgical clinical trials to improve our practice for patients of the future while maintaining our commitments to the current patient at the bedside?

Table 48.1 Key ethical points in surgical trials

Historic breeches in **ethical conduct** in the study of human subjects led to the creation of national and international ethical codes that are mandatory in development and execution of surgical clinical trials.
There are unique barriers to conducting **surgical clinical trials**, as compared to medical trials. For a surgeon to participate in such research, there are surgeon-specific, patient-specific, and community-specific ethical issues that must be considered.
Clinical equipoise is the concept of uncertainty over the ideal treatment approach when considering available options among the surgical community and is required to develop and conduct surgical clinical trials.
Appropriate **study design** to minimize risk, respect autonomy, provide appropriate comparison (if indicated), and address key surgical questions that could change clinical practice is key in the ethics of surgical trials.
Informed consent is an integral part of ethical study conduct (autonomy).
It is the duty of the surgeon to take care of the patient (**beneficence**) while minimizing harm (**non-maleficence**) and respecting the patient's wishes (**autonomy**), ultimately serving the community (**justice**). To do this, one must have the data to make informed treatment decisions. Therefore, surgeon participation in clinical trials promotes clinical ethics.

In this chapter, we begin by exploring the historic breeches in ethical codes that led to the creation of national and international guidelines in human experimentation. [5–7] From there, we compare and contrast the process and barriers in the development of medications with those of the implementation of novel surgical techniques. Next, we explore the idea of clinical equipoise as the foundation on which we justify creation of and enrollment in surgical clinical trials. Even if equipoise is established, there remains controversy in the ethics of trial design including the utilization of placebo (or sham surgery), which we explore [8, 9]. We then consider patient autonomy as it relates to informed consent for participation in trials. Lastly, we shift to discuss the practice of evidence-based medicine and the balance of ethical principles to serve both individuals and society (Table 48.1).

48.2 Search Strategy

A systematic search in the National Library of Medicine (pubmed.gov) from inception to May 15, 2020 was conducted. Searches were not restricted by language or study type. References of the included articles were also searched manually. The search terms included "ethics and surgical clinical trials," "ethics and surgical research", "ethics and emergency surgery research," "equipoise and surgical trials," "ethics and placebo-controlled surgical trials", and "ethics and sham surgery." The most relevant articles were selected for inclusion.

48.3   Discussion

48.3.1   Ethical Standards in Clinical Trials: A Historical Perspective

National and international codes of conduct for the study of human subjects have been created to guide the ethical development of clinical trials. While these guidelines are now widely recognized and accepted, they originated from necessity in response to historic, atrocious human experimentation that grossly violated ethical principles [5–7]. During World War II, Nazi physicians conducted medical experimentation on unwilling, vulnerable populations with flagrant disregard to the concepts of beneficence or non-maleficence. In the aftermath of the war, when these crimes were acknowledged, the Nuremberg Code was created. This policy delineates the minimum standards necessary in the conduct of human trials where voluntary participation is required (autonomy); potential benefits are maximized while minimizing risk (beneficence and non-maleficence); and the study is stopped if clear harm is appreciated (non-maleficence) [5]. The World Medical Association further refined these international regulations in the Declaration of Helsinki in 1964 [3, 6, 10]. A decade later, gross neglect of these standards were again acknowledged in the United States where over the course of decades, black patients living in poverty were unwillingly and unknowingly subjected to experimentation with anticipated serious morbidity by the researchers. Physicians withheld available therapy to treat syphilis to study long-term effects of untreated disease with known harm to the subjects. This atrocity led to the drafting of the Belmont Report, which emphasizes the standards of incorporating and balancing the ideals of justice, autonomy, beneficence, and non-maleficence in all trials involving human subjects. These experiences ultimately led to current practices with respect to these codes and external regulation of clinical trials by institutional review boards. [3, 7, 10, 11]

48.3.2   Clinical Trials in Medicine and Surgery

With this history and these guidelines in mind, one can begin to consider how to approach the goal of scientific research to improve clinical practice and treatment options. On the spectrum of treatment advancement, one must appreciate the difference between new drug development and development of novel surgical techniques. Typically, randomized controlled trials are conducted to determine safety and efficacy of new medications. Then, these data are reviewed by the United States Food and Drug Administration where drug approval decisions are made. However, this routine, rigorous testing and outside approval method are neither standard nor required in surgery. Rather, novel techniques are often pioneered by individual surgeons, sometimes based on data from animal or human studies. New procedures are then carried out in a number of patients, a case series may be published, and, most times in the absence of clinical trials, this new method may become widespread and perhaps widely adopted [10, 12]. Thus, as opposed to medical clinical trials, trials in surgery usually occur after techniques have been extensively adopted in the community [13]. Ashton et al. describe this phenomenon as "dissemination first, evidence later." [12].

This spread of innovative techniques as treatment options for patients without data supporting their efficacy, or defining their risk, creates a barrier to further study that is unique to surgery. The techniques that have already been adopted may be believed to offer benefit, bringing into question the clinical need for further study. Some surgeons believe that conducting a trial in this circumstance may deprive patients from the benefits of this technique, while subjecting them to risk and potentially creating a burden on society where resources must be diverted to the study: conceptually questioning beneficence, non-maleficence, and justice [3, 13]. Despite these concerns, belief in efficacy of a practice and the ability to generate evidence supporting that practice do not always coincide. As an example, ligation of the internal mammary artery to treat angina used to be a common practice. Physiologically, this procedure would be expected to divert blood flow to the coronary arteries and relieve symptoms; however, when subjected to study, this procedure was found to be ineffective, despite its popularity [3, 14]. Thus, pursuing the actual evidence changed practice, and ultimately led to better patient care with respect to ethical principles. As such, Adibe et al. and Burger et al. propose that perhaps there should be a change in the process where surgical trials could be conducted *before* widespread dissemination [10, 13].

Unique to surgeons are barriers both in starting and in completing clinical trials. In fact, Mouw et al. report that once a trial has started, the rate of trial completion is higher in medical trials than in surgical trials (55.51% versus 39.49%, $p < 0.001$), and being a surgical trial is an independent risk factor for early trial discontinuation (OR 1.25 $p = 0.041$) [15]. One contributor to these findings is poor or slow enrollment. Though the reasons for this are multifactorial, this brings to light a key element: equipoise [15].

48.3.3 The Concept of Clinical Equipoise

Equipoise occurs when there is uncertainty over the ideal treatment approach when considering available options. In order to ethically conduct a study, one must have equipoise [3]. When equipoise is applied to treating surgical patients, one must acknowledge that it is multi-faceted. Here, we discuss this in the context of equipoise per the surgeon, per the clinical community (clinical equipoise), and per the patient.

Surgeons typically have strong opinions about which treatments are best for their patients (no personal equipoise) [16]. While some surgeons may call for a trial to evaluate a surgical approach because they feel there is equipoise, other surgeons may feel that one approach is unquestioningly better than the other and hence do not condone the study. Some of the roots of this go as deep as surgical residency. Surgical training is structured such that we learn to operate and how to make surgical decisions in an apprenticeship-model where our mentor's and our institution's practices are dogma [13, 17]. As such, surgical approach and surgical decision-making may be quite different between two well-trained surgeons, and these surgeons may feel strongly that their personal practice best serves the patient, despite the lack of evidence either way [12, 13]. These strong feelings of individuals have led to the failure of trials to reach enrollment targets to obtain statistical study power, have slowed trial enrollment, and have led to selection bias of participating patients [18]. For example, the lack of personal equipoise for individual surgeons led to the early discontinuation of the Stenting and Angioplasty with Protection in Patients at High Risk for Endarterectomy (SAPPHIRE) trial that was designed to compare outcomes of carotid endarterectomy and carotid stenting [12]. Similarly, lack of personal equipoise led to slow enrollment and highly selected patients enrolled on the American College of Surgeons Oncology Group (ACOSOG) Z0011 trial. This study compared outcomes of breast cancer patients with limited axillary disease on sentinel lymph node biopsy during breast conserving therapy: comparing those who underwent completion lymphadenectomy or no additional axillary surgery. The slow, selected enrollment led to criticisms on the universal applicability of the study findings and recommendations [16].

In the age of evidence-based medicine, however, the surgeon must transcend their data-less opinions in order to find the truth. Without data, one runs the risk of depriving patients of optimal treatment (beneficence) and ultimately harming patients (non-maleficence) throughout their surgical career despite the surgeon's good intentions. Clinical equipoise requires the investigator to not know which treatment is better. As such, it serves as the ethical basis for any clinical trial. In this way, it is the avenue down which an individual, opinionated surgeon may put aside personal belief that is lacking evidence in order to pursue data on optimal treatments of current and future patients (justice) [13]. From data generated through the application of clinical equipoise to support trials, the historic, common, invasive practices of extracranial-intracranial arterial bypass for stroke and arthroscopic knee debridement for osteoarthritis were found to be non-therapeutic and were abandoned [13]. Additionally, surgical clinical trials in breast cancer have revolutionized breast cancer care by improving oncologic outcomes and reducing morbidity over the last century [19].

In the pursuit of data to optimize patient care, at least one more point of view must be considered: the patient's. Even in the context of clinical equipoise, the patient may prefer one treatment over the other. Sometimes this is secondary to marketing of a new technique or approach [3]. Patients may seek surgeons who exclusively perform the preferred intervention. Or if on trial, the patient may elect to cross-over treatment arms, which poses a potential barrier in trial completion and interpretation [12]. Yet, this underscores the key ethical principle of autonomy, which must be respected and balanced with other ethical principles in clinical research.

48.3.4   Ethics of Study Design

Once one has ethically assessed whether a study is indicated, the next question is
one of design- both ethical and practical. How can the study be structured such that
it addresses the question at hand to gather relevant and potentially practice-changing
data to further medicine (justice and beneficence) while maximizing benefit as well
as minimizing risk (non-maleficence) and respecting the choices and personhood of
the participants (autonomy)? With so many different, and at times competing, factors to consider, this must be approached in a thoughtful manner. Ashton et al. propose a detailed, phased plan of key components to consider at the interface of ethics
and surgical clinical trials. They describe the intimate relationship of ethics and
clinical trials at four key phases of the surgical trial: trial initiation, trial design, trial
conduct, and data analysis and reporting [12].

One integral step to this approach is determining the appropriate comparison to
make. Ethical questions arise as one considers options of comparing a surgical
approach with another surgical technique, with a surgical placebo (sham surgery),
with a non-operative medical treatment, or with no intervention [8]. When two operative interventions are compared that are felt to be therapeutic, clinical equipoise is
the key element that must be present to ethically proceed with the trial. As the practice of laparoscopic cholecystectomy became routine, a trial comparing outcomes
of laparoscopic and open cholecystectomy began. With time, however, the trial was
discontinued early; even without clear data, the belief that laparoscopic cholecystectomy was superior became widespread throughout the surgical community. Thus,
ethically, it was felt that the trial could not continue (loss of clinical equipoise) [17].

Beyond innovative techniques, another research interest in surgery is de-
escalating therapy to reduce morbidity (non-maleficence) but maintain therapeutic
outcomes. Once an intervention has been accepted and there are data to support its
value, there are ethical issues to consider in de-escalation. Angelos et al. describe
key components that should be incorporated into a non-intervention surgical trial to
make it ethically sound, using the specific example of non-operative therapy for
early-stage thyroid cancer [20]. These include ensuring that the goal of the research
is both valuable in a social and scientific context; the study design is appropriate to
achieve these endpoints with independent review apart from the researchers; there
is fair patient selection without targeting vulnerable populations and with appropriate informed consent to participate; and the study is designed for minimization of
personal risk while maximizing societal and perhaps personal patient benefit as privacy is maintained [20].

Interestingly, there is quite a bit of controversy over study types comparing surgery to a non-operative intervention or no intervention with respect to the role of the
placebo effect [10, 21]. Some have proposed that the invasiveness itself of a surgical
procedure may carry with it a placebo effect that alters patient outcomes, irrespective of the technical aspects of the procedure. This could potentially skew study
outcomes toward inappropriately favoring a non-therapeutic surgical approach over
medical therapy or no therapy at all [22, 23]. To that end, the study design that

carries the highest level of evidence and is considered the gold standard in clinical trials is the randomized, blinded, placebo-controlled study [13]. The concept of surgical placebo poses unique problems and ethical concerns to the surgeon. To provide an invasive intervention with no known or postulated therapeutic component, the surgeon puts the patient at risk for complication with no expected personal benefit to the patient. This is at its root distinct from medication trials where the placebo "sugar pill" poses no real threat [3]. Though the level of risk may vary based on the design of the sham operation, no surgery is without risk of complication. Therefore, the surgeon must carefully weigh these individual risks to the patient (non-maleficence) with the potential benefit of generating the data to form guidelines for future patients (justice and beneficence). Some investigators are proponents of utilization of the surgical placebo-control arms under specific situational contingencies [8, 23, 24]. This type of trial design may be appropriate when there is clinical equipoise, the clinical question potentially offers value to patient care, there is no standard data-supported other surgical intervention to compare, the potential value of the knowledge gained outweighs the risk of placebo where that risk is minimized, and the patient knows placebo is an option and consents to it [8, 23, 24]. Others argue that sham surgery is not ethical, as there are typically alternative study designs that could lead to the same conclusions without putting patients in the placebo group at the same level of risk of a nontherapeutic procedural intervention [9]. Additionally, there is an unquestioned intimate relationship between a surgeon and their patient where trust is key. Some argue that in performing non-therapeutic surgery where the patient is blinded to the intervention, the surgeon violates that trust by misleading the patient (issues of autonomy) [3].

48.3.5   Informed Consent: Patient Autonomy

Along with clinical equipoise, voluntary informed consent in trial participation represents another cornerstone of ethical clinical research and is a key concept in both the Nuremberg Code and the Belmont report. [3, 5, 7] The surgeon must appropriately engage the patient in conversation regarding the study design: treatment arms, therapeutic options, potential risks and benefits, and randomization if appropriate. Patients can then knowingly and willingly enroll in trials, accepting treatment based on the study design. With these open and honest discussions, surgeons can circumnavigate the aforementioned issues of violating the patient's trust through deception [3]. One pitfall of trial participation is the common misconception of the patient that by participating in a study, they are personally going to benefit from the study intervention, despite the lack of evidence and presence of equipoise [25]. Although this idea of "therapeutic misconception" is prevalent, one can again address this by having truthful and detailed discussions with patients who are making decisions to consent about the reality of the treatment arms [10]. In this way, the patient can be appropriately informed about trial participation and have the opportunity to voluntarily participate.

But what about clinical trials in surgical emergencies where time is of the essence, and patients may be too ill to provide informed consent to participate in a trial? Patients who present in this way are particularly vulnerable. Yet, when clinical equipoise is present and data are needed to better treat patients globally, Doig et al. argue that there are situations where study enrollment without initial consent is appropriate, citing the Closed or Open after Laparotomy (COOL) study which examines outcomes of patients who undergo primary as opposed to delayed primary abdominal fascial closures in emergent laparotomies [11]. In this study, identification of potential patient participants could only be made in the operating room at a time when the patient could not consent. The requirements for recruitment to waive upfront consent were that immediate intervention is required secondary to a serious threat; there must be clinical equipoise; risk and benefit of the experimental arm is appropriately weighed; the participant does not have decision-making capacity to consent; another appointed decision-maker cannot be consulted because of emergency timing needed to intervene; and the patient has no prior directive related to participation. After initial enrollment, there was opportunity for delayed consent of the patient or the surrogate decision maker. [11] This approach centers on justice and potential benefit and non-maleficence for patients of the future to whom these data could be applied; however, there remains disagreement around the ethical issues in waiving consent in regards to patient autonomy, even in these emergency situations [21].

48.3.6 Evidence Based Medicine and Need for Surgical Trials

Without sound data to treat patients, we cannot always know whether we are serving them or doing them harm. Evidence based medicine is described as "the conscientious, explicit, and judicious use of current best evidence in making decisions about the care of individual patients…[by] integrating individual clinical expertise with best available external clinical evidence from systematic research." [26] To contribute to the data we use to make evidence-based decisions, one must participate in trials. Some argue that it is a surgeon's ethical duty to their patients to participate in clinical trials; continuing to perform a surgery that may put patients at risk without benefitting them because "that's how we were trained" is contradictory to the oath we took to first do no harm [3, 4, 13, 22]. However, in approaching these studies, one must consider all of the facets of clinical ethics and weigh them in an effort to best serve the patient at the bedside and the patients in the future.

48.4 Case Discussion

To care for the patient with breast cancer who has had a complete clinical response to neoadjuvant therapy with the option of trial enrollment to study non-operative management, the aforementioned ethical concepts must be considered [2]. First, there is uncertainty within the breast oncology clinical community as to whether patients benefit from surgical intervention when they have no evidence of residual invasive disease; hence, there is clinical equipoise that justifies the study of no surgical intervention. With surgery as part of the breast cancer treatment algorithm, patients typically have excellent oncologic outcomes, but they are at risk of morbidity associated with surgical intervention. Trial enrollment for no surgical intervention could eliminate that surgical risk; however, we do not understand the potential oncologic risk a patient takes on by forgoing surgery (weighing beneficence and non-maleficence). Through this study of individual patients, our understanding of breast cancer treatment could change. With that, new treatment guidelines could be created to improve the outcomes of breast cancer patients of the future (justice). But we must make the risks to the individual participants clear. There must be an open, honest, and detailed discussion with the patient regarding the standard surgical interventions and trial enrollment with non-operative therapy. To enroll in the trial, the patient must voluntarily give informed consent, and may withdraw at any time (autonomy). Lastly, in an effort to do no harm, if preliminary results suggest poor outcomes in patients in the trial compared to those undergoing standard therapy, one must have a low threshold to discontinue the study (non-maleficence). In this case, after appropriate counseling, the patient elected to enroll on the trial with active surveillance for breast cancer rather than pursue surgical intervention.

48.5 Concluding Remarks

Ethical considerations in surgical clinical trials are vast. Clinical equipoise is necessary to ethically move forward in studying differential outcomes of two interventions (or non-intervention). In study design, one must take into account how a trial could change the practice of medicine and surgery to improve outcomes of patients in the future (beneficence and justice) and weigh this against potential harm for trial participants (non-maleficence). One of the key concepts in ethical study enrollment is appropriate informed consent of the participants (autonomy). A balance among these ethical principles should be pursued as we strive to understand and optimize surgical interventions and ethically designed surgical clinical trials can benefit our patients and advance the surgical field.

48.6 Selected References

- Adibe OO, St Peter SD. Equipoise, ethics, and the necessity of randomized trials in surgery. Arch Surg. 2012;147(10):899–900. doi:https://doi.org/10.1001/archsurg.2012.1796
  - A concise summary of the importance of clinical trials in surgery highlighting some of the barriers that surgeons face in conducting these trials.

- Angelos P, Hartl DM, Shah JP, et al. Ethical issues in non-intervention trials for thyroid cancer. Eur J Surg Oncol. 2018;44(3):316–320. doi:https://doi.org/10.1016/j.ejso.2017.03.002

  - A surgeon's reflection on historical ethical issues in clinical trials, problems related to surgical placebo, the necessity of equipoise in surgical clinical trials, and the importance of skepticism and pursuing evidence to treat surgical patients.

- Burger I, Sugarman J, Goodman SN. Ethical issues in evidence-based surgery. Surg Clin N Am. 2006;86(1):151–168. doi:https://doi.org/10.1016/j.suc.2005.10.003

  - A thoughtful exploration of the interface between ethics and evidence-based medicine in surgery with a focus on the ethical considerations in surgical trial design.

References

1. National Comprehensive Cancer Network: Breast Cancer (Version 4.2020). 2020. Accessed 13 July 2020. https://www.nccn.org/professionals/physician_gls/pdf/breast.pdf
2. Clinical Trials. Eliminating surgery after systemic therapy in treating patients with HER2 positive or triple negative breast cancer. Accessed July 13, 2020. https://ClinicalTrials.gov/show/NCT02945579
3. Angelos P, Hartl DM, Shah JP, et al. Ethical issues in non-intervention trials for thyroid cancer. Eur J Surg Oncol. 2018;44(3):316–20. https://doi.org/10.1016/j.ejso.2017.03.002.
4. Askitopoulou H, Vgontzas AN. The relevance of the Hippocratic oath to the ethical and moral values of contemporary medicine. Part I: the Hippocratic oath from antiquity to modern times. Eur Spine J. 2018;27(7):1481–90. https://doi.org/10.1007/s00586-017-5348-4.
5. Permissible medical experiments. In: Trials of war criminals before the Nuremberg military tribunals under control council law no. 10. Volume II. U.S. Government Printing Office; 1949. p. 181–4.
6. World Medical Association. World medical association declaration of Helsinki: ethical principles for medical research involving human subjects. JAMA. 2013;310(20):2191–4. https://doi.org/10.1001/jama.2013.281053.
7. The National Commission for the Protection of Human Subjects of Biomedical and Behavioral Research. The Belmont report: Ethical principles and guidelines for the protection of human subjects of research. 1979. Accessed April 13, 2021. https://www.hhs.gov/ohrp/sites/default/files/the-belmont-report-508c_FINAL.pdf.
8. Beard DJ, Campbell MK, Blazeby JM, et al. Considerations and methods for placebo controls in surgical trials (ASPIRE guidelines). Lancet. 2020;395(10226):828–38. https://doi.org/10.1016/s0140-6736(19)33137-x.
9. Polgar S, Ng J. Ethics, methodology and the use of placebo controls in surgical trials. Brain Res Bull. 2005;67(4):290–7. https://doi.org/10.1016/j.brainresbull.2015.06.028.
10. Burger I, Sugarman J, Goodman SN. Ethical issues in evidence-based surgery. Surg Clin N Am. 2006;86(1):151–68. https://doi.org/10.1016/j.suc.2005.10.003.
11. Doig CJ, Page SA, McKee JL, et al. Ethical considerations in conducting surgical research in severe complicated intra-abdominal sepsis. World J Emerg Surg. 2019;14:39. https://doi.org/10.1186/s13017-019-0259-9.

12. Ashton CM, Wray NP, Jarman AF, Kolman JM, Wenner DM, Brody BA. Ethics and methods in surgical trials. J Med Ethics. 2009;35(9):579–83. https://doi.org/10.1136/jme.2008.028175.
13. Adibe OO, St Peter SD. Equipoise, ethics, and the necessity of randomized trials in surgery. Arch Surg. 2012;147(10):899–900. https://doi.org/10.1001/archsurg.2012.1796.
14. Cobb LA, Thomas GI, Dillard DH, Merendino KA, Bruce RA. An evaluation of internal-mammary-artery ligation by a double-blind technic. N Engl J Med. 1959;260(22):1115–8. https://doi.org/10.1056/nejm195905282602204.
15. Mouw TJ, Hong SW, Sarwar S, et al. Discontinuation of surgical versus nonsurgical clinical trials: an analysis of 88,498 trials. J Surg Res. 2018;227:151–7. https://doi.org/10.1016/j.jss.2018.02.039.
16. Spillane AJ, Mann GB. Surgeon knows best versus breast cancer surgical clinical trial equipoise: a plea for the sake of future trials. ANZ J Surg. 2017;87(3):111–2. https://doi.org/10.1111/ans.13831.
17. Meakins JL. Innovation in surgery: the rules of evidence. Am J Surg. 2002;183(4):399–405. https://doi.org/10.1016/s0002-9610(02)00825-5.
18. Donovan JL, de Salis I, Toerien M, Paramasivan S, Hamdy FC, Blazeby JM. The intellectual challenges and emotional consequences of equipoise contributed to the fragility of recruitment in six randomized controlled trials. J Clin Epidemiol. 2014;67(8):912–20. https://doi.org/10.1016/j.jclinepi.2014.03.010.
19. Throckmorton A, VanderWalde L, Brackett C, et al. The ethics of breast surgery. Ann Surg Oncol. 2015;22(10):3191–6. https://doi.org/10.1245/s10434-015-4751-5.
20. Angelos P. Ethical issues of participant recruitment in surgical clinical trials. Ann Surg Oncol. 2013;20(10):3184–7. https://doi.org/10.1245/s10434-013-3178-0.
21. Kottow MH. Clinical and research ethics as moral strangers. Arch Immunol Ther Exp. 2009;57(3):157–64. https://doi.org/10.1007/s00005-009-0027-8.
22. Boyle K, Batzer FR. Is a placebo-controlled surgical trial an oxymoron? J Minim Invasive Gynecol. 2007;14(3):278–83. https://doi.org/10.1016/j.jmig.2006.12.006.
23. Savulescu J, Wartolowska K, Carr A. Randomised placebo-controlled trials of surgery: ethical analysis and guidelines. J Med Ethics. 2016;42(12):776–83. https://doi.org/10.1136/medethics-2015-103333.
24. Horng S, Miller FG. Ethical framework for the use of sham procedures in clinical trials. Crit Care Med. 2003;31(3, Suppl):S126–30. https://doi.org/10.1097/01.ccm.00000549606.49187.67.
25. Miller FG, Brody H. A critique of clinical equipoise. Therapeutic misconception in the ethics of clinical trials. Hast Cent Rep. 2003;33(3):19–28. https://doi.org/10.2307/3528434.
26. Sackett DL, Rosenberg WM, Gray JA, Haynes RB, Richardson WS. Evidence based medicine: what it is and what it isn't. BMJ. 1996;312(7023):71–2. https://doi.org/10.1136/bmj.312.7023.71.

Chapter 49
Introducing New Techniques, Technology, and Medical Devices

Kelly C. Landeen (iD), Fabien Maldonado (iD), and Alexander Langerman (iD)

Abstract Introducing new procedures, technologies, and medical devices to one's practice inherently presents a surgeon with ethical dilemmas regarding their safety and efficacy. This chapter provides an overview of the history of surgical innovation and how new medical devices and surgical procedures are regulated, with discussion on ethical dilemmas surgeons may face as they expand their armamentarium of surgical techniques. Above all, this chapter aims to encourage innovation that is safe and appropriate, and to equip surgeons for the decision-making and discussions that should accompany surgical innovation.

Keywords Innovation · Research · Regulation · Learning curve · Informed consent

K. C. Landeen
Department of Otolaryngology – Head and Neck Surgery, Vanderbilt University Medical Center, Nashville, TN, USA
e-mail: Kelly.Landeen@vumc.org

F. Maldonado
Departments of Thoracic Surgery, Department of Pulmonology, Center for Biomedical Ethics and Society, Vanderbilt University Medical Center, Nashville, TN, USA
e-mail: Fabien.Maldonado@vumc.org

A. Langerman (✉)
Department of Otolaryngology – Head and Neck Surgery, Department of Radiology and Radiological Sciences, Center for Biomedical Ethics and Society, Vanderbilt University Medical Center, Nashville, TN, USA
e-mail: Alexander.Langerman@vumc.org

© The Author(s), under exclusive license to Springer Nature Switzerland AG 2022

V. A. Lonchyna et al. (eds.), *Difficult Decisions in Surgical Ethics*, Difficult Decisions in Surgery: An Evidence-Based Approach,
https://doi.org/10.1007/978-3-030-84625-1_49

687

Case

Imagine that you are a surgeon who specializes in sleep surgery within the field of otolaryngology. You are very intrigued by a new surgical technique that has been developed to treat obstructive sleep apnea (OSA). The procedure includes implanting a new, static device into the pharyngeal wall, which increases overall anterior-posterior (AP) diameter of the pharynx. It has been approved by the Food and Drug Administration (FDA) for use in adults who meet specific clinical criteria for OSA and have failed other treatments.

You are a talented surgeon who has completed all your residency and fellowship training, but you have not yet performed this specific procedure. You have attended several lectures, undergone extensive online training, and have interacted with the device itself on numerous occasions. Your department chair, who is a huge proponent of the device and whose spouse helped to develop it, is very eager for you to begin performing the surgery. It has undergone one clinical trial, which demonstrated overall safety and efficacy in a cohort of 100 patients.

Finally, the perfect patient comes in who meets all the necessary criteria and who you think is a good candidate for the surgery. He even has a great insurance plan that will cover the entire global fee of the surgery and postoperative period.

Much time is spent discussing the new device with the patient, and you explain in detail how it works and how it could improve his OSA. He is very interested, as his poor sleep has led to high blood pressure and is negatively affecting his quality of life. Yet he is a nervous gentleman and worries about the risks of something 'experimental.' He finally asks you if you have done this before, and how your other patients have done after the surgery. What do you say?

49.1 Introduction

We once believed the earth was flat, we were the center of the universe, and disease was caused by imbalances in our body fluids. Only after the ridicule and persecution of scientific pioneers have these theories been debunked. Major advancements in medicine are no different and have nearly always been met with resistance. Yet medical advancements carry the weight of human life, and a healthy dose of caution is both necessary and appropriate.

The dangers of medical advancement lie in large part within the unknown. We often stand on the shoulders of giants who have come before us, and only hear about the successes and breakthroughs. We hear much less about those giants whose experiments went poorly. Historically we as a people have been fearful of new things and have rejected scientific breakthroughs that could save lives; yet it is also true that 'new' does not always equal 'better.' The unforeseen risks of new devices,

Table 49.1 Principles of Medical Ethics and their Applications in Surgical Innovation

Beneficence	• New surgical procedures and devices may improve outcomes • Morbidity and mortality may be reduced • Cosmesis may be improved
Nonmaleficence	• There is a learning curve associated with new techniques, and complication rates may be higher when a surgeon is learning • We do not know all of the long-term complications of new
Autonomy	• Transparency is vital, and a surgeon must communicate lack of experience, potential for unforeseen complications, and conflicts of interest • Consent in these patients may never be truly informed due to the unknowns
Justice	• Patient selection for new procedures and devices should be fair

the inexperience of a surgeon with a new procedure, and the inability to predict outcomes all hang in the balance of novel breakthroughs in surgery. Nevertheless, much of the oversight in surgical innovation comes from surgeons themselves, and this responsibility is not to be taken lightly.

In this chapter we will discuss the ethical dilemmas inherent in surgical innovation, how innovation is regulated today, and the important role that a surgeon plays in ensuring the ethical administration of care when it comes to new technologies, procedures, and devices (see Table 49.1).

49.2   Search Strategy

A thorough literature review was performed to investigate the ethical considerations in surgical innovation. Using PubMed® (National Library of Medicine, 1996), searched terms included "surgical ethics," "surgical innovation," "medical device regulation," "surgical regulation," and "surgical transparency." For historical examples of medical advancements, this search was expanded to include sources found via the Encyclopaedia Brittanica, Inc. (15th edition, 2010), which was accessed online. Further research into current regulation of medical devices and pharmaceuticals included thorough review of the United States Food and Drug Administration (FDA) current policies, as outlined on the organization's governmental website.

49.3   Discussion

49.3.1   Medical Advancements in History

When Ignaz Semmelweiss, a Hungarian physician in Vienna in 1847, proposed handwashing between obstetric cases as a method to reduce puerperal fever, he was met with outcry. Physicians everywhere were skeptical, offended, and hostile.

Despite demonstrating reduced mortality in his practice, he was mocked and shamed by the western medical community for decades [1]. Yet around the world, a very few others were noticing similar patterns. Due to worsening mental illness, Dr. Semmelweiss was committed to an asylum in 1865, where he tragically died from injuries after being beaten by the institution's guards. It wasn't until germ theory gained more traction with the breakthroughs of John Snow, Louis Pasteur, and Joseph Lister that the medical community posthumously accepted Semmelweiss' theories on hand washing [2]. Today he is regarded as one of the first proponents of germ theory and a pioneer of surgical antiseptic technique [3].

Skepticism about new medical advancements, however, is often warranted and should give pause to practitioners. Consider the lobotomy procedure, which was developed in the 1930s as a surgical means to ameliorate symptoms in mentally ill patients prior to the advent of antipsychotics. It involved drilling or driving a pick into the frontal lobe of the brain in order to sever neural connections thought to cause overstimulation, excess emotions, and psychiatric symptoms. There were multiple variations, and lack of oversight meant that surgeons had vast liberty to develop new techniques and modify the procedure as they saw fit. Regardless of the variation, the lobotomy was met with both enthusiasm and skepticism [4]. While it could be successful in calming patients, it often left them with debilitating functional disabilities requiring institutionalization. Other serious side effects included brain hemorrhage, seizures, and death. Possibly the most famous lobotomy was performed on Rosemary Kennedy, the 23-year-old, intellectually handicapped sister of President John F. Kennedy. The procedure left her incapacitated, partially paralyzed, and barely able to speak; she was institutionalized until her death at age 86 [5]. Lobotomies were gradually outlawed in various countries, but not before over 40,000 lobotomies had been performed in the United States alone, well into the 1970s [4].

Medical devices are a prime example of how 'new' is not always 'better.' When a device is approved for the market, it has likely only been tested in a small cohort of patients. The long-term outcomes are still to be determined. One study found that first-generation gastric bands had a complication rate of nearly 20%, which was reduced to 10% in second-generation models [6]. This demonstrates that despite a shaky start, the industry was able to learn from post-market surveillance and adjusted the device accordingly to make it safer.

In addition to dangerous surgery, there is also the possibility of fraud. There are many historical examples of medical scams. In the 1900s Harry Hoxsey, a man with an eighth-grade education and no medical training, made a living by vast sales of tonics that reportedly cured cancer. As expected, these remedies have now been proven ineffective and he has been discredited [7]. In the 1920s and 1930s John Brinkley falsified his medical degree and touted a 'miracle cure' for male impotence by surgical xenotransplantation of goat testicles into humans; he too was ultimately discredited, but not before he had performed fraudulent surgeries on countless men and women and earned over $12 million [8]. Even as recently as 2019, Italian surgeon Paulo Macchiarini, who performed highly dangerous tracheal transplants, falsified his data despite unfortunate results and deaths. He was ultimately sentenced to 16 months in prison [9].

This is in contrast to physicians like Semelweiss and Snow who went against the teachings of the time to pioneer innovation for the betterment of society. Dr. Ernest Armory Codman was the first physician to keep his peers accountable and to establish the importance of long-term follow up of surgical outcomes. He spearheaded hospital reform at the turn of the twentieth century by developing his End Results System. He kept track of his patients after he operated on them and monitored them for at least one year, often longer, and identified adverse outcomes, which he published in a book. He also attempted to audit other surgeons and monitored their patients, believing that all outcomes should be publicized to the community. Dr. Codman ruffled many feathers in his efforts and was often viewed as rude, overreaching, and misguided. He was reviled by the medical community for daring to question its "successes and practices" and was even fired from Massachusetts General Hospital. Although he died in relative anonymity, he forever changed accountability in modern healthcare by being a founder of what would become the American College of Surgeons and the Joint Commission on Accreditation of Healthcare Organizations. His End Results System ultimately paved the way for surveillance epidemiology and regulatory oversight [10].

As we learn and grow as a medical community, we continue to make incredible strides in surgical advancement by way of persistent innovation and the development of new technologies. The coming of the digital age, minimally invasive surgery, laser procedures, and implantable devices has made the field of surgery almost unrecognizable from what it was even 20 years ago.

49.3.2 Modern Medical Oversight

In order to explore the ethics of modern surgical advancements, it is important to understand how innovation is regulated. In the case of surgical technique, formal regulation does not currently exist. This is because surgery uses known anatomic landmarks to help guide the improvisation necessary to navigate a targeted pathology. No two patients are alike, and different approaches are used based on intraoperative findings and decisions. There are also variations in region, practice environment, and physician preference. Historically, surgical innovation has resulted from the endeavors of a few well-respected individuals who have shared their knowledge with the medical community for critique and adaptation [11]. The mentorship model of medicine means that an accepted technique or practice is then shared with trainees and adapted for their own personal use.

The lack of regulatory oversight in surgery has been deemed an ethical 'grey zone,' as there are significant improvements in patient care that can be made with this ability to refine techniques, but they are not risk-free [12]. For example, enthusiastic acceptance of laparoscopic cholecystectomy in the 1990s, while overall reducing morbidity and mortality, was associated with an increase in injury to the common bile duct [13]. There is no review board or advisory committee that vets every surgical method practiced and procedural variation. It is interesting to note that the distinction between a 'new' surgical technique and a 'minor variation' in an established procedure is not clearly defined, and so it is often unclear which new procedures necessitate human subject experimentation with oversight by an institutional review board (IRB).

We have limited objective data on surgeries due to the narrative nature of operative reports; medications, on the other hand, are categorically logged by time, dosage, and administration method. Procedural 'data' as it exists is often a subjective account in the form of an operative report and is often lacking the detail necessary to catalogue the nuances of the intervention [14]. A surgeon's outcomes can and should be monitored. Surgeons practicing risky maneuvers are, and should be, subject to institutional review and malpractice suits. Ultimately, however, it is up to surgeons to operate ethically, and to maintain honesty with patients and with themselves on their limitations of known and novel procedures.

49.3.3 The Role of the Food and Drug Administration in Regulating Medical Devices

The FDA was specifically designed for oversight of pharmaceuticals. Medications must undergo several stages of clinical trials both before and after they are approved for use in the general population (see Fig. 49.1). They are also classified based on their risks and benefits and labeled with any warnings deemed appropriate. This process takes several years, and only in rare instances is approval expedited [15].

While not as clearly delineated as the pharmaceutical regulation process, the FDA must also approve the sale of any new medical devices including diagnostic tests, implants, and instruments. This starts with classifying the risk of the device.

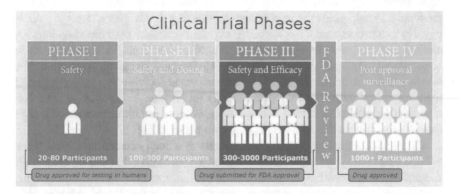

Fig. 49.1 Clinical trial phases. (https://www.ildcollaborative.org/resources/phase-iii-ipf-clinical-trials (public domain))

	% of Medical Devices	Examples	Potential Risk Level	Subject to
Class I Devices	47%	Toothbrushes, oxygen masks, elastic bandages	Low to none	"General" controls to ensure device safety and effectiveness once manufactured
Class II Devices	43%	Orthopedic and spine implants, IV pumps, ultrasound equipment	Potentially pose more risk	"General" control + "Special" controls (labeling, testing and performance standards)
Class III Devices	10%	Cardiac pacemakers, implantable defibrillators, coronary stents	Potential for adverse outcome	Premarket approval since they typically support or sustain life or are implanted in the body

Exempt – If a device falls into a generic category of an exempted Class I device, a premarket notification application and FDA clearance is not required before marketing the device in the U.S. However, the manufacturer is required to register its establishment and generic product with the FDA.

Examples: Manual toothbrushes and stethoscopes, mercury thermometers, bedpens

Fig. 49.2 FDA medical device classification. (https://healthtrustpg.com/thesource/clinical-connection/checks-and-balances/ (public domain))

All devices are classified from Class I (least risk to patient) to Class III (most risk to patient) based on indications and intended use (see Fig. 49.2). The manufacturer may classify their device based on FDA data and classification of existing similar devices or may request a formal classification by the FDA for a fee. The FDA may re-classify the device upon review [16].

A device may not be marketed within the United States until it has been approved or cleared by the FDA. Class III devices, or class II devices for which no existing device similar in safety and efficacy exists, must be approved through a process known as pre-market approval, which typically requires clinical trial data. Interestingly, more than 90% of devices on the US market are only 'cleared' by the FDA through the 510(k) pathway, with the FDA merely agreeing with the manufacturer that the device is as safe and effective as at least one other marketed device, or so-called 'predicate' device [17, 18]. This pathway does not generally require human clinical trial data, and post-marketing surveillance, while recommended, is in practice rarely requested. Finally, there are regulatory exemptions that do not require a 510(k) submission. This includes almost all Class I and many Class II devices [19]. Importantly, there is the possibility for abuse of the system by comparing a new medical device to an obsolete, or even dangerous, predicate with little or no clinical data. Introduction of these new devices instead relies upon the integrity of the device manufacturer, presuming that the company has done its due diligence.

Even in the case of new devices requiring pre-market approval, the level of clinical evidence is limited compared to that required of pharmaceuticals [17]. One example of this is the Essure implantable coil, a permanent birth control device implanted in the fallopian tubes. Placement is minimally invasive and can be done in the office setting. This class III device underwent one clinical trial before it was given premarket approval in 2002. Only 25% of patients in the clinical trial were followed for 2 years, and none were followed beyond that timeframe; the device was also not directly compared to other permanent sterilization methods such as tubal ligation. Unfortunately, postmarket studies demonstrated high rates of complications including chronic pelvic pain, allergic reactions, autoimmune responses, and unintended pregnancies. These complications often led to removal of the device, which sometimes resulted in the unique complication of retained metal fragments after attempted removal [20]. After public outcry, scrutiny, and lawsuits, the manufacturer did eventually remove the device from the market, but it was never formally recalled.

Furthermore, once a device is on the market, there is no required surveillance. The FDA monitors the ongoing safety and efficacy of medical devices via an online system for adverse event reporting called MedWatch. This system is also utilized to monitor pharmaceuticals, biologics, cosmetics, and food products after they are approved [21]. Both exempt and approved devices must be registered with the FDA for continued surveillance. Yet this system relies heavily on the voluntary participation of the manufacturer and the practitioners using these devices. Once again, appropriate oversight and the task of monitoring outcomes often falls to physicians.

How does the current process relate to the new medical device you are interested in implanting in your patient as presented in the case at the beginning of this chapter? There was one study demonstrating the safety and efficacy of the implant, which was approved by an IRB and performed by the manufacturer. The device has been approved by the 510(k) pathway as submitted by the manufacturer, which demonstrated that the device was similar to existing hypoglossal nerve stimulators. The new device you intend to implant, however, works by a different mechanism and is implanted in a different location within the neck than the previously approved device—so are they truly correlated? Was the comparison of these two devices enough to prove that your new implant is safe and effective?

49.3.4 Transparency in Surgical Innovation

As history has shown, and modern oversight reminds us, surgical advancement must go hand in hand with communication and transparency. Uncharted territory must be navigated carefully, with diligence on the part of the surgeon to ensure that these advancements are as safe and effective as they can be in their early stage of development and acceptance, that the patient is aware of the known and unknown risks, and that any conflicts of interest are acknowledged.

49.3.5 Research Vs Innovation

What is the difference between innovation and research? Surgical research is not clearly delineated from innovation, but research is typically regarded as generating generalizable knowledge by way of formal testing. For example, Dr. Semmelweiss was innovative in his identification of handwashing to reduce puerperal fever. When he practiced this intervention between his procedures and analyzed the results in his patients, he was performing research. He did not have the help of IRBs, as we do today, to help determine what is deemed human subjects research. A surgeon should always ask him- or herself if a given procedure should be performed on a patient without external oversight. If there is any question, it is reasonable to reach out to the IRB at that institution and get help in this determination. Yet IRBs are often composed largely of researchers, with few clinicians, so these committees may not be equipped to handle questions about the appropriateness of a novel surgical technique. Ideally, alternative avenues would be available, such as an innovation oversight committee, although these rarely exist and are not broadly institutionalized. In the absence of such resources, a good place to start would be to discuss a proposed innovation with colleagues who have expertise in your area and can provide a second opinion on feasibility and appropriateness.

Knowing the difference between research and innovation is important, not only for appropriate regulation but also for discussions with patients. Think like a patient for a moment. Would you like to be treated with cutting edge surgical techniques and breakthrough therapies? The answer is probably yes. Would you like to be a research study participant for an experimental surgical technique that hasn't been done before? Maybe not. Patients want cutting edge treatments, but they do not want to be the guinea pig. They want new, but not *that* new.

For this reason, transparency is always of the utmost importance when discussing a new procedure or device with a patient. Your sleep apnea device is new and innovative, but is it experimental? One study has shown it is safe and effective, but is that enough? It is up to you to be open with your patient about the limited data on this device, and to advise him that although this is not part of a clinical trial, it is still new. Now more than ever, patients want to be informed and to be a part of medical decision-making [22]. When it comes to new technologies, patients want to know— does it work [23]? Do the benefits outweigh the risks? What are the risks?

49.3.6   The Learning Curve and Surgical Training

Because patients want to be informed, communication is key. This requires an ongoing dialogue between a physician and a patient, which begins as early as the initial clinic evaluation.

The first important aspect of transparency comes from the surgeon's ability to discuss his or her own inexperience with the patient. Every new skill or technique is associated with a learning curve. Surgeons go through many years of residency training in existing procedures. Yet the training continues after residency, and even a skilled surgeon who has been practicing for years may inevitably struggle with adaptation of a new technique. This does not necessarily mean it is unsafe for a surgeon to attempt a new procedure, but it is not without risks. One cohort study in endonasal craniopharyngioma resection identified a distinct learning curve; after performing 20 cases there was a significant reduction in major neurological complications and overall better outcomes [24]. Yet for a physician to reach that point where outcomes improve, the procedure must be performed on those first few patients. The most important thing a surgeon can do is be up front about lack of experience and share with the patient that it is a procedure he or she is still learning.

This can be a tough discussion to have with a patient; while it is important to be truthful, it is also important to not cause undue alarm. The ethical thing may in fact be to provide reassurance on experiences that the surgeon *does* have and compare that to the new procedure while still being transparent about the lack of procedure-specific experiences.

When discussing with your patient, you can reference the countless surgeries you have already performed in the head and neck and the years of training you have undergone. It may be worthwhile to discuss other sleep apnea implants you have used, such as the hypoglossal nerve stimulators to which this new device was compared in order to seek FDA approval. You may tell the patient [1] yes, it is different, and you are still learning, [2] there will be a learning curve, and you will have to adapt what you already know to this new scenario, but [3] you are confident in your existing abilities, your knowledge of this anatomy, and your adaptability. It is possible to be transparent without sowing fear in your patient.

An attending surgeon may not be the only one learning in the operating room. Another important disclosure is whether any trainees will be present. Education for residents on new surgical techniques may be just as important as that of the attending; it shifts their learning curve earlier, to a time when they have oversight and can seek help from an attending if needed. One study showed that transitioning to endoscopic tympanoplasty, while simultaneously educating residents on the procedure, maintained good surgical outcomes with similar results to the conventional microscopic method [25]. Trainees are important for the structure of academic medicine and for our healthcare system in general, but their involvement should not be hidden from the patient. Always disclose whether fellows, residents, or medical students will be involved in patient care. The topic of surgical education is lengthy and complex; it is covered in more detail in Chaps. 11, 12, 13, 14, and 15.

49.3.7   *Disclosing Potential Conflicts of Interest*

Patient care comes first and should be the primary concern of any procedure. Disclosure to the patient must also incorporate any conflicts of interest the surgeon has, whether they be financial, personal, or professional. For example, if a surgeon developed a device and gets a fee for every time it is used, that is a financial conflict of interest that should be disclosed. If the surgeon's spouse is a sales representative for the device, that should be disclosed. Academic conflicts of interest without direct financial gain may be present as well. The surgeon could be under pressure from his or her department to perform the new procedure. Performing this surgery could be the tipping point toward a promotion in academic rank. Successful new procedures could lead to more acceptance of research grants and further surgical innovation.

Some bias may be present in the data a surgeon relies on due to conflicts of interest that occurred before the surgeon was even involved. For example, the main clinical trial that established safety and efficacy of the first hypoglossal nerve stimulator that was released to the market in 2016 was funded entirely by the device manufacturer [26]. It is unlikely that every surgeon now performing implantation of these devices discloses, or is even aware of, this historical financial conflict of interest that brought the device to market.

Other conflicts of interest extend to the relationship between the institution and industry. For example, the device company could provide payments or non-monetary gifts to the institution for performing the procedure. Institutions can also negotiate contracts with companies in which they sell certain patient data or demographics to device companies, which can help in advertising their products. Academic institutions also often enjoy broadcasting these new surgical techniques, which improves their reputation and attracts new patients to their healthcare network. This is termed the "halo effect," in which excellence in one aspect of healthcare leads to a perception that the same institution delivers high quality care across the board, although this is not always the case [27]. Regardless of the type of disclosure, the important takeaway is that transparency is key in all physician-patient communication. For more information on surgical communication and transparency, see Chap. 5.

Now consider if there is anything you should disclose to your patient about the new device you are considering. You were not directly involved in the development or sale of the device, but your boss' spouse is one of the creators. You feel like your chairman will respect you more if you participate in groundbreaking surgeries. You may get more research funds or even a promotion. You are eager to build an exciting practice, and this surgery could help you forge ahead in your academic career. If your patient were to have a negative outcome and then find out that you were pressured into it, his trust in you would be devastatingly broken.

As such, it is worthwhile to disclose your close relationship to the device creators; note that this may be a conflict of interest, but it may also be an asset. You can disclose your conflicts to the patient while also providing reassurance of your confidence in the device and your advantageous connections to the manufacturers, if those relationships do exist. If something were to go wrong, your patient is aware that you, and he, can potentially help to problem solve with the manufacturers and improve the device. This helps to create buy in from the patient and demonstrate that you are in this together. Again, honesty is the answer here. Be transparent and know that up-front communication is easier and can be a major asset, whereas trying to rehabilitate a broken patient-doctor relationship is often too little, too late.

49.3.8   Informed Consent

At this point you have already begun an open, honest discussion with the patient about the intended procedure. The next step is to discuss the risks and benefits of the procedure and to obtain written, informed consent from the patient.

The best way to discuss the risks and benefits of a new procedure is typically to discuss the alternatives. How does the new procedure compare to the gold standard? When discussing with your patient, you can compare this treatment to existing surgeries for OSA, to the implantable hypoglossal nerve stimulator, and to non-surgical treatments such as CPAP.

Many new techniques in surgery are meant to improve cosmesis rather than morbidity and mortality, so in these instances it is particularly important to highlight the differences between procedures and why they are performed. For example, a minimally invasive technique may reduce the appearance of a surgical scar, but if used in a cancer case it may not provide the best visualization and there is a risk of incomplete resection and persistent cancer.

Keep in mind that this patient's informed consent may not truly be as "informed" as it would be for a more established procedure. This is because at the early stages of development of new procedures and devices, we have very little information on the efficacy and long-term outcomes. Surgeons must explain what they know, but they must also explain the limits of their knowledge. If only a handful of patients have undergone the procedure, there may be unforeseen consequences that have not yet been encountered.

For this reason, the post-surgical care and monitoring of patients is of the utmost importance. This responsibility often falls to surgeons, as Dr. Codman told us over 100 years ago. We cannot simply perform a new surgery, or any surgery for that matter, and hope things go well; it is our duty to ensure close clinical follow up that is appropriate for each patient and procedure performed. Keeping tabs on your patients by way of close clinical follow up is the surgeon's version of stage IV clinical trials, or postmarket surveillance, that is performed for pharmaceuticals.

The ability to safeguard the health of patients is why physicians are often held to a higher standard. The ethics of when, why, how, and on whom to operate ultimately fall to the surgeon. The patient's care is entrusted to the practitioner, not just for the few hours they are in the operating room, but for weeks, months, and even years after the surgery is performed. This is why the American College of Surgeons' pledge is to "pursue the practice of surgery with honesty and to place the welfare and the rights of my patient above all else." [28].

49.3.9   The Principles of Bioethics: A Case Review

Let's return to our new hypothetical sleep apnea device. When we started, your patient was asking you about your outcomes in the procedure, and how other patients you've implanted have fared. But of course, you've never done this procedure before. Taking into account our detailed analysis within this chapter, what ethical considerations are there in this patient discussion?

This new device demonstrates **beneficence** by its ability to improve quality of life in people who have failed CPAP trial. Your patient may have an improvement in his hypertension and quality of life, which are very important to him. The procedure can also be an alternative to more painful procedures and does not require daily use like CPAP, which your patient failed. However, most surgeries do not work for everybody, and since it is a new device, it is difficult to prove the long-term efficacy of the device, and its overall benefit is not certain. There is no way to know the long-term effects of the device, because it simply has not been studied yet. The benefits may outweigh the risks for now, but we cannot know if the scales will tip unfavorably toward risk as time goes on.

Speaking of risks, this device requires a surgical implantation. An implanted foreign body carries inherent risk of infection, biofilm formation, and rejection. Avoiding these risks as much as possible is the important consideration of **nonmaleficence**. Since it is being implanted into the pharynx, there is also a risk of damage to important neurovascular structures, changes in swallowing, globus sensation, and difficulty breathing. You must disclose all of this to the patient. Again, since this is a new device, the risks we do not know are just as important to discuss. There are devices that were once thought perfectly safe that became problematic years later, and as such we cannot know exactly what long-term risks exist. We must first do no harm, and in this case, you must acknowledge that harm may exist without our knowledge or may arise in the future.

You also have not done this procedure before, and any surgery being performed without experience carries the possibility of complications. It is important to share with the patient that you are still learning. You can highlight the many surgeries you have performed in this anatomical location, citing completion of your training and several years of practice. Your knowledge of anatomy is adaptable to the new procedure and will help guide your decision-making in the operating room. Yet ultimately, this is something you have not done. Furthermore, you will have a resident with you helping you through the case. Residents are vital to our healthcare system, and sharing with your patient how and why your resident will be assisting is important for him to understand your judgment and to build trust.

The patient must know all of this in order to make an informed decision and exercise his or her **autonomy** as outlined in the declaration of Helsinki [29]. You should outline the known and unknown risks so that the patient can be as informed as possible. You also must keep any preconceived notions, bias, or influence out of the discussion, and disclose any conflicts you have. Your department chair is eager for you to begin these implantations, and his wife's role as device creator may have an influence on that. Disclosing this relationship to the patient is important. Fortunately, it also demonstrates your close working relationship with the device manufacturers and may be helpful in the future if the patient has questions for them. Additionally, having an implanted device requires quite a bit of motivation from the patient, who may need to return for frequent postoperative visits and long-term monitoring. You must make sure your patient is willing to put in this work to ensure safety and appropriate monitoring.

Unfortunately, this device is not available for everyone. The principle of **justice** ensures that the new device is distributed in as fair a way as possible. There are already limitations on who can be implanted, as patients must have first failed CPAP trial and must have a BMI <40. This patient has great health insurance that will cover the cost of the procedure, device, and postoperative follow up appointments. Could this make you see the patient as a more favorable candidate? It is important to be self-aware and to ensure that your medical decision-making is not swayed by reimbursement practices. On the other hand, this patient is very motivated. The responsible thing is to implant this device in motivated patients who can reliably make it to appointments and be monitored appropriately. Yet despite an equal distribution of the device, there will inevitably be unforeseen disparities and adverse outcomes.

Ultimately, the conversation with this patient needs to be factual, and it needs to be honest. The details of these discussions, the importance of transparency when considering new medical devices, and the four tenets of bioethics can all be drawn back to those simple, yet vital, characteristics of the discussion.

In this hypothetical scenario, your honesty with the patient about the device and your own inexperience, combined with your confidence in your abilities as a surgeon, engendered trust and created an open patient-physician relationship in which he could share his concerns and you could address them together. The patient underwent implantation of this new device without any major complications; at his postoperative visit he felt significant improvement in his sleep quality, while data from a repeat sleep study confirmed improvement in his sleep apnea.

49.4   Conclusion

Surgical innovation is a necessity, but history has shown us that it can be met with resistance that can either hinder necessary progress or keep important safety measures in check. New procedures always carry inherent risks. The development of new technologies and devices is regulated by the FDA, but ultimately much of the decision-making, patient safety, and ethical decisions come down to the surgeon. There is minimal oversight of the development of new surgical techniques, and so surgeons must keep themselves and their colleagues accountable. Our own field must self-regulate, and we must be able to classify what is novel enough to necessitate the appropriate clinical research prior to attempting a procedure on unsuspecting patients.

Throughout all stages of innovation, the surgeon must be transparent. This includes selecting the appropriate patients for new procedures and devices, disclosing the surgeon's own lack of experience and personal conflicts of interest, obtaining consent that is as informed as possible, and keeping up with postsurgical outcomes to monitor for unanticipated complications.

A concept that pervades new medical technologies is the unknown—the risks we cannot foresee, the learning curve associated with new procedures, and the lack of data available. As such, the unknowns must be discussed at length with the patient; they are arguably just as important as the knowns. Yet the field of surgery is continually changing, and a surgeon should not be afraid to embrace the unknown. We can continue to innovate as long as we do so with integrity and accept the ethical responsibility that befalls us to maintain the beneficence, nonmaleficence, autonomy, and justice of our patients.

49.5   Selected References

- Semmelweiss. Br Med J. 1893;1:26. doi:https://doi.org/10.1136/bmj.1.1671.26

  - Historical entry highlighting the work done by Dr. Ignaz Semmelweiss several decades earlier. He had been ridiculed and died in anonymity. The BMJ attempts to rebuild his reputation posthumously and credits him with initiating practices that by then had begun to take root in medicine and paved the way for the then widely accepted germ theory of disease

- Caruso JP, Sheehan JP. Psychosurgery, ethics, and media: a history of Walter Freeman and the lobotomy. Neurosurg Focus. 2017;43(3):E6. doi:https://doi.org/10.3171/2017.6focus17257

  - The history of the lobotomy procedure: its creation, intentions, and outcomes.

- Weil M. Rosemary Kennedy, 86; President's Disabled Sister. *Washington Post.* January 8, 2005; page B06. Accessed July 2020. https://www.washingtonpost.com/wp-dyn/articles/A58134-2005Jan8.html

  - Obituary for Rosemary Kennedy, one of the first victims of the surgical procedure lobotomy as treatment for mental retardation.

- Public Warning Against Hoxsey Cancer Treatment. Food and Drug Administration. U.S. Dept Health, Education, Welfare. Vol 74. April 4, 1956.

  - The FDA response to Harry Hoxsey's peddled anti-cancer tonics, discrediting him as a charlatan and warning the public about his fraudulent claims.

- Brown K, Solomon MJ, Young J, Seco M, Bannon PG. Addressing the ethical grey zone in surgery: a framework for identification and safe introduction of novel surgical techniques and procedures. ANZ J Surg. 2019;89:634–638. doi https://doi.org/10.1111/ans.15104

  – A review of surgical training and the process of developing new techniques, typically developed without oversight and passed from teacher to student with alterations and adjustments. This is termed an 'ethical grey zone' in which innovation can lead to improvement, but is not regulated and, if left unchecked, may be dangerous. The authors compare surgical training to the highly regulated pharmaceutical industry and propose possible regulatory methods with safety checkpoints and mandatory reporting of outcomes.

- Development & Approval Process: Drugs. FDA. 28 October 2019. Accessed February 12, 2021. https://www.fda.gov/drugs/development-approval-process-drugs. Classify Your Medical Device. FDA. 20 February 2020. Accessed February 12, 2021. https://www.fda.gov/medical-devices/overview-device-regulation/classify-your-medical-device. Premarket Notification 510(k). FDA. 13 March 2020. Accessed February 12, 2021. https://www.fda.gov/medical-devices/premarket-submissions/premarket-notification-510k

  – The above sources from the FDA website outline current policy in the regulation and oversight of medical devices and pharmaceuticals. Specific attention is paid to the 510 k pathway for medical device approval, in which safety and efficacy are compared to other devices in order to get approval, allowing for potential abuse if the new device has any significant variation from the predicate.

- Angelos P. Ethics and surgical innovation: challenges to the professionalism of surgeons. Int Jour Surg. 2013;11(S1):S2–S5. doi:https://doi.org/10.1016/s1743-9191(13)60003-5

  – An overview and evaluation of current methods in surgical innovation with emphasis on the evolution of informed consent, potential conflicts of interest, and the learning curve associated with new techniques. While innovation is important, ther is potential for unprofessionalism. The onus is on surgeons to act altruistically and provide checks and balances in their own practices when considering new surgical techniques.

- Strollo PJ, Soose RJ, MaurerJT, et al. Upper-Airway Stimulation for Obstructive Sleep Apnea. New Engl J Med. 2014;370:139–149. doi:https://doi.org/10.1056/NEJMoa1308659

  – Original investigation into the safety and efficacy of the hypoglossal nerve stimulator Inspire® which came to market in 2016. This research was funded entirely by the device manufacturer and highlights the importance of following funding to ensure no conflicts of interest exist.

References

1. Semmelweiss. Br Med J. 1893;1:26. https://doi.org/10.1136/bmj.1.1671.26.
2. Elliot GF. The germ-theory. Br Med J. 1870;1:488–9. https://doi.org/10.1136/bmj.1.489.488-a.
3. Nakayama DK. Antisepsis and asepsis and how they shaped modern surgery. Am Surg. 2018;84(6):766–71. https://doi.org/10.1177/000313481808400616.
4. Caruso JP, Sheehan JP. Psychosurgery, ethics, and media: a history of Walter freeman and the lobotomy. Neurosurg Focus. 2017;43(3):E6. https://doi.org/10.3171/2017.6focus17257.
5. Weil M. Rosemary Kennedy, 86; President's Disabled Sister. *Washington Post*. January 8, 2005; page B06. Accessed July 2020. https://www.washingtonpost.com/wp-dyn/articles/A58134-2005Jan8.html.
6. Beitner MM, Ren-Fielding CJ, Fielding GA. Reducing complications with improving gastric band design. Surg Obes Relat Dis. 2016;12(1):150–6. https://doi.org/10.1016/j.soard.2015.08.520.
7. Public Warning Against Hoxsey Cancer Treatment. Food and Drug Administration. U.S. Dept Health, Education, Welfare. Vol. 74. April 4, 1956.
8. Lapkin A. The Bizarre history of a bogus doctor who prescribed goat gonads. National Geographic Family. July 15, 2016. Accessed February 12, 2021. https://www.nationalgeographic.com/news/2016/07/documentary-interview-medicine-science/.
9. Day M. Disgraced tracheal transplant surgeon is handed 16 month prison sentence in Italy. BMJ. 2019;367:16676. https://doi.org/10.1136/bmj.16676.
10. Ernest Armory Codman. Wikipedia. Wikimedia Foundation. 10 May 2020. Accessed 22 July 2020. https://en.wikipedia.org/wiki/Ernest_Amory_Codman.
11. Riskin DJ, Longaker MT, Gertner M, Krummel TM. Innovation in surgery: a historical perspective. Ann Surg. 2006;244(5):686–93. https://doi.org/10.1097/01.sla.0000242706.91771.ce.
12. Brown K, Solomon MJ, Young J, Seco M, Bannon PG. Addressing the ethical grey zone in surgery: a framework for identification and safe introduction of novel surgical techniques and procedures. ANZ J Surg. 2019;89:634–8. https://doi.org/10.1111/ans.15104.
13. van de Graaf FW, Zaimi I, Stassen LPS, Lange JF. Safe laparoscopic cholecystectomy: a systematic review of bile duct injury prevention. Int J Surg. 2018;60:164–72. https://doi.org/10.1016/j.ijsu.2018.11.006.
14. van de Graaf FW, Lange MM, Spakman JI. Comparison of systematic video documentation with narrative operative report in colorectal cancer surgery. JAMA Surg. 2019;154(5):381–9. https://doi.org/10.1001/jamasurg.2018.5246.
15. Development & Approval Process: Drugs. FDA. 28 October 2019. Accessed February 12, 2021. https://www.fda.gov/drugs/development-approval-process-drugs.
16. Classify Your Medical Device. FDA. 20 February 2020. Accessed February 12, 2021. https://www.fda.gov/medical-devices/overview-device-regulation/classify-your-medical-device.
17. Premarket Notification 510(k). FDA. 13 March 2020. Accessed February 12, 2021. https://www.fda.gov/medical-devices/premarket-submissions/premarket-notification-510k.
18. Rathi VK, Ross JS. Modernizing the FDA's 510(k) pathway. N Engl J Med. 2019;381(20):1891–3. https://doi.org/10.1056/nejmp1908654.
19. Medical Device Exemptions 510(k) and GMP Requirements. FDA. 8 Fevruary 2021. Accessed February 12, 2021. https://www.accessdata.fda.gov/scripts/cdrh/cfdocs/cfpcd/315.cfm.
20. Walter JR, Ghobadi CW, Hayman E, Xu S. Hysteroscopic sterilization with Essure: summary of the U.S. Food and Drug Administration actions and policy implications for Postmarketing surveillance. Obstet Gynecol. 2017;129:10–9. https://doi.org/10.1097/aog.0000000000001796.
21. MedWatch: The FDA Safety Information and Adverse Event Reporting Program. FDA. 10 February 2021. Accessed February 12, 2021. https://www.fda.gov/safety/medwatch-fda-safety-information-and-adverse-event-reporting-program.
22. Angelos P. Ethics and surgical innovation: challenges to the professionalism of surgeons. Int Jour Surg. 2013;11(S1):S2–5. https://doi.org/10.1016/s1743-9191(13)60003-5.

23. Benz HL, Saha A, Tarver ME. Integrating the voice of the patient into the medical device regulatory process using patient preference information. Value Health. 2020;23(3):294–7. https://doi.org/10.1016/j.jval.2019.12.005.
24. Kshettry VF, Do H, Elshazly K, et al. The learning curve in endoscopic endonasal resection of craniopharyngiomas. Neurosurg Focus. 2016;41(6):E9. https://doi.org/10.3171/2016.9FOCUS16292.
25. Li B, Asche S, Yang R, Yueh B, Fina M. Outcomes of adopting endoscopic Tympanoplasty in an academic teaching hospital. Ann Otol Rhinol Laryngol. 2019;128(6):548–55. https://doi.org/10.1177/0003489419830424.
26. Strollo PJ, Soose RJ. MaurerJT, et al. upper-airway stimulation for obstructive sleep Apnea. New Engl J Med. 2014;370:139–49. https://doi.org/10.1056/NEJMoa1308659.
27. Brown EG, Anderson JE, Burgess D, Bold RJ. Examining the "halo effect" of surgical care within health systems. JAMA Surg. 2016;151(10):983–4. https://doi.org/10.1001/jamasurg.2016.1000.
28. American College of Surgeons. Statements on Principles. April 12, 2016. Accessed September 23, 2020. https://www.facs.org/about-acs/statements/stonprin.
29. WMA Declaration of Helsinki – Ethical Principles for Medical Research Involving Human Subjects. World Medical Association. 9 July 2018. Accessed February 14, 2021. https://www.wma.net/policies-post/wma-declaration-of-helsinki-ethical-principles-for-medical-research-involving-human-subjects/.

Chapter 50
Uterus Transplantation

Anji Wall (ID) **and Giuliano Testa** (ID)

Abstract As a non-life-saving, temporary transplant intended for the specific purpose of enabling women with absolute uterine factor infertility to carry and deliver their own pregnancy, uterus transplantation (UTx) has engendered substantial ethical debate from its earliest stages of pre-clinical research. Currently in the phase of clinical trials, research protocols require graft hysterectomy (in the absence of complications necessitating earlier removal) at the earlier of five years or delivery of a second pregnancy, to minimize the risks of long-term immunosuppressive therapy, given that there is no off-setting medical benefit to retaining the uterus after achieving the goal of delivering a healthy baby. A novel dilemma has arisen in the context of UTx recipients who do not wish to undergo graft hysterectomy as required under these protocols. This dilemma pits respect for the recipient's autonomy against the transplant team's obligations to avoid unnecessary harm and to maximize the benefit of medical interventions. This chapter addresses the unique ethical challenge presented—how should the transplant team navigate patient preferences to defer or not undergo graft hysterectomy?

Keywords Uterus transplantation · Graft hysterectomy · Informed consent Research ethics · Surgical ethic

A. Wall (✉) · G. Testa
Annette C. and Harold C. Simmons Transplant Institute, Baylor University Medical Center, Dallas, TX, USA
e-mail: anji.wall@bswhealth.org; Giuliano.Testa@bswhealth.org

© The Author(s), under exclusive license to Springer Nature Switzerland AG 2022
V. A. Lonchyna et al. (eds.), *Difficult Decisions in Surgical Ethics*, Difficult Decisions in Surgery: An Evidence-Based Approach,
https://doi.org/10.1007/978-3-030-84625-1_50

705

Case

A 34-year-old female is three years status post uterus transplantation from a living unrelated donor. She had no complications from the operation and has had one successful live birth. She is currently in the second trimester of pregnancy with a second child. The fetus is developing appropriately, and the uterus transplant recipient has not had any pregnancy related complications. In her prenatal visits, the UTx team has discussed the need to remove the graft after this pregnancy because they limit the number of pregnancies for recipients to two and have a graft recipient time limit of five years so as to avoid the risks associated with long term immunosuppressive medications. The recipient has stated numerous times that she is not yet ready for a graft hysterectomy. The medical team is struggling to navigate this disagreement.

50.1 Introduction

Uterus transplantation (UTx) is a surgical procedure that combines the fields of solid organ transplantation and assisted reproductive technology (ART). Currently, UTx is only performed under research protocols in the United States. UTx is truly a process rather than a procedure, with success defined as a healthy live birth. To achieve success, UTx recipients undergo transplantation, induction of immunosuppression, embryo transfer, pregnancy, and cesarean section. As an experimental surgical procedure that is both an organ transplant and an assistive reproductive technology, the ethical questions surrounding uterus transplantation are numerous and the frameworks used for addressing ethical issues are drawn from each of these fields [1]. From the organ transplant standpoint, ethical questions include how to elicit appropriate informed consent for deceased and living uterus donation, if living donation meets the requirement of nonmaleficence and beneficence and how to justly allocate the limited supply of donor organs [2, 3]. From an assisted reproductive technology perspective, questions have arisen about if the risks and benefits of the procedure are appropriately balanced, if the alternative options of surrogacy or adoption should be preferred from both a risk/benefit perspective and from a justice perspective, and the extent to which we should respect reproductive autonomy in the setting of UTx [4–7]. Finally, from the perspective of an experimental surgical procedure, ethical concerns include determining the best approach for informed consent given the multitude of unknowns about the procedure, deciding how to balance the individualized UTx recipient care with research protocols, and determining how to maintain transparency of clinical trial results [8, 9]. While all of these ethical questions are important in uterus transplantation, this case specifically deals with the question of how to address the conflicting recommendation of the UTx team for the Utx recipient to undergo a graft hysterectomy versus the UTx recipient's desire to keep the graft. Analysis of this specific ethical question requires utilization of research and clinical ethics frameworks. Using the seven requirements of ethical

Table 50.1 Ethical principles and application to the case

Ethical principle	Example of application to the case
Respect for autonomy	The UTx recipient did not want to undergo graft hysterectomy and had decision-making capacity so if she maintains this position, the principle has priority over other considerations.
Respect for enrolled research subjects	Because this is a research trial, the UTx recipient is also protected by human subjects' research regulations which require that human subjects have the authority to withdraw from studies if they chose to do so. The UTx recipient could elect to keep the uterus and withdraw from the research trial.
Nonmaleficience	Both the proposed procedure, graft hysterectomy, and the alternative of keeping the graft and staying on immunosuppression have risks of harm.
Beneficence	Since both options have the risk of harm to the UTx recipient, this must be balanced with the potential benefits. The benefit of graft hysterectomy is the withdrawal of immunosuppression and the mitigation of long-term risks. There is no medical benefit to keeping the graft in place but there might be a perceived psychological benefit.

research developed by Emanual and colleagues, the two that are most pertinent to this care are ensuring a favorable risk benefit ratio and respect for enrolled subjects with a specific focus on the right of the participant to withdraw from the research trial [10]. The underlying clinical ethical principles most relevant to this case are respect for autonomy, nonmaleficence and beneficence [10]. In this chapter, we use the research and clinical ethics principles described here to analyze and resolve the case of disagreement about the graft hysterectomy procedure (see Table 50.1).

50.2 Search Strategy

A search was conducted in PubMed using the search terms: Uterus transplantation and ethics; Uterus transplantation and informed consent; Uterus transplantation and reproductive autonomy; Vascular Composite Allotransplantation and ethics; Research ethics; Ethics and assisted reproductive technology; Surgical ethics. Years searched were 2000–2021.

50.3 Historical Perspectives on Uterus Transplantation

Uterus transplantation is the only medical option for women with absolute uterine factor infertility (AUFI) who desire to experience pregnancy and child birth. Proof of the concept of UTx as a procedure to restore fertility began in small animal studies. The first successful live birth after UTx in an animal model was in a mouse in 2003 [11]. The first large animal study to achieve successful UTx was a sheep model in Columbia which resulted in 3 of 12 sheep achieving pregnancy and subsequent successful live births [12]. Non-human primates were the next step in animal research on UTx. The first non-human primate study of UTx was in baboons, in which 20% of the subjects reestablished menstruation [13]. An allogenic UTx performed on a baboon from a living donor achieved greater than 12-month graft survival but did not result in a live birth [14]. The first non-human primate UTx to result in a live birth was in a macaque monkey in Japan [15]. This team performed a study of allogenic UTx in macaques and were able to achieve resumption of menstruation but no pregnancies in a subsequent cohort [16].

The first successful human uterus transplant was reported in 2014 in Sweden, with a baby born from a UTx recipient who had received a uterus graft from a living donor [17]. In 2016, the first successful live birth after a deceased donor UTx occurred in Brazil [18]. The first live birth after living donor UTx in the United States was reported in Dallas [19]. To date, more than 60 UTx have been done worldwide and more than 20 live births have been delivered [20, 21].

50.4 Technical Aspects of Uterus Transplantation

Uterus transplantation begins with the donation of a uterus graft. The uterus graft is procured either from a deceased or living donor. The deceased donor procurement can either be done in a similar fashion to other abdominal organs, where warm dissection is followed by flush and then extraction, or through a workflow similar to living donor procurement, where the uterus is removed prior to cold flush of the other organs [18, 22]. The living donor operation is done either through a lower midline laparotomy or with a minimally invasive approach [23, 24]. The most technically challenging aspect of the living donor uterus procurement is dissection of the uterine vessels as they run deep into the pelvis very close to the ureters. The robotic donor hysterectomy technique allows for excellent visualization of the vessels and the ureters, and uterus can be extracted through the vagina, so the donor has only a few small incisions for the robotic ports [23]. The UTx recipient procedure is done through a lower midline incision with exposure of the external iliac arteries and veins bilaterally and the vaginal cuff. The donor uterine arteries and veins are anastomosed to the recipient external iliac arteries and veins, respectively in an end to side fashion, bilaterally. The donor vagina is anastomosed to the recipient vagina in an end to end fashion.

50.5 The Process of Uterus Transplantation

Uterus transplantation is a process rather than a single procedure. First, potential recipients are screened for medical and psychological suitability [24]. Following evaluation, potential recipients must go through in vitro fertilization (IVF) and have a minimum number of high-quality embryos, as determined by the transplant program prior to listing for UTx. After listing, the recipient either schedules and undergoes UTx from a living donor or is placed on the waiting list for deceased donor UTx. Following the transplant, uterus function is first demonstrated by return of menstruation, which should occur by 90 days post transplantation [25]. The next step for recipients is to undergo embryo transfer (ET), which can be done as early as thre months post UTx. The timing of ET depends on immunosuppression regimen, infection risk and graft stability [26]. If embryo transfer is successful, recipients carry the pregnancy to viability and deliver via cesarean section. If there are medical contraindications to a subsequent pregnancy or the recipient does not desire a subsequent pregnancy, a graft hysterectomy can be done at the time of delivery or in the post-partum period. If the recipient desires a second pregnancy, the uterus remains in place and the process of embryo transfer proceeds again when she is medically and psychologically ready, within the confines of the center-specific policy on maximum graft-recipient time [26].

50.6 The Unique Characteristics of Uterus Transplantation

The aim of UTx is to restore normalcy by transplanting a uterus from a deceased or a living donor to a woman with congenital or acquired absence of the uterus. The uniqueness of UTx is evident even in comparison to transplants like hand and face. The latter aim at restoring normalcy in everyday functions. They make the recipients closer to "normal" by been able to use their hand instead of a prosthesis and going out in public without psychological trauma. Uterus transplant restores normalcy for one unique function: reproduction; its aim is the birth of the child. It is a transplant that is not intended to replace function indefinitely, since the lack of the uterus does not cause any physical functional deficits. It is, therefore, a temporary transplant that will be removed once one or two babies have been delivered. The alternative pathways to parenthood, adoption and surrogacy, do provide the couple with a family but do not offer the "normal" experience of pregnancy and delivery.

50.7 An Overview of Ethical Issues Raised in Uterus Transplantation

Even during the human pre-clinical phase, the ethical debate about UTx was intense. Questions were raised regarding its necessity since valid alternatives for parenthood already existed. Specifically, the ethical analysis of the necessity of uterus transplantation focused on the ethical principles of nonmaleficence, doing no harm, and beneficence, or ensuring an appropriate balance of risks and benefits. Is uterus transplantation harmful to women both psychologically and physically? Are the myriad potential and unknown risks of uterus transplantation outweighed by the potential benefit of gestational motherhood? [3, 27] Specific beneficence related questions were also raised regarding performing a procedure to allow a woman to carry her own pregnancy when the transplanted uterus could not transmit the same sensation of a "normal" uterus, making the experience of pregnancy absent [4]. In the context of non-maleficence and risk-benefit ratio for the living uterus donor, many questioned if the risks are justified since UTx is not a life-saving procedure. In addition, when family members are potential donors, there were concerns expressed about the potential for coercion to donate [28, 29].

The role of reproductive autonomy in uterus transplantation has also been addressed in ethical discourse. For example, the alternative option of adoption is often characterized as superior: why would a woman undergo UTx with all of the associated risks when so many children are awaiting adoption? [30] In addition, some question if uterus transplantation can be conceptualized in a similar way to other ART because it is so much more complex than other ART procedures like IVF [4, 31]. Additional concerns include the fear that the option of uterus transplantation will perpetuate the notion of a woman's worth being linked to child-bearing [29, 32].

Distributive justice concerns about access to uterus transplantation have been discussed as well. From a financial standpoint, why would society invest limited financial resources, especially when provided by a government, for a non-life saving transplant when many life-saving procedures are underfunded and need financial support? [28, 33]

Research ethics concerns, especially vulnerability to the therapeutic misconception being a primary example have also been described in ethical discourse about UTx. Would women with AUFI overestimate the benefits and underestimate the harms of UTx, thereby undermining their ability to make an autonomous decision or truly participate in informed consent? Even more fundamentally, with uterus transplant being a novel procedure with unknown risks and potential complications for all parties involved, recipient, child and donor, there were concerns about how to design a proper informed consent process for UTx clinical trial participation.

Some of these questions have been fully or partially answered with data from clinical trials. For example, there is greater certainty regarding the potential benefit of UTx with the successful births of many children following UTx in different parts of the world [20, 21]. Much more information is now available regarding the type and incidence of complications for all parties involved, allowing for a more appropriate informed consent[23, 34, 35]. Case reports of pregnancy during UTx also reveal that recipients have the same sensations as described in "normal" pregnancies and gain significant value from the gestational experience [36].

While all of the ethical challenges with UTx warrant significant attention, the purpose of this chapter is to address the unique ethical challenge presented in the case—how should the transplant team navigate patient preferences to defer or not undergo graft hysterectomy?

50.8 Case Discussion: Addressing Conflicts Over Graft Hysterectomy

In the Dallas UtErus Transplant Study (DUETS), the UTx team at Baylor University Medical Center in Dallas performed 20 uterus transplants, 18 from living donors and two from deceased donors. This study resulted in the first live birth after UTx in the US and has now reported 12 live births following UTx [19, 37]. The DUETS team has anecdotally found that UTx recipients often feel reluctant to part with the uterus after the delivery of a child or children, when the transplanted uterus has exhausted its intended function.

As mentioned above, uterus transplant is designed to be a temporary transplant. Most of the existing UTx protocols have a time limit, after which a graft hysterectomy is performed because of the known side effect of the immunosuppressive medications and the need to limit the uterus transplant recipient's exposure. Most of the UTx research protocols have a graft-recipient time limit of five years [26]. And, it is possible that despite a technically successful uterus transplant, the subsequent embryo transfers will not materialize into a pregnancy within that timeframe, resulting in an unsuccessful transplant. Importantly, although a second pregnancy is discussed as an option with potential UTx recipients, this possibility is incumbent upon the absence of complications suffered during the first pregnancy or complications suffered because of the immunosuppression. No matter the reason—because of reached time limit, complicated pregnancy or immunosuppressive complications—a conflict arises when the wish of the uterus transplant recipient to retain the uterus collides with the medical opinion or time limitation of the transplant team recommending removal.

This is a new, interesting scenario previously unknown to the field of transplantation. If anything, the opposite has happened in hand transplantation where some patients have asked to have their newly transplanted limb removed because they are not achieving their desired quality of life with the transplanted hand. There are different reasons why the recipient of a uterus transplant would want to retain the uterus: the wish to have a pregnancy in a case in which the five years have gone by without success; the wish to have a second pregnancy; the wish not to depart from the new feeling of wholeness that the presence of the uterus has given. The latter is peculiarly important because restoring "anatomical normalcy" per se is not the purpose of uterus transplant; UTx is a means to achieve pregnancy and delivery of a healthy child or children.

Nonetheless it is understandable how a woman born without an essential organ would feel "whole" after its transplant. There is plenty of evidence that the congenital lack of the uterus and consequent lack of menstrual periods is a reason for adolescent trauma [38]. This trauma is intensified when women with AUFI try to navigate relationships and plan their families. The wish to retain the transplanted uterus, whether for psychological or purely functional reasons can be very strong in UTx patients. On the other hand, the desire to remove the transplanted uterus so as to protect the long-term well-being of the recipient is also a defensible and reasonable position for the transplant team.

The ethical challenge that the transplant team is facing is that the recipient is opting for a choice that will cause harm and has no medical or reproductive benefit. Respecting her autonomous choice conflicts with their obligation to avoid unnecessary harm as well as their obligation to maximize the benefit of medical interventions and minimize the risks. This ethical dilemma is made more challenging because this patient underwent UTx in the context of a research trial, so the results are even more intensely scrutinized by regulatory bodies and by peer review of research publications. From a research ethics perspective, the two underlying benchmarks most applicable to this care are ensuring a favorable risk benefit ratio and respect for enrolled subjects with a specific focus on the right of the participant to withdraw from the research trial [10].

Starting from the principle of respect for autonomy for surgical patients and respect for the enrolled subjects from a research ethics framework, in UTx research trials, each potential recipient is informed of the risks and benefits as well as the process of UTx and gives her informed consent for the procedure at the beginning of the process but also provides informed consent for each independent procedure that is subsequently performed (e.g., cervical biopsies, stricture revision, cesarean section). So, while the recipient consented to the whole process up front, she is given the opportunity to refuse interventions throughout the process. In addition, beyond the right to refuse any given intervention, research participants also have the right to withdraw from research trials altogether which could be an option for this research participant.

If the UTx recipient refuses to consent to the graft hysterectomy, as is a real possibility in the case presented at the start of this chapter, how should the transplant team respond? There are a variety of options for the team when faced with this situation. At the one extreme, the transplant team can agree with the recipient's new autonomous decision and leave the uterus in place. By putting respect for autonomy and respect for enrolled subjects first, the research team will be infringing on the competing ethical principles of non-maleficence, beneficence and ensuring a favorable risk-benefit ratio in research studies. The risk of not performing graft hysterectomy is related to the long-term risks of immunosuppression treatment (e.g., cancer and infectious complications), which will be necessary to maintain graft viability. The team could allow the patient to keep the graft but recommend withdrawal of immunosuppression which will almost certainly result in graft rejection and ultimately result in the need for graft hysterectomy. Therefore, to maintain the viability of the uterus, the team must continue prescribing the immunosuppressive medications needed to avoid rejection. One option in this case is to remove the patient from the research protocol to respect her decision to not undergo graft hysterectomy and transfer her clinical care to another physician. While UTx is novel procedure there is precedent for the transfer of post-transplant immunosuppression from the transplant surgical team to a medical team in other solid organ transplants. Despite this precedent, it would be very unlikely for another physician to be comfortable taking over the care of a UTx recipient who underwent a procedure in the research trial and still has the graft in place. Realistically, the care of the UTx recipient would certainly remain with the research team as finding a physician willing to take over management would be almost impossible.

At the other extreme, the transplant team could utilize the initial consent of the recipient, refuse to accept her new decision and proceed with graft hysterectomy, acting in a way that minimizes the harm of ongoing immunosuppression. While this option is in line with minimizing long term harms, it risks the physical and psychological harms associated with graft hysterectomy and it infringes on respect for autonomy and respect for enrolled subjects. Moreover, practically speaking, the team cannot force the UTx recipient to have a surgery she refuses to undergo. Given that the uterus is within the recipient and removal requires a surgical procedure, the recipient has a stronger claim to the uterus then the medical team and it is far-fetched to propose that the team would ever be empowered to remove the uterus, even if leaving it may mean causing harm to the mother.

While the theoretical option of keeping the uterus in place and transferring the care of a UTx patient to another physician would practically solve the dilemma of non-abandonment, it does not solve the dilemma of resolving the conflicting views of the parties involved. As we will discuss below, neither extreme option is desirable, and the ideal situation is to develop a conflict resolution process with a third-party involved to bring the transplant team and the UTx recipient to a consensus.

Before getting to the point of total disagreement and having to decide on who has the ultimate claim on what happens to the transplant uterus, the transplant team and recipient have an opportunity to come to an agreement about the graft hysterectomy through conflict resolution. The DUETS protocol addresses the need for graft hysterectomy at the conclusion of childbearing or at 5 years post-transplant as part of the initial informed consent process. In addition, the discussion of timing of graft hysterectomy or desire for a second pregnancy is revisited in the first trimester of the first pregnancy. In our updated protocol, we include our clinical psychologist in the discussions about the timing of graft hysterectomy and the potential for a second pregnancy so she can help the recipients navigate these decisions. From our experiences, we believe that the discussions about graft hysterectomy must happen at multiple time points and should include a third party, ideally the transplant team psychologist or psychiatrist who understands the patient's emotional attachment to the uterus and underlying motivations for her decisions. It is essential that the team explores the recipient's reasons for not wanting to proceed with the graft hysterectomy. We have found that recipients not only have an emotional attachment to the graft and feel a sense of loss when it is removed, but that they also have strong personal preferences about the timing of graft hysterectomy. For example, some do not want their graft removed at the time of delivery because they will always associate that loss with the birth of their child. By having multiple conversations about graft hysterectomy with recipients, involving the team psychologist or psychiatrist, and giving recipients decisional authority over the timing of the graft hysterectomy, the possibility of an agreement to proceed with graft hysterectomy is more likely than not. If the recipient continues to refuse the graft hysterectomy, the conflict resolution process can help the team and UTx recipient navigate the best resolution when it comes to management of immunosuppression and graft surveillance going forward.

50.9 Case Conclusion

In this case, with the involvement of the team psychologist, the UTx recipient agreed to undergo graft hysterectomy as was recommended by the team. She elected to have the procedure done post-partum so that it was not associated with the timing of the birth of her second child.

50.10 Concluding Remarks

Uterus transplantation is a novel surgical procedure that allows women with AUFI to have the opportunity to carry and deliver their own child. The alternatives to UTx, adoption and surrogacy, result in parenthood but do not offer the experience of gestation. The unique features of UTx—quality of life transplant, temporary nature, and goal of childbirth—all contribute to the myriad of ethical issues associated with this procedure. In this chapter, we address one specific ethical issue that we have identified in the DUETS UTx clinical trial, the disagreement between a UTx recipient and the transplantation team about graft hysterectomy. While UTx recipients provide consent for "all" elements of UTx prior to their inclusion in the clinical trial, they also provide individual consent for each procedure that happens. They may agree to graft hysterectomy at the outset and change their minds later in the clinical course. Ultimately, the recipient has the final say and must consent to a graft hysterectomy. However, it is the role of the transplant team to navigate this difficult decision and encourage the patient to undergo graft hysterectomy.

50.11 Selected References

- Arora KS, Blake V. Uterus transplantation: ethical and regulatory challenges. J Med Ethics. 2014;40:396–400. https://doi.org/10.1136/medethics-2013-101400.
  - This article highlights several of the ethical questions about uterus transplantation, including living versus deceased donation and uterus graft allocation.
- Johannesson L, Testa G, Flyckt R, et al. Guidelines for standardized nomenclature and reporting in uterus transplantation: an opinion from the United States Uterus Transplant Consortium. Am J Transplant. 2020;20:3319–25. https://doi.org/10.1111/ajt.15973.
  - This manuscript provides guidance on standardizing both the terminology and outcomes reporting for uterus transplantation which is essential to a new field in order to ensure consistency and transparency to patients.

- Johannesson L, Wall A, Putman JM, Zhang L, Testa G, Diaz-Garcia C. Rethinking the time interval to embryo transfer after uterus transplantation—DUETS (Dallas UtErus Transplant Study). BJOG. 2019;126:1305–9. https://doi.org/10.1111/1471-0528.15860.

  - This manuscript argues that the amount of time that a recipeint has the uterus graft in place should be minimized in order to decrease immunosuppression exposure and the ensuing risks of cancer and infections.

- Testa G, Johannesson L. The ethical challenges of uterus transplantation. Curr Opin Organ Transplant. 2017;22:593–7. https://doi.org/10.1097/mot.0000000000000467.

  - This manuscript provides an overview of ethical issues associated with uterus transplantation when the field was in the very early stages and prior to the first reported successful uterus translant in the US.

- Testa G, McKenna GJ, Bayer J, et al. The evolution of transplantation from saving lives to fertility treatment: DUETS (Dallas UtErus Transplant Study). Ann Surg. 2020;272:411–7. https://doi.org/10.1097/sla.0000000000004199.

  - This manuscript details the procedural and patient care evoluation of uterus transplantation during the largest clinical trial of uterus trnaslant in the world. It specifcally details how failures were addressed and how each case was a learing experience for the next.

- Wall A, Johannesson L, Testa G, Warren AM. Two cases of pregnancy following uterine transplant: an ethical analysis. Narrative Inq Bioeth. 2020;10:263–8. https://doi.org/10.1353/nib.2020.0074.

  - This manuscript is the first case series that describes how uterus transplant recipients actually experience pregnancy and childbirth. In these two cases, the UTx recipients felt that they had 'normal' pregnancy experience and that they gained significant personal value from their pregnancies.

References

1. Horvat M, Iltis A. What are good guidelines for evaluating uterus transplantation? AMA J Ethics. 2019;21:E988–95. https://doi.org/10.1001/amajethics.2019.988.
2. Bruno B, Arora KS. Uterus transplantation: the ethics of using deceased versus living donors. Am J Bioeth. 2018;18:6–15. https://doi.org/10.1080/15265161.2018.1478018.
3. O'Donovan L, Williams NJ, Wilkinson S. Ethical and policy issues raised by uterus transplants. Br Med Bull. 2019;131:19–28. https://doi.org/10.1093/bmb/ldz022.
4. McTernan E. Uterus transplants and the insufficient value of gestation. Bioethics. 2018;32:481–8. https://doi.org/10.1111/bioe.12523.
5. O'Donovan L. Pushing the boundaries: uterine transplantation and the limits of reproductive autonomy. Bioethics. 2018;32:489–98. https://doi.org/10.1111/bioe.12531.

6. Testa G, Johannesson L. The ethical challenges of uterus transplantation. Curr Opin Organ Transplant. 2017;22:593–7. https://doi.org/10.1097/mot.0000000000000467.

7. Lotz M. Uterus transplantation as radical reproduction: taking the adoption alternative more seriously. Bioethics. 2018;32:499–508. https://doi.org/10.1111/bioe.12490.

8. Petrini C, Gainotti S, Morresi A, Nanni CA. Ethical issues in uterine transplantation: psychological implications and informed consent. Transplant Proc. 2017;49:707–10. https://doi.org/10.1016/j.transproceed.2017.02.013.

9. Arora KS, Blake V. Uterus transplantation: ethical and regulatory challenges. J Med Ethics. 2014;40:396–400. https://doi.org/10.1136/medethics-2013-101400.

10. Emanuel EJ, Wendler D, Grady C. What makes clinical research ethical? JAMA. 2000;283:2701–11. https://doi.org/10.1001/jama.283.20.2701.

11. Racho El-Akouri R, Kurlberg G, Brannstrom M. Successful uterine transplantation in the mouse: pregnancy and post-natal development of offspring. Hum Reprod. 2003;18:2018–23. https://doi.org/10.1093/humrep/deg396.

12. Ramirez ER, Ramirez Nessetti DK, Nessetti MBR, et al. Pregnancy and outcome of uterine allotransplantation and assisted reproduction in sheep. J Minim Invasive Gynecol. 2011;18:238–45. https://doi.org/10.1016/j.jmig.2010.11.006.

13. Enskog A, Johannesson L, Chai DC, et al. Uterus transplantation in the baboon: methodology and long-term function after auto-transplantation. Hum Reprod. 2010;25:1980–7. https://doi.org/10.1093/humrep/deq109.

14. Johannesson L, Enskog A, Molne J, et al. Preclinical report on allogeneic uterus transplantation in non-human primates. Hum Reprod. 2013;28:189–98. https://doi.org/10.1093/humrep/des381.

15. Kisu I, Mihara M, Banno K, et al. A new surgical technique of uterine auto-transplantation in cynomolgus monkey: preliminary report about two cases. Arch Gynecol Obstet. 2012;285:129–37. https://doi.org/10.1007/s00404-011-1901-2.

16. Kisu I, Mihara M, Banno K, et al. Uterus allotransplantation in cynomolgus macaque: a preliminary experience with non-human primate models. J Obstet Gynaecol Res. 2014;40:907–18. https://doi.org/10.1111/jog.12302.

17. Brannstrom M, Johannesson L, Bokstrom H, et al. Livebirth after uterus transplantation. Lancet. 2015;385:607–16. https://doi.org/10.1016/s0140-6736(14)61728-1.

18. Ejzenberg D, Andraus W, Baratelli Carelli Mendes LR, et al. Livebirth after uterus transplantation from a deceased donor in a recipient with uterine infertility. Lancet. 2019;392:2697–704. https://doi.org/10.1016/s0140-6736(18)31766-5.

19. Testa G, McKenna GJ, Gunby RT Jr, et al. First live birth after uterus transplantation in the United States. Am J Transplant. 2018;18:1270–4. https://doi.org/10.1111/ajt.14737.

20. Jones BP, Saso S, Bracewell-Milnes T, et al. Human uterine transplantation: a review of outcomes from the first 45 cases. BJOG. 2019;126:1310–9. https://doi.org/10.1111/1471-0528.15863.

21. Testa G, McKenna GJ, Bayer J, et al. The evolution of transplantation from saving lives to fertility treatment: DUETS (Dallas UtErus Transplant Study). Ann Surg. 2020;272:411–7. https://doi.org/10.1097/sla.0000000000004199.

22. Testa G, Anthony T, McKenna GJ, et al. Deceased donor uterus retrieval: a novel technique and workflow. Am J Transplant. 2018;18:679–83. https://doi.org/10.1111/ajt.14476.

23. Johannesson L, Koon EC, Bayer J, et al. DUETS (Dallas UtErus Transplant Study): early outcomes and complications of robot-assisted hysterectomy for living uterus donors. Transplantation. 2021;105:225–30. https://doi.org/10.1097/tp.0000000000003211.

24. Testa G, Koon EC, Johannesson L, et al. Living donor uterus transplantation: a single center's observations and lessons learned from early setbacks to technical success. Am J Transplant. 2017;17:2901–10. https://doi.org/10.1111/ajt.14326.

25. Johannesson L, Testa G, Flyckt R, et al. Guidelines for standardized nomenclature and reporting in uterus transplantation: an opinion from the United States Uterus Transplant Consortium. Am J Transplant. 2020;20:3319–25. https://doi.org/10.1111/ajt.15973.

26. Johannesson L, Wall A, Putman JM, Zhang L, Testa G, Diaz-Garcia C. Rethinking the time interval to embryo transfer after uterus transplantation—DUETS (Dallas UtErus Transplant Study). BJOG. 2019;126:1305–9. https://doi.org/10.1111/1471-0528.15860.

27. Olausson M, Johannesson L, Brattgard D, et al. Ethics of uterus transplantation with live donors. Fertil Steril. 2014;102:40–3. https://doi.org/10.1016/j.fertstert.2014.03.048.

28. Shapiro ME, Ward FR. Uterus transplantation: a step too far. Am J Bioeth. 2018;18:36–7. PMID: 30040573

29. Horsburgh CC. A call for empirical research on uterine transplantation and reproductive autonomy. Hast Cent Rep. 2017;47(Suppl 3):S46–9. https://doi.org/10.1002/hast.795.

30. Castellon LAR, Amador MIG, Gonzalez RED, et al. The history behind successful uterine transplantation in humans. JBRA Assist Reprod. 2017;21:126–34. https://doi.org/10.5935/1518-0557.20170028.

31. Williams NJ, Scott R, Wilkinson S. The ethics of uterus transplantation. Bioethics. 2018;32:478–80. https://doi.org/10.1111/bioe.12530.

32. Blake VK. Financing uterus transplants: the United States context. Bioethics. 2018;32:527–33. https://doi.org/10.1111/bioe.12506.

33. Zaidi D. Re-evaluating the ethics of uterine transplantation. J Clin Ethics. 2017;28:212–6. PMID: 28930707

34. Johannesson L, Kvarnstrom N, Molne J, et al. Uterus transplantation trial: 1-year outcome. Fertil Steril. 2015;103:199–204. https://doi.org/10.1016/j.fertnstert.2014.09.024.

35. Ramani A, Testa G, Ghouri Y, et al. DUETS (Dallas UtErus Transplant Study): complete report of 6-month and initial 2-year outcomes following open donor hysterectomy. Clin Transpl. 2020;34:e13757. https://doi.org/10.1111/ctr.13757.

36. Wall A, Johannesson L, Testa G, Warren AM. Two cases of pregnancy following uterine transplant: an ethical analysis. Narrative Inq Bioeth. 2020;10:263–8. https://doi.org/10.1353/nib.2020.0074.

37. Johannesson L, Testa G, Putman JM, et al. Twelve live births after uterus transplantation in the Dallas UtErus Transplant Study. Obstet Gynecol. 2021;137:241–9. https://doi.org/10.1097/aog.0000000000004244.

38. Jarvholm S, Johannesson L, Brannstrom M. Psychological aspects in pre-transplantation assessments of patients prior to entering the first uterus transplantation trial. Acta Obstet Gynecol Scand. 2015;94:1035–8. https://doi.org/10.1111/aogs.12696.

Chapter 51
Cancer Patients Paying Hefty Prices for Newest Treatments: Case of High Intensity Focused Ultrasound (HIFU) Ablation of Prostate Cancer

Ciro Andolfi ⓘ, Scott J. Hunter ⓘ, R. Matthew Galocy, and Arieh L. Shalhav

Abstract High-Intensity Focused Ultrasound (HIFU) has recently emerged as an alternative therapeutic option in patients with clinically localized prostate cancer, who are a better fit for focal treatment. As is the case for many surgical innovations, the absence of long-term efficacy and safety outcomes creates the pretext for insurance companies to deny coverage, limiting access to only those who can afford out of pocket payment. Guided by a sample clinical scenario, in this chapter we offer an analysis of a range of ethical concerns associated to the lack of coverage of new technologies, as well as a step-by-step approach to surgical decision making.

Keywords Prostate cancer · Surgical innovation · High intensity focused ultrasound · HIFU · Medicare · Insurance coverage · Clinical trial · Social justice Patient autonomy

C. Andolfi (✉) · R. M. Galocy · A. L. Shalhav
Section of Urology, Department of Surgery, The University of Chicago Medical Center, Chicago, IL, USA
e-mail: mgalocy@surgery.bsd.uchicago.edu; ashalhav@surgery.bsd.uchicago.edu

S. J. Hunter
Section of Neuropsychology, Department of Psychiatry and Behavioral Neuroscience, Institutional Review Board, Biological Sciences Division, The University of Chicago Medical Center, Chicago, IL, USA
e-mail: shunter@yoda.bsd.uchicago.edu

© The Author(s), under exclusive license to Springer Nature Switzerland AG 2022

V. A. Lonchyna et al. (eds.), *Difficult Decisions in Surgical Ethics*, Difficult Decisions in Surgery: An Evidence-Based Approach,
https://doi.org/10.1007/978-3-030-84625-1_51

719

Clinical Case

Mr. P, a 64-year-old man with an elevated serum prostate-specific antigen (PSA), received news that his pelvic MRI showed a lesion localized to the right lobe of the prostate with a high probability for cancer. No extra-capsular extension or regional lymph nodes involvement was noticed. The prostate biopsy revealed intermediate-risk disease with a Gleason score (GS) of 7 (4+3). Patient's stage was T2N0. After learning about his diagnosis, Mr. P was told that there were three possible validated treatment choices: (1) Surgical resection with radical prostatectomy; (2) Regional radiation therapy; and (3) Active Surveillance (AS). In view of the patient's age and excellent baseline health status, the surgeon recommended radical prostatectomy. However, Mr. P showed some concern about this procedure. Specifically, he worried about a potential deterioration of his erectile function and urinary continence. In addition, he was not willing to enroll in AS, due to the inconvenience of frequent regular follow-up and biopsies. Considering Mr. P's preference for a focal therapy, the surgeon told him that he was also a suitable candidate for High-Intensity Focused Ultrasound (HIFU) ablation, a new treatment option with minimal invasiveness, promising outcomes, and fewer complications than surgery or radiation therapy. Nonetheless, he was also cautioned about the need for more robust evidence on long-term efficacy, and the lack of coverage by healthcare insurances, including Medicare. After inquiring about the surgeon's level of experience and preliminary results, Mr. P commits to this novel approach, deciding to pay out of pocket to undergo HIFU prostate hemi-ablation.

51.1 Introduction

Depending on tumor stage and life expectancy, the European Association of Urology (EAU) and the American Urological Association (AUA) generally recommend radical prostatectomy, External Beam Radiation Therapy (EBRT) and AS as standard treatment options for patients with localized prostate cancer. HIFU has recently emerged as an alternative therapeutic option in patients with clinically localized prostate cancer, who are a better fit for focal treatment. HIFU prostate ablation uses a transrectal probe to deliver ultrasound to the targeted lesion, inducing local thermal damage and coagulative necrosis. As the energy is delivered transrectally, the rectal mucosa is often actively cooled to prevent local injury and recto-urethral fistula. Given that no portion of the device penetrates tissues, HIFU is a truly noninvasive therapy, and the low rates of adverse effects such as erectile dysfunction and urinary incontinence make it a more attractive option than EBRT among patients with localized, intermediate-risk disease (GS 7).

Unfortunately, the absence of long-term oncological outcomes remains a major limitation and pretext used by insurance companies to deny coverage. Therefore, men hoping to avoid some side effects of prostate cancer treatment must pay thousands of dollars for a procedure whose long-term effects are still unknown. The data available so far suggest that HIFU has fewer negative side effects than surgery or radiation and gives selected patients another valuable management option, beyond just actively watching their cancer. However, while the continuing debate regarding patients' treatment options has created an opportunity for HIFU, it has also increased the risk of the procedure's benefits being overstated, leading patients with low-risk disease (GS 6) to get a treatment that they do not need. Finally, HIFU requires a complex set of skills to be performed appropriately, urging the need for validated credentialing and privileging processes.

In this chapter we will focus on the major issues that physicians can face during surgical decision making with patients eligible for innovative yet-uncertain treatments, particularly challenging the core ethical principles, such as beneficence, nonmaleficence, respect for autonomy, and social justice. We will refer to the case of Mr. P as an example of how to address those issues without compromising or influencing patient's choice. In addition, we will review relevant literature on the interdependence between surgical innovation and healthcare coverage.

51.2 Search Strategy

A literature search using the search engines PubMed and Medline was performed with limitation to the English language and the years 2005–2020. The search terms utilized were *prostate cancer, HIFU, surgical innovation, Medicare, CMS, CED, insurance, reimbursement, coverage, clinical trial, clinical registry*, and *out of pocket*. We selected 19 articles for review.

Table 51.1 The four-box model approach (adapted from Jonsen [1])

Medical indications	Patient preferences
• Medical problem • Treatment goals • Treatment options • Likelihood of success • Possible complications	• Aware of risks • Understands benefits • Decisional capacity • Personal preferences • Surrogates
Quality of life	**Contextual features**
• Baseline functionality assessment • Independence and lifestyle • Expected recovery time • Possible long-term and permanent deficits resulting from treatment	• Conflicts of interest • Financial gain/interests • Economic burden • Professional biases • Research conflicts

51.3   Discussion

Surgical decision making is a process requiring absolute respect to the ethical principles of beneficence, nonmaleficence, patient autonomy, and social justice. This is even more critical in surgical innovation, where the surgeon's desire to push the envelope must be counterbalanced by the responsibility of ensuring patient safety (see Chap. 49). Jonsen et al. [1] developed a general model called the four-box approach (see Table 51.1) to provide physicians with a practical guide to making ethical decisions, which is applicable in most clinical scenarios. This decision-making tool includes four major areas: (a) Medical Indications; (b) Patient Preferences; (c) Quality of Life; and (d) Contextual Features. With particular emphasis to the last topic, below we review all four areas and see how to use them in our clinical case.

51.4   Medical Indications

Medical Indications is the physician's clinical judgment aiming to provide the most appropriate treatment to the patient. The ethical principles behind this clinical process are beneficence and nonmaleficence. Beneficence primarily means to cure or improve patient's health. Nonmaleficence means to provide care to the patient in ways that prevent further injury. Relevant questions to be asked in this respect are: *What are the goals of treatment? What are the probabilities of success of various treatment options and how can harm be avoided?* From a more radical but aggressive approach such as prostatectomy to the least invasive AS, the surgeon presented to Mr. P the entire spectrum of available options, including HIFU. Still, cancer resection being the primary goal, the surgeon recommended surgical prostatectomy.

51.5   Patient Preferences

Patient Preferences are the choices that reflect the patient's own experience, beliefs, and values as informed by the physician's recommendations. Respect for patient autonomy, by acknowledging his moral right to choose and follow his own plan of life and actions, is the guiding ethical principle of this topic. Relevant questions to be asked are: *Has the patient been informed of the benefits and risks of treatment recommendations? Does the patient have the capacity to decide, and if so, what are his preferences for treatment? If the patient lacks decision making capacity, who is the surrogate decision maker that will be making healthcare decisions for him?* Although in theory the goals of both patient and doctor should align, patients sometimes refuse the recommendations doctors provide. Listening to patient preferences is the foundation of trust, and necessary for a better doctor-patient relationship. Patients who collaborate with their physicians to reach a shared healthcare decision have greater confidence in their doctor, and express greater satisfaction with their care. By contrast, Mr. P. seemed equally concerned about the risk of incontinence and erectile dysfunction, diverting his interest away from prostatectomy and EBRT.

51.6   Quality of Life

Clinical factors such as relatively young age and good general health status led the surgeon to consider his patient a good candidate for surgery. However, the ethical dimension of patient care must include not only appropriateness of interventions (beneficence) and respect for patient's preferences (autonomy) but also the improvement or preservation of quality of life (beneficence as satisfaction). To do so, the use of objective assessment measures such as quality of life questionnaires is of great help to properly evaluate preoperative baseline function and provide postoperative estimates for each treatment options. Relevant question to be asked in this respect are: *Do quality of life assessments raise any questions that might contribute to a change of treatment plan? What are the ethical implications of improving or enhancing a patient's quality of life?* In our case, Mr. P. not only showed particular interest in preserving urinary continence and sexual function, but the use of specific questionnaires such as International Prostate Symptom Score (IPSS) and Sexual Health Inventory for Men (SHIM) revealed optimal performance, likely to be affected with prostatectomy. We can't stress enough the importance of inquiring patients about their personal preferences and expectations.

51.7   Contextual Features

The fourth topic contains external items that are not part of the clinical workup, such as professional, legal, and financial implications. In the case of HIFU, lack of insurance coverage represents a major obstacle leading to a series of controversies and ethical debacles, such as fairness to healthcare access, voluntary consent to research, and risk of coercion [2–4]. Relevant questions to be asked in this respect are: *Are there any financial factors creating conflicts of interest in the clinical decision? Is patient's enrollment in clinical research free of constrains?* Medical device companies attempting to market a new treatment device in the U.S. often make the erroneous assumption that obtaining clearance from the Food and Drug Administration (FDA) is the final step. In fact, going through the FDA regulatory process is only the halfway point. Healthcare coverage is a key component in making new medical technology available to most patients, but the complex path to reimbursement can take years and many companies don't make it through, failing to produce revenue as patients would have to pay out of pocket for a procedure with no clear evidence on long-term outcomes. As recent decades have witnessed accelerated advances in medical technology, many complex medical, economic, and social issues have been raised about lack of coverage and patient accessibility.

51.8   The Responsibility of Funding Innovative Treatment Options

The FDA plays an important role in determining how new technologies are used, given its regulatory responsibilities: conducting premarket reviews of new products to ensure their safety and effectiveness, administering good manufacturing process requirements, and performing post-market surveillance [5–7]. However, a much bigger hurdle is obtaining medical codes to facilitate reimbursement from public and private payers. In recent years, insurers have had a significant impact because of their coverage and payment determinations. Because few patients can pay for their health care directly, third-party payers play a central role in determining how new medical technologies are used [8, 9]. Technology manufacturers rely on insurance reimbursement to create a favorable climate for selling their products, while health providers depend on this reimbursement to offset the costs of incorporating new products into their medical practices [2, 10–12]. Insurer coverage policies and payment rates are tied to procedure codes. If a new procedure involves more costly equipment, is more difficult to perform, or requires more skill than current procedures, new codes are a necessary precondition for securing a higher payment rate. New codes also spur insurers to consider whether the new procedure should be covered. These are difficult decisions even when there is a rich body of evidence about the impact of new technologies on health outcomes. When new devices do not fit into established insurance categories, when they attract attention because of their cost, or when they are used for new indications, reimbursement plays an extremely important role. Insurer coverage and payment processes not only determine whether current technologies will be made available to patients, but they also create a climate that can provide incentives or disincentives for manufacturers to innovate in the first place [2, 8–13].

Medicare, because it has a major role in public policy and is a very large payer, has come under pressure to find ways to reconcile the tension between strict evidence-based coverage standards and being rapidly responsive to innovation and emerging technologies. The need to address this tension led to a series of decisions over the past decade in which Medicare payment has been linked to a requirement for prospective data collection. Therefore, the Center for Medicare Service (CMS) chose to link coverage decisions to prospective clinical studies with a Coverage with Evidence Development (CED) program [6, 14]. However, this policy raises many concerns, such as the lack of a defined rationale behind new treatment eligibility and the possible "coercive" link between insurance coverage and research study participation [2, 10, 14–20]. Currently, whether CED is recommended depends on both the characteristics of the technology (is it expected to have a positive net benefit?) and the range of authority of the purchasing institution (can they ensure that the research is properly conducted?), with no clear criteria or formal guidelines. This lack of guidance causes concern that CED could slow innovation by creating a disincentive to develop new products for conditions for which the evidence base is not well developed. Formal protocols for CED should be accompanied by a clear statement defining type of study design and data required to provide evidence development and reduce uncertainty. Designing the necessary clinical research, getting funding, and implementing a scheme in a time frame that is consistent with the needs of clinicians, patients, and other decision makers is challenging. Short-term studies are not desirable given the considerable investment in evidence development, while long-term schemes are also not desirable given the costs and risks involved. Additionally, physicians are not usually paid for data collection and reporting, which may affect the quality of the data and lead to bias. Compliance with data collection may be weak and the monitoring of the study poor also because of limited clinical staff availability. On the other end, stakeholders can influence decisions around the conduct of CED decisions. For example, manufacturers may pressure the initiation of a study and relevant conflicts of interest arise when they play a role in the funding, data collection, and evaluation of a research protocol. Therefore, patients who are not aware of what a CED scheme entails, may be distrusting and assume that the primary objective is cost containment, rather than a genuine effort to support early access to innovations and clinical research. Identifying and counselling potential participants, and obtaining consent requires considerable effort and if patients are not adequately informed, they may decline to participate or prematurely withdraw. The legislative language underpinning Medicare promising coverage for all care deemed "reasonable and necessary" does not imply a right or entitlement to coverage for interventions that do not meet the evidentiary standard established by Medicare itself. So, many have questioned whether it is ethical to restrict access to new technologies only to patients paying out of pocket or willing to participate in registries and clinical trials, and to withhold a potentially beneficial innovation from a subset of patients who cannot participate (see Chap. 49). Certainly, requiring that clinical data be placed in a research registry to receive covered treatment would not infringe on the right to covered medical care, as all patients and their physicians who would prefer the treatment in question would have access to it. However, as patients must be willing to participate in a research investigation to qualify for reimbursement, it is debated whether their study enrollment should be considered voluntary and free of coercion.

51.9 Concluding Remarks

Over the years, public and private insurers have had the expectation that if they are to pay for medical services within a covered benefit category, then those services must be medically necessary. Such coverage usually ends up excluding treatments and technologies that are considered experimental. Often, emerging therapies such as HIFU fall somewhere in the middle—past the point of being experimental, but with uses so new that in many cases medical societies have not issued consensus guidelines on their use—creating a dilemma for payers and a social justice controversy for patients and providers. The CED policy presents a creative initiative from Medicare with the potential of filling the gap between no evidence and no coverage. Health insurances instituting a CED policy should take steps to develop transparent and accountable criteria defining standards for new treatments eligibility; describe the rationale for the choice of registry or clinical trial as the vehicle for evidence development; and ensure adherence to ethical requirements.

51.10   Selected References

- Carter D, Merlin T, Hunter D. An ethical analysis of coverage with evidence development. Value Health. 2019;22(8):878–883. https://doi.org/10.1016/j.jval.2019.02.011

  – Sometimes a government or other payer is called on to fund a new health technology even when the evidence leaves a lot of uncertainty. One option is for the payer to provisionally fund the technology and reduce uncertainty by developing evidence. This is called coverage with evidence development (CED).

- Felgner S, Ex P, Henschke C. Physicians' decision making on adoption of new technologies and role of coverage with evidence development: a qualitative study. Value Health. 2018;21(9):1069–1076. https://doi.org/10.1016/j.jval.2018.03.006

  – When new medical technologies enter the market, their time of adoption is a key point in patient care, as evidence and experience regarding their utilization often differ in their extent. With the aim of maximizing patient benefit and reducing risks, many new technologies can lead to better outcomes in patients' treatment and diagnosis; however, there might be uncertainty regarding their effectiveness and risks because at the time of market approval only little or no evidence may be available.

- Sorenson C, Drummond M, Burns LR. Evolving reimbursement and pricing policies for devices in Europe and the United States should encourage greater value. Health Aff. 2013; 32(4):788–796. https://doi.org/10.1377/hlthaff.2012.1210

  – Policy makers and other stakeholders in Europe and the United States are increasingly concerned with getting better value from investments made in technological innovations. One potential solution is to rely more heavily on studies of the effectiveness and costs of new technologies to inform coverage, reimbursement, and pricing decisions.

Conflict of Interest All authors have no conflicts of interest to disclose.

References

1. Jonsen AR, Siegler M, Winslade WJ. Clinical ethics: a practical approach to ethical decisions in clinical medicine. 8th ed. McGraw-Hill Education; 2015.
2. Varabyova Y, Blankart CR, Greer AL, Schreyögg J. The determinants of medical technology adoption in different decisional systems: a systematic literature review. Health Policy. 2017;121(3):230–42. https://doi.org/10.1016/j.healthpol.2017.01.005.
3. Bénard A, Duroux T, Robert G. Cost-utility analysis of focal high-intensity focussed ultrasound vs active surveillance for low- to intermediate-risk prostate cancer using a Markov multi-state model: cost-utility analysis of F-HIFU vs AS. BJU Int. 2019;124(6):962–71. https://doi.org/10.1111/bju.14867.
4. Emberton M. Translating cost-utility modelling into the real world—the case of focal high-intensity focussed ultrasound and active surveillance. BJU Int. 2019;124(6):900–1. https://doi.org/10.1111/bju.14918.
5. Van Norman GA. Drugs and devices. JACC Basic Transl Sci. 2016;1(5):399–412. https://doi.org/10.1016/j.jacbts.2016.06.003.
6. Rothery C, Claxton K, Palmer S, Epstein D, Tarricone R, Sculpher M. Characterising uncertainty in the assessment of medical devices and determining future research needs. Health Econ. 2017;26(S1):109–23. https://doi.org/10.1002/hec.3467.
7. Raab GG, Parr DH. From medical invention to clinical practice: the reimbursement challenge facing new device procedures and technology—part 1: issues in medical device assessment. J Am Coll Radiol. 2006;3(9):694–702. https://doi.org/10.1016/j.jacr.2006.02.005.
8. Raab GG, Parr DH. From medical invention to clinical practice: the reimbursement challenge facing new device procedures and technology—part 2: coverage. J Am Coll Radiol. 2006;3(10):772–7. https://doi.org/10.1016/j.jacr.2006.02.028.
9. Sorenson C, Drummond M, Burns LR. Evolving reimbursement and pricing policies for devices in Europe and the United States should encourage greater value. Health Aff. 2013;32(4):788–96. https://doi.org/10.1377/hlthaff.2012.1210.
10. Cappellaro G. Diffusion of medical technology: the role of financing. Health Policy. 2011;100:51–9. https://doi.org/10.1016/j.healthpol.2010.10.004.
11. Raab GG, Parr DH. From medical invention to clinical practice: the reimbursement challenge facing new device procedures and technology—part 3: payment. J Am Coll Radiol. 2006;3(11):842–50. https://doi.org/10.1016/j.jacr.2006.02.027.
12. Sorenson C, Drummond M, Wilkinson G. Use of innovation payments to encourage the adoption of new medical technologies in the English NHS. Health Policy Technol. 2013;2(3):168–73. https://doi.org/10.1016/j.hlpt.2013.05.001.
13. Martelli N. New French coverage with evidence development for innovative medical devices improvements and unresolved issues. Value Health. 2016;19:17–9. https://doi.org/10.1016/j.val.2015.10.006.
14. Tunis SR, Pearson SD. Coverage options for promising technologies: medicare's 'coverage with evidence development'. Health Aff. 2006;25(5):1218–30. https://doi.org/10.1377/hlthaff.25.5.1218.
15. Carter D, Merlin T, Hunter D. An ethical analysis of coverage with evidence development. Value Health. 2019;22(8):878–83. https://doi.org/10.1016/j.jval.2019.02.011.
16. Felgner S, Ex P, Henschke C. Physicians' decision making on adoption of new technologies and role of coverage with evidence development: a qualitative study. Value Health. 2018;21(9):1069–76. https://doi.org/10.1016/j.jval.2018.03.006.
17. Miller FG, Pearson SD. Coverage with evidence development: ethical issues and policy implications. Med Care. 2008;46(7):746–51. https://doi.org/10.1097/MLR.0b013e3181789453.
18. Trueman P, Grainger DL, Downs KE. Coverage with evidence development: applications and issues. Int J Technol Assess Health Care. 2010;26(1):79–85. https://doi.org/10.1017/s0266462309990882.

19. Walker S, Sculpher M, Claxton K, Palmer S. Coverage with evidence development, only in research, risk sharing, or patient access scheme? a framework for coverage decisions. Value Health. 2012;15(3):570–9. https://doi.org/10.1016/j.jval.2011.12.013.
20. van de Wetering EJ, van Exel J, Brouwer WBF. The challenge of conditional reimbursement: stopping reimbursement can be more difficult than not starting in the first place! Value Health. 2017;20(1):118–25. https://doi.org/10.1016/j.jval.2016.09.001.

Index

© The Editor(s) (if applicable) and The Author(s), under exclusive license to
Springer Nature Switzerland AG 2022
V. A. Lonchyna et al. (eds.), *Difficult Decisions in Surgical Ethics*, Difficult
Decisions in Surgery: An Evidence-Based Approach,
https://doi.org/10.1007/978-3-030-84625-1

Printed in the United States
by Baker & Taylor Publisher Services